HISTOLOGY

Slide Atlas
A slide atlas of Histology, based on the contents of this book, is available. In the slide atlas format, the material split into volumes, each of which is presented in a binder, together with numbered 35mm slides of each illustration. Further information can be obtained from:

Gower Medical Publishing
Middlesex House
34-42 Cleveland Street
London W1P 5FB, UK

Gower Medical Publishing
101 Fith Avenue, New York
NY 10003, USA

HISTOLOGY

Alan Stevens MBBS FRCPath

Senior Lecturer in Histopathology, University of Nottingham Medical School

Consultant Histopathologist to Trent Regional Health Authority

James Steven Lowe BMedSci BMBS MRCPath

Reader in Pathology, University of Nottingham Medical School

Consultant Neuropathologist to Trent Regional Health Authority

with contributions by

the late Paul R. Wheater BA BMedSci BMBS

H. George Burkitt BDSc MBBChir FRACDS

Gower Medical Publishing • London • New York

Distributed in the USA and Canada by:
J B Lippincott Company
East Washington Square
Philadelphia PA 19105
USA

Distributed in the UK and Continental Europe by:
Gower Medical Publishing
Middlesex House
34–42 Cleveland Street
London W1P 5FB
UK

Distributed in Australia and New Zealand by:
Harper and Row (Australia) Pty Ltd
PO Box 226
Artarmon
NSW 2064
Australia

Distributed in Southeast Asia, Hong Kong, India and Pakistan by:
Harper and Row (Asia) Pte Ltd
37 Jalan Pemimpin 02–01
Singapore 2057

Distibuted in Japan by:
Nankodo Company Ltd
42-6 Hongo 3-chome
Bunkyo-Ku
Tokyo 113
Japan

Library of Congress Cataloging in Publication Data:
Available on request

British Library Cataloguing in Publication Data:
Stevens, Alan
    Histology
    I. Title   II. Lowe, James
    611
    ISBN 0-397-44633-0

Project Manager:	Lindy van den Berghe
Design:	Marie McNestry
	Richard Prime
Illustration:	David McElwaine
	Linda Payne
	Marion Tasker
Line artists:	Lee Smith
	Robert Wilkins
Production:	Susan Bishop
Index:	Nina Boyd
Publisher:	Fiona Foley

Typeset on Apple Macintosh ®
CRC output by the Last Word
Text set in New Baskerville; legends and tables set in Helvetica
Colour reproduction by Bright Arts in Hong Kong
Produced by Mandarin Offset
Printed in Hong Kong

This book is dedicated to the memory of

Paul Richard Wheater

(28th December 1951 to 7th September 1989)

who was involved in the conceptualisation of this book and
produced some of the early photomicrographs.

His tragic illness and early death cast a shadow over an otherwise
joyful enterprise.

His friendship, enthusiasm, photographic skills and ebullient
humour are sadly missed.

PREFACE

We have written this book for the new generation of students of medicine and human biology who demand a detailed but readable textbook of medically relevant histology to complement teaching they receive in cell biology, anatomy, and pathology.

There has been a sad perception among students that histology is tedious and boring, with the result that they don't bother to learn. One reason is that histology tends to be taught in isolation at an early stage of most courses and the detailed study which is required appears excessive. Another unfortunate reason is that histology has been neglected in many faculties, with teaching often delegated to staff with no real interest in the subject. Times are changing. While it was once possible for students to get by with a superficial knowledge of histology, advances in biology and medical practice now make this impossible.

Histology has never been such an important part of the medical and biology curriculum as it is today. The teaching of biochemistry and physiology increasingly revolve around the new discipline of cell biology and so a knowledge of cellular histology is of paramount importance. Thanks to new technology, histology has also become a central part of the practice of clinical medicine. More and more, diagnosis of disease rests on the histological examination of small samples of tissue which are now obtainable from virtually every part of the body by safe painless techniques of biopsy.

An understanding of the causes, mechanisms and effects of disease is increasingly dependent on a knowledge of histology.

Students are often dissatisfied with present histology textbooks. The main complaints are that textbooks are difficult to read, are either overburdened with detail of animal histology (not always relevant to man) or are pictorial atlases lacking substance. Importantly, many students feel that histology textbooks give little to indicate the clinical importance of the subject and the relevance of histology to biology.

Today's students demand books which are easy to read yet sufficienctly detailed to satisfy examination requirements. In this book we have addressed the problems of presenting a modern view of human histology in a compact form. The text has a 'user-friendly' layout representing the best of contemporary design, material is presented in a variety of visually attractive ways, and two theme sections on practical histology and clinical relevance run throughout.

The Practical Histology sections are generally at the end of each chapter on a green tint background and aim to show students what they can expect to see using routine sections with a class microscope. These supplement the main chapters in which histological features are demonstrated using a variety of special techniques not normally available in practical microscopy classes.

The Clinical sections are on a blue tint background and relate closely to adjacent sections on normal histology. These aim to show how important diseases are based on altered structures and hence the clinical relevance of histology.

As working histopathologists with a responsibility for teaching students we feel well-equipped to present a balanced view of histology which is relevant to human biology and clinical practice. Students only have a short time to assimilate an immense amount of knowledge and we hope our efforts in this book ease the way.

AS, JSL Nottingham 1991

ACKNOWLEDGEMENTS

We wish to thank the Laboratory staff of the University Department of Histopathology, Queen's Medical Centre, Nottingham, for the skill and patience with which they have produced the sections which we have photographed for this book. In particular we are grateful to Ian Wilson, Angela Crossman, Janet Palmer, Leanne Ward and David McQuire for paraffin sections, Neil Hand for acrylic resin sections, Ken Morrell and his team for immunocytochemical preparations, and Janet Palmer for enzyme histochemical preparations.

We owe a particular vote of thanks to Trevor Gray who has spent many hours searching out suitable material for transmission and scanning electron microscopy, and is responsible for all of the electron micrographs in this book.

Mr Bill Brackenbury photographed all the gross specimens, and also provided us with many of the very low magnification photomicrographs.

Dr H George Burkitt, a friend and former colleague, wrote the original draft of Chapters 6 and 7; we hope that our editing of his material has retained the flavour of his original contribution.

Many professional colleagues at Queen's Medical Centre contributed suitable tissue for processing and subsequent photomicrography. Dr J. Wendy Blundell supplied the arteriograms in Chapter 16 and sections of the conducting system of the heart in Chapter 8. Dr Ian Leach also supplied much material on the heart for Chapter 8, and Dr Peter Furness kindly allowed us to use one of his electron micrographs showing the polyanionic sites in the glomerulus. Dr Jane Zuccollo provided us with much material relating to human foetal and neonatal histology, and Dr Mark Stephens supplied us with a rare slide of an early human implantation site. Dr Mark Wilkinson provided some sections for Chapter 9, and gave valuable advice. John Mulligan, Philip Dawes and Lynette Newberry were instrumental in our obtaining a wide range of well-preserved human tissues for use in this book. Jocelyn Germaine of the London Hospital kindly made available some of the material used in the section on teeth in Chapter 10.

Professor R. John Mayer helped greatly with aspects of cell biology, in particular new ideas about the acid vesicle system.

We are particularly grateful to Dr Keith Robson who, on so many occasions, bravely held the fort and did our work whilst we were involved in writing this book, and to Isabella Streeter and Linda Dewdney who spent many hours at the word processor knocking our text into shape.

Finally, we would like to thank all of the staff of Gower Medical Publishing who have been involved in the production of this book. Lindy van den Berghe edited our bursts of verbosity with considerable skill and insight, and bullied us very sweetly into meeting our deadlines; her insight into students' requirements had a profound influence on our style of writing and illustration. Claire Ginzler was responsible for word processing our edited manuscripts. Marie McNestry is largely responsible, with Richard Prime, for the design and visual impact of the book, and Marie's team of artists, particularly David McElwaine, Lynda Payne and Marion Tasker, created beautiful and informative artworks from our often rough originals. Fiona Foley directed the orchestra with a deft touch, using a combination of flattery, cajolery and sterness, ideally tuned to the prevailing circumstances. It has been a considerable pleasure to work with them all.

ABOUT THIS BOOK

Considerable thought has gone into designing this book to meet the requirements of students of histology who have a limited time to assimilate information, yet need to take in a maximum of detail in one sitting without re-reading portions of text or becoming fatigued. Many features of this book have been designed to maximise flow of information.

Chapter content

Whilst being a comprehensive coverage of human histology, the content of chapters is arranged slightly differently to that in older textbooks of histology to reflect the integration and emphasis that is now occurring in modern medical and human biology courses.

Main text

The type faces used have been chosen for clarity and legibility. The text has been divided up by headings and the liberal use of paragraph breaks to help the assimilation of material.

Caption text

The caption text is, in general, not repetitive of the main text and is designed to be read when referenced from the main text. This serves two purposes: firstly it maintains the flow of information, and secondly it provides a refreshing break from reading the main text. For this reason many of the captions are used as the vehicle to put over complex pieces of information, especially those pertaining to three dimensional structure.

Photomicrographs and electronmicrographs

We have tried to make this textbook uncluttered by omitting information that the student is unlikely to use. In the belief that it is more important for students to grasp the arrangement and structure of tissues rather than to engage in a mental exercise working out sizes from magnifications, we have departed from the practice of giving magnifications for each of the micrographs. Instead, we have given physical dimensions of important structures when they are described and feel that this lessens the perceived burden of students reading the text.

In a similar manner, only the name of special staining methods is usually given in captions, and more details can be found in the Glossary of Techniques and Stains.

CLINICAL SECTIONS

We hope that the examples we have chosen illustrate the vital role that an understanding of histology will play in later studies of human biology and disease. These sections are an important part of the book as they also provide a mental break in reading, and physically lighten the look of pages.

PRACTICAL HISTOLOGY SECTIONS

Many students give up on microscopy because they feel that they cannot see what they have just read about. In most cases this is entirely appropriate, as what you can see is determined by the material in class histology slides. The practical histology sections are designed to put histology into a classroom teaching perspective and hopefully lessen the anxiety of the students who feel that they cannot use a microscope.

Feedback

The authors welcome comments from teachers and students who have used this book for their courses and personal study; in particular, whether the content and method of presentation of material satisfy their requirements. We will endeavour to incorporate suggestions into subsequent editions, and hope that teachers and students will take this opportunity to have an input into the creation of this valuable teaching resource. Enjoy!

CONTENTS

1. HISTOLOGY: DON'T SWITCH OFF!

HISTOLOGY IS A CENTRAL BIOLOGICAL AND MEDICAL SCIENCE

Histology is the study of the structure of biological material and the ways in which individual components are structurally and functionally related.

It is central to biological and medical science since it stands at the crossroads between biochemistry, molecular biology and physiology on the one side, and disease processes and their effects on the other.

Samples of human biological material can be obtained from many areas of the body by quick, safe and painless techniques, for example via:
• needles into solid organs;
• endoscopic tubes into the alimentary tract or body cavities,
• special flexible cannulae along blood vessels.

Accessible tissues such as the skin, mouth, nose, etc. can be sampled using a scalpel (Fig. 1.1).

Knowledge of normal histological appearances is essential if abnormal diseased structures are to be recognized.

This is an exciting period in histology, for we are now able to explore the physiological and molecular basis of biological structures through the development of techniques that allow us to examine the chemical molecular make up of living tissues down the microscope. It is now becoming clear why various biological structures are shaped and arranged as they are.

An understanding of histology is vital to comprehend biochemical and physiological processes, and to gain insight into how abnormalities of structure lead to disorders of function and biochemistry, and result in disease.

HISTOLOGY WAS ONCE EMPIRICAL

The study of histology began with the development of simple microscopes and techniques for preparing thin slices of biological material to make them suitable for examination. Despite their simple equipment, and somewhat inadequately prepared material, early histologists learnt a surprising amount about the structure of biological material.

Such studies led Virchoff to propound his **cellular theory** of the structure of living organisms that established the cell as the basic building block of most biological material.

In those early years a vocabulary of histology was developed, on light microscopic analysis of cells accompanied by

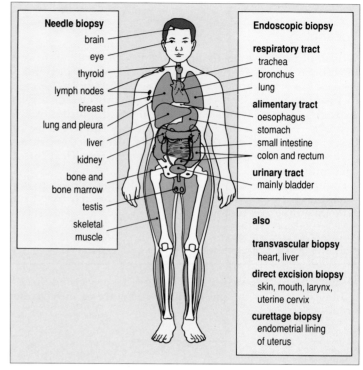

Fig. 1.1 Histology in diagnostic medicine.
It is now possible to obtain small samples from many areas of the body by various techniques. Histological examination of such samples is an increasingly important and direct way of diagnosing disease.

a limited understanding of cell physiology and function.

Collections of cells having similar morphological characteristics were described as forming **tissues** and these were subdivided into four types.
• Epithelial tissues described cells which covered surfaces, lined body cavities or formed glands such as salivary glands.
• Muscular tissues described cells with contractile properties.
• Nervous tissues described cells forming the brain, spinal cord, and nerves.
• Connective tissue described cells that produced extracellular matrix and served to link or support other specialized tissues by forming tendons, bones, or fatty tissue.

MODERN HISTOLOGY IS A PRECISE SCIENCE

Modern investigative techniques have now revolutionized our understanding of cells. The techniques of protein sequencing, molecular genetics (with the ability to analyse and dissect the genetic code) and cloning of cells in culture have also given unprecedented insight into the working of cells.

Vocabulary

Whilst improvements in knowledge and understanding have been matched in other sciences by the rapid emergence of new vocabularies, this has not always been the case in histology. For many years the terms and classifications that originated from early histological studies were retained. With every new discovery about the structure of living material, attempts were made to force the new information into an old, often inappropriate, classification of cells and tissues.

Fortunately, this rigid histological dogma is now giving way to a more exciting and functional approach based on understanding cell biology.

CELLS ARE BASIC FUNCTIONAL UNITS

Modern knowledge confirms Virchoff's correctness in ascribing the cell as the basic unit of structure of most living organisms.

Cells vary considerably. Arising from a single fertilized egg, each cell develops structural attributes to suit its functions through the process of **differentiation**, and is a considerably more sophisticated and complex unit than was formerly suspected.

Molecular biology has shown that cells of diverse morphological appearance can be grouped together because of common functional attributes or interactions.

Some cells are adaptable. It has also become apparent that even in the adult there are populations of highly adaptable, uncommitted cells, which can modify both their structure and functional activity to adapt to changing environmental demands. This facility is of vital importance in adaptation to internal or external stress, and is commonly seen in disease processes (e.g. replacement of damaged heart muscle by strong fibrous tissue following a heart attack).

The general structural and biological properties of cells are discussed in Chapter 2 and many of their specialized functional attributes in Chapters 3, 4 and 5.

CELLS ARE NOW CLASSIFIED ACCORDING TO FUNCTION

It is now possible to classify cells into groups based on their main function. The groupings which will be used in this book are **epithelial cells**, **supporting cells**, **contractile cells**, **nerve cells**, **germ cells**, **blood cells**, **immune cells**, and **hormone secreting cells** (Fig. 1.2).

Cell group	Epithelial cells	Support cells	Contractile cells	Nerve cells	Germ cells	Blood cells	Immune cells	Hormone-secreting cells
Example	gut and blood vessel lining, covering skin	fibrous support tissue, cartilage, bone	muscle	brain	spermatozoa, ova	circulating red and white cells	lymphoid tissues (nodes and spleen)	thyroid and adrenal
Function	barrier, absorption, secretion	organize and maintain body structure	movement	direct cell communication	reproduction	oxygen transport, defence	defence	indirect cell communication
Special features	tightly bound together by cell junctions (see Chapter 3)	produce and interact with extracellular matrix material (see Chapter 4)	filamentous proteins cause contraction (see Chapter 5)	release chemical messengers onto surface of other cells (see Chapter 13)	half normal chromosome complement (see Chapters 17 & 18)	proteins bind oxygen, proteins destroy bacteria (see Chapter 6)	recognize and destroy foreign material (see Chapter 7)	secrete chemical messengers (see Chapter 15)

Fig. 1.2 Modern functional cell classification.

It is important, however, to recognize that a cell may have several functions and be a member of more than one cell class, for example:
- many of the hormone-producing cells are also epithelial in type, being tightly bound together by specialized junctions to form a gland;
- many immune cells are also blood cells;
- some support cells are also contractile.

The structural and functional specializations delineating each type of cell group are broadly outlined in Chapters 3, 4 and 5, and discussed in more detail throughout the book.

TISSUES ARE FUNCTIONAL ARRANGEMENTS OF CELLS

A **tissue** is an assembly of cells that are arranged in a regular formation.

This term usefully describes simple arrangements of cells termed **simple tissues** (e.g. cartilage). However, most apparently distinct tissues contain a mixture of cells, extracellular matrix and cell products with different functions, which may be termed **compound tissue** (Fig. 1.3). For example, 'nervous tissue' contains nerve cells (neurones), support cells (astrocytes), immune cells (microglia) and epithelial cells (ependyma).

The concept of simple and compound tissues is useful in descriptive histology, but for brevity the unqualified term tissue is used to imply either type.

Support cells, not 'connective tissue'

The one exception to the acceptable use of the term tissue is the old expression 'connective tissue', used historically to describe a wide range of living material containing cells associated with a dominant extracellular matrix component, whose the oretical function was to act as a supporting stroma serving more highly specialized cell types.

The original group of 'connective tissues' included cell/matrix combinations such as bone, cartilage, tendon, fibrous tissue, bone marrow and blood, and adipose tissue.

It has also been traditional to use the term 'loose areolar connective tissue' to describe tissue that is partly made up of support cells that produce an extracellular matrix, but also contains cells belonging to the immune system (e.g. lymphocytes and macrophages), nerve cells, and blood vessels.

In this book the term 'connective tissue' has been avoided because it underemphasizes the structural organization involved in such highly developed tissues. Instead, the concept of **support cells** is used, which emphasizes the importance of interactions between extracellular matrix and cells.

Support cells and their specializations are discussed in Chapter 4, while bone, tendons and ligaments are discussed in Chapter 14.

CELLS FORM ORGANS AND SYSTEMS

An **organ** is an anatomically distinct group of tissues, usually of several types, which perform specific functions, for example, heart, liver and kidney.

The term **system** has two uses:
- It describes cells with similar function but widely distributed in several anatomical sites, for example, the specialized hormone-producing cells scattered in the gut and lung (diffuse endocrine system), which cannot be an organ as they do not form an anatomically distinct mass.
- System also describes a group of organs, which have similar or related functional roles, for example, the tongue, oesophagus, stomach, intestines, exocrine pancreas and rectum are components of the alimentary system, and the kidney, pelvicalyceal system, ureters and bladder are part of the urinary system.

The relationships between cells, tissues, organs and systems are shown in Fig. 1.3.

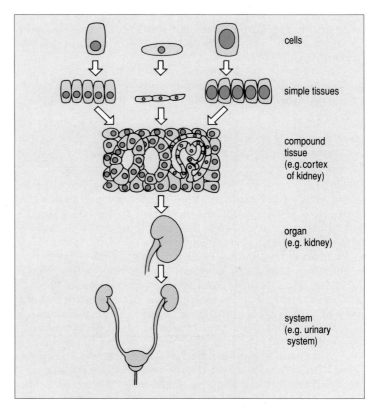

Fig. 1.3 Cells, tissues, organs and systems.

CELL HISTOLOGY IS
ALIGNED TO CELL BIOLOGY

Until recently the only way to look at the fine structure of individual cells (cell histology) was by using electron microscopy. This is now complemented by the increasing use of immunohistochemical methods, which use antibodies to specific cell constituents to visualize details within cells at the light microscopic level that are not visible by other techniques.

In addition it is now possible to stain specific DNA and RNA sequences by the technique of *in situ* hybridization, thereby gaining fundamental insight into the molecular mechanisms of cells.

A clear understanding of the fine structure and molecular organization of cells greatly improves comprehension of biochemical and physiological processes.

This overlap between structure, physiology and biochemistry is now acknowledged by the term **cell biology**.

SYSTEMS HISTOLOGY IS
ALIGNED TO ANATOMY

Study of the arrangement of different tissues at the microscopic level (systems histology) gives insight into the structure and function of organs and systems. This type of study is an extension of anatomy and is often termed microscopic anatomy for this reason.

The study of systems histology is an important component of human biology and in most curricula is taught alongside normal anatomy.

HISTOLOGY IS ESSENTIAL FOR
UNDERSTANDING PATHOLOGY

Pathology (understanding disease processes) accounts for nearly half of the study required by medical practitioners irrespective of their specialization, and from its earliest beginnings has always been intimately linked to a study of systems histology and microanatomy.

In most curricula, however, pathology is taught at a later stage than histology, so that by the time students are studying diseases they have forgotten normal histology.

This is unfortunate as most disease processes are associated with histological abnormalities, and in clinical practice a histological diagnosis is the mainstay of modern medicine, as the following examples illustrate.
• A 35-year-old accountant has an episode of jaundice (goes yellow) and blood tests reveal that this is due to a viral infection of the liver (viral hepatitis). He recovers, but on follow-up 6 months later further blood tests suggest that there is continuing liver damage.

His physician therefore removes a piece of his liver through a needle (biopsy) so that it can be examined histologically.

Such an examination will reveal the pattern of liver cell damage and indicate whether the disease is progressive with a poor outlook, or on the other hand is restricted and has a good prognosis.

Thus interpretation and understanding of this disease requires knowledge of the microanatomy of the liver.
• A 20-year-old student develops kidney failure and the cause is not apparent on blood tests or radiology. The renal physician therefore removes a piece of kidney via a needle so that the diagnosis can be made by histological examination.

Special staining methods highlight subtle structural abnormalities by light microscopy (Fig. 1.4), while electron microscopy provides valuable information about abnormalities at a subcellular level.

On the basis of the abnormalities which are revealed, the renal physician can institute appropriate treatment.

Clinical management of this patient requires knowledge of the microanatomy of the kidney. Assessment of progress, and the effect of treatment are monitored by repeated biopsy.
• The classification of tumours (cancer) is based on histology, and accurate histological assessment of tumours is the cornerstone of modern cancer treatment.

For example, a 15-year-old girl has swollen lymph nodes in her neck. A surgeon removes one so that it can be

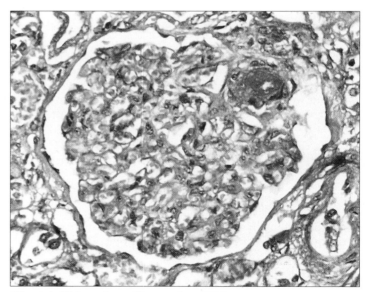

Fig. 1.4 Kidney (paraffin section, MSB stain).
Micrograph showing a section of kidney from a patient with kidney failure. The special stain shows the nature and location of the main abnormality.

examined histologically, and microscopy reveals that the swelling is caused by a form of cancer.

The treatment given to the girl depends on the histological type of the tumour (i.e. is it derived from muscle, lymphoid cells, endocrine cells?). This is answered by the histological reports which in describing cellular morphology and differentiation, reveals the precise type of tumour.

TECHNIQUES USED IN HISTOLOGY AND CELL BIOLOGY

High resolution light microscopy

Light microscopy uses thin sections of tissue to study cell morphology, which are usually obtained as follows.
• The tissue is immersed into a preservative solution (**fixative**), which cross-links or precipitates proteins and prevents degradation. The most common routine fixatives use **formaldehyde** in the form of formalin solution.
• The tissue is then **embedded** into a firm medium for cutting into thin sections, and this is most commonly done by removing water with alcohols and impregnating the tissue with **paraffin wax**.
• The tissue is then cut into sections (conventionally 5–8 μm thick) on a **microtome**.
• To see cellular details the tissue sections are immersed in **dyes** which stain different structures. The most common is the combination of **haematoxylin and eosin (H&E)**, although many specialized dye-impregnation methods can be used to highlight different cell structures.

Resolution of structures by light microscopy is of the order of 0.2 μm, but in routine practice with paraffin sections, this is seldom better than 0.6 μm.

Tissues may also be embedded in **acrylic or epoxy resins**, which allow much thinner sections to be cut than with paraffin wax, with the possibility of resolving finer structural details. These are increasingly used in histology, and examples will be used in this book where appropriate (see glossary of techniques and stains).

Other light microscopy techniques (i.e. phase contrast microscopy, interference contrast microscopy) use optical properties of non-stained cells to visualize structure.

Transmission electron microscopy

Use of an electron beam instead of light allows resolution of structures as small as 1 nm in well prepared tissues.

Tissue preparation for electron microscopy demands the use of special fixation of very small (less than 2 mm) tissue fragments, the most common fixative containing **glutaraldehyde**. In addition, because specimens are subjected to an electron beam in a vacuum, they need to be embedded in a robust material, the most common being **epoxy resin**.

Sections for electron microscopy have to be thin to allow good resolution and prevent scattering of electrons, being typically 0.1 μm thick (ultrathin sections). They are stained for electron microscopy by immersion in a solution containing a heavy metal (uranium or lead).

The use of electron microscopy allows the study of subcellular morphology and is a widely used routine method of morphological study.

Scanning electron microscopy

Scanning electron microscopy uses solid pieces of tissue rather than sections and allows the perception of three-dimensional views of the surface of cells or tissues (Fig. 1.5).

A small piece of fixed tissue is dried and **coated in gold**. An electron beam then scans the specimen and electrons produced from the surface are used to reconstruct a fine three-dimensional representation of the surface (see Figs 6.3 b, 6.16 b, 10.10, 10.11 & 10.38 e).

If living cells are frozen and then fractured there is a tendency for the fractures to open cells along membranes and distinct planes, which can then be studied using the scanning electron microscope. This technique of **cryofracture** provides information about the surface features of cell membranes.

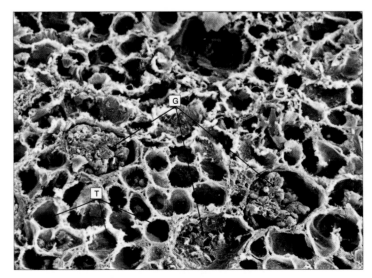

Fig. 1.5 Kidney (scanning electronmicrograph).
This scanning electronmicrograph shows the components of the cortex of the kidney, which are largely glomeruli (G) and tubules (T). At a higher magnification more surface details are evident (see Fig. 16.11).

Histochemistry

Certain dyes have affinity for specific chemical groups in molecules and these are used to localize substances in histological preparations.

Lipids. As lipids are dissolved out of paraffin-processed material, their detection is only possible if sections are prepared by freezing and cutting on a cryostat, followed by immersion in lipid soluble dyes such as **Sudan-black** or **Oil-red-O**.

Polysaccharides such as glycogen can be detected by a staining method called the **Periodic acid Schiff (PAS)** technique. Periodic acid is applied to sections to oxidize glucose residues in glycogen to aldehydes. Schiff reagent (a colourless bleached dye called **fuchsin**) is then applied and reacts with the aldehydes to produce purple fuchsin, (see Fig.4.11).

Specific enzymes. Detection of a specific enzyme in a tissue can be performed by incubating sections of fresh tissue in a reaction mixture containing the specific enzyme substrate, co-factors and a visualizing agent. An intense coloured product develops at the site of enzyme activity.

This technique (**enzyme histochemistry**) can be used to show the localization of a vast number of enzymes including acid and alkaline phosphatases, dehydrogenases and ATPases, and is routinely used to detect abnormalities in certain diseased tissue, particularly muscle (see Fig. 14.4).

Autoradiography

If tissues are provided with radioactively labelled metabolites, cells which take up the metabolite can be detected by dipping sections in a photographic emulsion and allowing the radioactivity to create silver grains in the emulsion.

This is termed autoradiography and is a powerful technique for studying cell function.

If radiolabelled thymidine (a DNA component) is incorporated, the autoradiograph will show cells that are actively dividing.

Immunocytochemistry

Immunocytochemistry uses antibodies to specific cell molecules to detect their presence in tissue sections.

Polyclonal antibodies to a substance are obtained by inoculating an animal (commonly rabbit or sheep) with the purified protein and harvesting serum.

Alternatively monoclonal antibody may be produced by inoculating a mouse and fusing suitable antibody-producing cells with immortal mouse myeloma cells to continually produce antibodies in tissue culture.

Immunofluorescence is an immunocytochemical technique in which the antibody is labelled with a fluorescent dye and its localization after staining is detected by fluorescence microscopy.

Immunoperoxidase methods. Immunofluorescence has been largely replaced by immunoperoxidase methods in which the location of antibody (primary antibody obtained from rabbit) is detected by a second antibody, which has been raised in another species.

This second antibody is linked to an enzyme called horseradish peroxidase, which can be developed as a coloured (usually brown) reaction product (see Fig.10.31b).

In contrast to immunofluorescent preparations, immunoperoxidase sections are permanent and can be viewed with a normal light microscope.

Cell culture

Cells may be grown in artificial media and this has facilitated analysis of structural and functional attributes of cells, particularly analysis of cell metabolism.

Although cell culture is still widely used as a research tool, its main use in hospital medical practice is in the growth of cells for subsequent analysis of chromosomes.

Cell fractionation

Cell fractionation techniques allow whole cells to be disrupted in a controlled manner. The different particles which result are then separated for functional or structural analysis. This is achieved by high speed centrifugation of disrupted cells in specialized solutions of known density.

Nuclei, mitochondria, endoplasmic reticulum, and ribosomes can all be isolated in relatively pure form in this manner.

2. THE CELL

Cells have many common features, which are independent of any specialized function (Fig. 2.1).

• An outer **membrane** surrounds each cell and separates it from its environment and from other cells.

• Cells are composed of a solution of proteins, electrolytes and carbohydrates (cytosol), divided up into specialized functional areas (organelles) by inner membrane systems.

• Their shape and fluidity are partly determined by the arrangement of internal filamentous proteins (**intermediate filaments**, **actin** and **microtubules**), analogous to scaffolding, which form the **cytoskeleton**.

The main membrane-bound organelles are:

• the **nucleus**, which contains the cellular DNA;

• **mitochondria**, which provide energy;

• **endoplasmic reticulum** (ER), which is involved in biosynthesis of protein and some lipids;

• **Golgi**, which is involved in processing biosynthetic products for incorporation into the cell or for secretion;

• **vesicles**, which act as temporary packages of material undergoing transport around the cell;

• **lysosomes**, which contain hydrolytic enzymes to digest macromolecules within the cell;

• **peroxisomes**, which contain enzymes involved in fatty acid metabolism.

CELL MEMBRANES

The outer membrane surrounding each cell and the membranes surrounding internal cellular organelles have a common basic structure of a lipid bilayer containing specialized proteins in association with surface carbohydrates.

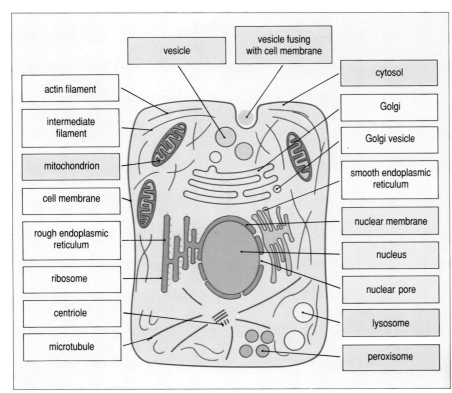

Fig. 2.1 Cell structure.
Diagram to show the main constituents of a cell and their distribution.

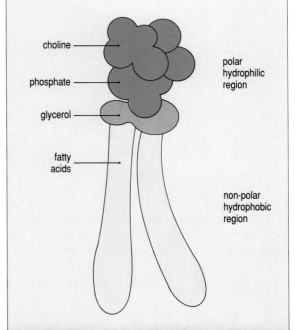

Fig. 2.2 Membrane phospholipid molecule.
Diagram of a membrane phospholipid molecule, which is the ma n com onent of cell membranes, and determines the fundamental properties of the cell membrane as a whole.

The most important determinant of membrane structure is the lipid component. Each type of membrane lipid molecule has one hydrophilic end and one hydrophobic end (Fig. 2.2), thus they are **amphipathic**.

Such lipids spontaneously form a bilayer in water with the hydrophobic ends forming an inner layer between the outwardly-directed hydrophilic groups. This basic structure of the cell membrane, into which membrane proteins are inserted (Fig. 2.3), confers important functional attributes.

• The membrane is a fluid, allowing lateral diffusion of membrane proteins and facilitating cell mobility.

• The polar lipid composition leads to differential permeability to different substances, being highly permeable to water, oxygen and small hydrophobic molecules such as ethanol, but virtually impermeable to charged ions such as Na^+ and K^+.

• Breaks and tears are spontaneously sealed as the polar nature of lipids eliminates free edges where hydrophobic groups would come into contact with the aqueous environment

• Membrane proteins are placed to perform functional roles in processes such as transport, enzymic activity, cell attachment and cell communication

Membrane lipids

Lipid forms 50% of the mass of cell membranes. There are three major types of lipid: phospholipids, cholesterol and glycolipids.

Phospholipids. There are four major phospholipids in the cell membrane: **phosphatidylcholine**, **sphingomyelin**, **phosphatidylserine** and **phosphatidylethanolamine**. These molecules make up about 50% of the lipid component and tend to surround membrane proteins, often specifically anchoring proteins with enzyme or transport functions.

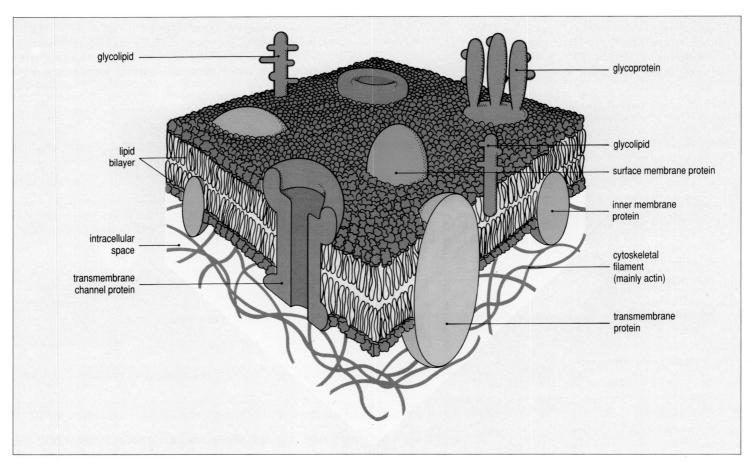

Fig. 2.3 Cell membrane structure.
The cell membrane is composed of a lipid bilayer with phospholipid hydrophobic groups facing inwards, and hydrophilic groups facing outwards. Protein molecules float within this basic structure with projecting carbohydrate groups being attached to glycolipids or proteins.

The composition of inner and outer lipid layers is not the same. For example, high concentrations of certain phospholipids in the inner face may be needed to complement the presence of an inner membrane protein because certain proteins need to be linked with specific phospholipids.

Cholesterol in cell membrane limits the movement of adjacent phospholipids and makes the membrane less fluid, but more mechanically stable.

Glycolipids are found only in the outer face of cell membranes with their associated sugars exposed to the extracellular space. The functional significance of this is not clear, but they may be involved in intercellular communication.

One of the most important membrane glycolipids is **galactocerebroside**, which is a major component of myelin, the fatty insulation layer around nerves (see Chapter 13). Another group of important glycolipids is the **gangliosides**, which constitute up to 10% of the lipid in nerve cell membranes.

Membrane proteins

Membrane proteins carry out most of the specialized functions of cell membranes and hence the types of protein encountered vary according to cell type. Membrane proteins:
- attach cytoskeletal filaments to cell membrane;
- attach cells to extracellular matrix (e.g. cell adhesion molecules);
- transport molecules in or out of cells (e.g. carrier proteins, membrane pump proteins, channel proteins);
- act as receptors for chemical signalling between cells (e.g. hormone receptors);
- possess specific enzymic activity.

Membrane proteins are able to diffuse laterally over the surface of the cell.

Membrane carbohydrates

Membranes have associated carbohydrate residues which are mainly confined to the surface directed away from the cytosol, being prominent in the luminal aspect of inner membrane systems as well as on the cell surface, where they have been termed the **glycocalyx**

Membrane carbohydrates can be demonstrated by staining with **lectins**, which are proteins extracted from plants with binding capabilities for specific carbohydrate groups.

Endocytosis and Exocytosis

Material from the extracellular space, as well as surface membrane, may be incorporated into the cell by invagination of the cell surface in a process termed endocytosis (Fig. 2.4). The invaginated cell membrane fuses to form an **endocytotic vesicle** or **endosome**, which is a small, sealed, spherical, membrane-bound body. The membrane and any material incorporated into such a vesicle can then be processed within the cell.

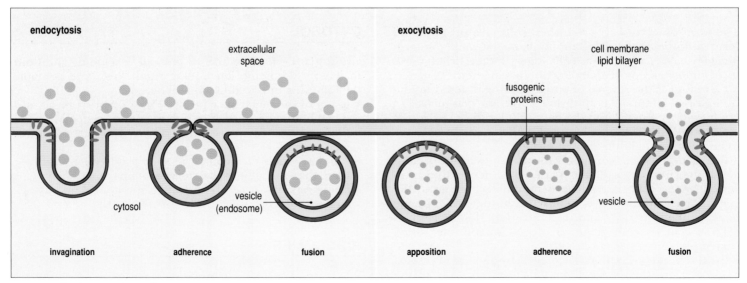

Fig. 2.4 Endocytosis and exocytosis.
It is currently thought that special proteins termed 'fusogenic proteins' mediate the process of membrane integration in endocytosis and exocytosis.

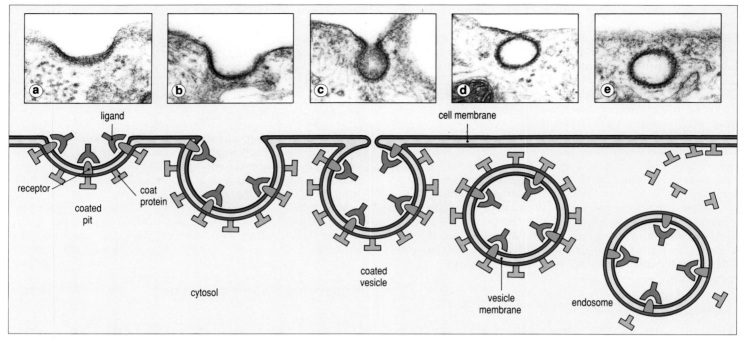

Fig. 2.5 Ultrastructure and diagrams of coated pit formation.

a A coated pit is braced by a coat of protein molecules and bears surface receptors that bind specific extracellular ligands. In most cases the coat protein (visible ultrastructually as a fuzzy membrane thickening) is **clathrin**, which forms an hexagonal lattice around the pit membrane.

b, c, d Assembly of the coat protein lattice drives progressive invagination of the pit to form a coated vesicle.
e Once internalized, the coat protein is shed and returns to the cell surface to form new coated pits.

This form of transport into cells is termed **receptor-mediated endocytosis** and is a feature of internalization of iron, low-density lipoprotein, and some growth factors.

The term **pinocytosis** is used when cells take up fluid and form endosomes about 150 nm in diameter, while the term **phagocytosis** is used when cells ingest large particles and form endosomes more than 250 nm in diameter.

Exocytosis is the reverse of endocytosis, and describes the fusion of a membrane-bound vesicle with the cell surface to discharge its contents into the extracellular space. Fusion of vesicles with the cell membrane also allows new membrane to be incorporated into the cell surface.

Pinocytotic vesicles constantly form at the surface of most cells, ingesting extracellular material, which is then processed by the cell, the vesicle membrane returning to the cell surface. Thus, there is a constant shuttle of membrane between cell surface and cell interior. These vesicles originate in specialized areas of cell membrane called **coated pits** (Fig. 2.5).

In certain cells, pinocytotic vesicles are used to transport material from the extracellular space on one side to the extracellular space on the other, thus allowing material to cross over a cellular barrier. This process is termed transcytosis.

CYTOSOL

Cytosol is the fluid matrix of the cell (excluding the fluid matrix inside membrane-bound organelles), and contains the following important components:
- much of the machinery involved in protein synthesis and metabolism (it is therefore rich in enzyme systems);
- filamentous proteins that form the cytoskeleton (see page 19);
- some products of metabolism such as glycogen and free lipid, for which it acts as a storage compartment or;
- numerous ribosomes, both free in the cytosol and associated with the cytosolic surface of rough ER.

RIBOSOMES

Ribosomes are small electron-dense particles, which impart a blue colour (basophilia) to the cytoplasm of protein-producing cells on light microscopy (Fig. 2.6).

Ribosomes synchronize the alignment of both messenger RNA and transport RNA in the production of peptide chains during protein synthesis.

Each ribosome is composed of a small subunit, which binds RNA, and a large unit, which catalyses the formation of peptide bonds. They are made up of specific ribosomal RNA as well as specific proteins. Ribosomal RNA is manufactured in the nucleolus (see page 12).

NUCLEUS

The nucleus is the largest single organelle in the cell and contains the cellular DNA (Fig. 2.7).

In light microscopic preparations nuclei are spherical or ovoid in shape, generally measuring 5–10 μm in diameter, stain with basic dyes such as haematoxylin (i.e. basophilic) and contain a smaller spherical structure, the nucleolus, which synthesizes ribosomal subunits.

Nuclei are bounded by two concentric membranes with different functional roles.
• The inner nuclear membrane contains specific membrane proteins that act as attachment points for filamentous proteins, which form a scaffolding to maintain the spherical shape. These filamentous proteins are **cytoskeletal proteins** (see page 19) and are termed **lamins**.
• The outer nuclear membrane bounds a space, the **perinuclear space**, which is continuous with the lumen of the ER; it may be associated with ribosomes in a similar manner to rough ER.

The nuclear membrane is perforated by numerous pores, which establish continuity between the cytosol and the chromatin lumen (Fig. 2.8).

Chromatin. The nucleus contains **DNA** wound around proteins called **histones** to form **nucleosomes**, which are regular repeating globular structures similar to beads on a string. The nucleosome string is then wound into filaments 30 nm in diameter, which form the structure of chromatin. Further condensation is possible during cell replication to form distinct **chromosomes** when chromatin forms large **looped domains** by attachment to DNA binding proteins.

Chromatin distribution is not uniform, reflecting varying degrees of unfolding corresponding to transcriptional activity.
• **Euchromatin** is seen as light-staining electron-lucent areas and represents actively transcribed cellular DNA.
• **Heterochromatin** is seen as dense-staining areas, often adjacent to the nuclear membrane, and is the highly condensed, transcriptionally inactive form.

Nucleolus

The nucleolus is a spherical area within the nucleus and measures 1–3 μm in diameter, increasing in size with active transcription. Inactive cells have indistinct nucleoli, while metabolically active cells have large or multiple nucleoli. In H&E preparations nucleoli stain blue-pink because of their affinity for both acidophilic and basophilic dyes.

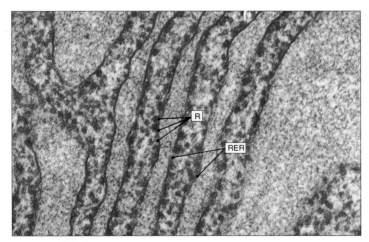

Fig. 2.6 Ribosomes.
Electronmicrograph showing ribosomes (R) visible as small electron-dense particles 20–30 nm in diameter. In the cytosol they are present either singly or in chains termed **polyribosomes**. They are also found attached to the cytosolic surface of ER where they are one component of rough ER (RER).

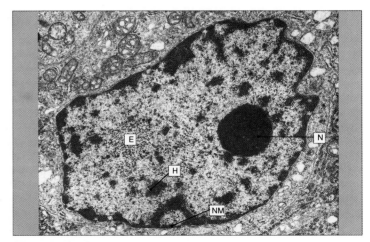

Fig. 2.7 Nucleus.
Electronmicrograph showing a typical cell nucleus. It is bounded by a double nuclear membrane (NM) The nucleolus (N) is clearly visible as an electron-dense circular area. Nuclear chromatin is divided into two types: heterochromatin (H) is dense-staining, while euchromatin (E) is light-staining.

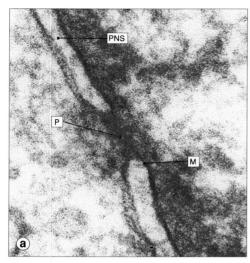

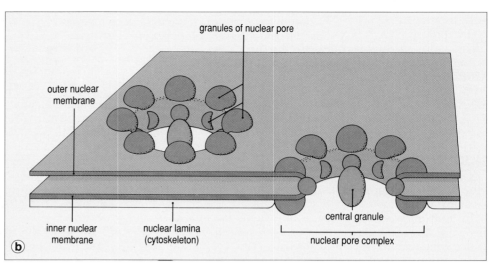

Fig. 2.8 Nuclear pore

a The double nuclear membrane (M) bounding the perinuclear space (PNS) is perforated by nuclear pores (P) which appear as gaps in transmission electronmicrographs.

b Structurally the pores are rimmed by eight protein complexes to form the nuclear pore complex shown in this diagram. The pores form channels, which allow diffusion of small molecules, but restrict movement of large molecules, between the cytosol and the nucleus.

Movement of some proteins into the nucleus is, however, desirable and it is currently thought that the nuclear pore complex recognizes and actively transports specific peptide sequences in proteins destined for the nucleus. In a similar fashion, large ribosomal subunits produced in the nucleus are probably actively transported into the cytosol.

The central granules of the pore complex are believed to be large proteins or components of ribosomes in transit between different cell areas.

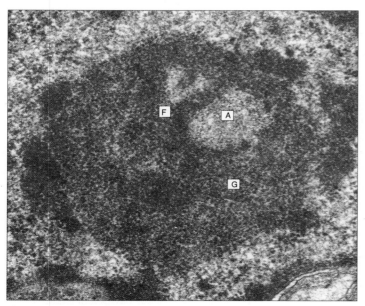

Fig. 2.9 Nucleolus.

Electronmicrograph showing the nucleolus from a cell actively producing protein. The pars amorpha (A), pars fibrosa (F), and pars granulosa (G) are clearly visible.

The nucleolus produces ribosomal RNAs, which are packaged with proteins to form ribosomal subunits and exported to the cytosol via the nuclear pore complexes.

By electron microscopy three regions of the nucleolus can be distinguished (Fig. 2.9).

• **Pars amorpha** (pale areas) correspond to large loops of transcribing DNA containing the ribosomal RNA genes. These so-called **nucleolar organizer regions** contain specific RNA binding proteins.

• **Pars fibrosa** (dense-staining regions) correspond to transcripts of ribosomal RNA genes beginning to form ribosomes.

• **Pars granulosa** (granular regions) correspond to RNA containing maturing ribosomal subunit particles.

Nuclear Lamina

The nuclear lamina is a network of protein filaments 20 nm thick that lines the internal nuclear membrane. It is composed of three proteins termed nuclear lamins A, B and C, which are organized into filaments and form a regular square lattice as a scaffold beneath the nuclear membrane.

It is thought that this nuclear lamina network interacts with nuclear membrane proteins and acts as a nuclear cytoskeleton, possibly interacting with chromatin in the spatial organization of the nucleus.

MITOCHONDRIA

Mitochondria are membrane-bound cylindrical organelles (Fig. 2.10) typically measuring 0.5–2 μm in length, which provide energy to cells through oxidative phosphorylation.

Mitochondria are believed to have evolved in human cells as symbiotic prokaryotic organisms similar to bacteria. In support of this hypothesis, each mitochondrion has its own DNA and systems for protein synthesis independent of the cell nucleus.

Each mitochondrion is constructed with two membranes, an outer membrane and an inner membrane. The two membranes define two inner mitochondrial spaces, the intermembranous space and the matrix space.

The outer membrane contains specialized transport proteins such as **porin**, which allow free permeability to molecules up to about 10 kD molecular weight, from the cytosol into the intermembranous space.

The inner membrane is highly impermeable to small ions due to a high content of the phospholipid **cardiolipin**.

This feature is essential to mitochondrial function as it permits the development of electrochemical gradients during the production of high energy cell metabolites.

The inner membrane is folded into pleats (**cristae**) thereby increasing its surface area, and is the location of respiratory chain enzymes, as well as ATP synthetase, which is responsible for energy generation.

The intermembranous space contains:
- metabolic substrates, which diffuse through the outer membrane;
- ATP generated by the mitochondrion;
- ions pumped out of the matrix space during oxidative phosphorylation.

The matrix space contains enzymes to oxidize fatty acids and pyruvate as well as for the citric acid (TCA) cycle. It also contains mitochondrial DNA and specific mitochondrial enzymes for mitochondrial DNA transcription.

The morphology of mitochondria varies with cell type.
- In cells with a high oxidative metabolism, mitochondria are commonly large and serpiginous.
- In cells secreting steroid hormones, such as those of the adrenal cortex, the cristae are tubular structures rather than flat plates.

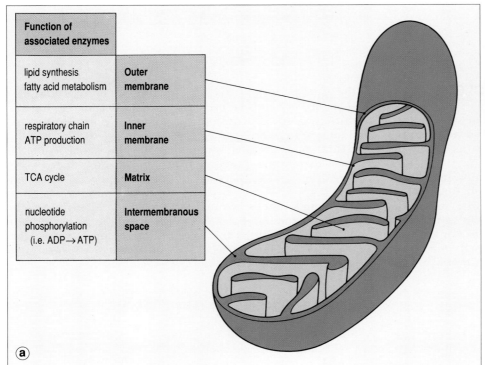

Function of associated enzymes		
lipid synthesis fatty acid metabolism	**Outer membrane**	
respiratory chain ATP production	**Inner membrane**	
TCA cycle	**Matrix**	
nucleotide phosphorylation (i.e. ADP→ATP)	**Intermembranous space**	

(a)

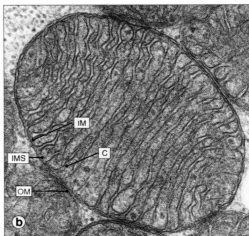

(b)

Fig. 2.10 Mitochondrion.
a Diagram of the structural organization of a mitochondrion accompanied by a table detailing the locations and functions of mitochondrial enzymes.
b Electronmicrograph of a mitochondrion. Note the outer membrane (OM), inner membrane (IM), intermembranous space (IMS), and cristae (C).

MITOCHONDRIAL CYTOPATHY SYNDROMES

Mitochondria contain their own special DNA, as well as a mechanism for transcription and translation to proteins that is independent of the rest of the cell. While many mitochondrial proteins are derived from this special DNA, a large number are also derived from nuclear DNA and are transported into the mitochondria from the rest of the cell.

Mitochondrial DNA is not inherited in the same way as cellular DNA, and in man the whole mitochondrial complement of a newly developing embryo is derived from mitochondria present in the ovum (i.e. are maternally derived); there is no paternal contribution.

Abnormal mitochondrial DNA can impair mitochondrial function and lead to defective cell functioning, which mainly results in structural abnormalities of muscle and the nervous system, and metabolic abnormalities derived from failure of oxidative metabolism. Such diseases are termed **mitochondrial cytopathies.**

Individuals can be considered to be mosaics of genetically different mitochondria. If a large number of abnormal mitochondria are inherited then it is likely that severe disease will develop, but if only a proportion are abnormal then the resulting disease may be less severe. The most common patterns of clinical disease are as follows.

• Muscle weakness, particularly affecting the extraocular muscles.

• Degenerative disease of the central nervous system, (e.g. loss of the optic nerve fibres, loss of cerebellar tissue, or degeneration of brain white matter).

• Metabolic disturbances, marked particularly by the development of abnormally high levels of lactic acid.

Such diseases may become manifest at any age from childhood into adult life and diagnosis can be assisted by muscle biopsy (Fig. 2.11), in which abnormal mitochondria can be seen in a large proportion of cases.

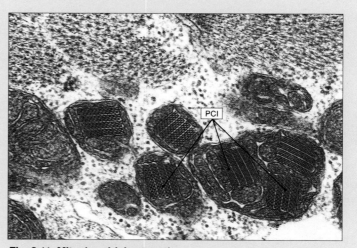

Fig. 2.11 Mitochondrial cytopathy.
Electronmicrograph of abnormal mitochondria in the muscle of a person with muscle weakness. Characteristic paracrystalline inclusions (PCI) are present, and are thought to be composed of excess mitochondrial protein, which accumulates as a result of the genetic abnormality (compare with Fig. 2.10b).

ENDOPLASMIC RETICULUM AND GOLGI

The ER and Golgi are two distinct regions of an intercommunicating membrane-bound compartment involved in the biosynthesis and transport of cellular proteins and lipids (Fig. 2.12).

They are arranged as deeply folded flattened membrane sheets or as elongated tubular profiles, their quantity depending on cellular metabolic requirements; little ER is present in metabolically inactive cells, but cells synthesizing and secreting protein-containing molecules contain vast amounts. Most cells have only a relatively small quantity of smooth ER with the exception of cells secreting or processing lipids.

Protein synthesis

Protein synthesis begins in the cytosol where messenger RNA attaches to free ribosomes, and translation produces the new peptide. The first portion formed is a **signal sequence,** which is different for proteins destined to remain in the cytosol and proteins destined for entry into membranes or for secretion.

Ribosomes producing peptides with the signal sequence for a membrane or secreted protein become attached to the surface of ER where the rest of the peptide is translated (Fig. 2.13).

Protein synthesis by rough ER results in either the attachment of membrane proteins to ER membrane, or retention of proteins destined for secretion or retention within the ER lumen. These newly made proteins then enter the smooth ER for transport to the Golgi.

Smooth endoplasmic reticulum

Smooth ER is a vital cell membrane system. As well as processing synthesized proteins it is the site of cell lipid synthesis, particularly membrane phospholipids. The lipid

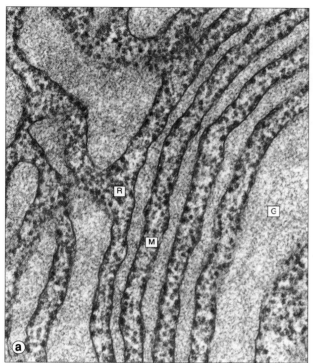

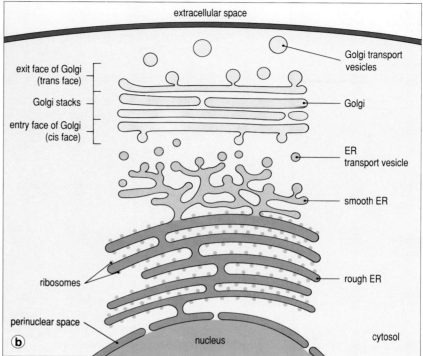

extracellular space

Golgi transport vesicles

exit face of Golgi (trans face)

Golgi stacks — Golgi

entry face of Golgi (cis face)

ER transport vesicle

smooth ER

ribosomes

rough ER

perinuclear space

nucleus

cytosol

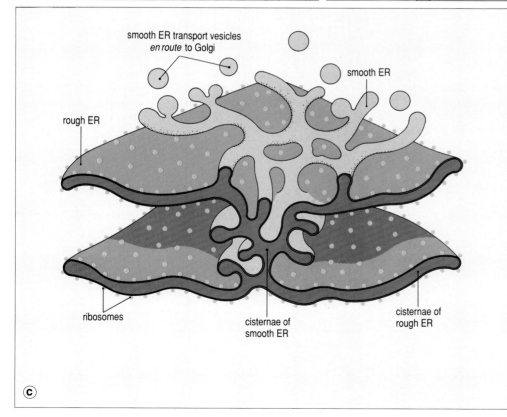

smooth ER transport vesicles *en route* to Golgi

smooth ER

rough ER

ribosomes

cisternae of smooth ER

cisternae of rough ER

Fig. 2.12 Endoplasmic reticulum.
a Electronmicrograph of rough ER, which is composed of sheets of membrane (M) studded with ribosomes (R) on its cytosolic surfaces. Granular material (G) within the ER lumen represents newly synthesized proteins.
b Diagram of the relationship between ER and Golgi. The lumen of rough ER is continuous with the perinuclear space and with the lumen of smooth ER, while the Golgi forms a separate membrane system. Communication between ER and Golgi is mediated by small vesicles of ER, which break off, move through the cytosol, and fuse with Golgi membrane.
c Diagram to show the spatial relationship between rough ER and smooth ER. Smooth ER cisternae are tubular.

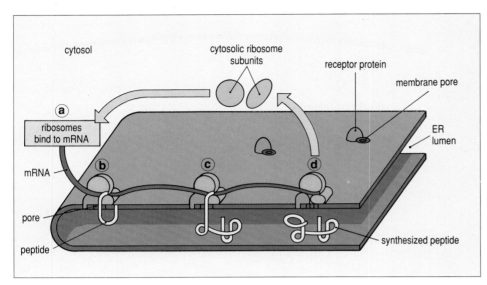

Fig. 2.13 Protein synthesis on rough endoplasmic reticulum.

a Free cytosolic ribosomes attach to messenger RNA and begin to produce a peptide.

b The ribosome attaches to a receptor on the ER membrane and the peptide is threaded into the ER lumen via a small protein-lined pore. At any one time several ribosomes may be transcribing the same messenger RNA strand.

c The original signal sequence that threads the peptide into the ER lumen is cleaved, and as the peptide is made it forms in the lumen. Some proteins (i.e. those destined to be integral membrane proteins) can also form directly within the ER membrane.

d After completion of peptide synthesis the ribosome detaches from the receptor protein and returns to the cytosolic free pool.

synthetic enzymes are located on its outer (cytosolic) face with ready access to lipid precursors.

Once synthesized and incorporated into the outer part of the smooth ER membrane lipid bilayer, phospholipids are flipped over into the inner part by specific transport proteins colloquially termed flipases.

Golgi

From the smooth ER, further processing of synthesized macromolecules takes place in the Golgi. To reach the Golgi, vesicles bud from the smooth ER and travel in the cytosol to fuse with its inner face. Membrane proteins are incorporated into the Golgi membrane while luminal proteins enter the Golgi space.

The Golgi membrane system has three important roles.
• Modification of macromolecules by the addition of sugars to form oligosaccharides.
• Proteolytic modification of peptides into active forms.
• Sorting of different macromolecules into specific membrane-bound vesicles for subsequent incorporation into a membrane, transport into the lumen of a specific membrane-bound organelle, or extracellular secretion.

To facilitate these three roles the Golgi is divided into three functional components (Fig. 2.14).

VESICLES

Vesicles are small spherical membrane-bound organelles. They are formed by the budding off of existing areas of membrane and have two main functions.

• They transport or store material within their lumina.
• They allow the exchange of cell membrane between different cell compartments.

The main types of vesicle are:
• cell surface-derived endocytotic (i.e. pinocytic or phagocytic) vesicle;
• Golgi-derived transport and secretory vesicles;
• ER-derived transport vesicles;
• lysosomes (see below);
• peroxisomes (see page 19).

The cellular distribution of these vesicles can be determined by immunohistochemical staining for specific vesicle-associated proteins or specific vesicle contents.

Acid vesicle system

A **lysosome** is a membrane-bound organelle with a high content of hydrolytic enzymes operating in an acid pH, which functions as an intracellular digestion system, processing either material ingested by the cell or effete cellular components. This definition encompasses a variety of membrane-bound organelles derived from slightly different sources and with different functional roles.

Lysosomes are now considered to be only one part of the **acid vesicle system**, a group of vesicles so-named because of their common **membrane H$^+$-ATPase**, which can decrease their luminal pH to 5. This low PH activates powerful **acid hydrolase enzymes**, which are derived from vesicles that bud from the Golgi.

The membrane proteins required for lysosomal function (particularly the membrane pump, which increases H$^+$ concentration to maintain the acid pH), are not present in

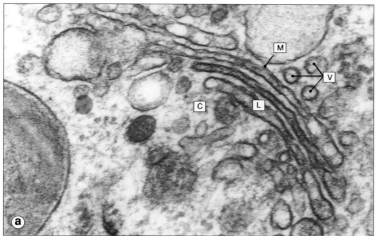

Fig. 2.14 Golgi.

a Ultrastructurally Golgi is seen as parallel stacks of membrane (M) delineating Golgi lumen (L) from the cytosol (C). Transport vesicles (V) can be seen *en route* from ER.

b Golgi has three functional parts: the nuclear-facing **cis face** receives transport vesicles from smooth ER and phosphorylates certain proteins; the central **medial Golgi** adds sugar residues to both lipids and peptides to form complex oligosaccharides; the **trans Golgi network** performs proteolytic steps, adds sugar residues, and sorts different macromolecules into specific vesicles, which bud off the trans face.

Sorting is performed by specific membrane receptor proteins, which recognize signal groups on macromolecules and direct them into correct vesicles.

New membrane lipid synthesized in the smooth ER makes its way into the cell membrane via the Golgi.

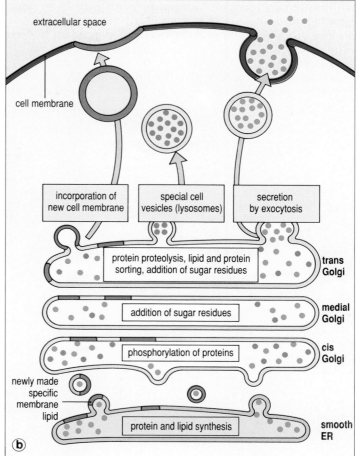

the initial **Golgi hydrolase vesicles**, (formerly called primary lysosomes), which appear as membrane-bound vesicles with a dense core measuring 0.2–0.4 μm in diameter (Fig. 2.15a).

A functional lysosome, fulfilling the definition of acid environment plus hydrolases, results from the fusion of hydrolase vesicles with endosomes (see Fig. 2.5) that do contain the correct membrane proteins, to form an **endolysosome** (formerly termed a secondary lysosome). Endolysosomes are larger than Golgi hydrolase vesicles, being 0.6–0.8 μm in diameter, but also have an electron-dense core (Fig. 2.15b). Endolysosomes can fuse with other endosomes derived from phagocytosis to form **phagolysosomes** and thereby particulate matter brought into the cell is digested.

In a similar fashion, effete organelles can be incorporated into intracellular membranes derived from ER and subsequently fused with an endolysosome to form an **autophagolysosome**; this enables old or damaged organelles to be recycled in a process termed autophagy.

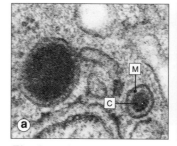
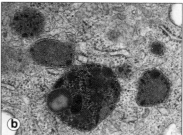

Fig. 2.15 Lysosomes.

a Electronmicrograph of Golgi hydrolase vesicles, which are bounded by membrane (M) and have electron-dense core (C) composed of acid hydrolase enzymes. The membrane of this type of vesicle does not contain H⁺-ATPase.

b Electronmicrograph showing several endolysosomes, which are produced by fusion of Golgi hydrolase vesicles with endosomes. Endolysosomes have a membrane containing H⁺-ATPase, which can reduce pH to activate the hydrolases.

Following digestion of material by acid hydrolases, indigestible amorphous and membranous debris may be seen in large membrane-bound vesicles, called **residual bodies.** The relationships between members of the acid vesicle system are shown in Fig. 2.16.

It is possible to demonstrate the presence of lysosomes by histochemical staining for acid hydrolases, the most reliable being the demonstration of acid phosphatases. Immunohistochemical reagents can also be used to detect specific hydrolases, for example cathepsin-B and β-glucuronidase.

Cells with a specific phagocytic function, such as certain white blood cells, have a well developed acid vesicle system.

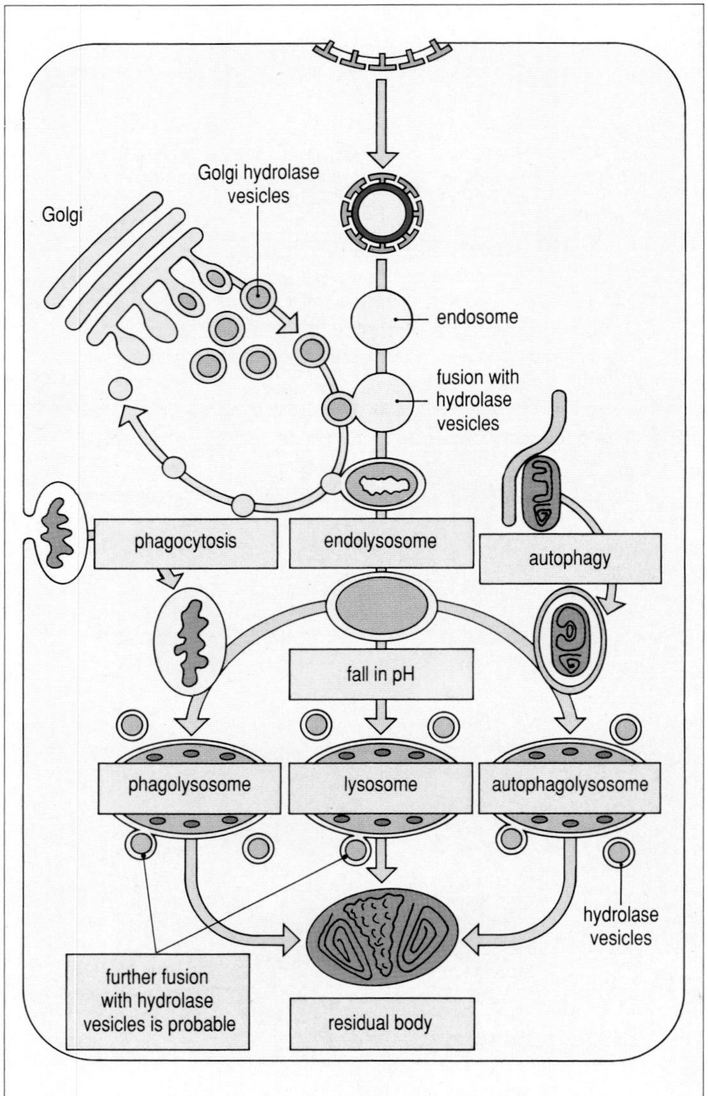

Fig. 2.16 Acid vesicle system.
Diagram of the relationships between the 'digestive' organelles of the acid vesicle system. Endosome forms from cell membrane and fuses with hydrolase-containing vesicles derived from the Golgi to form endolysosomes. The special Golgi membrane which forms the hydrolase vesicles is recycled back to the Golgi.

LYSOSOMAL STORAGE DISORDERS

In the acid vesicle system there are more than 30 defined and specific acid hydrolases, which not only degrade abnormal large molecules, but also recycle or process normal cell constituents.

Genetic defects in the production of specific acid hydrolases lead to an inability to degrade specific classes of molecule, which then accumulate in the acid vesicle system. Most of these defects are inherited as single gene autosomal recessive traits.

- **Lysosomal glycogen storage disease** (acid maltase deficiency) leads to the accumulation of glycogen, which cannot be broken down (Fig. 2.18).
- **Tay-Sachs disease** results from a deficiency in an enzyme degrading one of the sphingolipids (hexoseaminidase-A deficiency). Huge amounts of lipid accumulate in lysosomes and lead to severe neuronal degeneration.

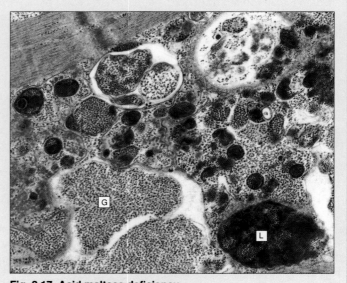

Fig. 2.17 Acid maltase deficiency.
Electronmicrograph showing glycogen accumulation (G) in muscle cytoplasm and also within lysosomal bodies (L).

Peroxisomes

Peroxisomes are small membrane-bound organelles containing enzymes involved in the oxidation of several substrates, particularly β-oxidation of very long chain fatty acids (C_{18} and above).

Ultrastructurally peroxisomes are small spherical bodies 0.5–1 μm in diameter with an electron-dense core, and occasionally a paracrystalline structure termed a **nucleoid**.

Several enzymes in peroxisomes oxidize their substrate and reduce O_2 to H_2O_2, while catalase, which is also present, decomposes H_2O_2 to O_2 and H_2O.

PEROXISOMAL DISORDERS

Several diseases are due to defects in the peroxisomal enzymes responsible for processing very long chain fatty acids, and are manifest by metabolic disturbances associated with acidosis, or with the storage of abnormal lipids in susceptible cells.

The most common example is **adrenoleukodystrophy**, in which impaired β-oxidation of fatty acids results in abnormal lipid storage in the brain, spinal cord and adrenal glands, leading to intellectual deterioration (dementia) and adrenal failure.

CYTOSKELETON

Several functions of the cell are maintained by a set of filamentous cytosolic proteins, the cytoskeletal proteins, of which there are three main classes depending on the size of their filaments.

Microfilaments (5 nm in diameter) are composed of the protein actin.

Intermediate filaments (10 nm in diameter) are composed of six main proteins, which vary in different cell types.

Microtubules (25 nm in diameter) are composed of two tubulin proteins.

These filamentous proteins become attached to cell membranes and to each other by anchoring and joining proteins to form a dynamic three-dimensional internal scaffolding in the cell. This scaffolding is in a continual state of assembly and disassembly, but periods of stability subserve specific functional roles such as maintaining cellular architecture, facilitating cell motility, anchoring cells together, facilitating transport of material around the cytosol and dividing the cytosol into functionally separate areas.

Actin

Actin accounts for about 5% of the total protein in most cell types. It is a globular protein (G-actin), which polymerizes to form filaments (F-actin) with all the actin subunits facing in one direction (polar filaments).

There are six molecular variants (isoforms) of actin, which have specific distributions in different cell types, for example isoforms restricted to smooth muscle or skeletal muscle.

Actin is an important component of the cytoskeleton for the following reasons.
• Actin filaments, in association with other proteins, form a layer (the **cell cortex**, Fig. 2.18) beneath the cell membrane. The actin is arranged into a stiff cross-linked meshwork by linking proteins, the most abundant being filamin. This meshwork resists sudden deformative forces, but allows changes in cell shape by reforming, which is facilitated by actin-severing proteins. The best characterized of these proteins is **gelsolin**, which breaks down actin networks in the presence of high cytosolic concentrations of free Ca^{2+} ions.
• Actin filament networks can provide mechanical support to the cell membrane by attachment to it via membrane anchoring proteins; the best characterized of these are **spectrin** and **ankyrin** in red blood cells (see Fig. 6.3c), but similar proteins are present in most other cells. In addition, actin can become linked to transmembrane proteins in specialized areas of the plasma membrane termed **adherent junctions** or **focal contacts** (see Figs 3.9 & 3.10), which are externally attached to other cells or extracellular structures; thus the actin filament network of one cell can become linked to other cells or structures.

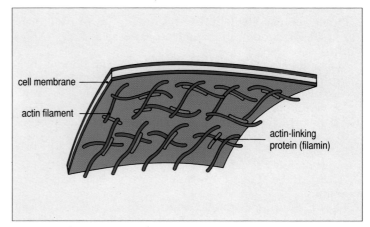

Fig. 2.18 Cell cortex.
The cell cortex is composed of a stiff, cross-linked meshwork of actin and actin-linking proteins, the most abundant being filamin. It forms a layer that lines the cytosolic face of the cell membrane.

- Actin filaments can form rigid bundles to stabilize protrusions of cell membrane termed microvilli (see Fig. 3.15). In these bundles, actin is associated with small linker proteins, the most abundant being **fimbrin** and **fascin**.
- In all cells, actin filaments interact with proteins called **myosins** to generate motile forces. Myosin is an actin-activated ATPase composed of two heavy chains and four light chains arranged into a long tail and a globular head. These myosin heads can bind to actin and hydrolize ATP to ADP. Sequential binding of myosin to individual actin subunits in F-actin causes the myosin to walk down the actin filament. As the actin filament is polar this generates a contractile force. Many of these contractile functions are transient, for example to produce the contractile force to separate dividing cells. In tissues specialized for contraction, this system is highly organized (see Fig. 5.1).

A modified form of myosin exists as monomeric structures without the long tail (**minimyosin**). This becomes attached to cell organelles and facilitates the transport of vesicles along actin filaments thus allowing organelles to move within the cell.

- Polymerization of actin filaments is probably responsible for the forces that drive local outgrowths of cell cytoplasm, such as spikes and ruffles, which are particularly evident in motile cells and cells undergoing migration in embryogenesis.

Microtubules

Microtubules are present in all cells except red blood cells. They are formed from two protein subunits (α and β tubulin), which polymerize in a head-to-tail pattern to form protofilaments. These are arranged into groups of 13 to form hollow tubes 25 nm in diameter (Fig. 2.19).

Other cellular elements are also made up of tubulin in the form of doublet or triplet tubules, such as centrioles and cilia (see below).

Microtubules are constantly polymerizing and depolymerizing in the cell and grow out from the microtubule organizing centre (see below). They are stabilized by associating with other proteins, (microtubule-associated proteins (MAPs)), which convert the unstable microtubular network into a relatively permanent framework. Microtubules are also stabilized by proteins that cap the growing end and prevent depolymerization.

Within the cell, microtubules have several important functions
- They form a network allowing transport around the cell via the attachment proteins **dynein**, which moves down a microtubule towards the cell centre, and **kinesin**, which moves up a microtubule towards the cell periphery. These attachment proteins are associated with the membranes of vesicles and organelles, and facilitate their movement

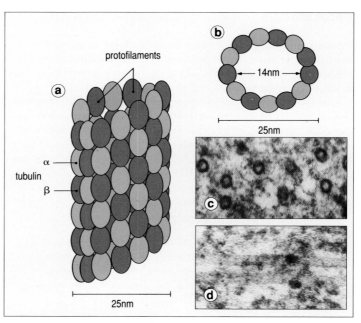

Fig. 2.19 Microtubules.
a Each microtubule is composed of 13 protofilaments of alternating α and β tubulin subunits. Microtubules are polar, with polymerization occuring at one end and depolymerization at the other. To stabilize their structure in cells, there are several microtubule-associated proteins (MAPs) such as Tau protein; in addition the ends of tubules may be capped by special stabilizing proteins, which prevent depolymerization.
b In cross-section each microtubule is 25 nm in diameter.
c Electronmicrograph showing the circular profiles of microtubules in cross section.
d Electronmicrograph showing the faint parallel lines of microtubules in longitudinal section.

around the cell. This process is particularly important in the transport of organelles down the long cell processes of nerve cells (see Chapter 13).
- They form a network (cytoskeleton) for membrane-bound cell compartments (e.g. they maintain the extended tubular arrangement of the ER).
- They form the cell spindle along which chromosomes are organized in cell division (see Fig. 2.23).
- They form the structural basis for specialized motile components of the cell, cilia (see Fig. 3.17).

Centriole

Microtubules originate in a special region of the cell (the **microtubule organizing centre**), which is a structure (the **centrosome**) based on an organelle composed of microtubules (the **centriole**, Fig. 2.20).

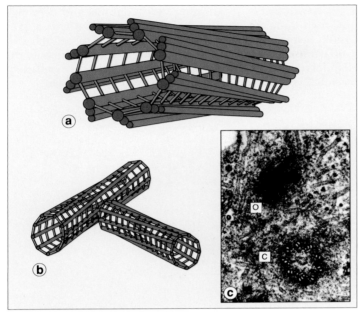

Fig. 2.20 Centriole.
a A centriole is composed of a cylindrical bundle measuring 0.2 x 0.4 μm composed of 9 microtubule triplets arranged together by linking proteins.
b In most cells, centrioles exist in pairs arranged at right angles to each other.
c In electron microscopic preparations, one centriole is usually visible in cross-section revealing the circular (C) arrangement of tubules, while its partner is cut either longitudinally or slightly obliquely (O).

Each centrosome consists of a pair of centrioles surrounded by an amorphous electron-dense area of cytoplasm, which acts as the nucleation centre for the polymerization of microtubules; these radiate from the centrosome in a star-like pattern called an **aster**. The protein forming the amorphous area is highly conserved in evolution and is present in both animal and plant cells. Each centrosome can act as the centre for about 250 microtubules.

The centriole has two roles in the cell.
• It organizes the cytoplasmic microtubular network in both normal and dividing cells.
• It organizes the development of specialized microtubules in motile cilia (see Fig. 3.17).

Intermediate filaments

Intermediate filaments are a group of filamentous cytoskeletal proteins comprising six main types, which have a specific distribution in different cell types (Fig. 2.21).

This restriction of distibution may be used for the histological assessment of cell types, using immunohistochemical staining for the various filaments. This is particularly useful when small samples of malignant tumour are being assessed to determine their likely site of origin.

The detection of cytokeratin argues strongly for an epithelial origin, while the presence of desmin would suggest a muscle derivation, and glial fibrillary acidic protein (GFAP) is only seen in specialized central nervous system tumours. Vimentin staining is least useful because it is expressed by many cell types and may be co-expressed in some cells with another more specialized intermediate filament.

Although intermediate filaments have several defined roles in cells as outlined below, detailed mechanisms of their function have not been elucidated unlike those of the other cytoskeletal proteins.
• Intermediate filaments are anchored to transmembrane proteins at special sites on the cell membrane (desmosomes and hemidesmosomes, see Figs 3.11 & 3.12) and spread tensile forces evenly throughout a tissue so that single cells are not disrupted.
• In epithelial cells of the skin, keratin intermediate filaments become compacted with other link proteins to form a tough outer layer (see Fig. 3.27) and hence have an important structural role as an impermeable barrier, as well as being the main constituent protein of hair and nail.
• In neurones, neurofilaments have long side-arms, which probably help to maintain the cylindrical architecture of nerve cell processes when subjected to lateral tensile forces in bending. They also anchor membrane **ion channel proteins** in place via a link protein ankyrin, to facilitate nerve conduction.
• When cells are damaged, the intermediate filament network, but not the microtubular or actin networks, collapses to form a perinuclear spherical ball associated with abnormal or damaged cellular proteins. It is possible that

Intermediate filament	Localization
cytokeratins	epithelial cells
desmin	muscle (smooth and striated)
glial fibrillary acidic protein (GFAP)	astrocytic glial cells
neurofilament protein	neurones
nuclear lamin	nucleus of all cells
vimentin	many mesodermal tissues

Fig. 2.21 Intermediate filaments.
Table showing the location of different types of intermediate filament.

in this situation the intermediate filaments act as a net to cocoon damaged cellular components in one spot for subsequent elimination by proteolysis. Following cell recovery, the intermediate filament network re-expands.

This phenomenon occurs in liver cells in response to persistent alcohol excess, when collapsed bundles of cytokeratin intermediate filaments (Mallory's hyaline) accumulate.
• In the nucleus, the nuclear lamins form a square lattice on the inner side of the nuclear membrane, which probably acts with other link proteins in organization of the nucleus.

CELL INCLUSIONS

Accumulations of products within certain cells may occur in the form of cytoplasmic inclusions.

Lipofuscin pigment appears as membrane-bound orange-brown granular material within the cytoplasm. Derived from residual bodies containing a mixture of phospholipids from cell degradation, lipofuscin is commonly referred to as 'wear and tear' pigment, as it becomes more prominent in old cells. It is particularly common in tissues from elderly persons, and is most evident in nerve, heart muscle and liver cells.

Lipid may accumulate as non-membrane bound vesicles, which appear as large clear spaces in the cytoplasm because paraffin wax processing dissolves out the fat. If the tissues are frozen and cut in a freezing microtome, the fat is stainable with certain dyes. Large fat vacuoles are a special feature of fat storage cells called adipocytes (see Fig. 4.20). Fat also accumulates in certain cells such as the liver in response to sub-lethal metabolic damage, the most common cause being alcohol ingestion.

Glycogen is a polymer and storage product of glucose and forms granules in the cell cytoplasm. Demands for energy are met by conversion of glycogen to glucose.

In certain cells, the presence of large amounts of glycogen causes pale staining or apparent vacuolation of cell cytoplasm. Glycogen can be stained by the PAS method and is also visible ultrastructurally as small granules in the cell cytoplasm (see Fig. 2.17).

CELL DIVISION

Mitosis

An essential feature of development is the ability of cells to divide and reproduce. In addition, death or loss of mature cells in the adult needs to be compensated for by growth of new cells.

Cells reproduce by duplicating their contents and dividing into two daughter cells. The phases of cell division are visible histologically and involve duplication of cellular cytoplasmic contents, duplication of DNA, separation of cellular DNA into two separate areas of the cell (**mitosis**, Figs 2.22 & 2.23) and finally cell division (**cytokinesis**).

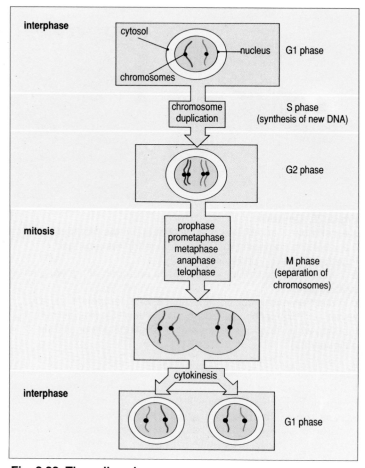

Fig. 2.22 The cell cycle.
The DNA of cells is only replicated during certain phases of a cell's growth pattern, which has been divided into several stages.

Cells which are not dividing are non-cycling or G_0 cells, while G_1 cells have just entered a phase of cellular growth. S phase cells actively synthesize DNA, G_2 cells have a double complement of cellular DNA and are resting prior to cell division, and M phase cells are in mitosis, which is composed of 5 stages.

The cell cycle is divided into two main periods: mitosis and interphase, which includes G_1, S and G_2 phases.

In most tissues only a small proportion of cells will be in the cell cycle, the majority being differentiated cells in a G_0 phase. Stem cells may be in a G_0 phase and only come to re-enter the cell cycle if there is a demand, for example following cell death.

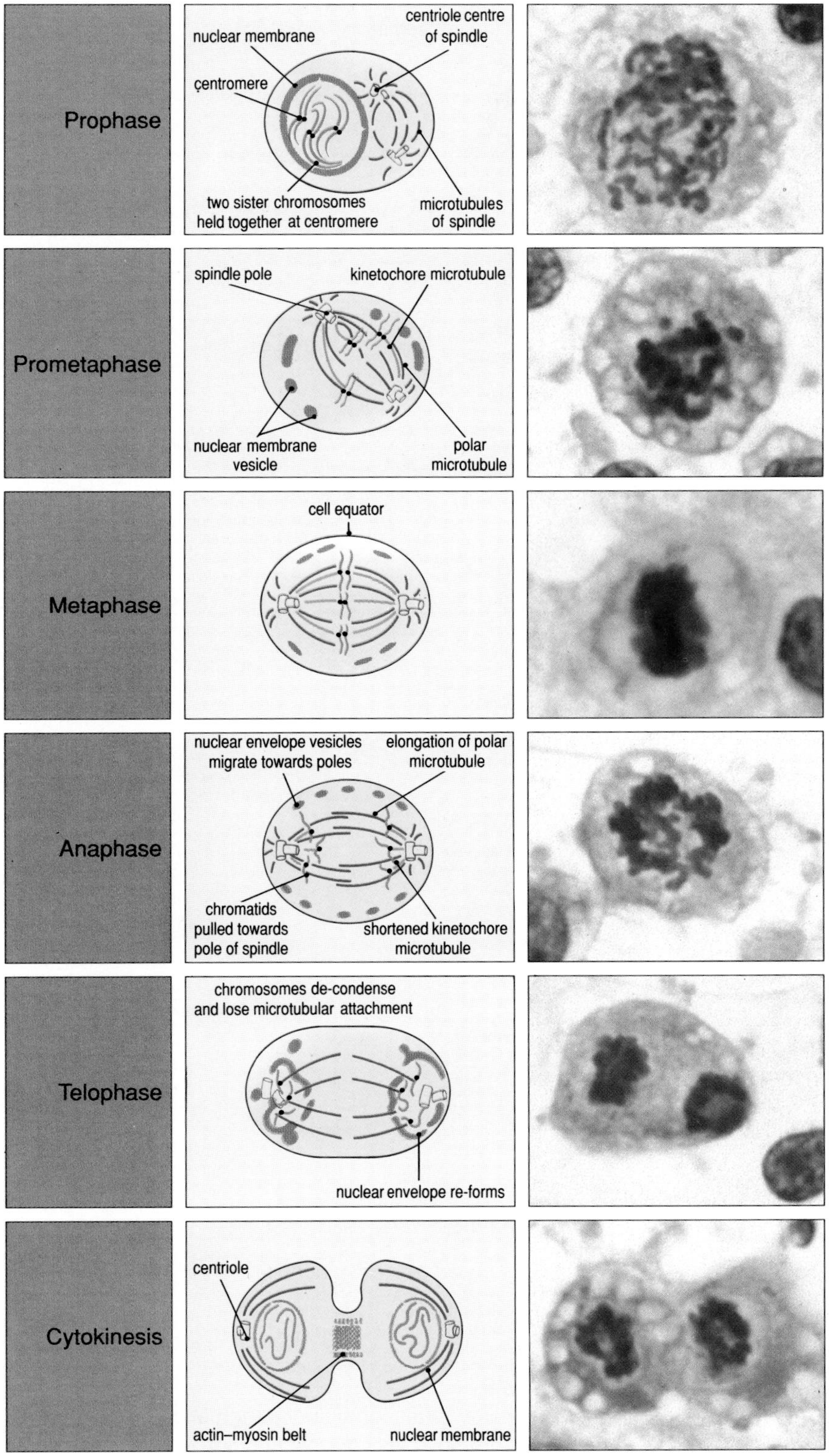
Prophase
nuclear membrane
centriole centre of spindle
centromere
two sister chromosomes held together at centromere
microtubules of spindle
Prometaphase
spindle pole
kinetochore microtubule
nuclear membrane vesicle
polar microtubule
Metaphase
cell equator
Anaphase
nuclear envelope vesicles migrate towards poles
elongation of polar microtubule
chromatids pulled towards pole of spindle
shortened kinetochore microtubule
Telophase
chromosomes de-condense and lose microtubular attachment
nuclear envelope re-forms
Cytokinesis
centriole
actin–myosin belt
nuclear membrane

Fig. 2.23 Mitosis.

The duplicated chromatin becomes condensed into parallel sister chromosomes imparting a coarse stippling to the nuclear region, which is associated with loss of the nucleolus.

The centriole replicates to form two microtubule organizing centres at opposite poles of the cell (the mitotic spindle), which is not visible by light microscopy.

The nuclear membrane breaks down to form small vesicles, allowing the microtubules of the spindle (see page 20) to interact with the chromosomes.

Each chromosome pair has an attachment site (kinetochore), which binds to spindle microtubules from each pole of the spindle (kinetochore tubules).The chromosome pairs move towards the centre of the spindle.

Movement of chromosomes along the microtubules leads to alignment of the chromosomes at the equator of the cell between the poles of the spindle.

The kinetochore attachments to the paired chromosomes separate and the chromosomes move to opposite poles of the spindle.

In late anaphase the spindle microtubules elongate causing elongation of the cell and further separation of the spindle poles.

The separated chromatids become separated from the kinetochore microtubules and the nuclear membrane reforms around each group of chromosomes.

The cell elongates further by elongation of the spindle microtubules.

This phase signals the end of mitosis.

Cleavage into two separate cells is produced by aggregation of an actin–myosin belt immediately beneath the equator of the telophase cell. The connecting region eventually separates with fusion of cell membranes to form two daughter cells.

At this stage a nucleolus appears in the dense chromatin mass in the newly formed nucleus.The cell now enters the G_1 phase of the cell cycle.

Not all cells are capable of division and several different populations of cells can be defined based on their capacity to divide and replicate.

- **Static cell populations** are cells which cannot divide, for example nerve cells and cardiac muscle cells.
- **Stable cell populations** do not normally divide, but can do so if cell loss occurs, for example liver cells.
- **Renewing cell populations** normally divide constantly to maintain themselves as a result of cell death, for example skin and gut lining cells, which are constantly shed, and blood cells, which have a short life span.

Once a new cell forms it may either differentiate into a mature cell type or divide again without differentiation to form uncommitted daughter cells, which may differentiate later. The uncommitted daughter cells, whose function is to provide a pool of cells to replenish a cell population, are called **stem cells**.

Several types of renewing cell populations are thought to originate from common stem cells, for example the different cells of the blood probably originate from a common haemopoietic stem cell, and enterocyte stem cells probably give rise to the different cell types lining the gut.

Following stem cell division, two types of cell may result; new stem cells to maintain the stem cell population, and **committed cells**, which differentiate along one cell line, but may still divide in what are termed **amplification divisions**.

A stem cell must reproduce itself each time it divides to maintain the stem cell population.

ANTI-CANCER DRUGS

Many drugs used to treat cancer act specifically on cells in the cell cycle (see Fig. 2.22), the aim being to remove abnormally growing cells.

Unfortunately these drugs act on normal body cells as well as cancer cells and have adverse effects particularly on renewing cell populations (see above), which depend on a high proportion of cells being in cycle.

Thus, blood cell production, hair production and gut-lining cell production are all impaired by the administration of such anti-cancer drugs.

MEIOSIS

Normal cells have two sets of complementary chromosomes derived from the maternal and paternal cells at fertilization and are therefore called diploid (i.e 2n) cells.

The germ cells (ova and spermatozoa), which are destined to fuse in fertilization to produce an embryo, have half the normal complement of chromosomes (i.e. are

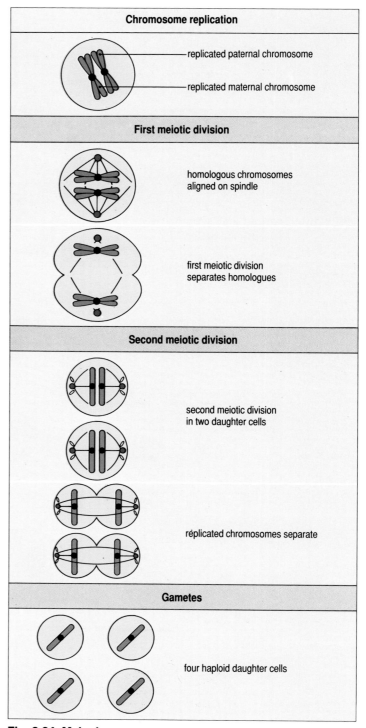

Fig. 2.24 Meiosis.
Meiosis results in the formation of four daughter cells, each with half the normal chromosomal complement (i.e. n, haploid).

haploid (n) cells), their production being achieved by a modified form of cell division, **meiosis**.

In meiosis (Fig. 2.24), complementary chromosomes become paired on the mitotic spindle following S phase of the cell cycle (see Fig. 2.22) with the maternal one attached to one pole and the paternal one attached to the opposite pole; the pole to which maternal and paternal derived chromosomes become attached is random for each chromosome.

This is in contrast to mitosis where complementary chromosomes do not align across the spindle.

Thus in meiosis, maternal and paternal complementary chromosomes are separated to opposite ends of the spindle by a first meiotic division. Once segregated in this way a second division (virtually identical to a mitotic division, see Fig. 2.23) separates replicated chromosomes. The result of meiosis is four daughter nuclei each containing one set of chromosomes.

PRACTICAL HISTOLOGY

General principles can be usefully applied when looking at cells either in cytological preparations or tissue sections to assess their activity, as outlined below.

Nucleus

A metabolically inactive cell has a compact round nucleus, which typically stains intensely as little chromatin is being transcribed. No nucleoli are visible as ribosome production is minimal.

A protein synthesizing cell has a large pale staining nucleus with large or multiple nucleoli, reflecting active transcription of chromatin. Similar nuclear changes are evident in cells in an active phase of multiplication (see Fig. 2.22).

A dead cell has a shrunken nucleus, which appears as an amorphous compact mass of intensely staining material. This later fragments into separate particles, and is completely lysed, leaving the cell devoid of any discernible nucleus.

Nuclear changes in cancer

A cell containing a very large nucleus relative to the amount of cytoplasm is generally in a phase of cell division. Cells with inappropriately large nuclei raise the suspicion of neoplastic change, for example cells on the surface of the cervix should have small nuclei unless there is abnormal cell growth such as that associated with the development of a cancer (see Fig. 18.00).

In any specialized cell type, all the nuclei in adjacent cells should be roughly the same size and have the same staining characteristics. In cancer however, nuclei vary in size and shape (**nuclear pleomorphism**) and commonly show dense staining chromatin in a coarse clumped pattern (**nuclear hyperchromatism**).

Cytoplasm

Examination of cell cytoplasm should concentrate on the intensity and distribution of acidophilic (pink) and basophilic (purple) elements.

A granular intensely pink-staining cytoplasm contains accumulations of organelles that take up acidic dye, which are usually mitochondria or secretory granules, (e.g. neurosecretory granules, or specialized granules, such as seen in white blood cells).

A diffuse purple tint to the cytoplasm indicates the presence of cytoplasmic RNA in the form of ribosomes, and thus active protein production.

Large non-staining areas are generally large secretory vacuoles, such as seen in cells secreting mucin. In some cell types they may represent fat.

Diagnostic Cytology

Cytology is the study of cellular form and refers to an important speciality in laboratory medicine, which concentrates on establishing the diagnosis of disease by examination of small numbers of cells.

Cells for examination are obtained from patients either by scraping the surface of epithelia (e.g. the cervix or gastric lining), aspirating solid tissues with a needle, or by collecting cells from body fluids, such as sputum or urine.

The ultimate aim is to detect abnormalities in cell structure that point to the development of disease. In clinical medicine the most important aspect is the recognition of changes which herald the development of cancer (**neoplastic changes**).

Epithelial cells form tightly cohesive sheets of cells called epithelia, which function mainly as:
- a covering or lining for body surfaces, for example skin, gut and ducts;
- the functional units of secretory glands such as salivary tissue and liver.

Epithelia are characterized by:
- cell adhesion mechanisms anchoring the cytoskeleton of each epithelial cell to its neighbours;
- cell adhesion mechanisms anchoring the epithelium to underlying or surrounding extracellular matrix materials.

Epithelial cells are further specialized to fulfil their specific role, which may be absorption or secretion, or to act as a barrier (see pages 32–41).

NOMENCLATURE AND CLASSIFICATION

The traditional nomenclature and classification of different types of epithelium is based on the two dimensional shape of cells as observed by early light microscopy, and ignores any specialized functional attributes. Thus the nomenclature now appears rather simplistic given the present detailed knowledge of the biology of these cells.

Traditional classification

The traditional classification is as follows.
- There are three main cell groups according to cell shape: **squamous** (flat plate-like, Fig. 3.1), **cuboidal** (height and width similar, Fig. 3.2), and **columnar** (height 2–5 times greater than width, Fig. 3.3).
- Epithelial cells form either a single layer in which all of the cells contact underlying extracellular matrix (**simple epithelium**), or several layers where only the bottom layer of cells is in contact with the extracellular matrix (**stratified epithelium**, Fig. 3.4).

Pseudostratified epithelium (Fig. 3.5) describes epithelial cells that appear to be arranged in layers, but are all in contact with the extracellular matrix. A **transitional epithelium** is a further special type of stratified epithelium which is restricted to the lining of the urinary tract (see Fig. 16.48), and varies between cuboidal and squamous depending on the degree of stretching.
- Epithelia are also grouped according to whether they are a surface or glandular component.

Limitation of traditional classification.

In the past, great emphasis was placed on the distribution of the different morphological types of epithelium and whether they were stratified or simple, surface or glandular; such classification is now outmoded. Although two epithelia may be described as cuboidal, their function and biology may be so different that it is misleading to equate them.

However, provided this limitation of nomenclature is realized, the use of a morphological classification of epithelia is still descriptively useful.

The traditional terms used to describe epithelia are found throughout this book, but are always qualified to give insight into their function.

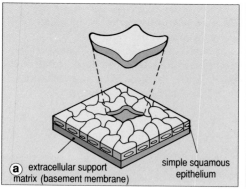

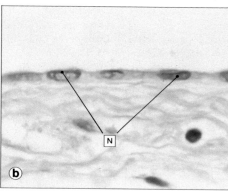

Fig. 3.1 Simple squamous epithelium.
a A simple squamous epithelium is composed of a single layer of cells, which are flat and plate-like.
b In histological sections, the nuclei (N) appear flattened and the cytoplasm is indistinct.

Although squamous refers to any flat epithelium, its use is restricted as many flat epithelia are given more specific names, the flat epithelium lining blood vessels being called endothelium, and that lining the abdominal and pleural cavities, mesothelium.

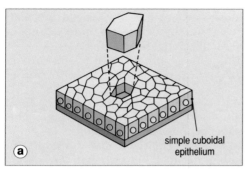

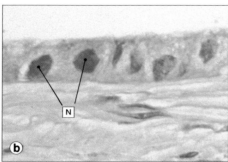

Fig. 3.2 Simple cuboidal epithelium.

a A simple cuboidal epithelium is composed of a single layer of cells whose height, width and depth are the same. Note they are not strictly cuboidal.

b In histological section, such cells usually have a centrally placed nucleus (N).

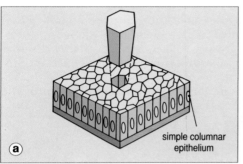

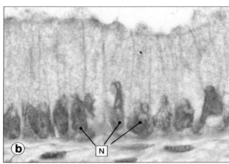

Fig. 3.3 Simple columnar epithelium.

a A simple columnar epithelium is composed of cells whose height is 2–3 times greater than their width.

b The nuclei (N) of columnar cells are basal and arranged in an ordered layer.

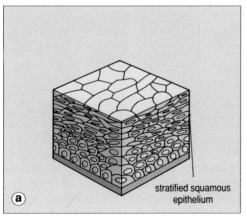

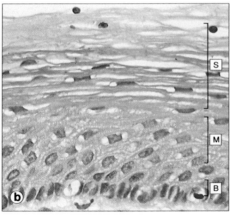

Fig. 3.4 Stratified squamous epithelium.

a A stratified epithelium is composed of several layers of cells such that cells high up in the epithelium are not in direct contact with the underlying extracellular matrix.

b Stratified squamous epithelium derives its name from the flattened (squamous) appearance of cells in the superficial part of the epithelium (S). Cells in the basal (B) and middle (M) layers of this type of epithelium are in fact pyramidal or polygonal and are not flattened. Nuclei in cells in the lower part of the epithelium are rounded, while higher up they assume an elliptical shape as the cells take on a flattened squamous morphology.

Fig. 3.5 Pseudostratified columnar epithelium.

a In a pseudostratified epithelium, several layers of nuclei suggest several layers of cells, but in fact all cells are in contact with the underlying extracellular matrix.

b Routine histological preparations show several layers of nuclei.

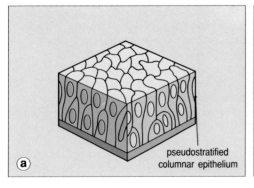

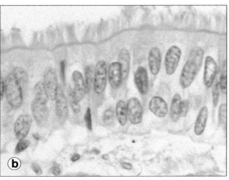

27

CELL ADHESION

The structural integrity of epithelium is maintained by adhesion of the constituent cells both to each other and to structural extracellular matrix.

These adhesions are mediated by cell membrane proteins acting as specialized **cell adhesion molecules**, and by specialized areas of cell membrane forming **cell junctions**. There are three types of cell junction: **occluding junctions** link cells to form an impermeable barrier, **anchoring junctions** link cells to provide mechanical strength, and **communicating junctions** allow movement of molecules between cells.

Occluding junctions

Occluding junctions have two main functions:
- prevention of diffusion of molecules between adjacent cells, thereby contributing to the barrier function of the epithelial cells in which they are present;
- prevention of lateral migration of specialized cell membrane proteins, thereby delineating and maintaining specialized cell membrane domains.

The occluding function is performed by intramembranous proteins (Fig. 3.6), which mediate the adhesion of adjacent cells.

Ultrastructurally an occluding junction is seen as a focal area of close apposition of adjacent cell membrane. This has lead to its alternative name of **tight junction**.

Occluding junctions are particularly well developed in the epithelial cells lining the small bowel, where they;
- prevent digested macromolecules from passing between the cells;
- confine specialized areas of the cell membrane involved in absorption to the luminal side of the cell.

Occluding junctions are also important in cells that actively transport a substance, for example the active transport of an ion, against a concentration gradient. In this situation occluding junctions prevent back diffusion of the transported substance (Fig. 3.7).

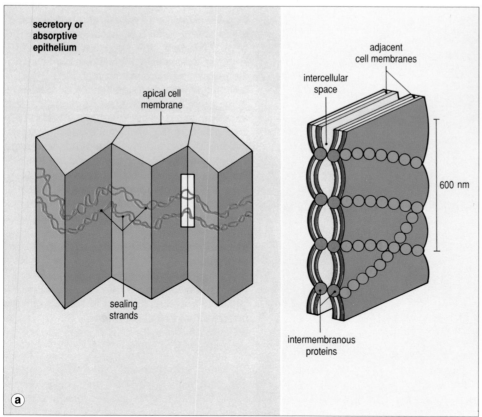

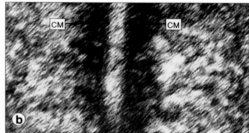

Fig. 3.6 Occluding junction–structure.
a Occluding junctions are particularly evident between epithelial cells that have secretory or absorptive roles. A collar of occluding junction is present between each cell, sealing individual cells into a tight barrier.

The intramembranous proteins that form these junctions are arranged as serpiginous intertwining lines (**sealing strands**), which stitch the membrane of adjacent cells together.

b An occluding junction is seen ultrastructurally as an area of close apposition of adjacent areas of cell membrane (CM) corresponding to the site of membrane attachment proteins.

joined throughout the walls 'sticking together'

Anchoring junctions

Anchoring junctions (Fig. 3.8) provide mechanical stability to groups of cells so that they can function as a cohesive unit, by linking the cytoskeleton (see page 19) between adjacent cells, as well as to supporting extracellular matrix.

Two separate classes of junction interact with different cytoskeletal filaments: **adherent junctions** and **focal contacts** link with the actin filament network, **desmosomes** and **hemidesmosomes** link with the intermediate filament network.

Adherent junctions link the actin filament network between adjacent cells (Fig. 3.9).

Focal contacts link the actin filament network of a cell to the extracellular matrix (Fig. 3.10).

Desmosomes connect the intermediate filament networks of adjacent cells (Fig. 3.11).

Hemidesmosomes connect the intermediate filament network of cells to extracellular matrix (Fig. 3.12).

Adherent junctions are most common towards the apex of adjacent columnar and cuboidal epithelial cells, where they link submembranous actin bundles into an adhesion belt. They are prominent in the cells lining the small intestine where they form a zone visible by light microscopy as an eosinophilic band (the terminal bar).

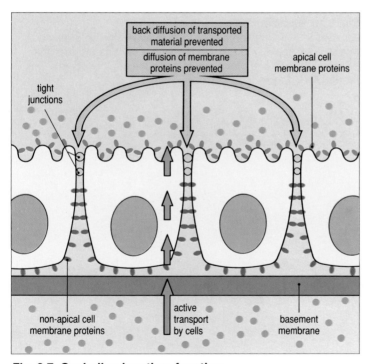

Fig. 3.7 Occluding junction–function.
Cells that transport molecules against a concentration gradient have occluding junctions to prevent back diffusion of the transported substance.

In addition, it is desirable to concentrate specialized cell membrane components into certain areas of the cell, for example a transport protein in the apical cell membrane.

Cells use occluding junctions to prevent lateral migration of specialized membrane proteins, thus establishing specialized membrane domains.

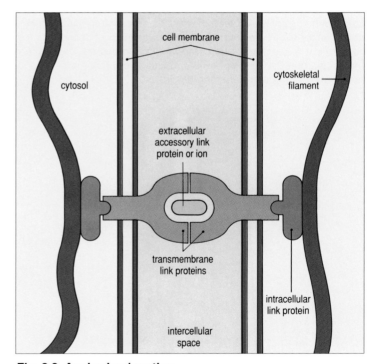

Fig. 3.8 Anchoring junction.
Diagram to illustrate the general structure of cell anchoring junctions.

Cytoskeletal filaments of adjacent cells are joined through intracellular link proteins, which attach the filaments to transmembrane link proteins. These can then interact with similar proteins on adjacent cells. The extracellular interaction may be mediated by additional extracellular proteins or ions, such as Ca^{2+}. Different (or multiple) link proteins and transmembrane proteins operate for the different classes of junction.

29

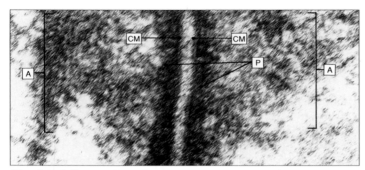

Fig. 3.9 Adherent junction.
Actin fibres in adjacent cells are linked by actin-binding proteins (α actinin and vinculin) to a transmembrane protein, which is one of a group of cell surface glycoproteins mediating cell adhesion (**cadherin**). The type in adherent junctions is E-cadherin, which links cells in the presence of Ca^{2+}.

Ultrastructurally, an adherent junction is a fuzzy plaque (P) of electron-dense material adjacent to the cell membrane (CM), corresponding to the location of α actinin and vinculin, into which actin filaments (A) are inserted. The intercellular junctional component (i.e. extracellular component of adjacent E-cadherin molecules and Ca^{2+}) is not visible, but is evident as a lucent area between the adjacent membranes.

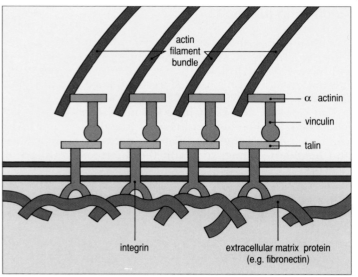

Fig. 3.10 Focal contact.
Bundles of actin filaments interact with actin-binding proteins (α actinin, vinculin and talin) to link with a transmembrane link protein, which is one of a class of cell adhesion molecules termed an **integrin** (see Fig. 4.9).

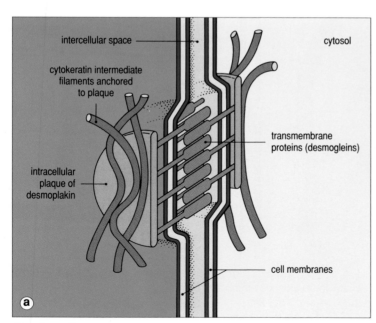

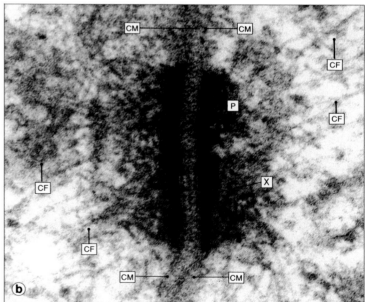

Fig. 3.11 Desmosome.
a Each desmosome consists of an intracellular plaque composed of several link proteins (the main types being desmoplakins), into which cytokeratin intermediate filaments (**tonofilaments**) are inserted. The cell adhesion is mediated by transmembrane proteins called desmogleins.

b The disc shaped adhesion plaques (P) in adjacent cells are seen as electron-dense areas into which cytokeratin filaments (CF) are inserted. The cell membranes (CM) between adhesion plaques are about 30 nm apart and there may be an electron-dense band between cells in some desmosomes (X).

In embryogenesis, adherent-type junctions transmit motile forces generated by the actin filaments across whole sheets of cells. They are thus essential in mediating the folding of epithelial sheets to form early organs in the embryo.

Desmosomes provide mechanical stability in epithelial cells subject to tensile and shearing stresses, and are particularly well developed in stratified squamous epithelium covering the skin.

Desmosomes are so characteristic of epithelial cells that their detection in malignant tumours of uncertain nature is indicative of an epithelial as opposed to a lymphoid or support cell origin.

A **junctional complex** describes the close association of several types of junction between adjacent epithelial cells and is a manifestation of the requirement for several types of epithelial cell attachment in order to maintain structural and functional integrity (Fig. 3.13).

DISEASE OF CELL JUNCTIONS–PEMPHIGUS

In pemphigus, the body produces abnormal antibodies to the proteins forming desmosome junctions in the skin; this prevents normal adhesion between the desmosomes. Affected people develop widespread skin and mucous membrane blistering as the desmosomal junctions between adjacent squamous cells of the skin fall apart.

Immunohistochemical staining can be used to demonstrate the abnormal antibodies adhering to the intercellular space between the diseased epidermal cells.

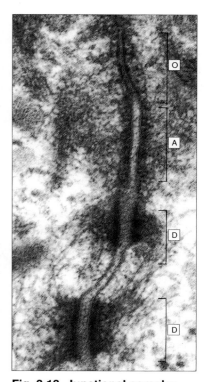

Fig. 3.13 Junctional complex.
A junctional complex is commonly seen towards the apex of cuboidal and columnar cells.

Immediately below the cell apex an occluding junction (O) is followed by an adherent junction (A), and below this by desmosomes (D).

This example is obtained from cells lining the small bowel where such complexes are well developed. In other epithelia, particularly those in which occluding junctions are not required, such fully developed complexes are uncommon.

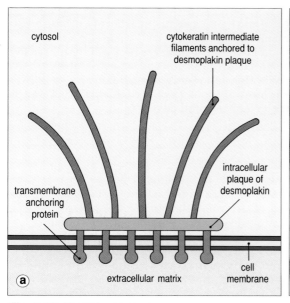
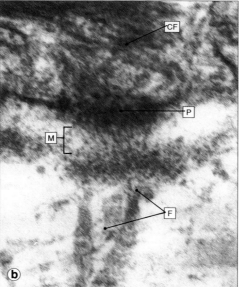

Fig. 3.12 Hemidesmosome.
a A hemidesmosome is similar to a desmosome except that it interacts with extracellular matrix rather than with an adjacent desmosome on another cell. In contrast to a desmosome, the cytokeratin filaments (tonofilaments) commonly terminate end-on rather than looping through.
b Ultrastructurally, a hemidesmosome consists of a dense plaque (P) composed of intracellular link proteins including desmoplakins, into which cytokeratin intermediate filaments (CF), are inserted. Linkage to the extracellular matrix (M) can be seen as a series of fine **anchoring fibrils** (F).

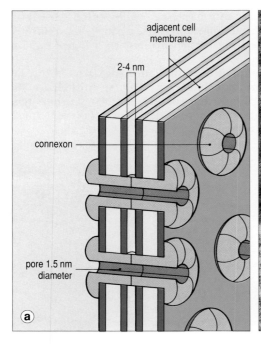
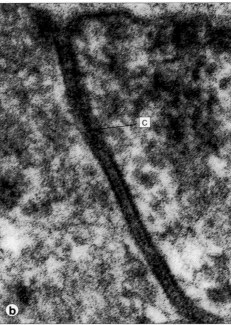

Fig. 3.14 Gap (communication) junction.
a Diagram showing a small part of a gap junction. Each junction is a circular patch studded with several hundred pores, each formed by six protein subunits traversing the cell membrane and termed a **connexon**. Pores on adjacent cells are aligned, allowing small molecules to move between cells.
b Ultrastructurally, a cross section of a gap junction is seen as a flat area of closely apposing cell membranes, between which the connexons (C) can just be seen as dot-like granules.

Communication junctions

Communication junctions (**gap junctions**) allow selective diffusion of molecules between adjacent cells and facilitate direct cell to cell comunication (Fig. 3.14).

Gap junctions are usually present at relatively low density in most adult epithelia, but are found in large numbers in embryogenesis, when they probably have a role in the spatial organization of developing cells.

Gap junctions are also important in cardiac and smooth muscle cells.

Basement membrane

Attachment of epithelial cells to underlying support tissues at hemidesmosomes and focal contacts is mediated by a specialized layer of extracellular matrix materials, the **basement membrane** (see Fig. 4.11). Basement membrane contains a special form of matrix protein called collagen, which is synthesized by the epithelial cells.

By light microscopy, basement membrane is just visible as a linear structure at the base of epithelia. It can be stained with the PAS technique.

CELL SURFACE SPECIALIZATIONS

The surface of epithelial cells is commonly modified to perform specialized functions.
• The main adaptation requirement is for increased surface area, which in different cell types is subserved by **microvilli**, **basal folds** and **membrane plaques**.
• The need to move substances over their surface is met by motile cell projections termed **cilia**.

Microvilli

Microvilli are finger-like projections of the cell surface (Fig. 3.15). Small microvilli are found on the surface of most epithelial cells, but are most developed in absorptive cells, such as kidney tubule cells and small bowel epithelium.

The shape of microvilli is maintained by a bundle of actin filaments, which form a core running through each villus and is anchored to the actin cortex of the cell. In epithelial cells of the small bowel, the actin core is also linked to the actin network of adherent junctions between adjacent cells.

Cell membrane covering microvilli is associated with specific cell surface glycoproteins and enzymes involved in the absorptive process. This cell surface specialization is just visible ultrastructurally as a fuzzy coating, but is much more evident when enzyme histochemistry or immunohistochemistry is used to detect specific proteins, such as lactase and alkaline phosphatase (see Fig. 3.19).

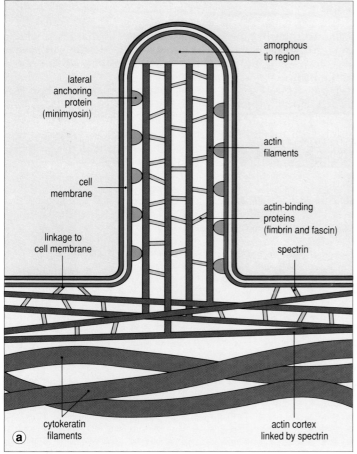

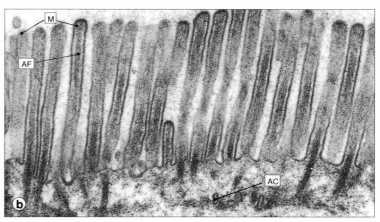

Fig. 3.15 Microvilli.

a Each microvillus is a finger-like extension of cell membrane, which is stabilized by a bundle of actin filaments held rigidly 10 nm apart by actin-binding proteins (fimbrin and fascin). The actin bundle is bound to the lateral surface of the microvillus by a helical arrangement of minimyosin molecules, which bind on one side to the actin and on the other to the inner surface of the cell membrane. The bundle is also adherent to the apex of the microvillus in an amorphous area of unknown composition, which may represent capping proteins for the actin filaments to prevent their depolymerization.

At the base of the microvillus the entering actin bundle is stabilized by the actin/spectrin cell cortex, under which are cytokeratin intermediate filaments.

b Electronmicrograph showing the surface of a cell lining the small bowel. Microvilli (M) form finger-like projections, each having an actin filament (AF) core that enters the cell and merges with the actin cortex (AC), which is also known as the terminal web.

Stereocilia are extremely long forms of microvilli and, despite their name, have nothing to do with true cilia (see below). They are found on epithelial cells lining the epididymis, and are the sensors of cochlear hair cells (see Chapter 13).

Basal folds

Basal folds are deep invaginations of the basal surface of cells (Fig. 3.16).

Basal folds are particularly evident in cells involved in fluid or ion transport, and are commonly associated with high concentrations of mitochondria, which provide the energy for ion and fluid transport.

The presence of basal folds and mitochondria imparts a striped appearance to the basal cytoplasm of such cells, giving rise to the descriptive term 'striated epithelial cells'.

Basal folds are seen in renal tubular cells (see Fig. 16.35) and in the ducts of many secretory glands.

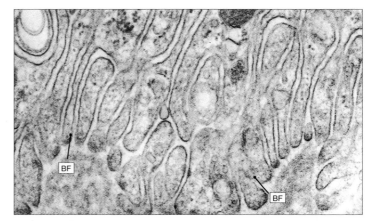

Fig. 3.16 Basal folds.
Electronmicrograph showing deep infolding of basal cell membrane (BF) of a distal tubule kidney cell. This facilitates cell membrane transport of ions by greatly increasing cell surface area.

Cell surface area can be similarly increased by folding of lateral cell membrane, which can be seen in some epithelial cells, particularly absorptive cells lining the gut.

Membrane plaques

Membrane plaques are rigid areas of the apical cell membrane found only in epithelium lining the urinary tract. They can fold down into the cell when the bladder is empty and unfold to increase the luminal area of the cell when the bladder is full.

Cilia

Cilia are hair-like projections, 0.25 μm in diameter, which arise from the surface of certain specialized cells and have a role in moving fluid over the surface of the cell or confer cell motility.

Each cilium is a highly specialized extension of the cytoskeleton and is composed of an organized core of parallel microtubules (the axoneme). These microtubules are bound together with other proteins to produce energy-dependent movement of the filaments, which results in beating from side to side (Fig. 3.17).

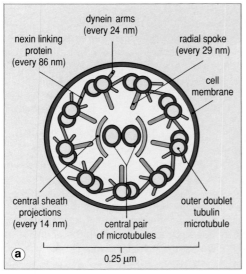

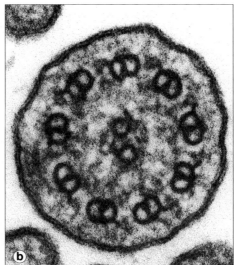

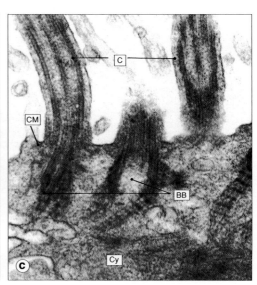

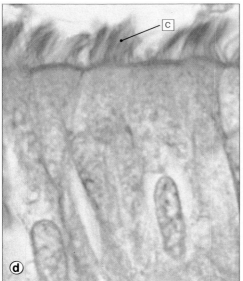

Fig. 3.17 Cilia.

a Diagram of a cross section of a cilium. The 9 outer doublet tubules are made of tubulin, while arms composed of the protein dynein occur every 24 nm down the length of the cilium and interact with adjacent doublets as a 'molecular motor' to produce bending. Links composed of another protein, nexin, are more widely spaced (every 86 nm) and hold the microtubules in position. Radial spokes extend from each of the 9 outer doublets towards a central pair of tubules at 29 nm intervals, while the central sheath projections are present every 14 nm and are thought to be involved in regulating the pattern of ciliary beating.

b Ultrastructural appearance of a cilium in cross section. Because the different constituent proteins are periodically spaced at different intervals along the length of the axoneme, not all are visible in any one plane of section.

c In longitudinal section, the base of each cilium (C) is seen to arise as a specialized derivative of the centriole (the basal body, BB). Here, the outer doublets of the cilium arise directly from the outer triplet of the centriole. This is in contrast to the microtubule organizing centre at the centriole, which is not in direct continuity with developing cytoplasmic microtubules. (CM, cell membrane; Cy, cytoplasm).

d Micrograph of a ciliated epithelium. Cilia (C) form a hair-like layer at the apical cell surface. As they are very fragile they may not be well preserved in poorly fixed or processed tissue.

Cilia are particularly evident in:
- epithelium lining the respiratory tract, where they move mucus over the cell surfaces (see Fig. 9.2);
- epithelium lining the fallopian tube, where they convey released ova to the uterine cavity (see Fig. 18.12).

A similar structure to that of cilia is found in the flagellum of spermatozoa (see Fig. 17.7).

CILIAL DEFECTS AND DISEASE

Genetic defects in genes coding for ciliary proteins give rise to uncoordinated or absent ciliary beating in ciliated epithelia. This causes the **immotile cilia syndrome**.

Ultrastructurally, elements of the cilia may be absent or abnormal (Fig. 3.18), and different individuals manifest different abnormalities, reflecting the genetic diversity of the condition.

There are several consequences of such an abnormality.
- In embryogenesis the defective cilia are unable to move cell layers correctly and the major organs do not assume their normal anatomical position, being commonly reversed with dextrocardia (right sided heart).
- Development of air sinuses in the skull, which is dependent on normal cilial action, is impaired.
- Failure of mucus removal from the lung results in recurrent and severe chest infections. Eventually, prolonged stagnation of secretions and recurrent bacterial infections lead to permanent dilation of the large air passages, which fill with stagnant infected secretions and lead to premature death.
- Infertility is common because ovum transport along the fallopian tube depends on normal ciliary function, and ciliary proteins make up the motile tail of spermatozoa.

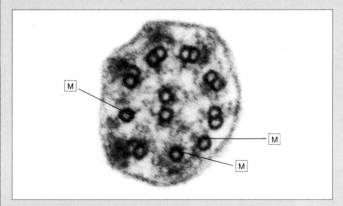

Fig. 3.18 Immotile cilia syndrome.
Electronmicrograph of cilia from a person with recurrent chest infections since childhood. The outer dynein arms are absent and there are abnormal single microtubules (M), which prevent normal motility. Compare with Fig. 3.17b.

Cell surface proteins

The surface of most epithelia is invested with a layer of protein, glycoprotein and sugar residues, which can be resolved ultrastructurally as an amorphous fuzzy coating to the cell membrane and, by virtue of the sugar content, is stainable by techniques such as the PAS method (see page 6). This coat is the **glycocalyx**.

Enzyme histochemical and immunohistochemical methods can be used to detect specific enzymes in this surface coat (Fig. 3.19), and it is apparent that epithelial cells at different sites have different functional attributes in terms of enzyme activity, despite similarities in their morphology.

SECRETORY ADAPTATIONS

Certain epithelial cells have structural specializations related to their role in the production and secretion of macromolecules, such as enzymes, mucins and steroids. In addition, epithelial cells can be adapted for the secretion and transport of ions.

Such cells are characterized by an expansion of their organelle systems, which are involved in the elaboration and secretion of macromolecules (see pages 36–37).

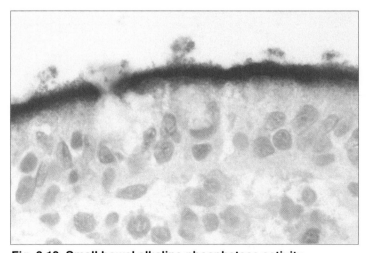

Fig. 3.19 Small bowel alkaline phosphatase activity.
The localization of cell membrane-associated alkaline phosphatase on the surface of epithelial cells lining the small bowel is shown. Note that the enzyme activity (demonstrated as a red stain deposit) is confined to the apical surface of the cells.

Protein-secreting epithelial cells

Although all cells contain the apparatus to produce structural proteins, certain cells are specialized to secrete a protein product and have the following characteristics.

• A well developed rough endoplasmic reticulum, which often results in purple coloration of the cytoplasm in H&E stained sections (see plasma cell, Chapter 7).

• Distinct polarity with basal rough endoplasmic reticulum, a supranuclear Golgi just visible as an ill-defined lucent area of the cytoplasm, and an apical zone containing granules filled with packaged protein ready for secretion by exocytosis. The staining characteristics of the apical portion of the cells depend on the nature of this protein (Fig. 3.20).

PRACTICAL HISTOLOGY

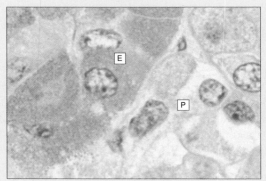

Fig. 3.20 Protein-secreting epithelial cells.
The cells shown in this micrograph are from the pituitary gland and are producing different peptide hormones, which impart different staining characteristics to the cells (eosinophilic (E), pale-staining (P)).

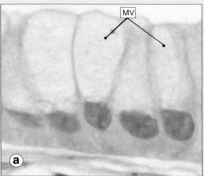

Fig. 3.21 Mucin-secreting epithelial cells.
a Micrograph of mucin-secreting surface epithelium showing the blue basal cytoplasm due to well developed basal endoplasmic reticulum, and the unstained vacuolated appearance of the apical cytoplasm due to large secretory vesicles of mucin (MV).
b Micrograph of mucin-secreting epithelial cells aggregated into a gland.

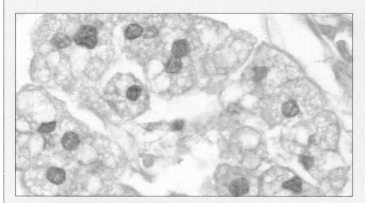

Fig. 3.22 Steroid-secreting epithelial cells.
According to their cytoplasmic composition, steroid-secreting cells vary in appearance in H&E stained sections from granular pink-staining cells, which contain many mitochondria and little lipid, to pale-pink staining and vacuolated cells, which contain abundant lipid and dilated smooth endoplasmic reticulum. The cells shown here are from the adrenal gland and have a pale and finely vacuolated appearance.

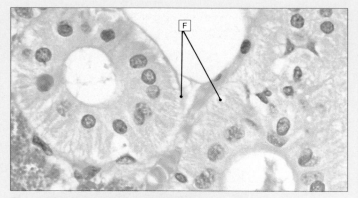

Fig. 3.23 Ion-pumping epithelial cells.
Micrograph of striated duct epithelial cells from salivary gland. Folding of the cell membrane (F) containing the active membrane protein produces a fine striped, appearance, while the large numbers of mitochondria impart a granular pink staining appearance to the basal part of the cell. Tight junctions are only visible ultrastructurally.

Mucin-secreting epithelial cells

Mucins (mixtures of glycoproteins and proteoglycans) have important functions in body cavities, for example as a lubricant in the mouth, as a lubricant in the vagina and as a barrier in the stomach.

Cells which produce and secrete mucin (Fig. 3.21) are characterized by the following features.
• A well developed basal rough endoplasmic reticulum makes the protein core of mucins and imparts a faint blue colour to the basal cytoplasm.
• A well developed supranuclear Golgi is the main site of protein glycosylation, but is not clearly visible by light microscopy.
• Large secretory vesicles of mucin at the cell apex impart an unstained vacuolated appearance to the apical cell cytoplasm.

Mucin-secreting cells may be part of a surface epithelium when they are termed **goblet cells**, for example in epithelia lining the gut (see Fig. 10.44), and respiratory tract (see Fig. 9.10).

In addition, mucin-secreting cells can be aggregated into specialized glands, for example in the genital tract, respiratory tract, and intestinal tract.

Steroid-secreting epithelial cells

Cells producing steroid hormones (Fig. 3.22) are mainly found in the adrenal gland, ovary and testis, and have the following characteristics.
• A well developed smooth endoplasmic reticulum (for lipid biosynthesis, see page 14), which gives the cytoplasm a granular pink appearance.
• Free lipid (lipids are the precursors of the steroid hormones) in vacuoles in the cell cytoplasm, which imparts a fine vacuolated appearance to the cells.
• Prominent mitochondria with tubular rather than flattened cristae. (Mitochondria are involved in the biosynthesis of steroids from lipid, but the functional significance of the tubular shape of their cristae is not clear).

Ion-pumping epithelial cells

Cells in the kidney tubules and in the ducts of some secretory glands transport ions and water, while acid-producing cells of the stomach transport H^+ ions (see Fig. 10.28).

Ion transport is mediated by membrane ion pumps; these use ATP as a source of energy for the exchange of ions between cytosol and extracellular space.

The structural specializations of ion-pumping epithelial cells (Fig. 3.23) are as follows.

• The cell membrane is folded to increase the active surface area of membrane containing the membrane protein that acts as the ion pump.
• Large numbers of mitochondria are closely apposed to the membrane folds to supply ATP.
• Tight junctions between the cells prevent back diffusion of pumped ions.

In cells of the intestine, gallbladder and kidney, the ion pumps move sodium and water from the apical surface to be absorbed, while in secretory glands, the cells move ions and fluid out of the apex of the cell, resulting in secretion of watery fluid (e.g. sweat).

Secretory mechanisms

There are four mechanisms of secretion of cell product by epithelial cells: merocrine, apocrine, holocrine and endocrine (Fig. 3.24).

Secretions from the apex of the cell onto a surface or into a lumen are termed **exocrine,** while secretions from the side or base of the cell, which enter the blood stream directly, are termed **endocrine**.

Glands

A gland is an organized collection of secretory epithelial cells. In many epithelia, secretion is performed only by occasional specialized cells (e.g. mucin-secreting goblet cells) scattered among other non-secretory cells (Fig. 3.25 a&b).

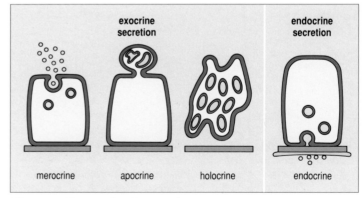

Fig. 3.24 Types of cell secretion.
Secretion of cell product may occur by exocytosis from the cell apex into a lumen (**merocrine** secretion); pinching off of apical cell cytoplasm containing cell product (**apocrine** secretion); shedding of the whole cell containing the cell product (**holocrine** secretion); or endocytosis from the cell base into the blood stream (**endocrine** secretion, see Fig. 15.1).

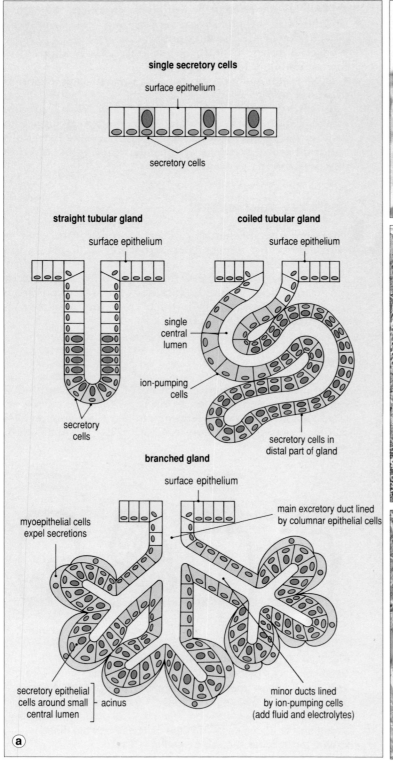

single secretory cells

surface epithelium

secretory cells

straight tubular gland

surface epithelium

secretory cells

coiled tubular gland

surface epithelium

single central lumen

ion-pumping cells

secretory cells in distal part of gland

branched gland

surface epithelium

myoepithelial cells expel secretions

main excretory duct lined by columnar epithelial cells

secretory epithelial cells around small central lumen

acinus

minor ducts lined by ion-pumping cells (add fluid and electrolytes)

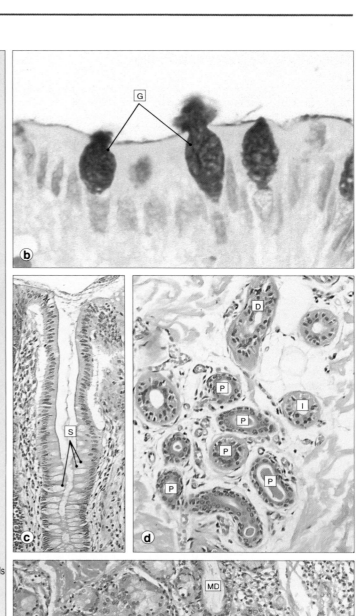

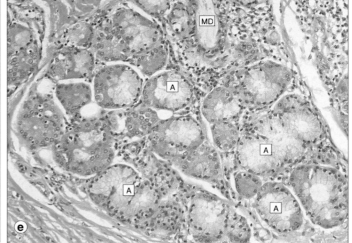

When more secretions are required, the surface area of secretory epithelium can be increased by invagination of the surface to form straight tubular glands (Fig. 3.25a&c) or by the formation of more complex coiled or branched glands, which may be divided into specialized zones for the secretion of different products (Fig. 3.25a&d).

The most structurally refined glands are those which have a branched architecture with secretory cells arranged in islands termed **acini** (Fig. 3.25a&e). Secretion from this type of exocrine gland is via a series of **ducts** lined by columnar epithelium with apical junctional complexes to prevent escape of the secretions (Fig. 3.26).

While most glands form part of other tissues (e.g. mucous glands in the respiratory tract), many are anatomically distinct (e.g. salivary glands, pancreas, liver).

Gland secretions are under hormonal and innervatory control, and all glands have a rich vascular supply to provide the necessary metabolites.

Neuroepithelial cells

Neuroepithelial cells are adapted to secrete chemical messenger substances into the extracellular space and blood.

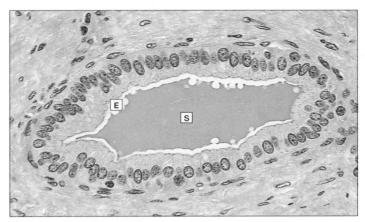

Fig. 3.26 Gland duct.
Ducts carry exocrine secretion from a gland and discharge it onto an epithelial surface or into a body cavity.

Ducts are lined by a tall columnar epithelium (E) and contain no specialized secretory cell. Note pink stained secretion (S) in the lumen.

Fig. 3.25 Secretory cells and glands.
a Diagram of secretory cells and glands.
b Alcian blue staining mucin in goblet cells (G) in a surface epithelium.
c H&E stained section showing a straight tubular colonic gland, which is typical of glands in the gut. Secretory cells (S) line straight tubules and discharge their mucin secretions onto the surface.
d H&E stained section of a sweat gland from the skin showing the arrangement of a coiled tubular gland. Secretory cells (S) are present in the distal part and there is zonation of secretory function, with an area of protein-secreting cells (P) being followed by an area of ion-pumping cells (I), which add fluid to the secretion in the lumen. The distal part of the lumen (D) has no secretory function, but is specialized for transporting secretions, having tight junctions to prevent back diffusion of ions; such tubules are termed ducts.
e H&E section of a branched gland showing the arrangement of secretory epithelial cells into acini (A), and main excretory duct (MD). The myoepithelial cells (see Fig. 5.10) are not readily visible at this low magnification.

BARRIER FUNCTION

An important function of many epithelia is as a barrier and this role is associated with certain specializations.
• Occluding junctions prevent diffusion of molecules between cells and therefore prevent diffusion of substances from one side of an epithelium to the other.
• The apical cell membrane of epithelial cells lining the urinary tract (i.e. transitional epithelium) contains a high proportion of sphingolipids. These not only form membrane plaques (see page 34), but are also believed to resist fluid and electrolyte movements from the cells in response to the osmotic effect of concentrated urine.
• Desmosomal and hemidesmosomal junctions provide a tight mechanical linkage between cells and extracellular matrix to resist shearing forces, and allow an epithelium to function as a mechanical barrier.
• Stratified squamous epithelial cells may undergo **keratinization**, a process in which the cytoskeleton of superficial cells of the epithelium becomes tightly condensed with other specialized proteins into a resilient mass. This results in cell death and the formation of a tough impervious and protective layer (**keratin**) from the remaining cell membranes and cytoplasmic contents (Fig. 3.27).

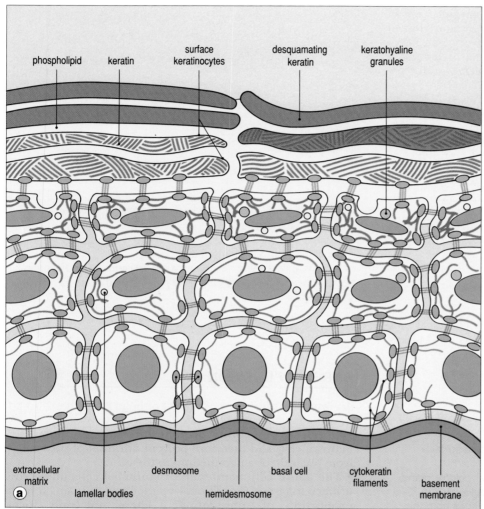

phospholipid keratin surface keratinocytes desquamating keratin keratohyaline granules

extracellular matrix

(a) lamellar bodies desmosome hemidesmosome basal cell cytokeratin filaments basement membrane

Fig. 3.27 Keratinization.

a Basal cells of keratinizing squamous epithelium are anchored by hemidesmosomes and desmosomes to basement membrane and adjacent cells respectively, and contain abundant cytokeratin intermediate filaments (tonofibrils). As the cells differentiate and move up the stratified epithelium they remain tightly bound by desmosomal junctions, but the cytokeratin proteins change from low molecular weight forms to higher molecular weight forms and the cells develop lamellar bodies.

Lamellar bodies are membrane-bound granules containing phospholipids, which are secreted by exocytosis into the extracellular space and form a lamellar sheet between cells in the upper epithelium. This is the main factor preventing water evaporation from the skin.

Keratinization begins when cells in the upper part of the epithelium switch off normal house-keeping genes and express genes coding for a variety of specialized proteins, which interact with the cytokeratin filaments and the cell membrane to produce a resilient and mechanically robust compact mass (**keratin**). Small granules (**keratohyaline granules**) contain some of these specialized proteins. A prominent protein (**involucrin**) associates with and thickens the cell membrane.

Keratinization ultimately transforms the cells into non-living proteinaceous material, which remains attached to underlying cells by existing anchoring junctions. The superficial cells are gradually lost to be replaced by cells beneath.

The surface keratin layer is mechanically strong, but flexible; it is relatively inert and acts as a physical barrier, particularly preventing ingress of microorganisms. The intercellular phospholipid renders the epithelium impermeable to water.

b H&E section of keratinized squamous epithelium. Note the purplish keratohyaline granules (KHG) and the absence of nuclei in the surface keratin layer (K).

c Keratinizing squamous epithelium stained to show involucrin (brown), which is only present in the upper keratinizing part of the epithelium.

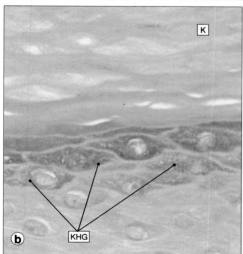

K

(b) KHG

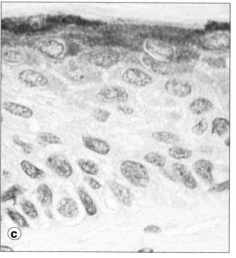

(c)

TUMOURS OF EPITHELIAL CELLS.

Cells may lose their normal growth control mechanisms and give rise to a tumour (**neoplasm**). Many such abnormal growths remain localized (**benign neoplasms**), but some grow into (invade) adjacent tissues and spread (metastasize) to other parts of the body (**malignant neoplasms**).

A malignant neoplasm arising from epithelial cells is termed a **carcinoma** (Fig. 3.28), while carcinoma derived from glandular epithelium is called an **adenocarcinoma** (Fig. 3.29).

In most cases, the cells of a carcinoma resemble those of their tissue of origin. The diagnosis of malignancy is based on the presence of **abnormal cytology** (see page 25), as well as by locating cells that have invaded other tissues.

In some cases, a carcinoma bears little resemblance to its cell of origin (**undifferentiated carcinoma**); such tumours commonly present with metastases and their site of origin may not be clear. In this situation it is essential to use immunohisto-chemistry and electon microscopy to confirm the diagnosis.

Finding desmosomal junctions by electron microscopy, or cytokeratin expression by immunochemistry, imply a diagnosis of carcinoma rather than a malignant tumour of lymphoid tissue or support cells.

Finding a specialized cell product by immunohistochemical techniques (see below) may help further by indicating for example a primary tumour in the thyroid (thyroglobulin) or prostate (prostate specific antigen).

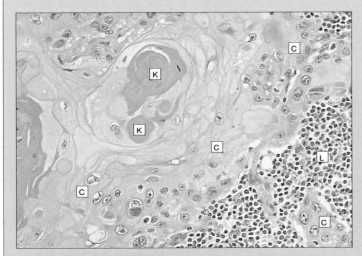

Fig. 3.28 Squamous cell carcinoma.
H&E section of lymph node containing normal lymphoid cells (L) and cancer cells (C), which are pink-staining and are associated with some keratinization (K), thus resembling normal squamous epithelium of the skin. This is squamous cell carcinoma and has spread from its origin in the skin via the lymphatic vessels.

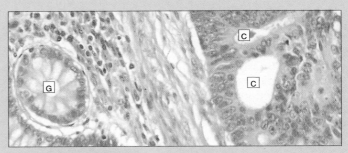

Fig. 3.29 Adenocarcinoma.
H&E section of colonic epithelium showing normal glandular epithelium (G) and carcinoma (C) forming gland-like structures (i.e. adenocarcinoma).

IMMUNOHISTOCHEMISTRY

Epithelial cells have the following characteristics detectable by immunohistochemical techniques (see page 6).
• Expression of the cytokeratin class of intermediate filament proteins. This is not a feature of other classes of cells, for example support cells or lymphoid cells.

• Expression of a class of cell surface glycoprotein (epithelial membrane antigen, EMA).
• Possession of a specialized stainable epithelial product by some epithelia, for example prostate-specific antigen and prostate-specific acid phosphatase in the ducts and acini of the prostate gland, thyroglobulin in cells of the thyroid gland, and γγ-enolase in cells of neuroendocrine lineage.

4. SUPPORT CELLS AND EXTRACELLULAR MATRIX

Support cells produce extracellular matrix materials, which are important for spatial organization and mechanical support in all tissues. They have the following common characteristics.
- Embryological derivation from **mesenchyme** (Fig. 4.1).
- Production of a variety of extracellular matrix materials.
- When mature, formation of sparsely cellular tissues in which matrix is the main component.
- Cell adhesion mechanisms that interact with extracellular matrix materials rather than other cells.

The support cells (see pages 50–52) are fibroblasts, chondrocytes, osteocytes, myofibroblasts and adipocytes. **Fibroblasts** secrete extracellular matrix components in most tissues, while **chondrocytes** secrete the extracellular matrix components of cartilage, and **osteocytes** secrete the extracellular matrix components of bone. **Myofibroblasts** secrete extracellular matrix components and also have a contractile function, and **adipocytes** store lipid.

In addition, support cells produce the specially organized extracellular matrix material that forms tissues such as the transparent cornea of the eye and tendons to anchor muscles.

A special adaptation of support cells is to store lipid in the form of adipocytes, which not only act as an energy store, but also have a cushioning and padding function.

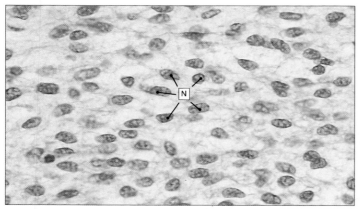

Fig. 4.1 Embryonic mesenchyme.
Mesenchyme is an embryonic tissue and may develop from any of the three germ layers. It is characterized by spindle-shaped cells with large nuclei (N), which develop into a variety of cell types in embryonic life, thus forming the family of support cells.

EXTRACELLULAR MATRIX

The extracellular matrix produced by most support cells is composed of two major materials: **glycosaminoglycans** (**GAGs**) and **fibrillar proteins**.

The general structure of support tissue is a scattered network of support cells producing an organized, abundant extracellular network of fibrillar proteins arranged in a hydrated gel of GAGs. Other cells (e.g. epithelial cells, contractile cells) are anchored to this tissue by cell–matrix anchoring junctions (see page 29).

Glycosaminoglycans (GAGs)

GAGs are large unbranched polysaccharide chains composed of repeating disaccharide units (70–200 residues). They have the following properties.
- A high negative charge because in all GAGs one of the repeating units is an amino sugar (N-acetylglucosamine or N-acetylgalactosamine), which is commonly sulphated (SO^{3-}), and in most GAGs the second sugar is uronic acid with a carboxyl group (COO^-).
- Strongly hydrophilic behaviour because they cannot fold into compact structures and therefore have a large permanently open coil conformation.
- Retention of positive ions (e.g. Na^+) together with water, thereby maintaining tissue architecture by virtue of an inherent turgor, which tends to prevent deformation by compressive forces.
- With the exception of hyaluronic acid, covalent attachment to proteins to form **proteoglycans**, which are huge molecules capable of maintaining a large hydration space in the extracellular matrix. The spatial organization and charge of proteoglycans facilitates selective diffusion of different molecules probably by allowing variation in pore size of the matrix gel. This is particularly important in the basement membranes of the kidney glomerulus (see Fig. 16.18).

GAGs can be divided into four groups according to their structure: hyaluronic acid; chondroitin sulphate and dermatan sulphate; heparan sulphate and heparin; keratan sulphate (Fig. 4.2).

Their varying tissue distribution probably reflects local requirements for specific pore sizes and charges in the extracellular matrix.

Glycosaminoglycan	Sulphation	Protein-linked	Distribution
Hyaluronic acid	no	no	cartilage, synovial fluid, skin, support tissue
Chondroitin sulphate	yes	yes	cartilage, bone, skin, cornea, arteries
Dermatan sulphate	yes	yes	skin, blood vessels, heart
Heparan sulphate	yes	yes	basement membrane, lung, arteries
Heparin	yes	yes	lung, liver, skin, mast cell granules
Keratan sulphate	yes	yes	cartilage, cornea, vertebral disc

Fig. 4.2 Glycosaminoglycans.
There are four main groups of glycosaminoglycans, which have different tissue distributions.

Sulphation causes the molecules to be highly negatively charged and contributes to their ability to retain Na^+ ions and water.

With the exception of hyaluronic acid, the glycosaminoglycans become linked to proteins to form proteoglycans.

The presence of specific types of glycosaminoglycan in different tissues confers special attributes to the extracellular matrix, particularly with regard to diffusion or binding of other extracellular substances.

Fibrillar proteins

The four major proteins that form fibrils in extracellular matrix are:
- collagen;
- fibrillin;
- elastin;
- fibronectin.

Collagen

Collagens are a family of closely related proteins and are the most abundant and important of the extracellular fibrillar proteins.

The main role of collagen is to provide tensile strength to tissues by forming **collagen fibres** (Fig. 4.3); in addition, one type of collagen forms the structural scaffold of **basement membranes** (see page 49).

Collagen fibres are constructed of precursor proteins (α chains) wound together to form rigid linear triple helix structures, which are then assembled into long filaments

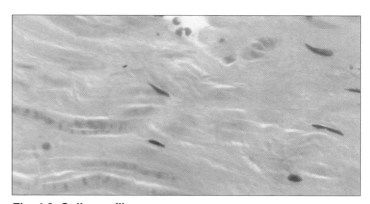

Fig. 4.3 Collagen fibres.
In H&E stained preparations collagen fibres appear as pink-stained material, which is often difficult to delineate from other structures that stain equally pink (e.g. support cells, walls of blood vessels). Special stains can be used to stain collagen (see Fig. 4.13), and immunohistochemical staining can also be performed for different molecular types of collagen, but is seldom used in the routine examination of tissues.

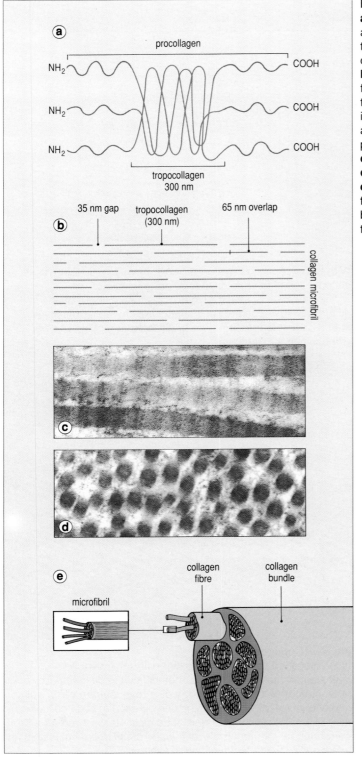

Fig. 4.4 Fibrillar collagen.
a Fibrillar collagen is formed from three polypeptide (α) chains, which are initially secreted with both amino and carboxyl terminal extensions to prevent collagen forming inside cells. Initial assembly of these chains is into a triple helix (**procollagen**).
b Cleavage of the amino and carboxyl extensions to leave the functional mid domains (**tropocollagen**) allows the molecules to align themselves into linear arrays to form long filaments. The individual collagen molecules are 300 nm long and are arranged with a 67 nm overlap between adjacent molecules. This gives rise to a periodicity of 67 nm.
c Electronmicrograph of collagen showing the periodicity of 67 nm.
d Electronmicrograph of collagen in transverse section.
e The initial filaments (collagen **microfibrils**) become arranged into **fibres**, and the fibres into larger **bundles** by tight cross-linking between adjacent molecules via lysine residues; this contributes to the mechanical strength of collagen fibres in tissues.

(Fig. 4.4). There are at least 20 types of α chain, which combine to produce different forms (Fig. 4.5).

Types I II and III collagen are arranged as rope-like fibrils and are the main forms of **fibrillar collagen**.
• **Collagen fibres** (type I collagen) resist tensile stresses in tissues, thus their orientation and cross linking varies according to the local environment.
• **Reticular fibres** (also called **reticulin**) are thin fibrils (about 20 nm in diameter) of type III collagen (Fig. 4.6). They form a loose mesh in many support tissues and are particularly evident in a zone beneath basement membranes, where they are thought to have a support function as part of the fibroreticular lamina (see Fig. 4.11c).
Reticular fibres can be considered as a fine scaffolding supporting specialized extracellular matrix components. In lymph nodes, spleen and bone marrow, reticular fibres form the main extracellular matrix fibres supporting the haemopoietic and lymphoid tissues. In parenchymal organs, such as the liver and kidney, reticular fibres form a network supporting specialized epithelial cells.

Type IV collagen assembles into a meshwork rather than fibrils and is restricted to basement membrane formation (see page 49).

Type VII collagen forms the anchoring fibrils of some basement membranes.

Although the main cells producing collagen are fibroblasts (see page 50), it can also be produced by other mesenchyme-derived cells of the support cell family, as well as by a variety of epithelial and endothelial cells, which produce the type IV collagen of basement membranes.

Type	I	II	III	IV	V	VI	VII	VIII	IX	X	XI
Morphology	large banded collagen fibre	small banded collagen fibre	small banded collagen fibre	sheet-like layers	thin fibrils	thin fibrils	short striated fibrils	uncertain	uncertain	uncertain	uncertain
Distribution	skin dermis, tendon, bone, ligaments, fascia, fibrous cartilage, cornea, loose fibrous tissue	hyaline and elastic cartilage, vertebral discs, vitreous of eye	blood vessels, parenchymal organs, bone marrow, lymphoid tissues, smooth muscle, nerves, lung, fetal skin	basement membranes, external laminae, lens capsule	basement membrane of placenta, smooth and skeletal muscle	ubiquitous	anchoring fibrils in basement membrane of skin and amnion	endothelium	cartilage	mineralizing cartilage	cartilage

Fig. 4.5 Molecular forms of collagen.

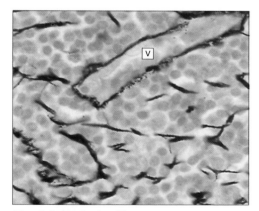

Fig. 4.6 Reticular fibres.
Reticular fibres cannot be seen in H&E sections, but can be stained by silver impregnation methods. In this micrograph, reticular fibres in a lymph node are seen as fine black lines, with lymphoid cells stained red in the background (V = vessel).

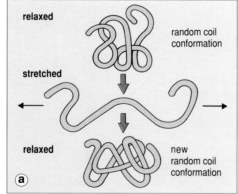

Fig. 4.7 Elastin.
a Elastin has a random coil structure in the relaxed state that can stretch, but re-forms as a different random coil on relaxation.
b Elastin molecules are covalently linked into arrays, which can reversibly stretch and recoil, and may be arranged as fibres or sheets.

Fibrillin

Fibrillin, a recently characterized fibril-forming glycoprotein, is the main component of **extracellular microfibrils** 8–12 nm in diameter, which are one constituent of elastic fibres (see Fig. 4.8). They are also found in the extracellular matrix of renal glomeruli (mesangium), the suspensory fibres of the lens, and in the spleen.

In addition, microfibrils are prominent in elastic-containing extracellular matrix, particularly in lung, skin and blood vessel walls.

Microfibrils mediate adhesion between different components of the extracellular matrix.

Elastin

Elastin is a hydrophobic protein, which assembles into filaments and sheets by cross-linking (Fig. 4.7) and is the main component of **elastic fibres.** Like collagen, elastin is produced by fibroblasts.

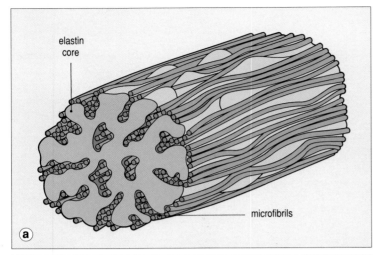

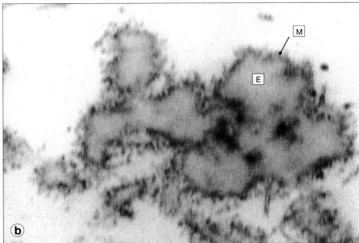

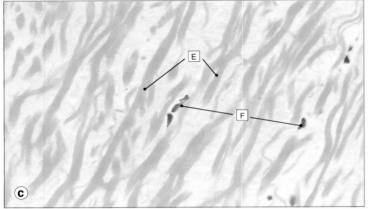

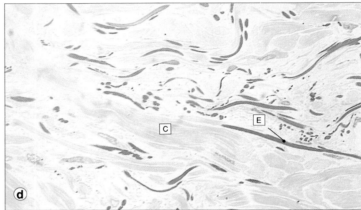

Fig. 4.8 Elastic fibre.
a Elastic fibres are composed of glycoprotein microfilaments (fibrillin) surrounding and organizing a core region of cross-linked elastin.
b Ultrastructurally, the elastin core appears as an electron-dense area (E) with microfilaments (M) arranged peripherally. The microfilaments are prominent in early formed elastic tissue, and

decrease in number with ageing.
c In H&E stained tissues, elastic fibres (E) stand out as glassy, bright pink-stained structures, taking up acidic dyes such as eosin with much greater avidity than collagen fibres. (F, fibroblast).
d Elastic fibres can be stained by special techniques. In this example, elastic fibres (E) in the dermis of the skin are stained blue by toluidine blue and contrast with the pale staining collagen (C).

Elastic fibres confer elasticity to tissues and allow them to recoil after stretching, being formed by the interaction of elastin and fibrillin. The fibrillin microfibrils appear to organize secreted elastin so that it is deposited between the microfibrils to form distinct fibres (Fig. 4.8). Elastic fibres are important constituents of many support tissues.

Fibronectin

Fibronectin is a multi-functional glycoprotein and exists in three main forms. These are:
- a circulating plasma protein;

- a protein that transiently attaches to the surface of many cells;
- insoluble fibrils forming part of the extracellular matrix, when fibronectin dimers cross-link to each other by disulphide bonds.

The functional importance of fibronectin stems from its ability to adhere to several different tissue components because it possesses sites binding collagen and heparin, as well as cell adhesion molecules.

Fibronectin is recognized by fibronectin receptor proteins in cell membranes, allowing cell adhesion to extracellular matrix. Such a fibronectin receptor is one of the

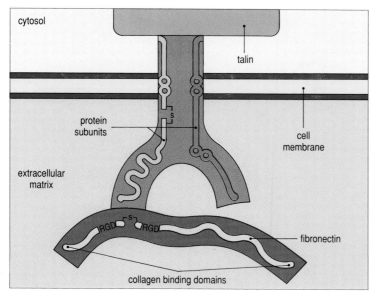

Fig. 4.9 Integrins.
Integrins are a class of cell adhesion molecule of which 16 have been functionally characterized. They are composed of two protein subunits.

The **fibronectin receptor** shown in the diagram is the best characterized of the integrin family, possessing a cytosolic domain binding to actin (via talin, and a recently described protein termed fibulin), a transmembrane domain, and extracellular domains binding to fibronectin. Thus, this molecule links the intracellular actin network with extracellular matrix at focal contacts (see Fig. 3.10). The laminin receptor (see below) is also one of the integrin family.

Integrins may bind to other cell surface proteins, thus acting as intercellular adhesion molecules (e.g. the platelet protein gp IIb/IIIa responsible for platelet fibrinogen-associated aggregation is an integrin). In addition, some integrins bind to extracellular matrix components and allow cell–matrix adhesion, the main extracellular matrix ligands being fibronectin, laminin, collagens, tenascin and thrombospondin.

class of cell surface receptors called **integrins** (Fig. 4.9). When tissues grow, fibronectin binds to cell surfaces via integrins and is thought to have an important role in organizing the subsequent deposition and orientation of early collagen fibrils through its collagen attachment sites.

Because fibronectin receptors are linked to intracellular actin, the orientation of the internal cytoskeleton of a cell influences the orientation of the extracellular matrix.

Extracellular structural glycoproteins

Several non-filamentous proteins, particularly laminin, entactin and tenascin, mediate interaction between cells and extracellular matrix.

Laminin

Laminin is a sulphated glycoprotein and is a major component of basement membranes. It is produced by most epithelial and endothelial cells, and is a cross-shaped molecule with binding sites for specific cell receptors (integrins), heparan sulphate, type IV collagen, and entactin (see below).

The multiple binding ligands for laminin make it a major extracellular link molecule between cells and extracellular matrix.

Entactin

Entactin is a sulphated glycoprotein that is a component of all basement membranes and binds with laminin. It is

thought to function as a link protein binding laminin to type IV collagen.

Tenascin

Tenascin is an extracellular glycoprotein involved in cell adhesion and is particularly expressed in embryonic tissue. It is thought to be important to cell migration in the developing nervous system

Basement membrane

Basement membranes are specialized sheet-like arrangements of extracellular matrix proteins and GAGs, and act as an interface between parenchymal cells and support tissues. They are associated with epithelial cells, muscle cells and Schwann cells, and also form a limiting membrane in the central nervous system.

Basement membranes have five major components: type IV collagen (Fig. 4.10), laminin, heparan sulphate, entactin, and fibronectin. With the exception of fibronectin, these are synthesized by the parenchymal cells. In addition, there are numerous minor and poorly characterized protein and GAG components.

Basement membrane has three main functions.
● It forms an adhesion interface between parenchymal cells and less specialized extracellular matrix, the cells having adhesion mechanisms to anchor them to basement membrane, while basement membrane is tightly anchored to the extracellular matrix of support tissues, particularly collagen. Where such an interface occurs in non-epithelial

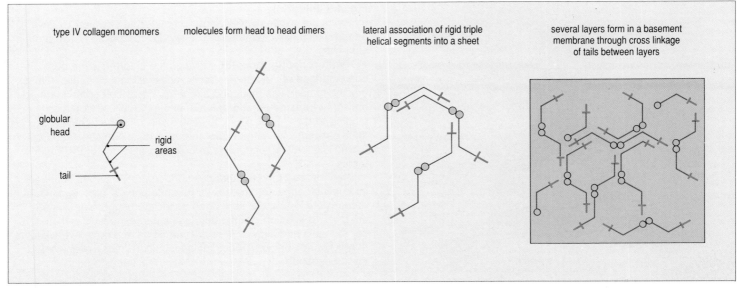

Fig. 4.10 Type IV collagen in basement membrane.
Type IV collagen molecules do not form filaments, but aggregate into a polygonal lattice. Separate sheets form a multi-layered structure, which acts as the skeleton for the rest of the basement membrane. This may be produced by epithelial cells as well as support cells.

tissues, for example around muscle cells, it is referred to as an **external lamina** as there is no basal surface.
• It acts as a molecular sieve (permeability barrier) with pore size depending on the charge and spatial arrangement of its component GAGs. Thus basement membrane of blood vessels prevents large proteins leaking into the tissues, that of the kidney allows urine production, but not protein loss from filtered blood, and that of the lung permits gaseous diffusion.
• It probably controls cell organization and differentiation by the mutual interaction of cell surface receptors and molecules in the extracellular matrix. These interactions are the subject of intense research, particularly in the investigation of mechanisms that might prevent the spread and proliferation of cancer cells throughout the body.
    The general structure of basement membrane has been well characterized (Fig. 4.11). Superimposed on this, minor protein and carbohydrate components are specific to certain tissues, thus renal basement membrane differs from that of the skin, for example.

CELL ADHESION TO EXTRACELLULAR MATRIX

The organization of cells into functional tissues and organs depends on the support functions of the extracellular matrix and the cells that produce it. While various types of intercellular junction tie cells together (see pages 29–30), the junctions between cells and the extracellular matrix are equally important in maintaining structural integrity.
    Junctions beween cells and extracellular matrix include the following.
• Hemidesmosomes (see Fig. 3.12) anchor the intermediate filament cytoskeleton of cells to basement membrane.
• Focal contacts (see Fig. 3.10) anchor the actin cytoskeleton to basement membrane. The interaction is mediated through the fibronectin receptor (see Fig. 4.9).
• Laminin receptors (see Fig. 4.9) anchor cells to basement membrane where laminin is a major component.
• Non-integrin glycoproteins (possessed by many cells) bind to collagen and other cell matrix components.

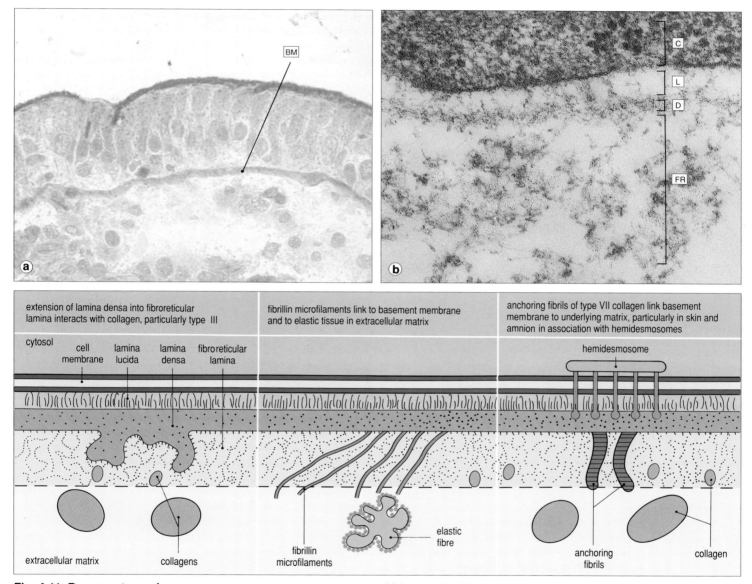

Fig. 4.11 Basement membrane.

a H&E preparations fail to show distinct basement membrane because it is only 0.05 μm thick and stains poorly; however, a high content of glycoprotein renders it stainable with PAS, when it appears as a faint magenta-stained line (BM).

Specific components of basement membrane can be detected with immunohistochemical staining, for example laminin and type IV collagen.

b By electron microscopy, basement membrane resolves into several layers (**laminae**). The **lamina densa** (D) is a dark staining band 30 – 100 nm thick. Between this and the attached cell (C) is a lucent zone, the **lamina lucida** (L), which is usually 60 nm wide. On the other side of the lamina densa is a rarified layer of variable thickness, **the fibroreticular lamina** (FR), which merges with fibrous proteins of the extracellular matrix. The structure seen by light microscopy with PAS and silver stains and referred to as basement membrane is a combination of all these laminae, but particularly the fibroreticular lamina.

The term **basal lamina** should strictly refer to the lamina densa as an ultrastructural feature. However, with the detection of specific basal lamina components by light microscopy using immunohistochemistry the terms basement membrane and basal lamina are commonly used interchangeably.

c The fibroreticular lamina anchors basement membrane to adjacent extracellular matrix by three main mechanisms, which vary according to site and are illustrated in this diagram.

SUPPORT CELL FAMILY

During embryogenesis, a proportion of developing mesenchymal spindle-shaped cells differentiate into the following types of support cells: fibroblasts, myofibroblasts, lipoblasts, osteoblasts, and chondroblasts.

The addition of 'blast' to the root name of a support cell indicates that the cell is actively growing or secreting extracellular matrix material. Support cells in a quiescent phase in tissues are indicated by the use of the suffix 'cyte' (e.g. fibrocyte, osteocyte, chondrocyte).

Fibroblasts, fibrocytes and fibrocollagenous tissue

Fibroblasts (Fig. 4.12) produce **fibrocollagenous (fibrous) tissue**, which is composed mainly of collagen fibres associated with GAGs, elastic fibres and reticular fibres (Fig. 4.13). Fibrocollagenous tissue is described as **loose** when collagen fibres are thin, haphazardly arranged and widely spaced, or **dense** when collagen fibres are broad and virtually confluent. The degree of organization and collagen orientation varies from site to site according to local tissue stresses.

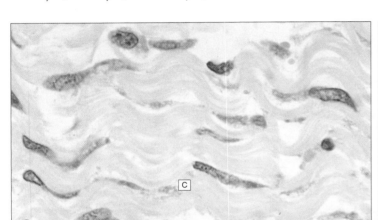

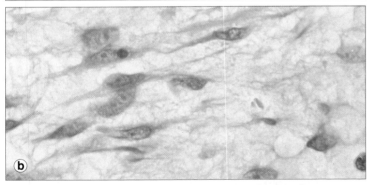

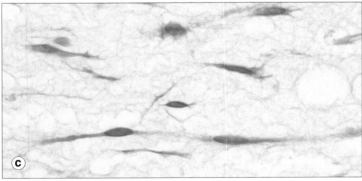

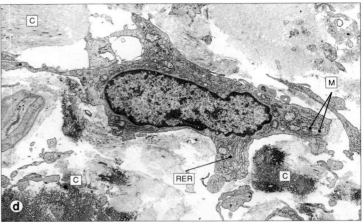

Fig. 4.12 Fibroblasts and fibrocytes.

a In the embryo, collagen-secreting cells develop from mesenchyme and appear as plump spindle-shaped cells separated by early secreted collagen (C), which stains pink in H&E preparations.

b In the adult, active collagen-secreting cells are called fibroblasts and are characterized by a large oval nucleus and large nucleolus, a tapering bipolar spindle-shaped morphology with small additional cell processes and basophilic cytoplasm reflecting active protein synthesis.

c Once collagen secretion has stopped the fibroblasts lose their voluminous basophilic cytoplasm and the nucleus shrinks reflecting non-transcription of DNA. The cells are now called **fibrocytes** to indicate this inactivity.

d Ultrastructurally, fibroblasts have a well developed rough endoplasmic reticulum (RER), Golgi, and secretory vesicles, reflecting active collagen secretion. Mitochondria (M) are numerous. Collagen fibres (C) are visible adjacent to the cells.

Fibroblasts also secrete elastic and reticular fibres, and when they form reticular fibres in lymphoid tissue and bone marrow, they have a highly branched stellate shape and are often called reticulum cells.

Highly organized dense fibrocollagenous tissue forms tendons and ligaments.

Fibrocollagenous tissue is the major support tissue in most organs, and has the following specific functions.

• Support of nerves, blood vessels and lymphatics; vessels and nerves are a conspicuous feature, particularly in loose fibrocollagenous support tissue.

• Separation of functional layers in organs and tissues (e.g. separation of mucosa from underlying tissues). Its loose arrangement and variable elastic content allow mobility and stretching.

• Support for transient and resident immune cell populations (i.e. macrophages, lymphocytes, plasma cells, mast cells).

• Formation of **fibrous capsule**, which surrounds most parenchymal organs, such as the liver, spleen and kidneys.

• Formation of **fibroadipose tissue**, which is a component of most tissues, by enclosing and blending with adipocytes.

Fibroblasts are extremently robust cells, and resist damaging stimuli that kill most other cell types, such as nerves, epithelial cells or muscle. They are important in tissue repair (see page 56).

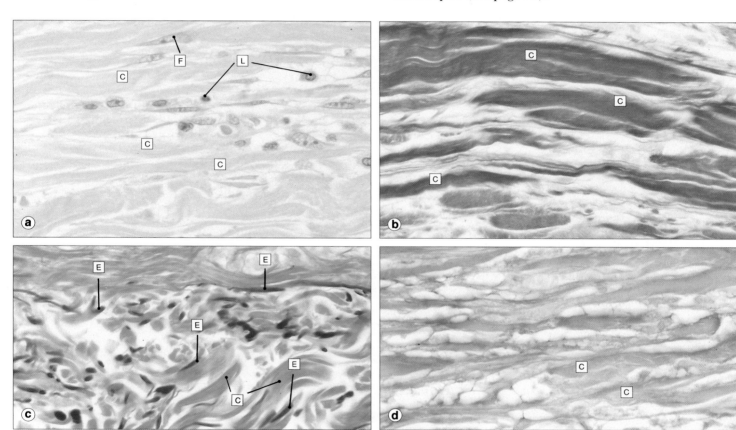

Fig. 4.13 Fibrocollagenous (fibrous) tissue.

a Fibrocollagenous tissue contains many extracellular matrix components with collagen fibres being predominant. Only collagen (C) is evident in H&E sections, staining light pink. Fibroblasts (F) are widely scattered and inconspicuous. Immune cells (i.e. lymphocytes (L), plasma cells, macrophages, mast cells) are occasionally found.

b The collagen fibres (C) in loose fibrocollagenous tissue can be stained by dyes with affinity for collagen (e.g. Van Gieson, shown here). The bundles are haphazardly arranged and of varying thickness.

c In most loose fibrocollagenous tissues elastic fibres are present, but are usually inconspicuous in H&E preparations. They are revealed by special stains (elastic stain) as wavy black-staining fibres (E), which contrast with the orange-stained collagen (C). Elastic fibres form a minor and variable component of most fibrocollagenous tissues.

d Stains for the GAG component of fibrocollagenous tissue reveal that the unstained areas of the H&E preparation are rich in this extracellular material (seen here stained blue with Alcian blue stain). (C, collagen). In contrast with loose fibrocollagenous tissue, dense irregular fibrocollagenous tissue has little space for GAGs and appears uniformly pink with few architectural features. Collagen-secreting fibroblasts are widely spaced and inconspicuous.

Myofibroblasts

Myofibroblasts resemble fibroblasts by light microscopy, but ultrastructurally contain aggregates of actin fibres associated with myosin to subserve a contractile function (see page 66). They are not prominent in support tissues, being found only in small numbers, and identifiable by immunohistochemical or ultrastructural methods.

Myofibroblasts develop during repair following tissue damage, and may originate either by proliferation of the normally inconspicuous tissue myofibroblasts, or possibly by differentiation of fibrocytes. They produce collagen and their contractile properties contribute to retraction and shrinkage of early fibrocollagenous scar tissue (see Fig. 4.22).

The myofibroblast can be considered as a bifunctional cell with the properties of a fibroblast as well as those of a smooth muscle cell, but in contrast to smooth muscle cells, myofibroblasts are not associated with an external lamina (see page 48)

Chondroblasts, chondrocytes and cartilage

Chondroblasts elaborate a special support tissue called **cartilage**.

Developing from embryonic mesenchyme, chondroblasts first appear as clusters of vacuolated cells with a rounded morphology. These contrast with the spindle-shaped cells of surrounding undifferentiated mesenchyme, which develop into fibroblasts and form a confining sheet of cells termed the **perichondrium**.

Chondroblasts contain abundant glycogen and lipid and their active synthesis of extracellular matrix proteins is indicated by their basophilic cytoplasm, which is due to a high content of rough endoplasmic reticulum (Fig. 4.14a).

Growth of cartilage results from proliferation of chondroblasts within established matrix (**interstitial growth**) and also by development of new chondroblasts from the perichondrium (**appositional growth**). After depositing cartilage matrix, chondroblasts become less metabolically active and have small nuclei with pale indistinct cytoplasm (i.e. they become **chondrocytes** (Fig. 4.14b).

Cartilage has two main extracellular components:
- fibrous proteins (predominantly type II collagen), which confer mechanical stability;
- abundant GAGs, which resist deformation by compressive forces.

The collagen fibres are thin and arranged in an interwoven lattice, which merges into the extracellular matrix of adjacent support tissues.

The major GAGs are hyaluronic acid, chondroitin sulphate and keratan sulphate, and these are mainly linked in large proteoglycan molecules to the collagen lattice.

Because of its high content of sulphated GAGs cartilage stains with basic dyes such as haematoxylin, which gives it a slightly blue colour in H&E preparations; this is particularly evident around the chondrocytes.

The arrangement of extracellular matrix in cartilage confers important properties.
- The tightly bound proteoglycans form a hydrated matrix with an inherent turgor that resists deformation by compressive forces.
- Small molecules can diffuse freely through the extracellular matrix.

There are three types of cartilage, hyaline cartilage, fibrocartilage and elastic cartilage, depending on its content of specific fibrous protein.

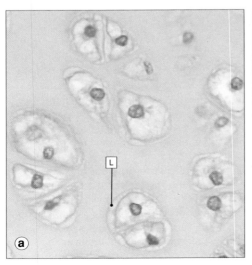

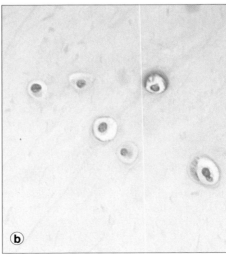

Fig. 4.14 Chondroblasts and chondrocytes.

a Chondroblasts are metabolically active and have large vesicular nuclei with prominent nucleoli. Their cytoplasm is pale and vacuolated because of a high lipid and glycogen content and tends to draw away from the extracellular matrix when fixed and embedded in paraffin, forming a space called a lacune (L).

b Chondrocytes are smaller than chondroblasts, having dense-stained nuclei and less cytoplasm, reflecting their low level of metabolic activity.

Types of cartilage

Hyaline cartilage contains type II collagen only (Fig. 4.15). It forms the temporary skeleton in fetal development until it is replaced by bone, the growing point in long bones in childhood, the articular surface in joints (see Chapter 14), and acts as a support tissue in the respiratory passages (see Fig. 9.8).

Fibrocartilage contains both type II and type I collagen (Fig. 4.16), and is a component of intervertebral discs, tendon attachments to bones, and the junctions between the flat bones of the pelvis (see Chapter 14).

Elastic cartilage contains elastic fibres in addition to type II collagen (Fig 4.17). It is located in the auricle of the ear, the walls of the external auditory canal and Eustachian tubes (see Chapter 14), and in the epiglottis of the larynx (see Fig. 9.6).

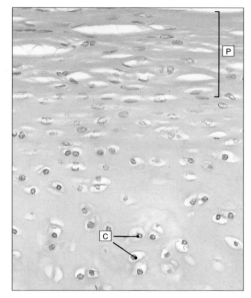

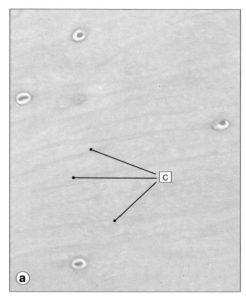

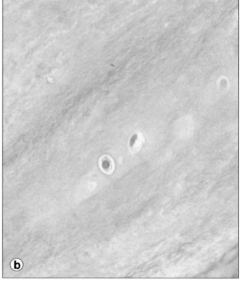

Fig. 4.15 Hyaline cartilage.
Hyaline cartilage from a child and therefore in a state of growth.

The perichondrium (P) is a layer of spindle-shaped fibroblasts with associated type I collagen, which merges with the outer layer of the pink-staining extracellular matrix of the hyaline cartilage. New chondroblasts develop from the perichondrium and allow appositional growth.

The chondroblasts show artefactual vacuolation, forming the characteristic lacunes around the cell bodies, and many in this sample are in small clusters (C), which will eventually move apart as the cells secrete extracellular matrix material during interstitial growth.

Hyaline cartilage is associated with perichondrium in most sites except when it lines joints.

Fig. 4.16 Fibrocartilage.
a In this H&E section of fibrocartilage, small inactive chondrocytes are dispersed in a pink-stained extracellular matrix in which coarse collagen fibres (C) are visible. These are type I collagen fibres, and merge with the type I collagen fibres in surrounding fibrocollagenous support tissue.
b The presence of Type I collagen is highlighted in this Van Gieson stained section of fibrocartilage in which it stains red.

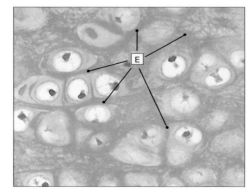

Fig. 4.17 Elastic cartilage.
The structural arrangement of elastic cartilage is similar to that of hyaline cartilage, with a perichondrial layer and chondrocytes set in an extracellular matrix, but differs because it contains elastic fibres.

These appear as bright pink-staining linear bundles running between cells (E), and confer great resilience and elastic recoil to the cartilage. The elastic fibres can be highlighted with special staining methods.

Osteoblasts and osteoid

Osteoblasts elaborate the support matrix of bone, **osteoid**, which subsequently calcifies to form bone.

Osteoid is composed mainly of type I collagen, which is associated with the extracellular GAGs, chondroitin sulphate and keratan sulphate. Two GAGs, sialoprotein and osteocalcin, appear to be unique to bone matrix and bind calcium, hence possibly having a role in bone mineralization. The cytology and structure of bone and its matrix are discussed in Chapter 14.

Adipocytes and adipose tissue

Adipocytes are characterized by their intracellular storage of fat. There are two types of fat-storing tissue, unilocular and multilocular adipose tissue.

Unilocular adipose tissue (**white fat**) develops from embryonic mesenchyme with the formation of spindle-shaped cells (**lipoblasts**) containing small fat vacuoles (Fig. 4.18). These mature into adipocytes, which store fat for use by other body tissues as a source of energy (Fig. 4.19).

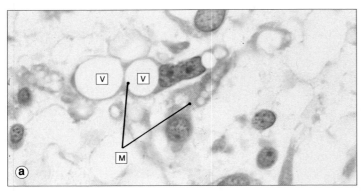

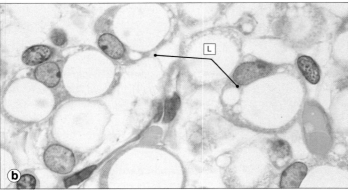

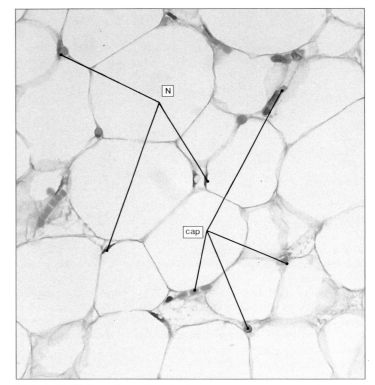

Fig. 4.18 Lipoblasts.
a In the fetus, the first indication of differentiation into a fat storing cell is when the spindle-shaped mesenchymal cells (M) accumulate fat in their cytoplasm in multiple small vacuoles (V).
b The vacuoles fuse to form a larger perinuclear vacuole and the cell is recognized as a maturing lipoblast (L), losing its spindle shape. With increased fat storage the cytoplasm becomes attenuated around a single huge lipid vacuole and the nucleus is displaced to one side.

Each developing lipoblast produces extracellular matrix material and a basement membrane forms around each cell.

Fig. 4.19 Unilocular adipose tissue.
Unilocular (white) adipose tissue cells (adipocytes) are 50–150 μm in size and polyhedral in shape.

In H&E stained preparations, as here, they appear as thin stringy wisps of cytoplasm surrounding an empty vacuole because embedding in wax involves immersion in lipid solvents, which remove all of the fat. Close examination reveals inconspicuous flattened nuclei (N) to one side of the cells.

Numerous fine arborizing capillary vessels (cap) transfer metabolites to and from the cells.

Ultrastructurally, adipocytes have prominent smooth endoplasmic reticulum and numerous pinocytotic vesicles, these being involved in lipid biosynthesis and transport. Each cell is surrounded by an external lamina and there is an extracellular matrix composed of reticular fibres (type III collagen).

Unilocular adipose tissue is the main form of fat storing cell in the adult, and is adapted both as a support tissue as well as an energy store as follows.
• It possesses receptors for growth hormone, insulin, glucocorticoids, thyroid hormones, and noradrenaline that modulate the uptake and release of fat.
• It has a rich capillary blood supply and is innervated by the autonomic nervous system. Local release of noradrenaline stimulates the release of stored fat into the blood.
• It is organized into pads by sheets of fibrocollagenous tissue at certain sites. These act as deformable shock-absorbing support tissues, particularly in the soles of the feet, the buttocks, around the kidneys and in the orbit around the eye.

Multilocular adipose tissue (**brown fat**) is most prominent in the newborn, its fetal development being separate from that of unilocular adipose tissue. Its function is to metabolize fat to produce heat in the neonatal period (Fig. 4.20).

Ultrastructurally multilocular adipose cells contain huge numbers of mitochondria in addition to lipid vacuoles; this correlates with their function of heat generation through mitochondrial metabolism of fatty acids.

The high mitochondrial density is responsible for both the eosinophilia seen histologically and the brown colour seen macroscopically, which gives this tissue its alternative name of 'brown fat'.

Multilocular adipose tissue does not usually persist in adult life and becomes lost during childhood, although small amounts may remain in certain sites (Fig. 4.21).

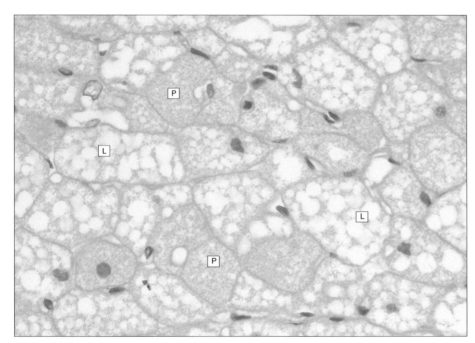

Fig. 4.20 Multilocular adipose tissue.
Multilocular adipose tissue is so-named because cells contain multiple small lipid droplets. It develops as clusters of plump eosinophilic cells differentiating from fetal mesenchyme, and has a restricted distribution, being concentrated in support tissues in the neck, shoulders, back, perirenal and para-aortic regions.

As shown in this micrograph, two populations of cells can be seen: lipid-rich cells (L) with a central nucleus and multiple small unstained vacuoles, and polyhedral-shaped cells (P) with a granular, pink-stained cytoplasm, a central nucleus and only occasional lipid vacuoles.

A capillary vascular supply together with thin fibrocollagenous septa divide the tissue into small lobules.

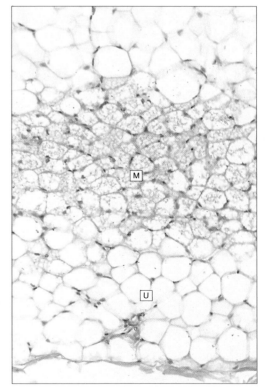

Fig. 4.21 Mixture of unilocular and multilocular adipose tissue.
Certain adipose tissue, particularly in the subcutaneous tissue over the back and shoulders, contains a mixture of both unilocular (U) and multilocular (M) adipose tissue.

GROWTH FACTORS AND SUPPORT CELLS

A number of polypeptide **growth factors** are known to modulate proliferation and differentiation of support cells by interacting with cell surface receptors, thereby affecting gene expression. Important members of this group are:

- platelet-derived growth factors;
- fibroblast growth factors (also termed heparin-binding growth factors);
- insulin-like growth factors;
- nerve growth factor.

These growth factors are secreted following damage to tissues (see below) and induce proliferation of support cells as well as development of new blood vessels. The support cells then repair damaged areas by secreting appropriate extracellular matrix.

TISSUE DAMAGE AND SUPPORT CELLS

Following tissue damage (e.g. by infection), the death of specialized cells can be rectified by regrowth only if the architecture of the support tissues (particularly basement membrane) is preserved; for example, epithelial cells lining the lung can regrow following some types of pneumonia.

If damage has been severe and the support tissue architecture is destroyed, such regrowth is usually not possible, and the area of dead tissue is repaired by the growth of non-specialized support tissue to form a **fibrous scar.**

Chemical mediators produced by damaged tissue attract phagocytic cells, such as neutrophils and monocytes (see page 73) from the blood into the tissue. These cells ingest the dead cells, while inactive support cells, particularly fibroblasts, are stimulated to proliferate by the secretion of growth factors (e.g. platelet derived growth factors and fibroblast growth factor).

The stimulated support cells are multipotential, and can differentiate into endothelial cells, myofibroblasts and fibroblasts, the damaged area becoming replaced by a mixture of these cell types, which form new blood vessels and lay down collagen. The resulting fibrocollagenous tissue is termed a **fibrous scar** (Fig. 4.22).

During this process of **healing by fibrous repair**, which is one of the basic responses to cell death in most body tissues, active fibroblasts assume a multipotential role and behave in a similar manner to the primitive mesenchyme from which they were derived, by differentiating into a variety of cell types.

Such an ability to transform into a variety of cell types in adult life to facilitate healing and repair is an important attribute of the support cell family.

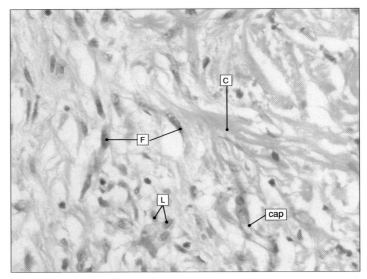

Fig. 4.22 Healing by fibrous repair.
Micrograph of the centre of a recent fibrous scar showing fibroblasts (F), capillaries (cap), collagen (C) and lymphoid/macrophagic cells (L).

TUMOURS OF SUPPORT CELLS

Support cells may form tumours which may be benign or malignant.

Usually these tumours resemble the cells of origin and contain specialized extracellular matrix; for example tumours of chondrocytes produce a cartilage-like ground substance, tumours of fibroblasts produce collagen. The malignant tumours are called **sarcomas** (Fig. 4.23).

support cell	benign tumour	malignant tumour
adipocyte	lipoma	liposarcoma
chondrocyte	chondroma	chondrosarcoma
fibrocyte	fibroma	fibrosarcoma
myofibroblast	fibrous histiocytoma	malignant fibrous histiocytoma
osteocyte	osteoma	osteosarcoma

Fig. 4.23 Tumours of support cells.

5. CONTRACTILE CELLS

Contractile cells are specially adapted to generate motile forces by the interaction of the proteins **actin** and **myosin** (**contractile proteins**).

There are four groups of contractile cell: muscle cells, myoepithelial cells, myofibroblasts and pericytes.
- **Muscle cells** are the main type and form **striated (voluntary) muscle, cardiac muscle,** and **smooth (involuntary) muscle.**
- **Myoepithelial cells** are an important component of certain secretory glands.
- **Myofibroblasts** have a contractile role in addition to being able to secrete collagen.
- **Pericytes** are smooth muscle-like cells that surround blood vessels.

Different arrangements of actin and myosin in each type of contractile cell, together with important structural adaptations, modulate and control contraction.

SKELETAL MUSCLE

Skeletal muscle cells form the structural basis of muscles (see Chapter 14), which are responsible for voluntary movement under the influence of the nervous system, and for maintenance of posture.

Structure

In embryogenesis, each skeletal muscle cell forms from the fusion of many hundreds of precursor cells (**myoblasts**), so in the adult each is a syncytium containing hundreds of nuclei, which are located just beneath the cell membrane.

Each skeletal muscle cell is a long thin cylindrical structure, typically 50–60 μm in diameter in an adult and up to 10 cm long depending on its location (Fig. 5.1).

In adult muscle, there is a resident population of muscle precursor cells (**satellite cells**), which can divide to form new muscle cells after tissue damage.

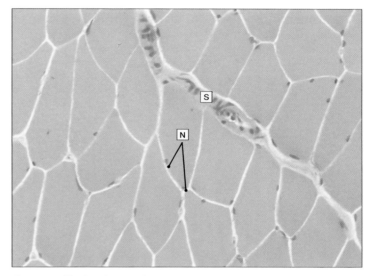

Fig. 5.1 Skeletal muscle.
In cross section skeletal muscle cells have a roughly hexagonal profile with individual cells moulded together. Nuclei (N) are arranged beneath the cell membrane. Fibrocollagenous septa (S) contain blood vessels.

In addition to contractile proteins, skeletal muscle cell cytoplasm contains numerous mitochondria, as well as abundant glycogen to provide energy.

Each muscle cell is surrounded by an external lamina (see page 48).

Terminology

Because of long usage, special terms are often used to describe skeletal muscle cell components; these are **sarcolemma** (cell membrane), **sarcoplasm** (cell cytoplasm), and **sarcoplasmic reticulum** (endoplasmic reticulum).

Structural and molecular basis of contraction

The contractile elements of skeletal muscle cells (**myofibrils**) are thin cylindrical structures 1–2 μm in diameter. They are composed of overlapping, repeating assemblies of thick (mainly myosin) and thin (mainly actin) filaments.

Any one muscle fibre has hundreds of myofibrils running parallel along its length, the alternating zones of thick and thin filaments giving rise to the descriptive term **striated muscle** (Fig. 5.2a). Ultrastructurally, the thick and thin filaments are held in place by plates of accessory proteins,

visible as lines, which divide the myofibrils into functional units called **sarcomeres** (Fig. 5.2b). Sarcoplasm, mitochondria, and other cellular elements are packed between the myofibrils.

There is a regular arrangement of contractile proteins within each sarcomere, with each thick filament being surrounded by six thin filaments (Fig. 5.2c&d). Contraction of muscle occurs as thick and thin filaments slide past each other (Fig 5.3), and is therefore accompanied by a decrease in the width of the light bands. The width of the dark bands remains unchanged.

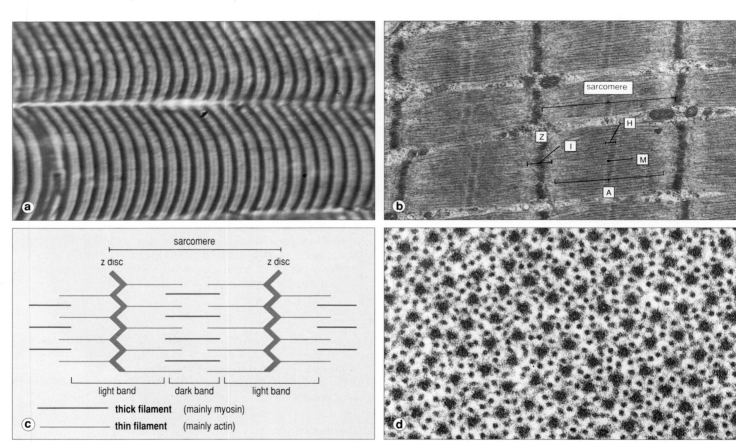

Fig. 5.2 Myofibrils.

a Individual skeletal muscle cells appear to have cross striations in longitudinal section due to the presence of stacks of myofibrils composed of alternating, overlapping zones of thick (dark stained) and thin (light stained) filaments.

b Ultrastructurally, several zones of staining can be discerned along myofibrils. The A (dark) band refers to the thick filament band and includes a zone where the thin filaments overlap the thick filaments. The H zone is a pale staining area in the centre of the A band and indicates where no thin filaments overlap the thick filaments. The I (light) band is the zone of thin filaments that does not overlap the

thick filaments, while the Z line is a dark band in the centre of the I band and the M line runs down the centre of the H band. The unit delineated between two Z discs is termed a **sarcomere**.

c Diagram to show the arrangement of filaments in a sarcomere. The thin filaments are composed mainly of actin, the thick filaments mainly of myosin.

d When viewed in cross section at the level of overlap between the A and I bands as in **b**, each myofibril is seen to have a regular spaced arrangement of thick and thin filaments, such that each thick filament is surrounded by six thin filaments arranged in an approximately hexagonal lattice.

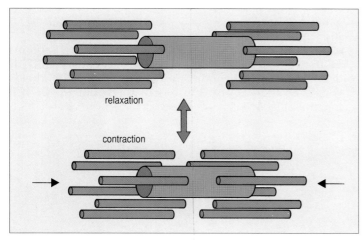

Fig. 5.3 Muscle contraction.
During muscle contraction the thin filaments of the myofibrils slide over the thick filaments. This is reversed on muscle relaxation.

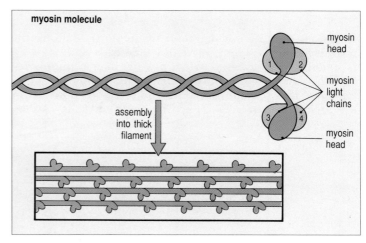

Fig. 5.4 Myosin molecule.
Each myosin molecule is composed of two tadpole-shaped heavy chains, the tails of which coil around each other, with four small light chains attached to the head portions.

The coiled, rod-like tail portions of many myosin molecules aggregate and pack together in a regular staggered array to form the filament, while the head portions project out in a regular helical pattern.

Thin filaments

Thin filaments are 8 nm in diameter and composed mainly of the protein actin. Each thin filament (F-actin) is formed by the polymerization of many single molecules of globular actin (G-actin). These actin filaments are polar, all G-actin molecules pointing in the same direction.

To form a complete thin filament, two actin filaments became attached by their tail ends to α-actinin in the Z line so that they face in opposite directions (i.e. away from the Z line).

Thick filaments

Thick filaments are composed mainly of the protein myosin (Fig. 5.4).

Like the actin filament, the myosin filament is polar. To form a complete heavy filament, two myosin filaments become attached by their tail ends so that they face in opposite directions (i.e. away from the M line). Different molecular types (isoforms) of myosin are present in different types of skeletal muscle fibre.

Accessory proteins

Skeletal muscle function depends on a precise alignment of actin and myosin filaments within each myofibril. This is achieved by **accessory proteins**, which link the different components and hold them in register with each other. These proteins can only be visualized using immunohisto-chemical techniques.

α **actinin** holds actin filaments in a lattice arrangement in the Z disc. Other Z disc proteins include **filamin**, **amorphin**, and **Z protein**.

Myomesin holds myosin filaments in a lattice arrangement in the region of the M line. Current models of the M line lattice suggest that additional, as yet uncharacterized, proteins are also involved.

Titin (**connectin**) is an extremely long elastic protein, which runs parallel to the filament array and links the ends of the thick filaments to the Z disc, maintaining their ends in register with the lattice of thin filaments.

Desmin filaments (one of the class of intermediate filament proteins), link adjacent myofibrils to each other and maintain their register. In addition, they link myofibrils to the cell membrane.

C protein is a myosin binding protein localized in seven stripes running parallel to the M band in the first half of the A band.

Contraction

In muscle contraction the actin filaments slide along the myosin filaments. This is driven by the heads of the myosin molecules, which bind to actin and, in a sequence of binding and release movements, 'walk' along the actin filament. This repetitive binding and release is powered by the hydrolysis of ATP (Fig. 5.5) and myosin can be regarded as an ATPase that is activated by the binding of actin.

Control of muscle contraction is achieved by proteins that bind to actin and prevent muscle contraction by blocking the myosin–actin interaction (Fig. 5.6). This is reversed by high concentrations of Ca^{2+} ions in the cell cytoplasm (Fig. 5.7).

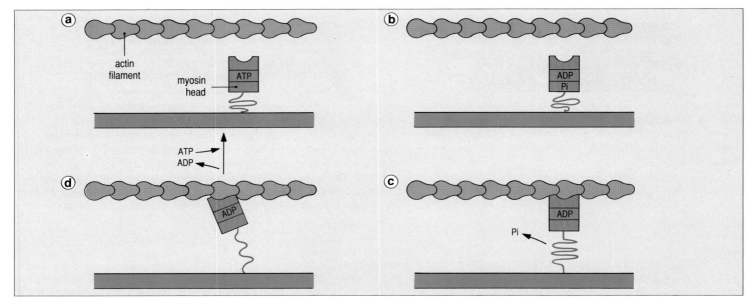

Fig 5.5 Use of ATP by myosin binding to actin.
A myosin molecule uses the energy of ATP to move along an actin filament.
a ATP bound to myosin is hydrolysed to ADP and phosphate (Pi).
b This causes myosin to bind loosely to actin.
c Pi is released and myosin binds tightly to actin.

d This binding initiates molecular folding of the myosin molecule to cause the movement of the molecule relative to the actin filament. ADP is released, fresh ATP binds, and the myosin returns to its non-attached state.

The cycle repeats and the myosin head 'walks' along the actin filament.

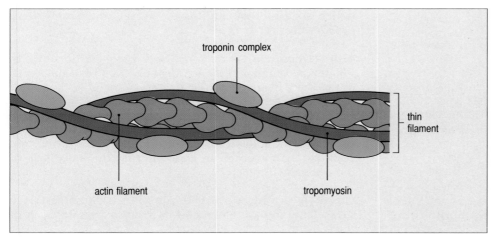

Fig. 5.6 Control of muscle contraction.
Tropomyosin is a long rod-like protein that winds around an actin filament to stabilize and stiffen it.

The troponin complex, which regulates the binding of actin to myosin, is attached to tropomyosin and composed of three separate polypeptides termed troponin T, I and C. Troponin T binds the complex to tropomyosin and positions the complex on the actin filament at the site where actin would bind to myosin. Troponin I physically prevents myosin binding to actin. Troponin C binds Ca^{2+} ions, which cause a conformational change in the troponin complex allowing myosin access to the actin filament.

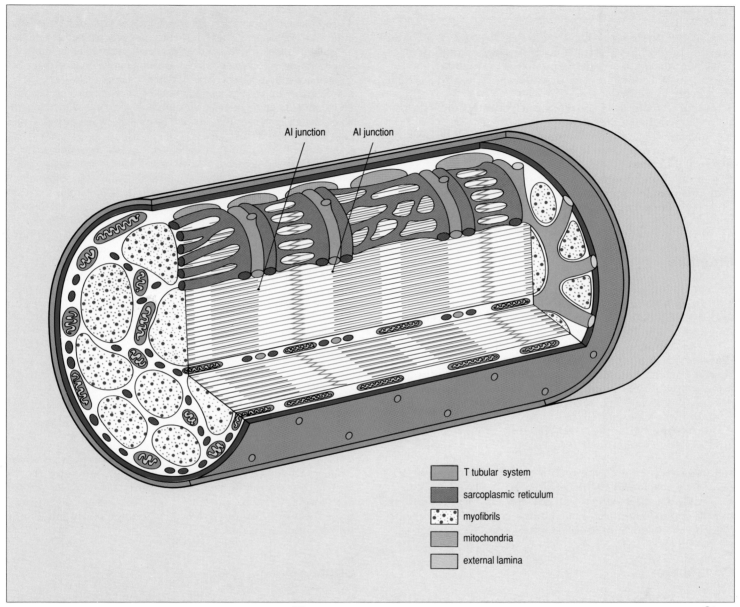

Fig. 5.7 Muscle cell excitation and intracellular Ca^{2+} ions.
Following a nerve signal, excitation of the muscle cell membrane is conveyed to the interior of the cell via a series of membranous channels (the **transverse tubular system or T tubules**), which extend from the muscle cell surface to surround each myofibril.

Running alongside each T tubule are two portions of **sarcoplasmic reticulum** called **terminal cisternae**, which contain a high concentration of Ca^{2+} ions and have electrically sensitive Ca^{2+} ion channels in their wall. Membrane excitation of the T tubule system causes these Ca^{2+} ion channels to open, thus allowing Ca^{2+} ions to flood into the sarcoplasm.

In the resting state muscle cells have little intracellular free Ca^{2+} ions, and a sudden increase in free cytosolic Ca^{2+} ions initiates muscle contraction.

Membrane pumps (Ca^{2+}-ATPase) in the sarcoplasmic reticulum pump the Ca^{2+} ions back into the sarcoplasmic reticulum rapidly (within about 30 msec) and stop contraction.

The close association of T tubules and sarcoplasmic reticulum form three tubules in cross section (a **membrane triad**).

In human muscle there is a membrane triad surrounding every myofibril in the AI junction region, thus there are two triads to each sarcomere.

61

CARDIAC MUSCLE

Like skeletal muscle, cardiac muscle is a type of striated muscle and is characterized by a similar arrangement of actin and myosin filaments to mediate contraction. The important differences between cardiac muscle and skeletal muscle are as follows.
- Cardiac muscle cells are mononuclear and much shorter than those of skeletal muscle.
- Long cardiac muscle fibres are produced by linking numerous cardiac muscle cells end to end via anchoring-type cell junctions.
- A population of stem cells, analogous to satellite cells of skeletal muscle (see page 57) is not present in cardiac muscle, hence regeneration following damage can not occur.

Structure

Instead of fusing to form syncytia as for skeletal muscle, (see page 57), cardiac muscle cells align into long chains and develop cell junctions, which anchor each cell to its neighbour (Fig. 5.8).

In the adult, a cardiac muscle cell is 15–20 μm in diameter and about 100 μm long with a centrally positioned nucleus. Intercellular junctions can be seen in light microscopic preparations as faint lines running transversely across fibres and are termed **intercalated discs**. These contain three types of cell junction.
- Desmosomal junctions tightly link adjacent cells via anchors involving the intermediate filaments (see Fig. 3.11).
- Adherent-type junctions anchor the actin fibres of the sarcomeres to each end of the cell (see Fig. 3.9).
- Communicating gap junctions (see Fig. 3.14) facilitate the passage of membrane excitation (communication) and thereby synchronize of muscle contraction.

Contraction

Contraction of cardiac muscle cells is regulated by cytosolic Ca^{2+} ion concentration in a manner virtually identical to that for skeletal muscle (see Figs 5.5&5.6) but:
- the cardiac muscle transverse (T) tubular system consists of much wider invaginations of the cell surface;
- sarcoplasmic reticulum associated with the T tubules is neither as regular nor as well organized as in skeletal muscle;
- the association of cardiac sarcoplasmic reticulum with T tubules takes the form of diads rather than triads, and is located in the region of the Z lines rather than the AI junction.

Fig. 5.8 Cardiac muscle.
a Cardiac muscle cells appear as elliptical or lobulated structures in transverse section. Their nuclei are centrally placed and have irregular shapes, and fibrocollagenous septa containing small blood vessels run between fibres. Between individual cardiac muscle cells there is a rich capillary blood supply.
b In longitudinal section, cardiac muscle appears as a series of anastomosing cords of cells, which branch and join with adjacent fibres at cell junctions (intercalated discs, ID), which are seen as pale lines in this PTAH stain.
c Ultrastructurally, cardiac muscle cells contain myofibrils with thick and thin filament systems virtually identical to those in skeletal muscle, but composed of different structural isoforms. Mitochondria are prominent and make up a much larger proportion of cell volume than in skeletal muscle. Several regions of the intercalated disc structure can be resolved showing desmosome-like junctions (D), adherent-type junctions (A), and in the lateral portions of the intercalated disc, prominent communicating gap junctions (G).
d Diagram of the structural arrangement of adjacent cardiac muscle cells. Cells are bound together by desmosomal junctions at interdigitating areas at the ends of adjacent cells to form the intercalated disc. Gap junctions facilitate transmission of the contractile stimulus between cells.

SMOOTH MUSCLE

Smooth muscle cells have a much less organized system of contractile proteins than striated skeletal and cardiac muscle cells. Forming the contractile portions of most hollow viscera (e.g. gut, urinary bladder, and uterus), as well as the contractile elements in blood vessel walls and secretory gland ducts, smooth muscle cells are found in situations requiring sustained slow or rhythmic contractions not under voluntary control.

Structure

Smooth muscle cells are typically spindle-shaped and, depending on site, vary in size from 20 μm (small blood vessels) to 400–500 μm (uterus). Each cell has a single, centrally located nucleus, which is elongated or elliptical in shape (Fig. 5.9).

In cross section, smooth muscle cells have polygonal profiles, but in longitudinal section appear as linear bundles.

Each smooth muscle cell is surrounded by an external lamina (see page 48) to which cell membranes adhere; small groups of cells are organized into bundles by fine collagenous tissue containing blood vessels and nerves.

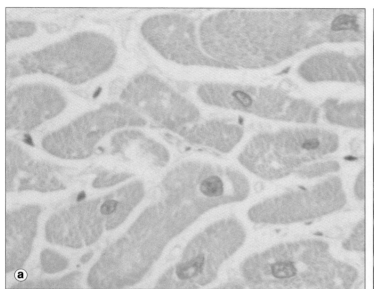

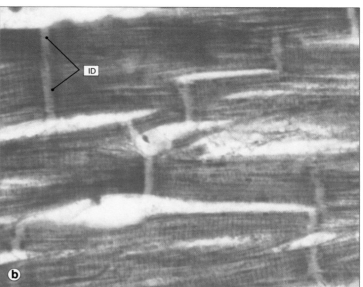

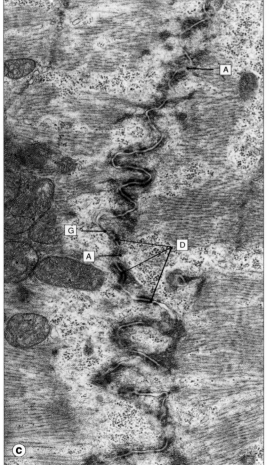

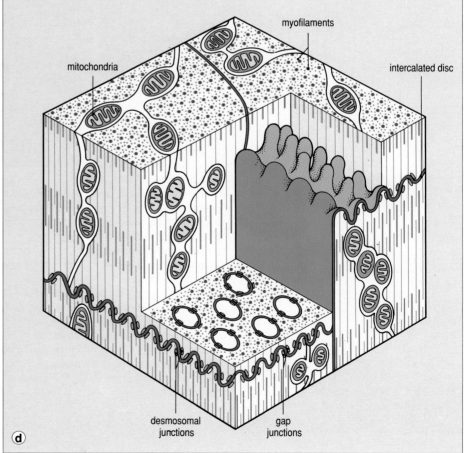

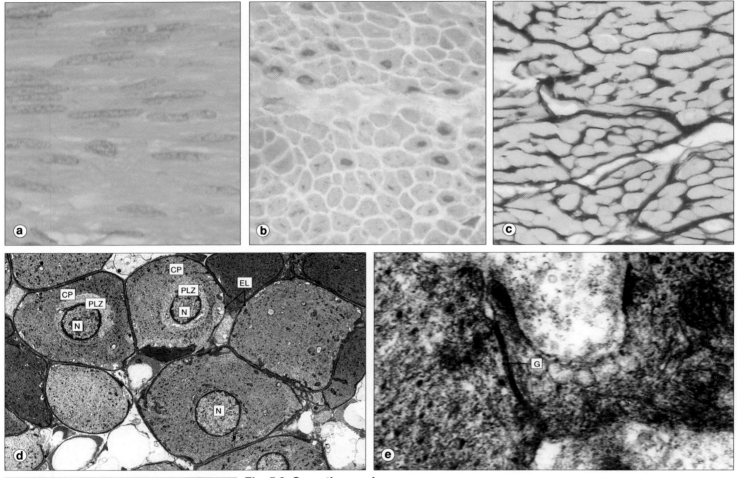

Fig. 5.9 Smooth muscle.

a In longitudinal section smooth muscle cells have abundant pink cytoplasm and are characterized by elongated centrally placed nuclei.

b In transverse section it is apparent that each cell has a polygonal profile and the centrally placed nuclei are evident.

c The external lamina surrounding each smooth muscle cell binds individual cells into a functional mass and is highlighted by silver staining, which detects type IV collagen and glycoproteins.

d Ultrastructurally smooth muscle cells are surrounded by an external lamina (EL) and have centrally placed nuclei (N). The irregularly arranged contractile proteins (CP) give rise to dense staining at the periphery of each cell, while mitochondria and other organelles are located in a perinuclear lucent zone (PLZ).

e Gap junctions (G) connect adjacent cells at defects in the external lamina.

f A terminal sac of the endoplasmic reticulum (ER) lies closely apposed toendocytotic vesicles (V) at the surface of the smooth muscle cell. The external lamina (EL) is visible.

Ultrastructurally, smooth muscle does not show the highly organized system of contractile proteins (i.e myofilaments) seen in striated muscle, but has an arrangement where bundles of contractile proteins criss-cross the cell and are inserted into anchoring points (**focal densities**). Focal densities are similar to adherent junctions and are studded around the cell membrane.

Tension generated by contraction is transmitted through the focal densities to the surrounding network of external laminae, thus allowing a mass of smooth muscle cells to function as one unit.

The abundant intermediate filaments of smooth muscle **desmin** are also inserted into the focal densities.

Energy is supplied by numerous mitochondria, which tend to be located, along with endoplasmic reticulum and other organelles around the nucleus in an area devoid of contractile filaments.

Although each smooth muscle cell is surrounded by an external lamina, this is deficient where the cells communicate with each other via **gap junctions**. These junctions, which are also termed **nexus junctions** in smooth muscle, are widespread and allow spread of membrane excitation between cells.

A characteristic feature of smooth muscle cells is the presence of numerous invaginations of cell membrane forming structures that resemble endocytic vesicles. It is thought that these invaginations function in a similar way to the specialized transverse (T) tubular system of striated muscle by controlling the entry of Ca^{2+} ions into the cell following membrane excitation. Terminal sacs of Ca^{2+} ion-containing endoplasmic reticulum terminate beneath the cell membrane close to these vesicles.

Contraction

The contraction mechanism of smooth muscle differs from that for striated muscle.
- Thin filaments of actin (an isoform specific to smooth muscle) are associated with tropomyosin (see Fig. 5.6) but, in contrast to striated muscle, there is no troponin.
- The thick filaments are composed of myosin, but of a different type to that in skeletal muscle and will only bind to actin if its light chain is phosphorylated; this phenomenon does not occur in skeletal muscle.
- Although Ca^{2+} ions in smooth muscle cells cause contraction as in striated muscle, the control of Ca^{2+} ion movements is different. In relaxed smooth muscle free Ca^{2+} ions are normally sequestered in sarcoplasmic reticulum throughout the cell. On membrane excitation, free

Ca^{2+} ions are released into the cytoplasm and bind to a protein called **calmodulin** (a calcium binding protein). The calcium–calmodulin complex then activates an enzyme called myosin light-chain kinase, which phosphorylates the myosin light chain and permits it to bind to actin. Actin and myosin subsequently interact by filament sliding to produce contraction in a similar way to that for skeletal muscle.
- Because the contractile proteins are arranged in a criss-cross lattice inserted circumferentially into the cell membrane, contraction results in shortening of the cell, which assumes a globular shape in contrast to its elongated shape in the relaxed state.

Innervation and functional arrangement

Unitary smooth muscle

Most smooth muscle is present in the walls of hollow viscera (e.g. gut, ureter, fallopian tube) where it is arranged in sheets with cells aligned circumferentially or longitudinally, with contraction resulting in reduction of the lumen diameter.

In these so-called **unitary smooth muscles**, cells tend to generate their own low level of rhythmic contraction, which may also be stimulated by stretch, and is transmitted from cell to cell via the gap junctions. Such smooth muscle is richly innervated by the autonomic nervous system (see Chapter 13), which increases or decreases levels of spontaneous contraction rather than initiates it *per se*.

Multi-unit smooth muscle

A second arrangement of smooth muscle is typified by that in the iris of the eye. Here, rather than simply modulating spontaneous activity, autonomic innervation precisely controls contraction, resulting in opening and closing of the pupil.

Similar neurally controlled or **multi-unit smooth muscle** is found in the vas deferens and some large arteries.

Secretory properties

Depending on its site, smooth muscle cells produce collagen, elastin, and other components of the extracellular matrix. Thus they have a support cell function as well as a contractile cell function. In most situations this support cell function is limited to manufacturing extracellular matrix to anchor the smooth muscle.

MYOFIBROBLASTS

Myofibroblasts are spindle-shaped cells that secrete collagen (i.e. fibroblast-like), but also have well defined contractile properties similar to those of smooth muscle (i.e. myoid).

In conventional histological sections myofibroblasts cannot be readily distinguished from fibroblasts, but immunohistochemical detection of their content of smooth muscle actin and desmin (not seen in fibroblasts), and ultrastructural demonstration of contractile proteins shows that they are distinct. Myofibroblasts lack an external lamina, in contrast to true smooth muscle cells.

In normal tissues, myofibroblasts are inconspicuous and commonly form an inactive population of cells, for example in the alveolar septa of the lung, and around the crypts of glands in the gut. They also form a sparse population in loose collagenous support tissue.

Following tissue damage, however, myofibroblasts become active and proliferate, and their role appears to be to repair defects resulting from tissue death. They secrete collagen to provide a firm scaffold to consolidate a damaged area (fibrous scar), and contract to reduce the physical size of the damaged area.

As well as being prominent in wound healing and in the normal processes of repair, myofibroblasts are also found in several diseases characterized by fibrosis of tissues, for example fibrosis of the lung following damage by immune-mediated diseases, atheroma in the lining of arteries (see Fig. 8.17), and cirrhosis of the liver (see Fig. 11.7). In these diseases the stimuli which cause myofibroblast proliferation are uncertain, but include local production of growth factors.

PERICYTES

Pericytes are spindle-shaped cells, which are found circumferentially arranged around capillaries and venules (see Fig. 8.21). They are surrounded by external lamina and, in normal tissues, show little cytoplasmic differentiation ultrastructurally, but contain actin and myosin immunohistochemically, suggesting a contractile function.

Following tissue injury pericytes proliferate and assume the role of primitive mesenchymal cells, being able to differentiate into myofibroblasts, as well as mesenchymal tissue, which develops into collagenous support tissue and new blood vessels.

MYOEPITHELIAL CELLS

Myoepithelial cells are found in exocrine glands including highly developed glands such as the breast, where they form a major population surrounding glandular acini and ducts, and squeeze secretions from the glandular lumina.

Myoepithelial cells are generally inconspicuous in routine H&E sections, appearing as a layer of flat cells running around acini and ducts. They have dark-stained rounded nuclei and clear or vacuolated cytoplasm.

Around acini, myoepithelial cells have a stellate, multi-processed morphology in three dimensions and form a contractile meshwork, which encloses secretory units of glands. Around ducts they are fusiform in shape and surround ductal cells in a manner analogous to barrel hoops.

Ultrastructurally myoepithelial cells contain contractile proteins arranged in a similar manner to that in smooth muscle and have numerous desmosomal connections with adjacent cells.

Immunohistochemically they can be detected by their content of the muscle-specific intermediate filament desmin (Fig. 5.10).

Myoepithelial cells are controlled by the autonomic nervous system and on stimulation contract and expel glandular secretions.

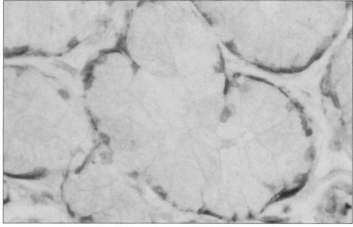

Fig. 5.10 Myoepithelial cells.
Myoepithelial cells in this section from salivary gland can be shown by an immunoperoxidase technique that demonstrates desmin, which is the muscle-specific intermediate filament and stains brown.

6. BLOOD CELLS

Blood has four major elements:
- **Red blood cells (erythrocytes)** transport oxygen from the lungs to the peripheral tissues.
- **White blood cells (leukocytes)** have a defensive role, destroying infecting organisms such as bacteria and viruses, as well as assisting in the removal of dead or damaged tissues.
- **Platelets (thrombocytes)** are the first line of defence against damage to blood vessels, adhering to defects and participating in the blood clotting system.
- **Plasma** is the proteinaceous solution in which the above mentioned cells circulate, and carries nutrients, metabolites, antibodies, hormones, proteins of the blood clotting system and other molecules throughout the body.

SITES OF BLOOD CELL FORMATION

The site of blood cell formation (**haemopoiesis**) changes several times during fetal development, the earliest sites being the yolk sac and then the liver (Fig. 6.1) and spleen. At 5 months, the fetal bone marrow begins to produce white cells and platelets, while red cell production by bone marrow starts later at around 7 months.

At birth, the bone marrow is the main site of red cell production and almost all bones in the body are involved.

As this only just meets normal requirements, any greater demand (e.g. due to excessive blood loss) results in increased haemopoietic activity by the liver and spleen; this is termed **extramedullary haemopoiesis**.

Over the next few years, with the rapid increase in bone size, the haemopoietic capacity of the bone marrow expands far beyond even emergency requirements, and so the haemopoietic bone marrow occupies less of the marrow space available. By skeletal maturity only the marrow of the vertebrae, ribs, skull, pelvis and proximal femurs is haemopoietic, the rest having been replaced by adipose tissue, although retaining its capacity to resume haemopoiesis should the need arise.

All cellular elements of the blood originate from a common progenitor stem cell, which differentiates to form stem cells giving rise to either red cells, white cells or platelets.

Bone marrow

Bone marrow occupies the spaces between the trabeculae of medullary bone (see Chapter 14), and consists of highly branched vascular sinuses and a reticulin scaffolding, with the interstices packed with haemopoietic cells (Fig. 6.2).

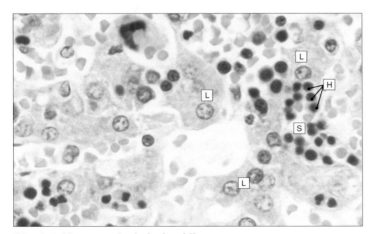

Fig. 6.1 Haemopoiesis in fetal liver.
Micrograph showing haemopoietic cells (H) in the sinusoidal spaces (S) between plates of liver cells (L) in a fetus.

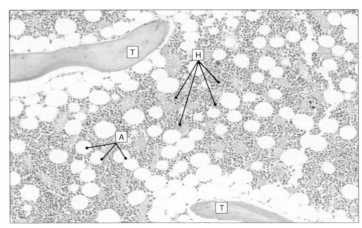

Fig. 6.2 Bone marrow.
Micrograph of decalcified vertebra showing haemopoietic bone marrow (H) in the spaces between the bony trabeculae (T) of the ilium. Some of the space is also occupied by adipocytes (A).

In addition to its haemopoietic function, the bone marrow, along with the spleen and liver, contains fixed macrophagic cells, which remove aged and defective red cells from the circulation by phagocytosis. It also plays a central role in the immune system, being the site of maturation of B lymphocytes, which produce antibodies (see Chapter 7).

Vasculature

Bone marrow is supplied by **medullary branches** derived from the nutrient artery of the bone, which pierces the cortical bone through a nutrient canal, giving off a series of small branches to the cortical and medullary bone.

This is augmented by smaller vessels from the muscle and periosteum surrounding the bone, which similarly penetrate the cortical bone.

The capillary network opens into a series of thin-walled **sinusoids**, which empty into a large central sinus, before leaving the bone as the **emissary vein** via the nutrient canal.

Endothelium

The bone marrow sinusoids are lined by flat cells (**endothelial cells**), which normally line blood vessels (see Fig. 8.20), and these lie on a discontinuous basement membrane.

The endothelial cells probably control the passage of all materials into and out of the haemopoietic compartment by endocytosis.

In places, their cytoplasm is so thin that the endothelial barrier is little more than the inner and outer layers of endothelial cell membrane; such sites may provide the exit route for mature blood cells into the circulation.

Support cells and extracellular matrix

Beyond the endothelium and its basement membrane is a discontinuous layer of support cells (**reticular cells**) with extensive branched cytoplasmic processes, which not only enclose well over 50% of the outer surface area of the sinusoid wall, but also ramify throughout the haemopoietic spaces. These cells synthesize collagenous reticular fibres (see Fig. 4.6), which along with the cytoplasmic processes, form a meshwork to support the haemopoietic cells.

By accumulating lipid, the reticular support cells may transform into the adipocytes found in bone marrow.

The extracellular matrix in the haemopoietic compartment contains coarse collagen fibres, as well as laminin and fibronectin, which facilitate adhesion of the haemopoietic cells to the marrow stroma. The associated proteoglycans, chondroitin sulphate, hyaluronic acid and heparan sulphate, may bind growth factors, which control haemopoiesis.

RED BLOOD CELLS

The **erythron** describes the whole mass of mature red cells (Fig. 6.3) and their progenitors. It functions as a dispersed organ, the number of red cells in the circulating blood being regulated to meet oxygen carrying needs, and the rate of red cell production varying with changing rates of their removal from the circulation.

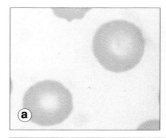
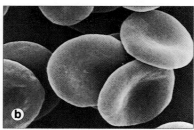
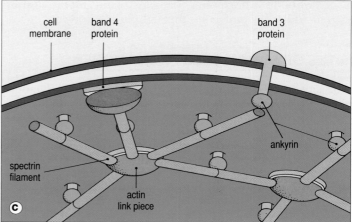

Fig. 6.3 Mature red cell.
a Typical appearance of a mature red cell in a stained smear of the peripheral blood. It is a biconcave-shaped disc 1.8 μm thick, and ranges from 7.5–8.7 μm in diameter, the size decreasing slightly with age. Its main cytoplasmic constituent is the protein complex **haemoglobin**, which results in its characteristic acidophilic staining property. Due to its biconcave shape which facilitates oxygen exchange, the centre of the cell appears pale.
b Scanning electronmicrograph showing the typical biconcave structure of a mature red cell.
c Diagram to illustrate the red cell cytoskeleton, which maintains its distinct shape. A filamentous skeleton of the protein spectrin is anchored to the cell membrane by three main proteins (band 3 protein, ankyrin, and band 4 protein), with short actin pieces, about 15 actin monomers long, linking spectrin to the band 4 protein. Other proteins are also involved, but have been omitted for clarity.

This behaviour is mediated by a number of factors, but particularly by the hormone **erythropoietin**, which adjusts red cell production to match oxygen demand. Erythropoietin is secreted mainly by the kidneys in adults, and by the liver in the fetus.

Red blood cells have a biconcave shape to maximize their surface area:volume ratio and thereby maximize oxygen exchange.

HEREDITARY SPHEROCYTOSIS

Hereditary spherocytosis is caused by an abnormal arrangement of the internal cytoskeleton of red cells. Normally the internal surface of the cell membrane is braced by cytoskeletal proteins via interactions between ankyrin and spectrin (see Fig. 6.3c). In hereditary spherocytosis, the ankyrin binding of spectrin is absent. As a result the red cell membrane is not braced and is easily deformed.

In hereditary spherocytosis red cells do not form their normal biconcave disc shape, but appear round and convex (Fig. 6.4). They are abnormally fragile and do not resist changes in osmotic pressure. This abnormally rapid breakdown of red blood cells is called **haemolysis**.

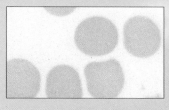

Fig. 6.4 Hereditary spherocytosis.
Micrograph showing the abnormal round convex-shaped blood cell of hereditary spherocytosis. Compare with Fig. 6.3a.

Erythropoiesis

Red cells are the terminal differentiated progeny of one cell line of pluripotent bone marrow stem cells, which is committed to erythropoiesis only. These unipotential stem cells are few in number and cannot be identified in bone marrow smears, but experimental red cell stimulation studies have shown that such cells have large nucleoli, many polyribosomes and large mitochondria. Differentiation of these stem cells into mature red cells is associated with:
- decreasing cell size;
- haemoglobin production;
- gradual decrease and eventual loss of all cell organelles;
- changing cytoplasmic staining, from intense basophilia due to large numbers of polyribosomes, to eosinophilia due to haemoglobin;
- condensation and eventual extrusion of the nucleus.

Along this path of differentiation, certain morphological cell types can be distinguished; **proerythroblast**, **basophilic erythroblast**, **polychromatic erythroblast**, **orthochromatic erythroblast** and **reticulocyte** (Fig. 6.5).

Red cells are formed in small **erythroblastic islands** consisting of one or two specialized macrophages surrounded by red cell progenitor cells.

The macrophages have long cytoplasmic processes, and deep invaginations to accommodate the dividing erythroid cells, which migrate outwards along the cytoplasmic process as they differentiate. When mature, the red cell contacts nearby sinusoidal endothelium and passes through its cytoplasm to enter the circulation.

Because it does not possess RNA, the mature red cell is unable to synthesize new enzymes to replace those lost during normal metabolic processes.

Diminishing efficiency of the ionic pumps is probably the main factor in red cell ageing, the cell becoming progressively less deformable, until it is unable to negotiate the splenic microcirculation and is removed by phagocytosis. Red cells have a lifespan of 100–120 days in the circulation.

The spleen, liver and bone marrow all dispose of aged and defective red cells, but their relative contributions under normal conditions is uncertain; the spleen appears to be the most active.

	Proerythroblast	Basophilic erythroblast (early normoblast)	Polychromatic erythroblast (intermediate normoblast)	Orthochromatic erythroblast (late normoblast)	Reticulocyte
	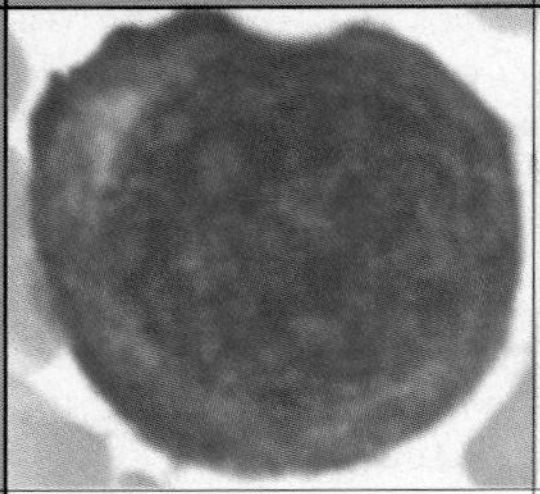	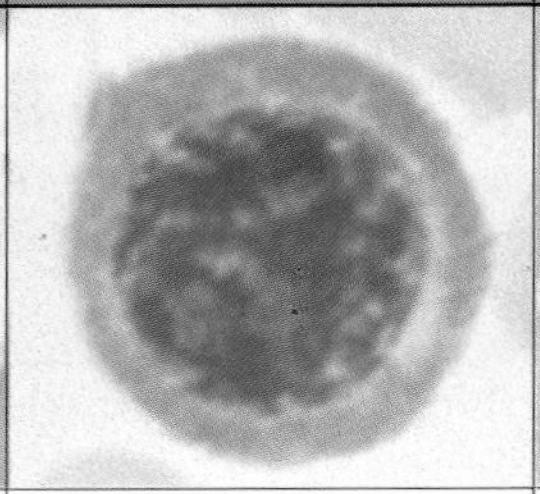	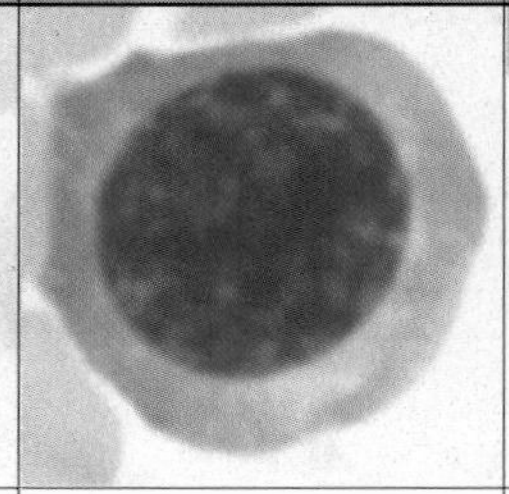	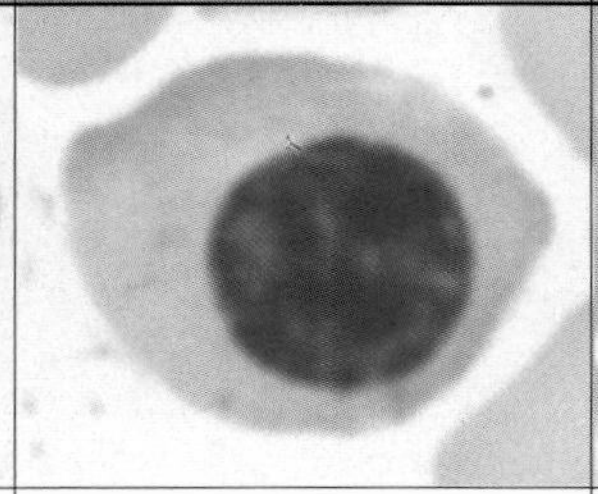	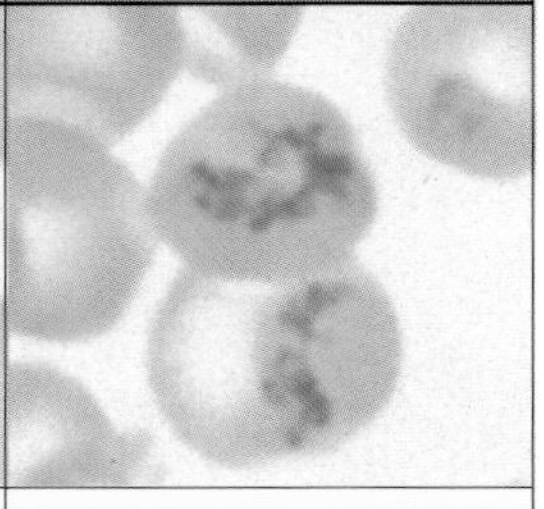
diameter	20–25 μm	16–18 μm	12–15 μm	10–12 μm	–
nucleus	large (80% of cell)	more condensed	condensed	extremely condensed, eccentrically located	absent
chromatin	fine and in clumps	in wheel spoke or clock face arrangement	clumps with more regular distribution	pyknotic	–
nucleoli	one or more, pale	variably identifiable	absent	–	–
cytoplasm	intensely basophilic (due to polyribosomes)	basophilic (due to polyribosomes)	polychromatic (combination of basophilia due to polyribosomes and eosinophilia due to haemoglobin)	more eosinophilic (due to increased haemoglobin content)	eosinophilic (due to haemoglobin)
organelles	plentiful, particularly polyribosomes	plentiful, particularly polyribosomes	reduction in number of organelles; haemoglobin formation commences	elimination of most, especially polyribosomes and mitochondria	remnants of organelles not easily visible with conventional stains, but can be demonstrated by supravital methods*
other features	contain ferritin (free and in lysosomes), divide into 8–16 cells	characteristic pale staining perinuclear halo	perinuclear halo still evident, cell replication complete	divides into smaller part containing nucleus (phagocytosed by macrophages), and larger part (passes through sinusoidal endothelium to enter circulation as a reticulocyte)	matures into red cell in 24–48 hours form 1% of circulating red cells, the proportion increasing when red cell demand increases, as shown in micrograph

*To demonstrate organelle remnants, fresh blood is incubated with brilliant cresyl blue or methylene blue dye (supravital staining); the remnants precipitate as blue reticular strands, hence the name reticulocyte

Fig. 6.5 Morphological stages in erythropoiesis.

ANAEMIA

The most common blood disorder is **anaemia** in which an inadequate haemoglobin supply causes weakness, pallor and sometimes breathlessness.

Anaemia may be the result of impaired red cell formation or excessive red cell destruction.

• The most common cause is deficiency of iron, which is essential for the formation of haemoglobin. Red cells are released into the circulation containing much less haemoglobin than normal, and are therefore pale-staining (**hypochromic**) and small (**microcytic**) (Fig. 6.6).

• Excessive red cell destruction usually occurs because the red cells are structurally abnormal and therefore more liable to damage whilst circulating: such cells are removed prematurely and in excess in the spleen causing anaemia (**haemolytic anaemia**). This can be due to a genetic abnormality of red cell structure and occurs in hereditary spherocytosis (see Fig. 6.4).

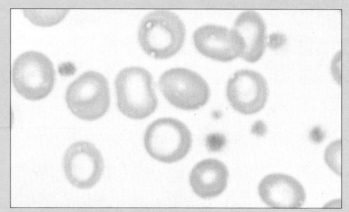

Fig. 6.6 Hypochromic, microcytic anaemia.
Micrograph of blood smear showing the hypochromic, microcytic red cells of iron deficiency anaemia. Compare with Fig. 6.3a.

WHITE BLOOD CELLS

White blood cells (leukocytes) are so-named because they are present in the white layer floating above the red cells when blood settles in a tube. White cells use the blood to transport them from the bone marrow to their major sites of activity in tissues, and their total number in peripheral blood is normally 4.0–11.0 x 10^9/litre.

Classification and nomenclature

There are five types of white cell, and their names and relative proportions in the circulation are as follows:
• neutrophils 40–75%;
• eosinophils 5%;
• basophils 0.5%;
• lymphocytes 20–50%;
• monocytes 1–5%.

If there is a requirement for increased activity of any one cell type in the peripheral tissues, the number and proportion of that cell type rises markedly.

Neutrophils, eosinophils and basophils are known as **granulocytes** because their cytoplasm contains prominent granules, and may also be referred to as **myeloid cells** because of their origin from bone marrow. Neutrophils are also commonly called **polymorphonuclear leukocytes** or **polymorphs** because of their multi-lobed nucleus.

Lymphocytes and monocytes are classed as white blood cells because they are a constituent of the blood and originate in bone marrow. They are found mainly in tissues such as lymph nodes and spleen. In the tissues, monocytes transform into macrophages, and basophils become mast cells.

Neutrophils

Neutrophils (Fig. 6.7) are highly motile, phagocytic cells. Their primary function is to ingest and destroy invading microorganisms. They play a central role in the early stages of the acute inflammatory response to tissue injury and are the major constituent of pus.

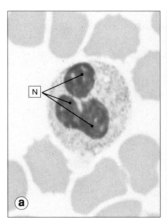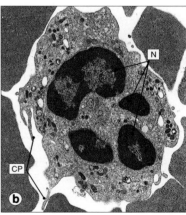

Fig. 6.7 Neutrophil.
a A mature neutrophil is 12–14 μm in diameter and has a characteristic multilobed nucleus (N), and pale-staining cytoplasm, in which only a few of the many granules it contains can be seen in a routine stain.
b Electronmicrograph of a neutrophil from the blood showing its characteristic multilobed nucleus (N), cytoplasmic processes (CP), and mixture of granule types within its cytoplasm. At this magnification, individual granule types cannot be identified.

Neutrophil granulopoiesis

A common unipotential stem cell type is believed to produce all three types of granulocyte, the first recognizable precursor being the **myeloblast**. The stages of subsequent maturation through **promyelocyte**, **myelocyte**, **metamyelocyte** and **band cell** are shown in Fig. 6.8.

Maturation from myeloblast to neutrophil takes about 7–8 days, and involves five cell divisions between myeloblast and metamyelocyte stages, after which no further multiplication divisions take place, and chemotactic ability, complement and Fc receptors are acquired.

Structurally mature neutrophils remain in the marrow for about 5 days and are then released into the blood. After circulating for about 6 hours, they migrate into the peripheral tissues where they survive for 2–5 days, unless destroyed earlier as a result of their phagocytic activity.

Loosely adherent to the sinusoidal endothelium in the bone marrow is a huge pool of stored neutrophils, which can be rapidly mobilized. Adrenergic stimuli cause a sudden outpouring of granulocytes from the bone marrow, leading to an increase in number of blood neutrophils (neutrophil leukocytosis).

If it is necessary to maintain a high blood neutrophil count, for example during bacterial infection, there is increased proliferation of the granulocyte precursors in the marrow.

Neutrophil nucleus

The characteristic neutrophil nucleus is composed of 2–5 distinct lobules, joined to one another by fine strands of nuclear material, the lobulation developing with cellular maturity. The chromatin is highly condensed reflecting a low degree of protein synthesis.

In females, about 3% of nuclei exhibit a small condensed nuclear appendage (drumstick chromosome), which represents the quiescent X chromosome (**Barr body**).

Neutrophil cytoplasm

Neutrophil cytoplasm contains three types (i.e. primary, secondary and tertiary) of membrane-bound vesicles (granules).

Primary granules are similar to lysosomes (see page 16) in other cells. They are the first granules to appear during neutrophil formation, but as the cell matures, their number falls with respect to secondary granules (see below), making them difficult to see with light microscopy. With electron microscopy, they are large and electron-dense.

As with lysosomes, primary granules contain acid hydrolases, but in addition they also contain antibacterial and digestive substances, most notably myeloperoxidase, which

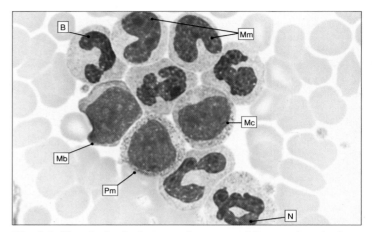

Fig. 6.8 Morphological stages in neutrophil granulopoiesis. Micrograph showing granulocyte precursors at various stages of maturation.

The **myeloblast** (Mb) is a large cell largely occupied by a nucleus in which nucleoli are prominent; its scanty cytoplasm contains a few granules.

The **promyelocyte** (Pm) contains more abundant cytoplasm and more primary granules; nucleoli are still present.

The **myelocyte** (Mc) shows early flattening or invagination of one face of the nucleus from which the nucleoli have disappeared. Its cytoplasm contains a mixture of a few primary granules and smaller secondary granules.

The **metamyelocyte** (Mm) shows more advanced invagination of the nucleus to a reniform shape, and a later stage, the **band** or **stab form** (B) has a horseshoe-shaped nucleus.

Increasing lobation of the nucleus produces the mature **neutrophil** (N), which features a multilobed nucleus and abundant cytoplasm containing small secondary granules.

can be detected by the peroxidase stain. Myeloperoxidase is therefore a useful light microscopic marker not only for these granules, but also in establishing cell lineage in the diagnosis of leukaemias (see page 77).

Secondary granules are specific to neutrophils and twice as numerous as primary granules. With a diameter of 0.2–0.8 μm (i.e. smaller than primary granules) they are barely visible with light microscopy.

Ultrastructural studies have shown secondary granules to be of variable size, shape and density and to contain substances involved in the mobilization of inflammatory mediators and complement activation. These substances are secreted into the extracellular environment.

Tertiary granules have only recently been described and contain enzymes (e.g. gelatinase) secreted into the extracellular environment. They also insert some glycoproteins into cell membranes, and this may promote cellular adhesion and hence may be involved in the phagocytic process. The stage at which tertiary granules develop is not known.

OTHER CYTOPLASMIC FEATURES

Alkaline phosphatase activity has long been recognized as a feature of neutrophil cytoplasm and has also been used as a marker for specific granules. It is found in a light fraction of neutrophil membranes and may constitute the contents of a fourth type of granule, described as a **phosphasome**.

The cytoplasm also contains various antioxidants to destroy potentially toxic peroxides, which may be generated during lysosomal activity.

OTHER ORGANELLES

Other neutrophil cytoplasmic organelles are sparse. There are only a few scattered profiles of rough endoplasmic reticulum and free ribosomes, and the remnants of the Golgi involved in granule packaging earlier in development. Mitochondria are also few, but provide about 50% of energy needs.

Neutrophils tend to operate in devascularized tissue where oxygen and glucose may be in short supply. They therefore contain abundant glycogen for anaerobic metabolism, which occurs mainly via the glycolytic pathway. Anaerobic metabolism also takes place via the hexose monophosphate shunt, but to generate microbicidal oxidants rather than for energy production.

Neutrophil phagocytosis

Phagocytosis (Fig. 6.9) is the process whereby cells ingest extracellular particles for destruction. Neutrophils have a role in the phagocytosis of bacteria and dead cells.

To reach an area of infection or tissue damage, neutrophils leave the circulation by adhering to endothelial cells by adhesion molecules expressed in response to local secretion of cytokines, and move through the endothelium and basement membrane.

Once in the support tissue, neutrophils respond to chemicals (**chemotaxins**), moving towards the highest concentration. Chemotaxins include degradation products of complement, products leaking from dead cells, and bacterial-derived polysaccharides in the extracellular space. Neutrophil motility is derived from assembly and disassembly of cellular actin filaments.

Neutrophils typically die soon after phagocytosis as this highly energy-dependent process uses up their glycogen reserve. When they die their lysosomal enzymes are released into the extracellular space, causing liquefaction of adjacent tissue. The collection of dead neutrophils, tissue fluid and abnormal material is termed **pus**.

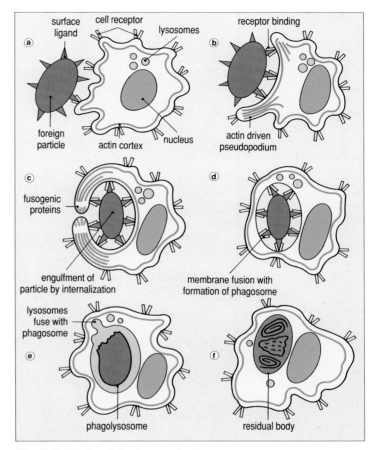

Fig. 6.9 Neutrophil phagocytosis.
a Neutrophils have membrane receptors, mainly for the Fc portion of antibodies, complement factors bound to foreign particles, and bacterial polysaccharides. Neutrophils do not phagocytose material to which they do not bind.
b As the first step in phagocytosis the neutrophil binds to the abnormal particle by its specific receptors. The cell pushes out pseudopodia to surround the particle, driven by assembly and disassembly of actin filaments.
c The pseudopodia fuse to completely enclose the abnormal particle and form an endocytotic vesicle. Special proteins probably allow final sealing of the membrane.
d The internalized particle in the endocytotic vesicle is called a **phagosome**.
e The phagosome fuses with neutrophil granules, particularly primary granules, which discharge their contents, exposing the particle to a potent mixture of lysosomal enzymes. If the particle is a bacterium, killing is enhanced by hydrogen peroxide and superoxide generated by the enzymatic reduction of oxygen by respiratory burst oxidase (RBO), a membrane enzyme.
f Foreign particle destruction is associated with formation of a residual body (see Fig. 2.16) containing degraded material.

EOSINOPHILS

Eosinophils have a bilobed nucleus and contain strongly eosinophilic granules (Fig. 6.10). They are phagocytic, with a particular affinity for antigen–antibody complexes, but have less microbicidal activity than neutrophils.

Circulating eosinophil numbers show a marked diurnal variation, being maximal in the morning and minimal in the afternoon. They increase greatly in many types of parasitic infestation, and protection against parasitic disease appears to be one of their main functions.

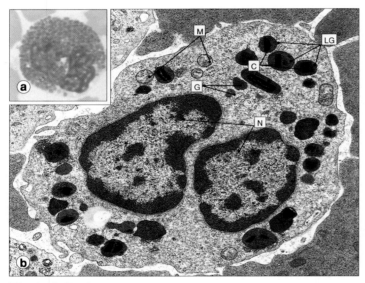

Fig. 6.10 Eosinophil.
a The eosinophil is 12–17 μm in diameter in blood films, and is easily recognizable by its large granules, which stain bright red. Most have a bilobed nucleus, but nuclear detail is often obscured by the numerous overlying, densely packed granules.
b Electronmicrograph of an eosinophil from blood showing its characteristic bilobed nucleus (N), scattered mitochondria (M) and cytoplasmic glycogen.

The characteristic granules (LG) are large and ovoid in shape (0.15–1.5 μm long and 0.3–1.0 μm wide), and contain a central electron-dense crystalloid (C) surrounded by a less dense matrix. In humans, the crystalloid has a cubic lattice structure and consists of an extremely alkaline (basic) protein called **major basic protein**, as well as other basic proteins, hydrolytic lysosomal enzymes and peroxidase, which has a different substrate specificity to the neutrophil myeloperoxidase.

Smaller granules (G), 0.1–0.5 μm in diameter, are also present in mature eosinophils and contain acid phosphatase and aryl sulfatase, which is eight times more concentrated than in other white cells and appears to be secreted in the absence of phagocytosis and degranulation.

Tissue (and sometimes blood) eosinophil numbers are also increased in certain allergic states, for example in the nasal and bronchial mucosae in hay fever and asthma, and in adverse reactions to drugs. However the role of eosinophils in allergic phenomena is not clear.

Eosinophil granulopoiesis

Eosinophils share a common progenitor with other granulocytes, their pathways of differentiation diverging after the myeloblast stage, but following comparable developmental stages.

Eosinophils are readily distinguishable from neutrophils at the early myelocyte stage by the appearance of their larger granules, most of which are eosinophilic, but a few are initially basophilic.

After production in the bone marrow, eosinophils are stored for several days before release into the circulation, where they remain for 3–8 hours before preferentially migrating to the skin, lungs and gastrointestinal tract. They may enter lung and gut secretions via lymphatics or by direct migration.

Eosinophils do not usually re-enter the circulation after migration, and their fate and lifespan are unknown.

Eosinophil phagocytosis and degranulation

Like neutrophils, eosinophils move chemotactically in response to bacterial products and complement components. They are preferentially attracted by substances released from mast cells, notably histamine and eosinophil chemotactic factor of anaphylaxis (ECF-A), as well as by activated lymphocytes (see Chapter 7).

All eosinophils have surface receptors for IgE (not found on neutrophils), which may be involved in the destruction of parasites. Only a few eosinophils have IgG Fc receptors, but these increase markedly in eosinophilia.

Phagocytosis involves the usual endocytotic process, but if the object is too large to be engulfed (e.g. a parasite), the eosinophil appears to release its granule contents into the external environment.

Eosinophils may function to localize the destructive effect of reactions causing secretion of mast cell granules (hypersensitivity allergic reactions) by:
- neutralizing histamine;
- producing a factor (eosinophil-derived-inhibitor), which is probably composed of prostaglandins E1 and E2, and is thought to inhibit mast cell degranulation.

Activated eosinophils inhibit vasoactive substances (e.g. leukotriene 3, formerly called SRS-A), which are produced by basophils and mast cells.

BASOPHILS AND MAST CELLS

Basophils are characterized by large, intensely basophilic, cytoplasmic granules, and are probably the precursors of tissue mast cells with which they have many structural and functional similarities (Fig. 6.11).

The granules of basophils and mast cells contain the sulphated proteoglycans, heparin and chondroitin sulphate, together with histamine and leukotriene 3.

Both basophils and mast cells have highly specific membrane receptors for the Fc segment of IgE produced in response to allergens (see Chapter 7). Exposure to allergen results in rapid exocytosis of their granules, thereby releasing histamine and other vasoactive mediators, and resulting in an **immediate hypersensitivity (anaphylactoid) reaction**. Such a reaction causes allergic rhinitis (hay fever), some forms of asthma, urticaria, and anaphylaxis.

Basophils are formed in the bone marrow, sharing a common precursor with the other granulocytes to the myeloblast stage. Development then proceeds through analogous stages to those of neutrophils and eosinophils. Their lifespan is unknown.

Mast cells reside in support tissues, especially those beneath epithelia, around blood vessels, and lining serous cavities. They are long lived and can proliferate in the tissues. In mucosae, but not in other sites, proliferation appears to depend on interaction with T lymphocytes.

LYMPHOCYTES AND PLASMA CELLS

In adults and older children lymphocytes are the second most numerous white cell in the blood, their numbers increasing in response to viral infections; they are the most numerous white cell in young children. There are two main types of lymphocyte, B and T, which perform different, but linked roles in the immune system (see Chapter 7).

Most circulating lymphocytes are small (Fig. 6.12), but about 3% are large, with a diameter of 9–15 μm. Their nuclei are ovoid or kidney-shaped with the dense chromatin typical of cells with little biosynthetic activity.

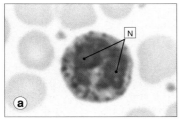
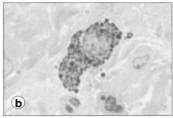
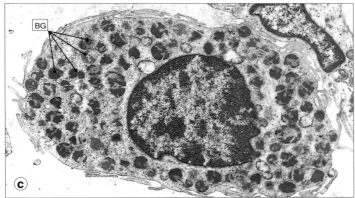

Fig. 6.11 Basophil and mast cell.
a The basophil is 14–16 μm in diameter. Its nucleus (N) is bilobed, the two lobes exhibiting marked chromatin condensation. The cytoplasmic granules are large, dark-blue staining, and often obscure the nucleus.
b Mast cells in tissues are ovoid or elongated spindle cells with a non-segmented nucleus. Their granule content imparts a diffuse purplish colour to the cytoplasm in H&E paraffin sections, unless special stains are used to demonstrate individual granules (as here). In thin resin H&E sections, the granules can be resolved by light microscopy.
c Ultrastructurally, mast cell granules (BG) are round or oval, membrane-bound and contain dense particles and less dense matrix. There is also a small population of smaller uniform granules found near the nucleus. Mast cell cytoplasm also contains free ribosomes, mitochondria and glycogen, while the cell membrane exhibits blunt, irregularly spaced surface projections.

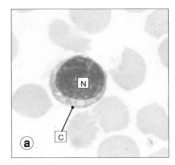
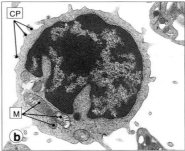

Fig. 6.12 Lymphocyte.
a In small lymphocytes, which have a diameter of 6–9 μm, the nucleus (N) occupies about 90% of the cell. The cytoplasm (C) appears only as a narrow rim and is slightly basophilic due to the presence of free ribosomes (RNA); rough endoplasmic reticulum is minimal.
b Ultrastructurally, lymphocyte cell membrane shows small cytoplasmic projections (CP), which appear as short microvilli with the scanning electron microscope, and are most numerous on B lymphocytes. Cytoplasm is sparse and contains only a few mitochondria (M) and occasional aggregates of glycogen.

Lymphocytes transform into active cells mediating the immune responses, particularly in specialized lymphoid tissues, the large lymphocytes in the blood representing such activated lymphocytes *en route* to the tissues.

Plasma cells

Plasma cells are a differentiated form of B lymphocyte and actively synthesize immunoglobulin.

Plasma cells form a small population in normal marrow and are usually seen in support tissues and specialized lymphoid organs. In health, they are not found in the blood.

Plasma cells are large and have an eccentrically located, round or oval nucleus with the chromatin coarsely clumped in a characteristic cart wheel or clock face pattern, reflecting active transcription.

Their cytoplasm is deeply basophilic due to its large content of ribosomal RNA in abundant rough endoplasmic reticulum. A well developed Golgi displaces the nucleus and is visible as a paranuclear halo.

MYELOMA

Myeloma is a malignant proliferation of a particular clone of plasma cells (Fig. 6.13) and occurs in bone marrow, either as a diffuse increase in plasma cells or as discrete tumours, which may be single or multiple.

The malignant plasma cells rarely spill over into the blood.

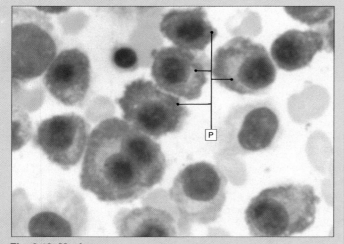

Fig. 6.13 Myeloma.
Micrograph showing a clump of plasma cells (P) aspirated from the bone marrow of a patient with myeloma.

MONOCYTES AND MACROPHAGES

Monocytes are the blood and bone marrow-located precursors of the macrophages found in tissues and lymphoid organs, and are members of a single functional unit, the **monocyte–macrophage system** (**mononuclear phagocyte system**). This system consists of the bone marrow precursors (**monoblasts** and **promonocytes**), circulating monocytes, and tissue macrophages, both free and fixed (**histiocytes**). Also included in this system are:

- Kupffer cells of the liver (see Fig. 11.2);
- sinus lining cells of the spleen and lymph nodes (see Chapter 7);
- pulmonary alveolar macrophages (see Fig. 9.14);
- free macrophages in synovial, pleural and peritoneal fluid;
- dendritic antigen-presenting cells (see Chapter 7).

Monocytes are large motile, phagocytic cells. In blood films they often show vacuolated cytoplasm (Fig. 6.14).

Ultrastructurally monocyte cytoplasm contains numerous small lysosomal granules and cytoplasmic vacuoles. The granules are electron-dense, homogeneous and membrane-bound, and are of two types. One type represent primary lysosomes and contain acid phosphatase, aryl sulfatase and peroxidase, and are analogous to the primary granules of neutrophils. The content of the other group of granules is not known. Numerous small pseudopodia extend from the monocyte, reflecting its phagocytic ability and amoeboid movement.

Monocytes respond chemotactically to the presence of necrotic material, invading microorganisms, and inflammation, and leave the blood to enter the tissues where they are called **macrophages**.

Monocyte numbers are depressed by corticosteroid administration.

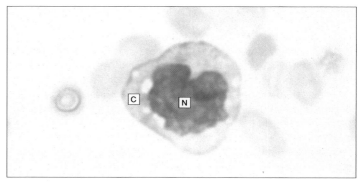

Fig. 6.14 Monocyte.
The monocyte is a large cell up to 20 μm in diameter with pale staining vacuolated cytoplasm (C), and an irregular nucleus (N), often with a deep indentation on one side.

Monocyte precursors

Two morphological monocyte precursors are recognized: the **monoblast** and the **promonocyte**. At least three cell divisions occur before the mature monocyte stage is reached.

Mature monocytes leave the bone marrow soon after their formation and there is no reserve pool. They spend about 3 days in the blood before migrating into the tissues in an apparently random fashion, and are then unable to re-enter the circulation.

WHITE BLOOD CELL ABNORMALITIES

Increased numbers of white cells appear in the peripheral blood in a variety of disorders, and provide a useful clue to the underlying disease. For example, there is:
- a considerable and sustained increase of circulating neutrophils in bacterial infections;
- an increase of circulating eosinophils in parasitic infestations and some allergies.

In both cases the white cells are qualitatively normal.

The most important and life-threatening disorders of white cells are the **leukaemias**, in which there is a malignant proliferation of the white cell precursors in the bone marrow. This produces vast numbers of white cells and their precursors, many of which spill over into the blood.

Leukaemias are classified according to the cell line involved (i.e. granulocytic, monocytic, lymphocytic) and also according to their degree of malignancy.
- In **chronic leukaemias** (Fig. 6.15a), the proliferating cells are partly or completely differentiated, for example, myelocytes, metamyelocytes band forms and neutrophils in granulocytic leukaemias. The diseases are slowly progressive.
- In **acute leukaemias** (Fig. 6.15b), the proliferating cells are the virtually undifferentiated precursor cells, for example, myeloblasts **in acute granulocytic leukaemia** and lymphoblasts in acute lymphoblastic leukaemia. Acute leukaemias are rapidly progressive.

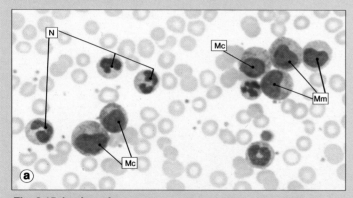

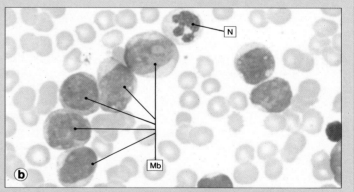

Fig. 6.15 Leukaemia.
a In this blood film from a patient with **chronic granulocytic leukaemia** there are increased numbers of mature white cells, mainly neutrophils (N), as well as precursor cells, mainly myelocytes (Mc) and metamyelocytes (Mm), which have escaped from the marrow into the blood.

b In this typical blood film from a patient with an **acute granulocytic leukaemia** the malignant cells are immature granulocyte precursors, mainly myeloblasts (Mb). Very few mature neutrophils (N) are being formed.

PLATELETS

Platelets (**thrombocytes**) are small disc-shaped anucleate cells (Fig. 6.16), and are formed by the cytoplasmic fragmentation of huge precursor cells (**megakaryocytes**) in the bone marrow. Platelets contain mitochondria, microtubules, glycogen granules, occasional Golgi elements and ribosomes, as well as enzyme systems for aerobic and anaerobic respiration. Their most conspicuous organelles however are their granules of which there are four types:

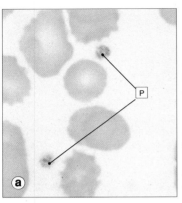
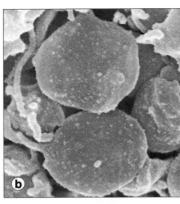

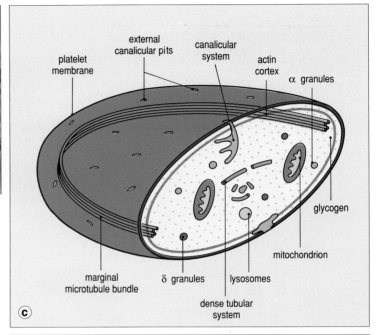

Fig. 6.16 Platelets.

a Platelets (P) are 1.5–3.5 μm in diameter in peripheral blood.

b Scanning electronmicrograph showing the smooth disc shape of an inactive platelet. The surface canalicular pores (see below) cannot be seen at this magnification.

c Diagram to illustrate platelet structure. Platelet cell membrane, which has a prominent glycocalyx that includes cell adhesion molecules for platelet adhesion, contains many external pits which connect a system of interconnected canalicular membrane channels with the external environment.

The cytoplasmic aspect of these membranes is associated with an actin cortex (see page 19). This canalicular system secretes the contents of the α granule, while the contractile proteins in the actin cortex (previously called **thrombosthenin**), are involved in clot retraction and extrusion of granule contents.

A well developed cytoskeleton incorporates a marginal band of microtubules arranged beneath the cell periphery; these depolymerize into component filaments at the onset of platelet aggregation.

Deep to the marginal band of microtubules and also scattered throughout the cytoplasm is the dense tubular system (DTS), consisting of narrow membranous tubules containing a homogeneous electon-opaque substance. Although histochemical studies have shown a platelet-specific isoenzyme of peroxidase within the DTS, the function of this system is poorly understood; there is some evidence that it may be the site of prostaglandin synthesis.

d Electronmicrograph of a platelet. The circumferential band of microtubules (MT), and elements of the dense tubular system (DTS), and canalicular system (CS) can be seen, as well as a selection of granules, including α and δ granules and some lysosomes(L).

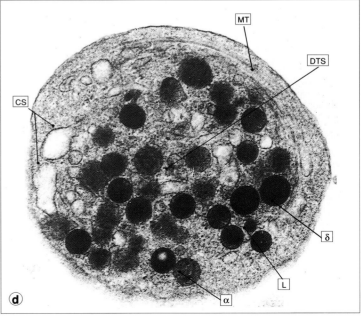

• α **granules** are variable in size and shape and contain three important groups of proteins (platelet exclusive proteins, coagulation factors and other proteins).

• **Dense granules** (δ **granules**) are electron-dense and appear to contain serotonin, which is not synthesized by platelets, but absorbed from the plasma.

• **Lysosomes** are membrane-bound vesicles containing lysosomal enzymes (e.g. acid hydrolases).

• **Peroxisomes** are few in number and have peroxidase (probably catalase) activity.

Platelets are essential to normal haemostasis, undergoing aggregation (Fig. 6.17) in the process.

Platelet function in haemostasis

Haemostasis is achieved by the steps outlined below.

• After loss of the lining endothelium of blood vessels, platelets adhere to collagen by interacting with glycoprotein receptors for Von Willebrand factor attached to collagen.

• Platelet actin, myosin and microtubules cause reversible platelet moulding and adhesion along a broad surface.

• Platelets then release the contents of their granules via the canalicular system in a secretion reaction. They also synthesize thromboxane. This is irreversible.

• Thromboxane, ADP and Ca^{2+} ions mediate adhesion of other platelets. Platelet phospholipids (with Ca^{2+} ions) activate the blood clotting cascade, leading to the formation of fibrin.

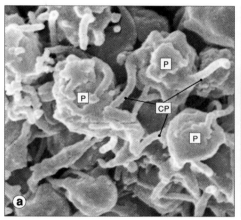
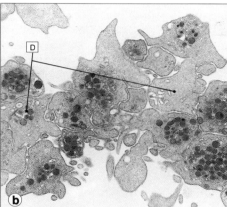

Fig. 6.17 Aggregating platelets.
a Scanning electronmicrograph of platelets (P) in the early stages of aggregation. They show extensive alteration in shape, becoming spherical. They also develop numerous long thin cytoplasmic processes (CP).
Compare with Fig. 6.16 b.
b Transmission electronmicrograph of aggregating platelets. Note the interlinking of some cytoplasmic processes (CP), and the decrease in granule numbers in some platelets (D). Compare with Fig. 6.16d.

PLATELET DISORDERS

Severe reduction in the number of platelets in circulating blood is called **thrombocytopaenia** and causes spontaneous bleeding because of the failure of platelets to seal over microscopic breaches resulting from minor trauma in vessel walls .

In the skin, this manifests as a reddish-purple blotchy rash, either small blotches (purpura) or larger bruise-like patches (ecchymoses).

Severe thrombocytopaenia may be solitary, for example idiopathic thrombocytopaenic purpura. It may also be part of a wider failure of haemopoietic bone marrow when it is associated with a reduction in the number of circulating neutrophils (neutropaenia) and red cells, for example when normal haemopoietic marrow is suppressed by tumour invasion in acute leukaemia (see Fig. 6.15b) or by drugs such as the cytoxic drugs used in cancer therapy.

Megakaryocytes

Megakaryocytes (Fig. 6.18) are the largest cells seen in bone marrow aspirates and produce platelets by cytoplasmic fragmentation.

The precursor of the megakaryocyte in the bone marrow is the **megakaryoblast**, which reduplicates its nuclear and cytoplasmic constituents up to seven times without cell division, each reduplication causing increased ploidy, nuclear lobulation and cell size.

Cytoplasmic maturation involves the elaboration of granules, vesicles and demarcation membranes (see below), and progressive loss of free ribosomes and rough endoplasmic reticulum. Megakaryocyte cytoplasm is divided into three zones.

• The **perinuclear zone** contains the Golgi and associated vesicles, rough and smooth endoplasmic reticulum, developing granules, centrioles and spindle tubules. It remains attached to the nucleus after platelet shedding

• The **intermediate zone** contains an extensive system of interconnected vesicles and tubules (the **demarcation membrane system, DMS**), which is in continuity with the cell membrane and has the function of delineating developing platelet fields (i.e. potential platelets), which like platelets, are uneven in size.

• The **marginal zone** is filled with cytoskeletal filaments and traversed by membranes connecting with the DMS.

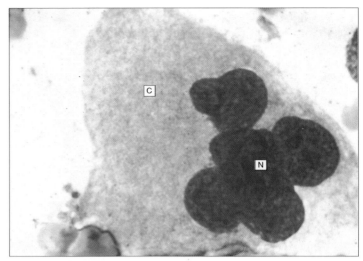

Fig. 6.18 Megakaryocyte.
Megakaryocytes are huge polyploid cells 30–100 μm in diameter, with a large irregular, multilobular nucleus (N) which contains dispersed chromatin, and is devoid of nucleoli. Their extensive cytoplasm (C) is filled with fine basophilic granules reflecting their profusion of cytoplasmic organelles.

With light microscopy, the cell margin is often difficult to define clearly due to the presence of numerous disaggregating platelets, cytoplasmic processes, ruffles and blebs.

7. IMMUNE SYSTEM

The body must constantly protect itself from a vast array of living organisms and other foreign bodies, which may gain access via the skin, gut, respiratory tract and other routes. This protection is provided by three mechanisms: surface protection, acute inflammation and the immune response.

Surface protection is provided by keratin in the skin, mucus in the respiratory and alimentary tracts, and by an acid environment in the vagina, thus these mechanisms are nonspecific.

Acute inflammation is an organized tissue response to foreign agents, whatever their nature, which are destroyed or neutralized by neutrophils that emigrate into the tissues from local blood vessels.

Acute inflammation is also a general response to tissue damage, invasion by organisms being only one cause. It is therefore nonspecific and proceeds in the same way whatever the initiating factor.

The immune response, in contrast to surface protection and acute inflammation is **specific** and targetted to chemical groups on invading or foreign agents.

The immune response is served by specialized tissues and cells, which form the **immune system**. This system depends on the recognition of exogenous materials as being foreign to the body, any foreign substance so recognized being known as an **antigen**.

Such recognition then activates the immune system to neutralize or destroy the antigen, with lymphocytes playing the central role.

The immune response is highly antigen-specific, but may employ the phagocytic cells of the nonspecific tissue defence system (see page 84) in initial antigen presentation or to effect final antigen destruction.

As most foreign agents are composed of many different antigens (i.e peptides, proteins, polysaccharides), the immune response may involve a combination of specific responses.

Mechanisms of the immune response

The immune response is served by several types of cell acting synergistically.
• Exogenous agents (commonly microorganisms) are first recognized as being foreign by **antigen-presenting cells (APCs)**, which constantly sample their local environment and are similar to macrophages. The exogenous agents are then broken down within the APCs into key components, which act as **antigens**.
• Specialized effector cells (**lymphocytes**) recognize the foreign antigens by specifically binding to them. Such lymphocytes then proliferate and mount an immune response.

There are two main types of immune response, cell-mediated immunity and humoral immunity, which usually work together in the elimination of a foreign agent.

Cell-mediated immunity is characterized by the joint action of lymphocytes and macrophages to destroy or neutralize the foreign agent.

Humoral immunity is characterized by the secretion of proteins (**antibodies**) by one type of lymphocyte. Antibodies neutralize foreign agents by specifically binding to the antigen.

While the immune response occurs in all body tissues, growth, maintenance and programming of immune cells takes place preferentially in the **lymph nodes, spleen, thymus gland** and **bone marrow**, which are the special organs of the immune system.

The special cells of the immune system are **T and B lymphocytes**, **macrophages** and **dendritic cells**.

LYMPHOCYTES

The two main types of lymphocyte (see Fig. 6.12) are T and B lymphocytes, or T and B cells.

B lymphocytes (B cells)

B cells:
- are derived from precursors in bone marrow;
- circulate in blood and through body tissues, and also populate specialized lymphoid organs;
- convert into **plasma cells**, which secrete specific **immunoglobulins** (**antibodies**, Fig. 7.1) when stimulated by appropriate antigen.

B cells, plasma cells and antibodies in the blood and body fluids are the basis of the **humoral response**.

All developing B cells have common genes coding for the production of immunoglobulins when they are called **germ line B cells**. During maturation, these genes undergo rearrangement to produce unique immunoglobulin proteins, which can specifically interact with antigen. In this way the diversity of the humoral immune response is generated. Cells that produce an immunoglobulin recognizing a normal body (self) antigen are thought to be eliminated during development.

Morphology

B cells that participate in the immune response mature from small inactive cells to large cells secreting immunoglobulin, their cytological appearance varying according to their activity.

Originating in the bone marrow, B cells develop their specialized attributes by maturing in peripheral tissues, the precise site being uncertain in man. In birds it is a structure called the Bursa of Fabricius, hence the origin of the term B (bursal) cells.
- **Inactive B cells** are small cells with barely discernible cytoplasm. The nucleus is rounded with compact chromatin reflecting a lack of DNA transcription.
- **B cells that have been stimulated to divide** as part of an immune response are larger than the inactive B cells and contain a moderate amount of basophilic cytoplasm. The nucleus is large with open vesicular chromatin and a visible nucleolus reflecting gene transcription.
- **Plasma cells** are antibody-secreting B cells, and therefore have cytological features that reflect their function as protein-secreting cells. Their cytoplasm is basophilic because of its high content of rough endoplasmic reticulum, and there is a clear area near the nucleus corresponding to the Golgi. The nucleus has an open chromatin pattern, said to resemble a clock face, and a large central nucleolus.

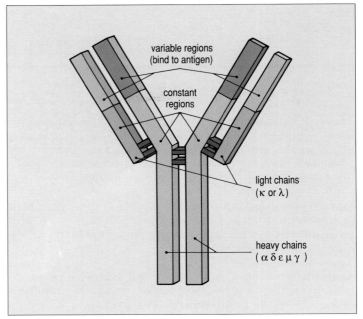

Fig. 7.1 Antibodies.
B cells are characterized by their ability to synthesize antibodies, which are glycoproteins designed to bind to specific antigens. Antibodies are also known as immunoglobulins, and fall into five different structural classes, IgG, IgA, IgD, IgM and IgE.

An antibody has two main components, immunoglobulin **light chains**, which may be either κ or λ in type, and immunoglobulin **heavy chains**, which may be either γ, α, δ, μ, or ε in type. The heavy and light chains have highly variable regions, which form the antigen-binding site, and constant regions, which form the main part of the molecule.

Antibodies may either circulate in the blood and body fluids, or remain bound to the surface of the B cell where they behave as antigen receptors, activating the B cell when the appropriate antigen is encountered.

T lymphocytes (T cells)

T cells are the second main type of lymphocyte and:
- are derived from bone marrow, but develop specialized attributes by maturing in the **thymus gland**;
- are divided into three main functional subsets (see below);
- circulate in the blood and through body tissues, and also populate specific areas of specialized lymphoid organs (see pages 86–100);
- secrete **lymphokines** (Fig. 7.2) when stimulated by antigen;

Lymphokine	Source	Target action
IL-1	antigen-presenting cell	activates TH cells
IL-2	TH cells	stimulates T cell proliferation
IL-3	TH cells	stimulates growth of haemopoietic cells
IL-4	TH cells	activates B cells, T cells, and mast cells
IL-5	TH cells	promotes proliferation and maturation of B cells
IL-6	TH cells/ macrophages	activates T cells and makes B cells secrete IgG
γ-interferon	TH cells	induces class II MHC expression and activates macrophages

Fig. 7.2 Lymphokines.
A major function of T helper (TH) cells is to synthesize proteins (lymphokines), which mediate local interactions between immune cells. Lymphokines are however not unique to lymphoid cells and are merely one subgroup of a family of secreted factors (**cytokines**), which usually act to influence the growth and differentiation of cells.

The most important lymphokines are the **interleukins** (IL) (see Fig. 4.9), which are all peptides or proteins that act on specific receptors on target cells.

• express surface proteins called **T cell receptors**, which are restricted to the surface of T cells, and recognize specific antigen in a similar way to that of antibodies.

Genetic mechanisms (T cell receptor gene rearrangement) generate the diversity of T cells needed to respond to different antigens.

Because T cells function by directing and recruiting other cells without secreting antibody they are described as being the basis of the **cell-mediated immune response**.

Morphology

As for B cells, the histological appearance of T cells depends on their activity (i.e. whether the cell is inactive, proliferating as part of an immune response, or actively secreting lymphokines).

• **Inactive T cells** are small cells with barely discernible cytoplasm. The nucleus is rounded with compact chromatin, reflecting a lack of DNA transcription.

• **T cells that have been stimulated to divide** as part of an immune response are larger than the inactive cells and have a moderate amount of basophilic cytoplasm. The nucleus is large with a convoluted appearance (in contrast to that of B cells) and an open vesicular chromatin pattern and a visible nucleolus, reflecting gene transcription.

• **Lymphokine-secreting T cells** have basophilic cytoplasm due to their high content of rough endoplasmic reticulum, and a large nucleus with a convoluted contour.

T cell subsets

There are several functional subsets of T cells: **T helper (TH) cells, cytotoxic T (TC) cells** and **suppressor T (TS) cells**. These subsets can be identified by their possession of different membrane protein and glycoprotein molecules.

TH CELLS

TH cells secrete lymphokines (see Fig. 7.2) and thereby help other lymphocytes perform their effector functions. Their assistance is necessary:

• to induce B cells to produce antibody;
• to activate macrophage defence systems (see page 84).

The main marker used to identify TH cells is the CD4 molecule.

TC CELLS

TC cells kill virus-infected and malignant cells. To become activated and carry out their cytotoxic functions, they need to interact with TH cells which modulate the immune response. TC cells express the CD8 cell surface marker.

TS CELLS

TS cells inhibit the response of TH cells and thus modulate the immune response.

As TS cells also carry the CD8 marker, TC and TS cells are often grouped together as suppressor/cytotoxic (TS/C) cells.

T cell receptors

T cells can also be subdivided according to the protein structure of their T cell receptors.

• αβ **receptors** are carried by about 90% of T cells, such cells expressing CD4 and CD8 markers.
• γδ **receptors** are carried by 10% of T cells, most of which do not express either the CD4 or CD8 markers. The role of these cells, which express other T cell markers, is not clear, but they appear to be important components of mucosal associated lymphoid tissues (see page 99). One major role is believed to be the recognition of certain antigens called **cell stress proteins**, which are expressed by damaged cells to facilitate the early elimination of such cells.

MACROPHAGES AND DENDRITIC CELLS

Macrophages and dendritic cells are monocyte-derived cells (see page 76), which become resident in the tissues, where they may assume a variety of morphological appearances as they differentiate to serve specialized roles.

• They may form a population of cells adapted mainly for phagocytosis; these cells (**fixed tissue macrophages** or **histiocytes**) remove or store material by assuming a rounded morphology with short broad pseudopodia, and contain large numbers of lysosomes.

• They may be stimulated by T cell-derived lymphokines (see Fig. 7.2) to secrete chemical messengers (**cytokines**), which control local cellular immune responses. Such **secretory-type macrophages** are large cells with voluminous pink-staining cytoplasm due to expansion of the Golgi and smooth endoplasmic reticulum. They are seldom seen in normal tissues, but are important in T cell-mediated immune responses, when they are termed **epithelioid cells** because of their superficial resemblance to epithelial cells.

• They may form specialized immune-surveillance cells (i.e **dendritic antigen-presenting cells, APCs**), which are characterized by elongated, ramified cell processes and a low content of lysosomal enzymes (Fig. 7.3).

Fixed tissue macrophages, secretory macrophages, epithelioid cells, and APCs, are often grouped together with blood monocytes to form the **mononuclear phagocytic system.**

Morphology and distribution

The morphology of macrophages is variable according to their site and function. The general structure and cytology of monocytes and macrophages is described on page 76.

Specialized macrophages are seen in the lung (alveolar macrophages, see Fig. 9.4), liver (Kupffer cells, see Fig. 11.3), brain (microglial cells, see Fig. 13.14) and skin (Langerhans cells, see Fig. 19.9).

Macrophages are an important component of the specialized organs of the immune system (see page 94). They are also particularly abundant in loose fibrocollagenous support tissue, which is found in most parts of the body (Fig. 7.4).

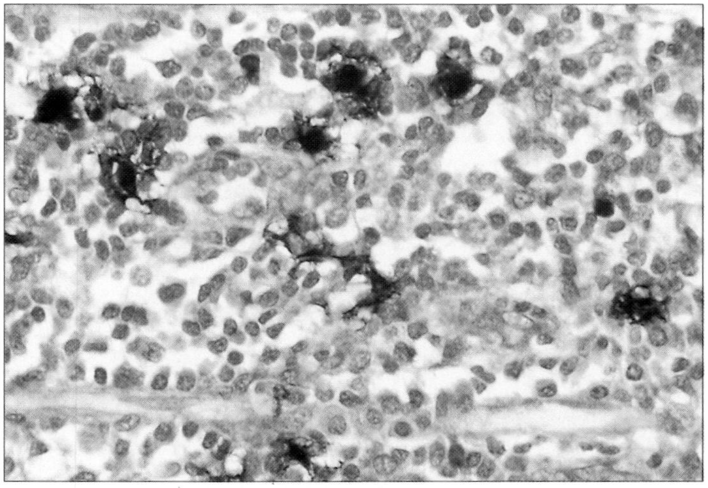

Fig. 7.3 Dendritic antigen-presenting cells.
Micrograph showing the ramifying cell processes of dendritic antigen-presenting cells from one area (paracortex) of a lymph node. The section is stained by an immunoperoxidase method, which detects a protein specific to this cell type.

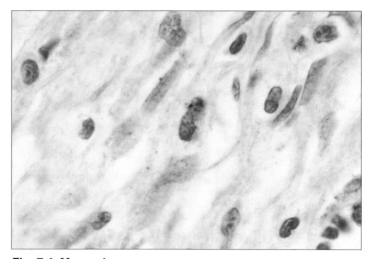

Fig. 7.4 Macrophages.
Macrophages are particularly abundant in the loose fibrocollagenous support tissue found in most organs. In this site they are adapted for major phagocytic activity, which is reflected by their high content of lysosomes. In H&E sections, normal macrophages are inconspicuous, but they may be detected by histochemical staining for acid phosphatase or immunochemical staining for lysosomal enzymes as here.

IMMUNOHISTOCHEMICAL IDENTIFICATION OF LYMPHOID CELLS

The many cytoplasmic and cell membrane proteins that characterize lymphocytes and related cells have been given names in an international system, which relates them to proteins (antigens) expressed at different phases of differentiation. These proteins are called **CD** (**Cluster of Differentiation**) molecules (Fig. 7.5).

Antibodies to CD molecules can be used to identify specific subtypes of lymphoid cell.

In addition to CD molecules, B cells can be identified by the presence of either the heavy or light chains of immunoglobulin.

CD molecule	Features	Location
CD1	formerly called T6, glycoprotein	cortical thymocytes, Langerhans' cells, interdigitating cells
CD2	corresponds to sheep red cell receptor	all T cells in early development
CD3	associated with T cell receptor proteins	T cells
CD4	glycoprotein, receptor for HIV1 virus	TH cells, macrophages
CD8	glycoprotein	T s/c cells
CD10	glycoprotein	pre-B cells, early forms of B cell, cells causing acute lymphoblastic (B cell) leukaemia in childhood (see Fig. 6.15)
CD19	glycoprotein	early forms of B cell
CD22	glycoprotein	all B cells
CD45	glycoprotein, known as leukocyte common antigen	many types of white cell, including T and B cells, and macrophages

Fig. 7.5 CD molecules.
Table outlining the features and locations of the most important CD molecules

The markers of lymphoid phenotype are extensively used in medical practice in the analysis and classification of tumours of the lymphoid cells termed **lymphomas**.

BONE MARROW

The bone marrow is the site of origin of B and T cell precursors, and of macrophages, and is discussed in detail on page 67.

THYMUS

The thymus is the site where immunologically naïve lymphocytes from the bone marrow differentiate into mature T cells. This involves differentiation into TH and Ts/c cells, and their proliferation to provide a continuous supply of T cells to lymphoid organs throughout the body.

During this process, the immunological system distinguishes self from foreign antigens and develops self tolerance.

The thymus is also an endocrine organ, secreting hormones and other soluble factors, which not only control T cell production, differentiation and maturation in the thymus, but also regulate T cell function and interactions in peripheral tissues. Although the nature and nomenclature of these substances is in a state of flux, because of the rapid advances being made in this field, there are at least three polypeptides with hormonal characteristics, namely **thymulin, thymopoietin** and **thymosin** $\alpha1$.

Normal thymic function is essential to the normal development of lymphoid tissues up to and even after puberty; thymectomy reduces the ability of the immune system to respond to newly encountered antigens.

The thymus is also an important site of haemopoiesis during fetal life.

Development

The thymus is the first lymphoid organ to develop, being derived from the endoderm and a small ectodermal element of the ventral wing of the third pharyngeal pouch on each side.

The thymus is unique among the lymphoid organs in having a supporting framework of epithelial cells (**epitheliocytes**), which are derived from the endoderm.

Structure

The thymus is a soft, lobulated organ lying in the superior and anterior mediastinum where its flattened shape

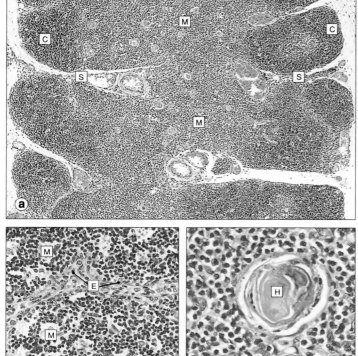

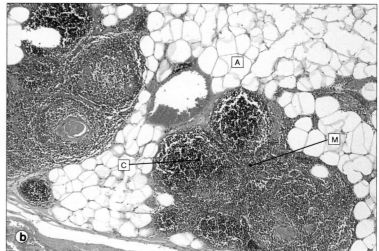

Fig. 7.6 Thymus.

a In the child the cortex (C) of the thymus is divided into lobules by fibrocollagenous septa (S) and is surrounded by adipose tissue of the mediastinum. The medulla (M) is less cellular.

b In the adult there is involution of the thymus with replacement by adipose tissue (A). The division into a cellular cortex (C) and less cellular medulla (M) is still apparent.

c The dominant feature of the thymic cortex is its content of a vast number of densely packed lymphocytes, which range in size

from small to large, depending on their activity.

Most if not all of the lymphocytes are in direct contact with epitheliocytes (E), which permeate the whole gland and act as a support framework. They are difficult to identify in the sea of lymphoid cells, but are visible where they surround blood vessels entering the gland.

Numerous macrophages (M) are scattered throughout the cortex and contain the phagocytosed debris of eliminated lymphocytes.

d The dominant feature of the thymic medulla is its epithelial component, the cells having large pale nuclei and abundant eosinophilic cytoplasm. Lymphocytes are less densely packed, than in the cortex, most being T cells probably *en route* to the circulation.

Hassall's corpuscles (H) are derived from epitheliocytes first appearing during fetal life and forming continuously thereafter. The process begins with the enlargement of a single medullary epitheliocyte, which then undergoes progressive degenerative changes characterized by nuclear disintegration and increasing cytoplasmic eosinophilia. Vacuoles appear in the cytoplasm, taking up the nuclear debris.

This process is repeated in nearby epithelial cells which form concentric lamellae around a central hyalinizing mass.

Hassall's corpuscles may grow as large as 100μm in diameter and undergo a variety of degenerative changes, becoming infiltrated by lymphocytes, macrophages and eosinophils; they may also show cystic change or calcification.

accords with the space left between surrounding structures.

At birth, the thymus is pinkish grey in colour and weighs 10–15g increasing to 30–40g by puberty. Thereafter it undergoes progressive involution and extensive fatty infiltration, and assumes a yellowish colour.

In the child, the thymic parenchyma is divided into an outer, highly cellular **cortex** and a pale-stained central **medulla.** The cortex is divided into irregular lobules 0.5–2.0 mm in diameter by fine septa extending in as far as the corticomedullary junction from a loose fibrocollagenous capsule. The less cellular medullary tissue forms a continuous central core. The thymus is composed of epitheliocytes, lymphocytes, macrophages and eosinophils (Fig. 7.6).

THYMIC EPITHELIAL CELLS (EPITHELIOCYTES)
The epitheliocytes form the stromal meshwork of the thymus, and have a variety of ultrastructural and immuno-histochemical features. At least four antigenically distinct cell types are recognizable, the **subcapsular cortical**, **inner cortical**, **medullary** and **Hassall's corpuscle** cells.

Thymic epitheliocytes have pale staining, oval nuclei and eosinophilic cytoplasm and can be readily identified in the medulla (see Fig. 7.6d). In the cortex, however their fine cytoplasmic extensions make them difficult to identify within the mass of lymphocytes.

With the electron microscope, typical desmosomes (see Fig. 3.11) are seen to bind the epithelial cells, which contain bundles of intermediate (cytokeratin) filaments.

Location. The arrangement of the epitheliocytes varies with their location in the thymus.
• Beneath the capsule, the epitheliocytes form a continuous layer, which is carried deeply into the thymus to invest the septa and vessels entering and leaving the organ.
• Within the cortex, the epitheliocytes form a sponge-like structure containing an extensive network of spaces, which becomes colonized by lymphocytes (see Fig. 7.6c).
• In the medulla, sheets of epitheliocytes converge to form a coarser, more solid structure with smaller interstices accommodating much smaller numbers of lymphocytes.
• Deep in the medulla, the epitheliocytes form bulky cords and whorls some of which contain lamellated structures (**Hassall's corpuscles,** see Fig. 7.6d).

Functions. In much of the thymic cortex, the epitheliocytes are in intimate contact with the lymphocytes, and completely enclose them by deep infoldings of surface membrane. Described as **thymic nurse cells**, these cells are thought to eliminate immature T cells that recognize self antigens.

Epitheliocytes also promote T cell differentiation, proliferation and subset maturation. In addition, they secrete at least three hormones and other substances, which regulate T cell maturation and proliferation within the thymus and other lymphoid organs.

THYMIC LYMPHOCYTES
Most thymic lymphocytes are T cells in various stages of differentiation. B cells are also present, but in smaller numbers. Although the term **thymocyte** is often used as a generic term for thymic lymphocytes, it strictly applies to immature lymphocytes of T cell lineage.

Clones of T cells are produced by cell division in the outer part of the thymic cortex and undergo maturation as they are pushed deep into the cortex towards the medulla.

In the medulla, the maturing T cells enter blood vessels and lymphatics to join the pool of circulating T cells. They subsequently populate peripheral lymphoid tissues, where they reach full immunological maturity.

Only a small minority of lymphocytes generated in the thymus are believed to reach maturity, these being clones of T cells with the ability to recognize foreign antigens. The rest of the lymphocytes are thought to recognize self antigens and are eliminated; this results in **immunological self tolerance**.

Although the thymus is usually considered to be a specifically T cell organ, occasionally mature B cells and B cell germinal centres, and rarely plasma cells, are found in the thymic medulla, particularly in children.

THYMIC MACROPHAGES
In the thymus there are several forms of macrophage including types with phagocytic and accessory immunological functions.

The cells responsible for removing dead lymphocytes are phagocytic mononuclear macrophages, which are found in the subcapsular cortex, and commonly contain nuclear and cytoplasmic debris (see Fig. 7.6c).

Macrophages containing relatively little phagocytosed material are common in the corticomedullary region and medulla, some taking the form of **dendritic interdigitating cells** (see page 84), which act as APCs for more mature T cells.

THYMIC EOSINOPHILS
Eosinophils appear in the thymus in fetal life and are usually present in childhood, sometimes in large numbers. They are uncommon after puberty. When present, eosinophils are located mainly in the support tissue of the septa, the medulla, and sometimes in Hassall's corpuscles.

Vasculature

The thymus receives its arterial supply via many small branches of the internal thoracic and inferior thyroid arteries, which enter the thymus mainly via the interlobular septa.

In the region of the corticomedullary junction the vessels give rise to small radially arranged arterioles and capillary loops to supply the cortex and medulla.

The cortical capillaries have continuous endothelium (see page 118), whereas those of the medulla and septa may be fenestrated.

At the corticomedullary junction, which is the site of lymphocyte migration into the thymus, the post-capillary venules have a taller endothelium.

Venous tributaries follow the course of the arterial vessels in the septa, some forming a plexus within the thymic capsule before draining via the thymic veins into the left brachiocephalic, internal thoracic and inferior thyroid veins.

The thymus receives no afferent lymphatics, but the medulla and corticomedullary area give rise to efferent lymphatics, which follow the course of the arteries and veins.

Blood–thymus barrier

Vessels entering and leaving the thymus are ensheathed by epitheliocytes, the intervening perivascular space containing support tissue, lymphoid aggregates and pericytes. There is thus a barrier between the blood and the thymic parenchyma comprising:
- capillary endothelium and basement membrane;
- perivascular support tissue;
- epitheliocytes and basement membrane.

Studies have shown that intravenously injected colloidal particles do not enter the extravascular spaces of the cortex and it is believed that this also applies to the ingress of antigens; thus the thymic cortex is an immunologically sequestered site. There is also evidence that if small amounts of material do enter the cortex they are rapidly phagocytosed by macrophages.

There appears to be no barrier to the entry of blood-borne material into the medullary extravascular spaces and it is probable that antigen is prevented from entering the cortex via the medulla by macrophages at the corticomedullary junction.

The blood–thymus barrier probably provides the essential environmental conditions for eliminating self–recognizing clones of lymphocytes; by excluding all foreign antigenic substances, the epitheliocytes are the only contact the lymphocytes have with the body's indigenous constituents (Fig. 7.7).

Involution

The thymus reaches its maximum weight at puberty, declining thereafter, so that in old age it may be so small as to be unrecognizable. Involution involves replacement of the gland by adipose tissue (fatty infiltration) and a decline in its lymphocyte content.

Fatty infiltration begins from birth onwards, but accelerates after puberty. Adipocytes increase in number in the perivascular compartment, and initially this is most apparent in the septa, thus involving the cortex first and then extending into the medulla (see Fig. 7.6b).

Lymphocyte depletion begins after one year of age and thereafter continues at a constant rate independent of puberty. It results in progressive collapse of the sponge-like epitheliocyte framework, which nevertheless remains intact, so that cords of epitheliocytes can be seen histologically even in the most atrophic thymic remnants. Such cells probably continue to secret thymic hormones into old age.

Despite the progressive decrease in their number with involution, thymic lymphocytes continue to differentiate and proliferate and thus maintain a continuing supply of T cells throughout life.

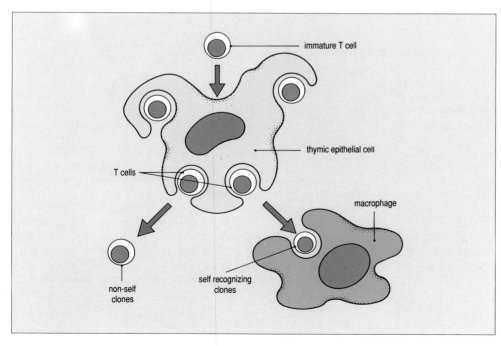

Fig. 7.7 Lymphocyte maturation in thymic cortex.
In the thymic cortex lymphocytes proliferate and are ensheathed by the processes of thymic epithelial cells. The T cells are in close contact with self antigens and non-self antigens are excluded by the blood–thymus barrier.

T cells which recognize self antigens are eliminated and phagocytosed by macrophages.

T cells which recognize non-self antigens leave the thymus to populate other tissues.

LYMPH NODES

Lymph nodes are small organs found in groups or chains at sites where lymphatic vessels draining an anatomical region converge to form larger lymphatic vessels, for example in the neck, axillae, groins, para-aortic area. They have two main functions.

• Phagocytic cells within the nodes act as nonspecific filters for particulate matter such as microorganisms and carbon, preventing them from reaching the general circulation.

• They provide an elegant mechanism whereby lymphocytes can interact with new antigens and APCs at an interface between lymph and the blood. Starting with only a small number of lymphocytes recognizing an antigen, lymph nodes facilitate proliferation of activated cells and thereby amplification of the immune response by forming clones of lymphocytes.

When relatively inactive, each lymph node is only a few mm in length, but this may increase greatly when functional demands are increased.

The cells of the lymph node can be divided into three functional types: lymphoid cells, immunological accessory cells, and non-immunologically active stromal cells.

Lymphoid cells

Lymphoid cells in lymph nodes include lymphocytes of all types and their derivatives; they originate in bone marrow, but increase in number in the thymus and other peripheral lymphoid tissues. Most of the lymphocytes enter the node via the blood, while a few enter via lymph draining from the tissues.

Immunological accessory cells

Immunological accessory cells comprise a variety of macrophages, including those with phagocytic antigen processing, antigen presenting, and nonspecific effector functions. These cells originate in the bone marrow and enter the peripheral tissues before reaching the lymph node in lymph. Many of the cells are part of the mononuclear phagocyte system and may subsequently return to peripheral tissues.

Non-immunologically active stromal cells

Non-immunologically active stromal cells comprise the lymphatic and vascular endothelial cells, and fibroblasts, which elaborate the stromal reticular framework. Many of the endothelial cells are highly specialized for interaction with lymphoid cells.

Structure

The lymph node is a bean-shaped organ with a fibrocollagenous capsule from which fibrous trabeculae extend into the node to form a supporting framework (Fig. 7.8).

The convex surface of the gland is penetrated by a number of **afferent lymphatic vessels**, which drain into the node, while at the hilum, there is a single **efferent lymphatic vessel,** which transports lymph towards larger collecting lymphatic vessels. In turn these vessels drain into more proximal nodes or chains of nodes, before entering the blood via either the thoracic duct or right lymphatic duct.

Lymph nodes contain three functional compartments (Fig.7.9).

These are:

• a network of endothelial-lined **lymphatic sinuses** continuous with the lumina of the afferent and efferent lymphatic vessels;

• a network of small blood vessels, including specialized post-capillary venules, where circulating lymphocytes enter the node;

• a parenchymal compartment composed of superficial cortex, paracortex and medulla.

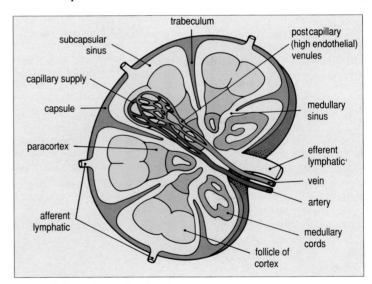

Fig. 7.8 Lymph node structure.
The bean-shaped lymph node has a hilum into which blood vessels enter, and from which efferent lymphatics emerge. It has an investing capsule.

Afferent lymphatic vessels penetrate the convex surface of the gland and drain into the sinus system.

The lymphoid parenchyma is divided into cortex, paracortex, and medulla.

The structural integrity of the lymph node is provided by a framework of reticulin fibres (see page 44), which are linked to the fibrous trabeculae. These fibres are most dense in the parenchymal compartment, but some fibres do traverse the lymphatic compartment where they are completely invested by endothelial cells.

Lymph node sinuses

Afferent lymphatics drain into a major **subcapsular sinus** running around the periphery of the lymph node, and from this sinus **cortical sinuses** pass down towards the medulla through the cortical cell mass.

Within the medulla, the dominant feature is a network of interconnected lymphatic channels called the **medullary sinuses**, which converge upon the efferent lymphatic vessel at the hilum.

On histological examination, only the larger channels, of the lymphatic compartment can be visualized. The cortical sinuses are generally difficult to see because of their highly convoluted shape and numerous fine extensions, which penetrate the cellular mass of the cortex.

The extremely thin and pale staining endothelial lining cells of the sinuses are almost impossible to identify with ordinary light microscopical staining methods.

Vascular compartment

The blood supply of a lymph node is the main route of entry of lymphocytes into the node, and also provides its metabolic needs.

One or more small arterial vessels enter the node via the hilum and then divide in the medulla into branches, which ramify into a capillary network corresponding to the cortical follicles and paracortex.

Within the paracortex, the **postcapillary venules** (see page 118) have a cuboidal endothelium bearing specialized cell receptors (lymphocyte-homing receptors), which are recognized by circulating lymphocytes and facilitate the passage of lymphocytes from the blood and into the lymph node. The post-capillary venules are often described as **high endothelial venules (HEVs)**.

The blood vessels of the superficial cortex and medullary cords are not thought to be specialized and do not appear to allow the exit of lymphocytes.

Small veins draining the node leave via the hilum.

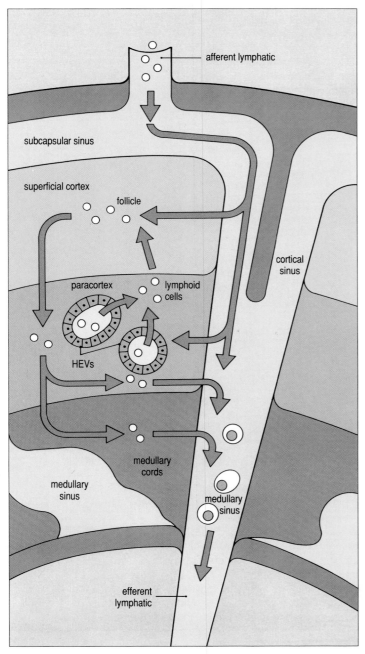

Fig. 7.9 Functional compartments of the lymph node.
Antigens, accessory cells and lymphocytes enter the lymph node via the afferent lymphatics, which drain into the subcapsular sinus, and thence into the cortical sinuses.

These antigens, accessory cells and lymphocytes may then enter the superficial cortex (composed of B cell follicles) or the paracortex (composed of diffuse sheets of T cells) or remain in the sinuses and leave the lymph node via the efferent lymphatic vessel.

The majority of lymphocytes enter the node from the blood via the high endothelial venules (HEVs), which are lined by a special endothelium bearing lymphocyte homing receptors.

Superficial cortex (lymphoid follicles)

The superficial cortex is characterized by densely staining spheroidal aggregations of lymphocytes (**lymphoid follicles**), their long axes oriented at right angles to the node capsule.

Some of the follicles (**primary follicles**) are of fairly uniform staining density; however most of the follicles responding to antigen have less densely staining **germinal centres** and are described as **secondary follicles**.

The lymphocyte population of the follicles consists predominantly of B cells, but there is a smaller population of Tн cells, macrophages and accessory cells.

B CELLS
B cells enter a lymph node via the HEVs of the paracortex and within a few hours many have migrated to the superficial cortex. If activated they proliferate and remain in the lymph node for an extended period as memory cells or plasma cells. In contrast, non-activated cells re-enter the

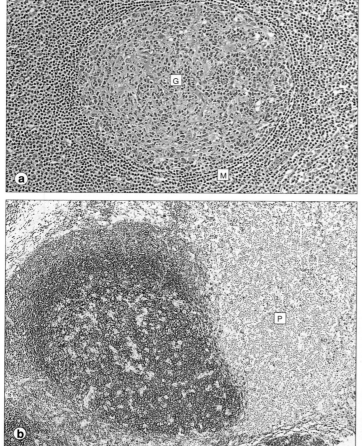

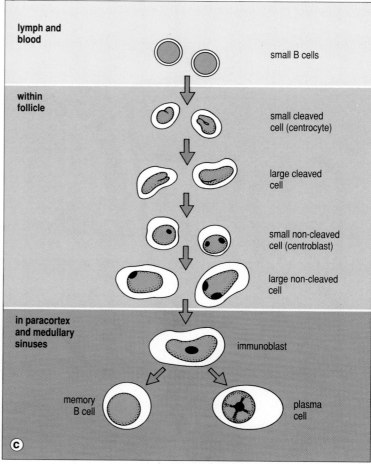

Fig. 7.10 Follicular B cells.

a Micrograph of an H&E stained secondary lymphoid follicle, which consists mainly of B cells. Small naïve B cells and a few T cells form the dark mantle zone (M), while the paler germinal centre (G) contains B cells in various stages of maturation. Accessory cells (see Fig. 7.11) are present, but are barely discernible at this magnification.

b Micrograph of an immunostained section of lymph node cortex using an antibody to B cells. The B cells stain brown in contrast

to the non-staining paracortex (P) which is rich in T cells.

c The maturation of B cells from small naïve cells to dividing cells responding to a specific antigen is associated with a distinct series of morphological changes.

From the small mature lymphocyte, the cell changes first into a centrocyte with a cleft nucleus, and then into a centroblast. This cell enlarges, leaves the follicle and migrates to the paracortex and medullary sinuses as an immunoblast, ultimately transforming into a plasma cell or a memory B cell.

general circulation within a matter of hours via the efferent lymph.

The primary follicles contain mainly naïve B cells and some memory cells. The secondary follicles on the other hand contain small naïve B cells peripherally and activated B cells in their germinal centres.

It is possible to identify several stages in the maturation of B cells in the follicles (Fig. 7.10). Activated B cells proliferate and mature and thereby produce an expanded population of identical cells recognizing the same antigen.

The activated B cells in the germinal centre are collectively called **follicle centre cells.** They are characterized by open nuclei, and have more cytoplasm and are less densely packed than the smaller, more peripheral follicular B cells; this explains the lower staining intensity of the germinal centres.

The proliferation and differentiation of antibody-secreting plasma cells is thought to result from T cell/B cell interaction in the paracortex, with the plasma cells then migrating directly to the medullary cords, where they are conveniently sited to secrete antibody into the efferent lymph.

GERMINAL CENTRE BORDERING CELLS

At the periphery of the germinal centres is a capsule-like structure of flattened stromal cells, which is open towards the node periphery.

The function of this pseudocapsule of so-called **germinal centre bordering cells** is obscure, but there is evidence that it prevents the entry of circulating T cells to the germinal centre. It has also been shown that activated lymphocytes entering a lymph node via afferent lymph pass into the germinal centres in large numbers, and this may explain why the pseudocapsule is open on one side.

ACCESSORY CELLS

A variety of immunological accessory cells are found in the superficial cortex, being derived from bone marrow and reaching the lymph node via the afferent lymph.

The description, nomenclature, phagocytic ability and immunological functions of immunological accessory cells remain controversial, but they all appear to play some role in antigen processing; this also applies to the accessory cells of the paracortex and medulla.

The main accessory cell types in the superficial cortex are:
- **sinus macrophages**, which are highly phagocytic cells of the subcapsular and cortical sinuses;
- **veiled cells**, which are so-named because of their veiled appearance on scanning electron microscopy; and are located mainly in the subcapsular sinuses;
- **tingible body macrophages**, which are so named because of their content of cellular debris, and are found within the germinal centres with an abundance of lysosomal enzymes;
- **marginal zone macrophages**, which constitute a morphologically diverse group of phagocytic cells located within the follicular interstitium immediately beneath the subcapsular sinus;
- **follicular dendritic cells**, which have numerous fine branching surface projections covered by electron-dense material, and are found in the superficial or **cap region** of the follicles.

Follicular dendritic cells retain antigen on their surface for many months. Their origin and immunological role is not fully understood and they appear to be in some form of continuity with germinal centre bordering cells.

These immunological accessory cells cannot be readily distinguished in H&E sections, but may be stained by immunochemical techniques for special macrophage markers (Fig.7.11).

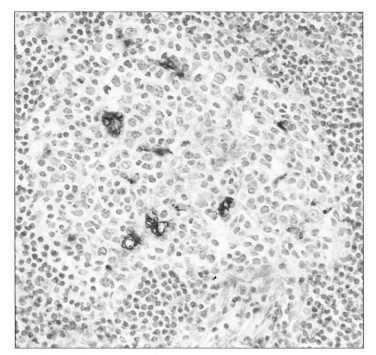

Fig. 7.11 Follicular accessory cells.
The follicular accessory cells are not easily distinguished in H&E sections, but can be stained by immunochemical techniques. This micrograph shows the tingible body macrophages stained brown by localizing a lysosomal enzyme, Cathepsin D.

Paracortex

The cell population of the paracortex consists of lymphocytes and accessory cells, which constantly traffic in and out of the region.

T CELLS

T (TH and TC/S) cells dominate the paracortex (Fig. 7.12), entering the node from the blood via the HEVs and leaving 6–18 hours later via the efferent lymphatic.

When activated, T cells enlarge to form **lymphoblasts**. These then proliferate to produce an expanded clone of activated T cells.

In a T cell dominated immunological response, the paracortex may expand into the medulla, producing a so-called **paracortical reaction**.

Activated T cells are then disseminated via the circulation to peripheral sites where much of their activity occurs.

ACCESSORY CELLS

Interdigitating cells are prominent in the paracortex and are one form of dendritic APC, being so-named because of their numerous cytoplasmic processes, which interdigitate with those of other cells. These cytoplasmic processes also make numerous contacts with other cell types in the vicinity.

There is some evidence that the veiled cells of the subcapsular sinuses and blood may be the precursors of the interdigitating cells.

Macrophages are also found in the paracortex and their cytoplasm is often seen to be packed with lipid (possibly engulfed cell membrane) and nuclear debris.

Medulla

The medulla contains mainly:
- larger blood vessels and their supporting trabeculae;
- cell-rich medullary cords;
- wide medullary sinuses (separating the medullary cords) through which lymph percolates towards the hilum from the cortex.

As in the cortex, the interstitial compartment of the medulla is supported by a framework of reticulin fibres, a small number of which traverse the sinuses.

PLASMA CELLS

The most common cells in medullary cords are plasma cells and their precursors. Plasma cells (Fig. 7.13) synthesize antibody, which is carried from the node to the general circulation via the efferent lymph. In addition, some mature plasma cells probably migrate from the node.

CLASSICAL MACROPHAGES

Classical macrophages are the main accessory cell type in the medulla, being located in the sinuses and deriving support from the traversing reticulin fibres.

Processing of lymph

Lymph draining into a lymph node via afferent lymphatics first enters the subcapsular sinus and then percolates through the cortical sinusoidal maze to drain into the medullary sinuses before leaving the node via the efferent lymphatics.

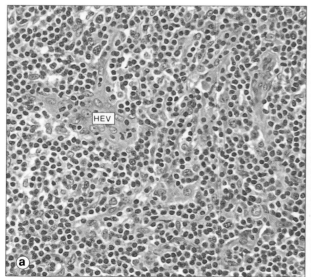

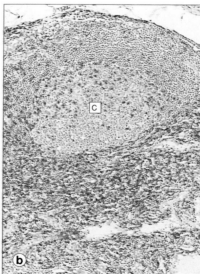

Fig. 7.12 Paracortex.
a Micrograph of lymph node paracortex showing sheets of T cells, which vary in morphology from small inactive cells to large cells representing activated, proliferating T cells. The high endothelial venules (HEV) are prominent, but accessory cells are inconspicuous even at high magnification.
b Micrograph of lymph node stained by an antibody technique that detects T cells. The paracortex stains brown (i.e. is T cell in nature), while the adjacent portion of cortical follicle (C) is not stained, being composed of B cells.

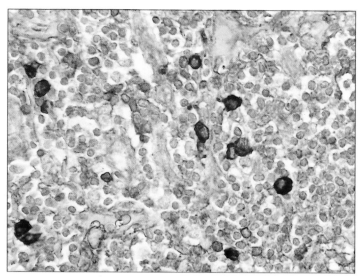

Fig. 7.13 Plasma cells in lymph node medulla.
Antibody-producing B cells (i.e. plasma cells) can be stained by immunochemical techniques for immunoglobulin light chains. This micrograph of a section stained for κ light chains highlights plasma cells (brown) in the medulla of a lymph node.

SPREAD OF CANCER TO LYMPH NODES

Cancerous cells may break off from primary tumours and enter lymphatic vessels, from where they migrate to lymph nodes. Once in the node they adhere to and proliferate in the sinuses (Fig. 7.14).

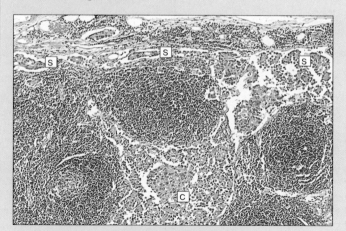

Fig. 7.14 Spread of cancer to lymph nodes.
Micrograph showing clumps of cancer cells from a carcinoma of the stomach in the subcapsular (S) and cortical (C) sinuses of a lymph node.

Some particulate matter is probably taken up from the lymph and disposed of by the phagocytic activity of the endothelial cells without evoking any immune response.

Antigens are phagocytosed and processed by various types of APC exposed to the lymph and are then transferred via the APC cytoplasmic extensions to sites where they may be encountered by lymphocytes.

Lymphocytes entering a lymph node in the afferent lymph constitute less than 10% of all of the lymphocytes entering the node except in the case of mesenteric nodes where they may constitute up to 30%. The rest of the lymphocytes gain entry via the high endothelial venules.

Activated lymphocytes pass through the endothelium of the subcapsular sinus and enter the germinal centres of the cortical follicles.

SPLEEN

The spleen lies in the left upper abdomen and in the adult weighs around 150 g, though this varies considerably with nutritional status and physical health, and gradually diminishes with age.

The two principal functions of the human spleen are:
- to mount a primary immune response to antigens in the blood;
- to act as a filter to remove particulate matter and aged or abnormal red cells and platelets from the circulation.

There are significant differences between the architecture of the spleen in different animals, and these have given rise to different descriptions of microanatomy. The following description is specific to the human spleen.

Structure

The spleen has a thin fibrocollagenous capsule from which short septa extend into the organ. These septa support an extensive meshwork of reticulin fibres, which scaffold the splenic parenchyma.

The reticulin framework is also attached to fibrocollagenous tissue associated with a branching arterial and venous network emanating from the splenic hilum. Such perivascular tissue does not form septa, but forms a sheath around the larger vessels.

Most of the spleen is composed of a vast array of sinusoids and vascular sinuses filled with blood (**red pulp**). An arborizing array of arteries (central arteries) associated with aggregates of lymphoid tissue is called **white pulp** (Fig. 7.15), and accounts for 5–20% of the total mass of the spleen.

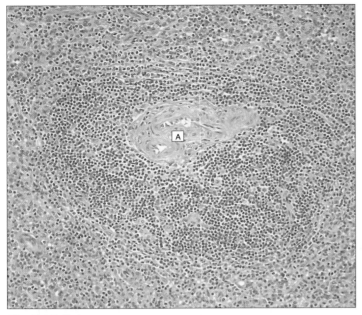

Fig. 7.15 Spleen.
Micrograph of an H&E stained section of spleen. The white pulp is seen as dense-staining aggregates of lymphoid cells adjacent to central arteries (A). The red pulp is less densely stained as it has fewer nuclei, and at this magnification it is not possible to distinguish between the various sinuses and parenchymal components.

Red pulp

The red pulp consists of loose support tissue scaffolded by reticulin fibres with several functional areas:

- capillaries, which terminate by draining into a fusiform-shaped macrophage-lined space, forming the **ellipsoidal (sheathed) capillaries** (see below);
- a parenchyma composed of stellate reticular support cells, which surrounds sponge-like cavities, through which blood from the sheathed capillaries slowly percolates;
- venous sinuses, which run adjacent to columns of parenchymal tissue and drain blood that has filtered through the parenchyma, as well as blood that has come directly from the sheathed capillaries (Fig. 7.16).

The sinuses are lined by flattened endothelial cells resting on a discontinuous basement membrane, which is interrupted by numerous narrow slits through which red cells squeeze. Phagocytic cells are closely associated with the walls of these sinuses.

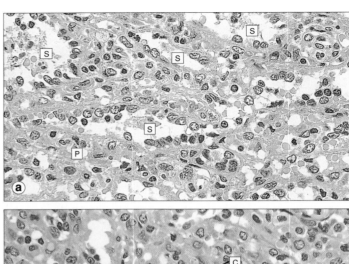

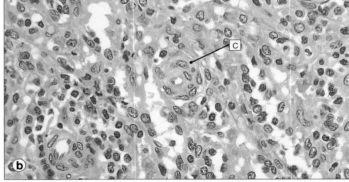

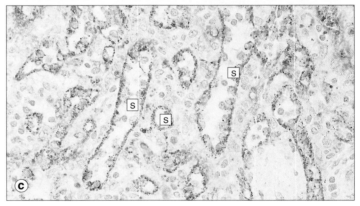

Fig. 7.16 Splenic red pulp.
a Micrograph of red pulp, which is composed of parenchymal areas (P) termed splenic cords, and sinusoids (S). The endothelial cells protrude into the sinuses.
b Micrograph of an ellipsoidal sheathed capillary (C), seen here in cross section.
c Micrograph of splenic red pulp venous sinusoids, which have been immunostained for the lysosomal enzyme cathepsin-D. This technique highlights in brown the abundant network of phagocytic macrophages associated with the walls of the venous sinusoids (S).

White pulp

The white pulp or splenic lymphoid masses are of two types, T cell and B cell. The functions of these two types of lymphoid tissue appear to be similar to those of the paracortex and superficial cortex of the lymph nodes, respectively (Fig. 7.17).

T CELLS

White pulp T cells, are mainly of the TH subset and form irregular masses around the central arteries. The central arteries are generally located at one side of the T cell area (Fig. 7.17).

At the periphery of the T cell zone is a narrow mantle zone of small lymphocytes enclosed by a broader **marginal zone**, in which less densely packed larger lymphocytes and dendritic APCs surround fine vascular channels with a reticulin scaffold.

In addition to these lymphoid areas associated with the central arteries, a significant number of B cell, T cell, and plasma cell aggregates are present in the splenic parenchyma.

B CELLS

White pulp B cells form follicles, which are usually located near an arteriole. In young people, many of the follicles have germinal centres, the proportion of such follicles diminishing with age.

Perilymphoid zones

The zone of red pulp immediately surrounding the T and B lymphoid masses is composed of a sparse reticulin scaffold and anastomosing fine vascular channels surrounded by dendritic APCs (marginal zone).

About 10 % of blood entering the spleen is believed to pass into this perilymphoid parenchyma from which it drains into the sinusoids or directly into the venous sinuses of the red pulp.

The function of the sinuses in the perilymphoid zones is not clear, but they may be a means of enhancing the interaction of APCs and splenic lymphoid immune responsive tissue with antigens that are blood-borne rather than tissue-based (e.g. circulating bacteria in septicaemia).

Vasculature

The arrangement of splenic blood vessels and sinusoids allows selective filtering of blood.

Central arteries run eccentrically in the white pulp of the spleen and give off:

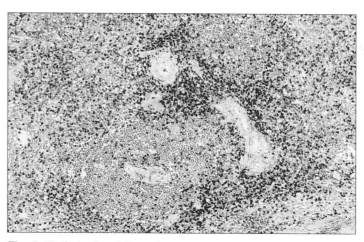

Fig. 7.17 Splenic white pulp.
Micrograph showing the white pulp of the spleen centred on the central artery. Immunostaining with antibody to detect T cells shows that the periarterial lymphoid cells are T cell in type (i.e. stain brown), but the follicle with the germinal centre is unstained because it is composed of B cells.

- leashes of arterioles and capillaries, which supply the white pulp;
- arterioles and capillaries that run directly into a system of marginal zone fine vascular sinusoids (Fig. 7.18).

The marginal zone sinusoids are arranged concentrically around the white pulp in the perilymphoid zone. In human spleen, perfusion studies have defined three concentric systems:

- the marginal zone network;
- the marginal sinuses;
- the perimarginal cavernous sinus.

The central arteries terminate in a series of straight arterial vessels, which are traditionally called **penicillary arteries**. These arteries are devoid of an investing layer of lymphoid cells and run in the red pulp. In turn, they give rise to arterioles and capillaries, which tend to leave the arterioles at right angles.

The splenic capillaries of the red pulp have a standard endothelial cell structure, which terminates abruptly in a fusiform arrangement of mononuclear phagocytes. They are described as ellipsoid sheathed capillaries (see Fig. 7.16b).

Most of the sheathed capillaries drain into the splenic parenchyma proper, which consists of a sponge-like network of spaces between stellate reticular cells (**splenic cords**). A small proportion of the sheathed capillaries also drain directly into the perimarginal cavernous sinuses.

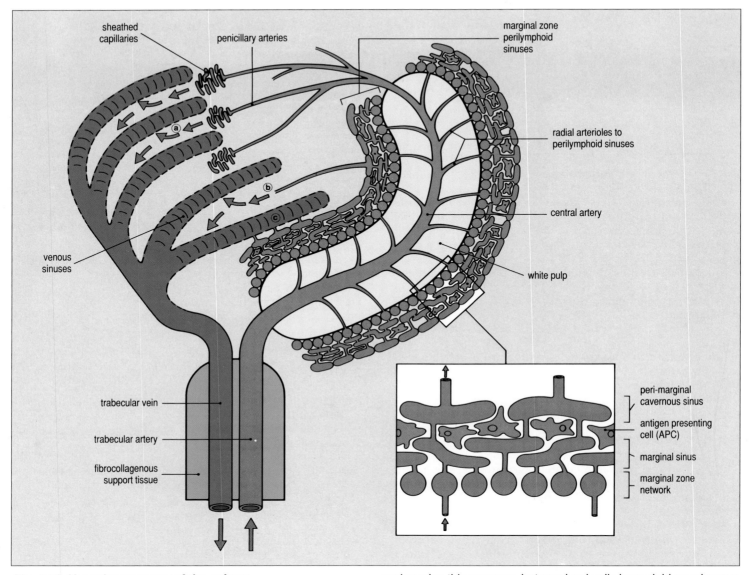

Fig. 7.18 Vascular anatomy of the spleen.

The spleen has two main functions. It removes aged and effete red cells from the circulation, and mounts an immune response to antigens circulating in the blood, particularly bacteria.

Blood enters the spleen in the splenic artery; this branches to form the trabecular arteries, which give rise to a series of central arteries surrounded by T cells.

In order to remove red cells, blood passes along the central arteries and then enters the red pulp through a series of specialized vessels (penicillary arteries and sheathed capillaries) to drain into the splenic parenchyma (splenic cords). The blood then percolates through spaces between the reticular cells forming the splenic cords, and squeezes through narrow slit spaces to enter the splenic venous sinuses. Normal red cells are deformable

and survive this passage, but aged red cells have rigid membranes and are lysed. Fragments of destroyed red cells are removed by phagocytic cells along the sinus walls.

Red cells leave the system via trabecular veins and enter the splenic vein. This pathway is the **open circulation (a)**.

A proportion of the splenic circulation enters small arterioles to reach a series of marginal sinuses, which run around the lymphoid sheaths. In this area blood comes into contact with dendritic antigen-presenting cells, and foreign antigens can be trapped and presented to appropriate lymphoid cells.

Most of the blood from the marginal sinuses enters the red pulp and then drains into the venous sinuses (**b**), but a small proportion passes directly into the sinuses and forms a **closed circulation (c)**.

SPLENECTOMY

Removal of the spleen is necessary:
- when it is ruptured following abdominal trauma;
- in some diseases, for example lymphomas;
- as part of some major operations, for example removal of the stomach for cancer.

Effects of splenectomy

The effects of removing the spleen highlight its main functions.

The blood film (Fig. 7.19) from a person who has had a splenectomy shows increased number of platelets and abnormal red cells with deformed shapes. In addition aged red cells contain blue staining particulate inclusions of degenerate cell material (Howell Jolly bodies).

These cells would normally be removed by percolation through the splenic cords and into the splenic sinuses.

Infection. Patients who have had a splenectomy are at risk of developing life-threatening bacterial septicaemia. The commonest organism involved is *Streptococcus pneumoniae*

The presence of *S. pneumoniae* in the blood would normally excite an immune response and prevent the development of an overwhelming infection, but in a person without a spleen the organism can circulate in the blood and reproduce.

Because the organism is in the blood it does not reach the immune surveillance systems provided by the lymph nodes.

It is therefore recommended that anyone undergoing a splenectomy is subsequently immunized against *S. pneumoniae*.

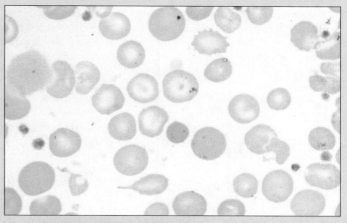

Fig. 7.19 Postsplenectomy blood film.
Micrograph of blood film from a patient following splenectomy. The red cells have bizarre shapes and in this field two of the cells contain small particulate blue staining inclusions (Howell Jolly bodies). Platelets are increased in number.

OPEN CIRCULATION

A system of filtering blood through the parenchyma (splenic cords) and then into the sinusoids is termed the **open circulation**, and is the main route of blood flow in the human spleen.

Blood percolates slowly through the spaces in the splenic cords and emerges through the slit-like openings in the walls of the sinusoids into the system of splenic venous sinuses and thence into the splenic veins.

CLOSED CIRCULATION

The closed circulation appears to be a minor component of human splenic blood flow. Blood from the perimarginal cavernous sinuses bypasses the slow route through the splenic parenchyma and enters the splenic venous sinuses instead. This provides a system for blood to pass rapidly through the spleen without filtration. In man a small number of capillaries arising from the central arteries also open directly into the venous sinuses.

MUCOSA-ASSOCIATED LYMPHOID TISSUE (MALT)

In addition to the mass of the peripheral lymphoid tissue encapsulated in the lymph nodes and spleen, the body contains an equally large amount of non-encapsulated lymphoid tissue, which is located in the walls of the gastrointestinal, respiratory and urogenital tracts.

This tissue is known as **mucosa-associated lymphoid tissue (MALT)** and takes the form of diffuse infiltrates or more discrete nodules; it provides immunological protection against invasion of the body via vulnerable exposed absorptive surfaces

The **gut-associated lymphoid tissue (GALT)** includes:
- the palatine, lingual, and pharyngeal tonsils (adenoids) (see page 125);
- mucosal nodules in the oesophagus;
- **Peyer's patches** in the small intestine (see page 159);
- lymphoid aggregations in the large intestine and appendix;

• a vast number of lymphocytes and plasma cells scattered throughout the lamina propria of the small and large intestines.

The **bronchus-associated lymphoid tissue (BALT)** is located beneath the mucosa of the large respiratory passages (bronchi) and shows close structural similarities with other forms of MALT.

In large aggregations of MALT, which are seen mainly in the tonsils and Peyer's patches, the lymphoid tissue is arranged into follicles, which often contain germinal centres, and are similar to those of the lymph nodes.

With immunohistochemical techniques, discrete B and T cell zones containing typical antigen-processing accessory cells can be identified and have functions analogous to those of the superficial cortex and paracortex of the lymph node, respectively.

The scattered lymphocytes in the lamina propria of the gut and respiratory tract are mainly B cells, some of which mature into antibody- secreting plasma cells. All classes of antibody are produced, but IgA predominates.

• IgA is secreted into the gut lumen in a form called secretory IgA, which is resistant to enzymatic digestion, and provides protection against pathogens before they breach the tissues.

• IgG and IgM are secreted into the lamina propria to deal with organisms eluding the surface protective mechanisms.

• IgE mediates the release of histamine from mast cells, which are present in large numbers in the lamina propria.

Peyer's patches

Peyer's patches, which number about 200 in the human, are large aggregations of MALT in the small intestine. They extend through the lamina propria and submucosa, and often bulge into the gut lumen.

The overlying epithelium of a Peyer's patch (dome epithelium) is characterized by cuboidal rather than tall columnar cells (see Fig. 10.25), and contains large numbers of intraepithelial lymphocytes. Goblet cells are absent.

Some of the epithelial cells exhibit numerous surface microfolds instead of the usual microvilli and have been designated **M cells**. These cells migrate from the mucosal crypts and function in the transfer of antigen between the lumen and the Peyer's patch.

Peyer's patch-mediated immune response

Antigen is taken up by macrophages and presented to B and T cells, to initiate an immune response as follows.

• IgA-secreting B cell precursors and memory cells appear to be stimulated in the Peyer's patches and travel via efferent lymphatics to mesenteric lymph nodes, where the immunological response is greatly amplified by cell division.

• Activated lymphocytes from the mesenteric lymph nodes then enter the circulation via the thoracic duct, and subsequently home in on the lamina propria of the gut.

• In the lamina propria the activated lymphocytes carry out their major effector functions, including final maturation into plasma cells and antibody secretion.

Unlike Peyer's patches, the lamina propria does not contain HEVs, and the mechanism by which Peyer's patch-derived lymphocytes recognize and home in on the gut lamina propria is unknown, but is thought to involve mutually attractive cell surface molecules called **addressins**. During lactation, Peyer's patch-derived B cells migrate to the breast where they mature into plasma cells and secrete IgA into the milk. Thus, the newborn is protected from the same potential ingested pathogens to which the mother is exposed.

A special subset of T cells in the Peyer's patches controls the differentiation of IgA-secreting B cell precursors and thus ultimately IgA secretion. The Peyer's patches themselves are not a site of significant IgA secretion.

Tonsils

Waldeyer's ring of pharyngeal lymphoid tissue comprises four groups of tonsillar tissue the largest being the **palatine tonsils**, which contain 12–15 deep tonsillar crypts lined by stratified squamous epithelium. These crypts frequently contain plugs of lymphocytes, bacteria and epithelial debris, which may become calcified.

The tonsils contain numerous lymphoid follicles with germinal centres, and the lymphoid tissue as a whole appears to have a similar cellular makeup to that of Peyer's patches. The epithelium overlying the tonsillar tissue contains T cells as well as dendritic APC s.

Bronchus-associated lymphoid tissue

The lymphoid aggregates of the respiratory tract are similar to those of the gut (i.e. Peyer's patches), but are generally smaller. They are covered by similar antigen sampling and transport M cells. As in the gut there are no afferent lymphatics, but efferent lymphatics drain lymph to the regional nodes.

Activated lymphocytes derived from the respiratory tract aggregations tend to home specifically to the respiratory mucosa.

PRACTICAL HISTOLOGY

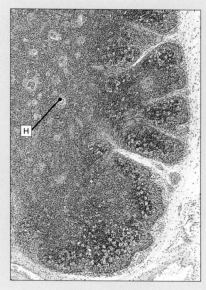

Fig. 7.20 Thymus.
Low power micrograph of thymus from a child. The gland is active with a dense staining cortex containing 'holes', which represent macrophages destroying self-recognizing clones.

Thymic epithelial cells stream down from the capsule and divide the gland into lobules.

The medulla contains numerous Hassall's corpuscles (H).

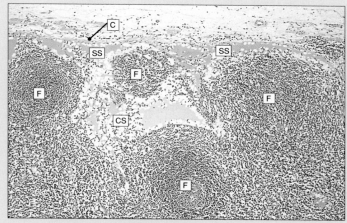

Fig. 7.21 Lymph node sinuses.
High power micrograph of a lymph node margin showing capsule (C), subcapsular sinus (SS), cortical sinus (CS) and follicles (F). The sinuses are filled with pink-staining protein-rich lymph.

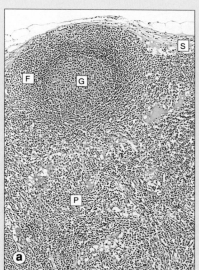

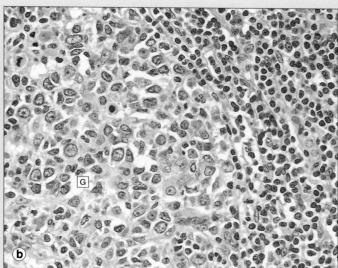

Fig. 7.22 Lymph node follicle.
a Low power micrograph of lymph node showing a follicle (F) with its germinal centre (G) and adjacent paracortex (P). The sinusoid (S) is indistinct, being filled with migrating lymphocytes.
b High power micrograph of the edge of a lymph node follicle showing a germinal centre (G) with a mantle zone. Note a variety of cells in the germinal centre; these are a mixture of developing B cells (see Fig. 7.10) and accessory cells. Accessory cells are very difficult to distinguish in H&E preparations (see Fig 7.11).

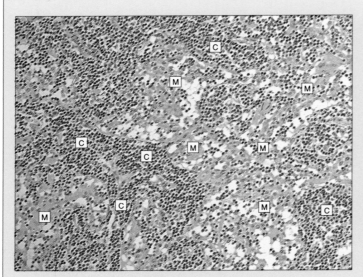

Fig. 7.23 Lymph node medulla.
High power micrograph of H&E stained lymph node medulla. The sinuses are not easily seen, but they may be identified by their content of pale-staining macrophages (M). Many of the lymphoid cells in the medullary cords (C) are plasma cells.

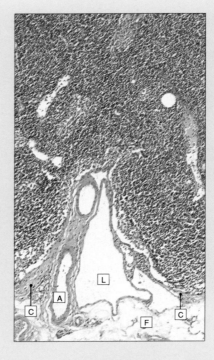

Fig. 7.24 Lymph node hilum.
Medium power micrograph of lymph node hilum showing the efferent lymphatic (L) and artery (A). The vein is not present in this plane of section.

The capsule (C) delineates the node from surrounding adipose tissue (F).

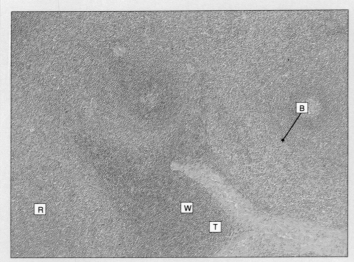

Fig. 7.25 Spleen.
Low power micrograph of spleen showing white pulp (W) and red pulp (R). Both B cell (B) and T cell (T) regions can be seen in the white pulp.

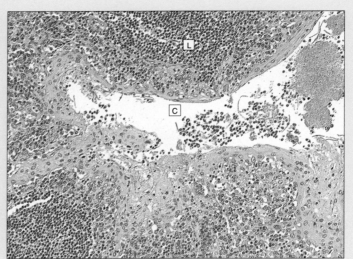

Fig. 7.26 Tonsil.
Medium power micrograph of a tonsil showing a tonsillar crypt (C) lined by squamous epithelium and surrounded by tonsillar lymphoid tissue (L). The crypt contains colonies of oral commensal bacteria, which is a normal finding.

8. BLOOD AND LYMPHATIC CIRCULATORY SYSTEMS

The main systems transporting oxygen, nutrients and waste materials from one part of the body to another are circulatory systems, in which substances are dissolved or suspended in liquid and carried from place to place in a system of tubes.

There are two main circulatory systems: the blood circulatory system and the lymphatic system.

• The **blood circulatory system** is the main method of transporting oxygen and carbon dioxide, nutrients and metabolic breakdown products, cells of the immune and other defence systems, chemical messengers (hormones), and many other important substances (e.g. blood clotting factors).

• The **lymphatic system** drains not only extracellular fluid from the tissues, returning it to the blood circulatory system after passage through lymph nodes, but also nutrients absorbed by the alimentary tract.

BLOOD CIRCULATORY SYSTEM

There are three types of blood circulatory system, the systemic, pulmonary and portal systems, two of which, the systemic and pulmonary circulations depend on a central pump, the heart, to push the blood around (Fig. 8.1).

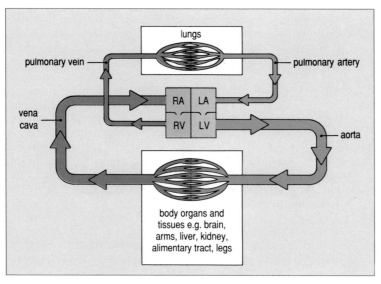

Systemic circulation

The systemic circulation transfers oxygenated blood from a central pump (the heart) to all of the body tissues (**systemic arterial system**) and returns deoxygenated blood with a high carbon dioxide content from the tissues to the central pump (**systemic venous system**).

Pulmonary circulation

The pulmonary circulation transfers deoxygenated blood with a high carbon dioxide content from a central pump (the heart) to the lungs (**pulmonary arterial system**) and transfers reoxygenated blood from the lungs back to the central pump (**pulmonary venous system**).

Portal systems

The portal systems are specialized vascular channels that carry substances from one site to another, but do not depend on a central pump. The largest portal system (hepatic portal venous) runs between the intestines and the liver (see page 118).

Fig. 8.1 Systemic and pulmonary blood circulations.
Diagram illustrating the main components and interrelationships of the systemic and pulmonary blood circulations.

The heart is a four-chambered pump central to both systems, and the direction of blood flow is indicated by arrows.

Blood vessels that transport blood **away** from the heart are called **arteries** (arterial systems) and those that take blood **towards** the heart are called **veins** (venous systems). The systemic venous and pulmonary arterial vessels carry deoxygenated blood; the pulmonary venous and systemic arterial vessels carry oxygenated blood.

In organs and tissues other than the lung the oxygenated blood gives up much of its oxygen and becomes deoxygenated; in the lungs deoxygenated blood is oxygenated. Gaseous exchange takes place in small, thin-walled vessels called capillaries.

HEART

The heart is a muscular pump with four chambers, two of which (**atria**) receive blood from the systemic and pulmonary venous circulations, while the other two (**ventricles**) pump blood into the systemic and pulmonary arterial circulations.

Anatomy

The wall of the heart has three layers.
• An outer **epicardium** (**visceral pericardium**) covered with flat mesothelial cells to produce a smooth outer surface (see below).
• A middle **myocardium** composed of specialized muscle (cardiac muscle), which is responsible for the pumping action of the heart.
• An inner smooth lining, the **endocardium**, in direct contact with the circulating blood.

Right atrium

The **right atrium**, which receives deoxygenated blood from the systemic venous circulation, has a relatively thick endocardium and a thin muscle wall, since it needs to contract only with sufficient force to push the blood a short distance into the right ventricle.

Right ventricle

The **right ventricle** has a thicker muscular wall than the right atrium because it pumps deoxygenated blood through the lungs (where the blood acquires oxygen, see Fig. 8.1) and then into the left atrium via the pulmonary veins.

Left atrium

The **left atrium** receives oxygenated blood from the pulmonary veins. It has a relatively thick endocardium and a thin muscle layer, since it contracts only with sufficient force to push the blood a short distance into the left ventricle.

Left ventricle

The **left ventricle** is the chamber with the thickest, most muscular, wall because it pumps oxygenated blood throughout the body with sufficient force to overcome the resistance of the walls of vessels of increasingly smaller bore, and then pushes the blood through the capillaries into the first components of the venous system. The left ventricle is therefore the chamber with the greatest oxygen demands, and the chamber most likely to fail.

Valves

During contraction of the ventricles (**systole**), blood is prevented from flowing back into the atria by the following two valves:
• the right atrioventricular (**tricuspid**) valve between the right atrium and right ventricle;
• the left atrioventricular (**bicuspid** or **mitral**) valve between the left atrium and left ventricle.

Similarly, to prevent blood flowing back into the two ventricles at the end of their contraction, there are valves between the ventricles and the large vessels into which they empty:
• the **pulmonary valve** between the right ventricle and its outflow vessel, the pulmonary artery;
• the **aortic valve** between the left ventricle and its outflow vessel, the aorta.

Fibrocollagenous skeleton

The heart has a fibrocollagenous skeleton, the main component being the **central fibrous body**, located at the level of the four cardiac valves.

Extensions of the central fibrous body surround the valves to form the **valve rings,** which support the base of each valve leaflet. The valve rings on the left side of the heart surround the mitral and aortic valves and are thicker than those on the right side, which surround the tricuspid and pulmonary valves.

A downward extension of the fibrocollagenous tissue of the aortic valve ring forms a fibrous septum between the right and left ventricles called the **membranous interventricular septum**. This is a minor component of the septum between the right and left ventricles, most of which is composed of cardiac muscle covered on both sides by endocardium. The membranous part is located high in the septal wall beneath the aortic valve.

Pericardial sac and epicardium

The heart is enclosed within a sac, the **pericardial sac**, which is composed of compact fibrocollagenous and elastic tissue, and lined internally by a layer of flat mesothelial cells, the **parietal pericardium**. This smooth mesothelial layer reflects over the outer surface of the heart to form the outer layer of the **epicardium**, which is sometimes called the **visceral pericardium.**

The pericardial cavity is the space between the parietal and visceral pericardial layers. It contains a small amount of serous fluid to lubricate the surfaces and permit friction-free movement of the heart within the cavity during its muscular contractions.

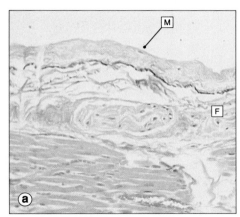

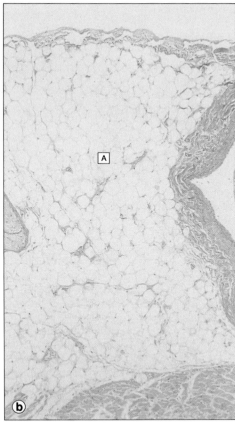

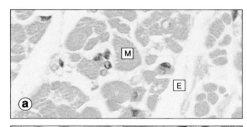

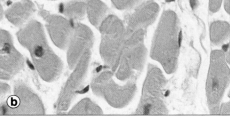

Fig. 8.2 Visceral pericardium (epicardium).

a Section of thin epicardium showing a narrow layer of fibrocollagenous tissue (F) containing elastic fibres (black), covered by flat mesothelial cells (M) identical to those of the inner surface of the parietal pericardium.

b Where the larger branches of the coronary arteries and veins run in the epicardium the fibrocollagenous layer is expanded by variable amounts of adipose tissue (A), which cushion the blood vessels, nerves and lymphatics and produce a thick epicardium.

Fig. 8.3 Myocardium.

a Micrograph of left atrial myocardium in approximate transverse section. The myocardial fibres (M) form an interconnecting network separated by loose fibrocollagenous tissue (the **endomysium**, E).

b Micrograph of left ventricular myocardium in approximate transverse section at the same magnification as **a**. The general structure is the same as left atrial myocardium, but the fibres of the left ventricle are thicker.

The epicardium forms the outer covering of the heart and has an external layer of flat mesothelial cells. These cells lie on a stroma of fibrocollagenous support tissue, which contains elastic fibres, as well as the large arteries supplying blood to the heart wall, and the larger venous tributaries carrying blood from the heart wall. The large arteries (coronary arteries) and veins are surrounded by adipose tissue, which expands the epicardium (Fig. 8.2).

The coronary arteries originate from the first part of the aorta just above the aortic valve ring and pass over the surface of the heart in the epicardium sending branches deep into the myocardium. This superficial location of the arteries is of great practical importance since it permits surgical bypass grafting of blocked arteries.

Myocardium

The bulk of the heart is **myocardium**, which is the contractile element composed of specialized muscle fibres called **cardiac muscle** (see Fig. 5.8d).

The amount of myocardium in the various chambers of the heart varies according to the workload of that chamber (Fig. 8.3).

● The left and right atria push blood into empty ventricles against minimal resistance during diastole and therefore have thin myocardial layers.

● The right ventricle pushes blood through the pulmonary valve and into the pulmonary arterial tree to the small vessels involved in gaseous exchange in the lungs, and then through the pulmonary venous system until it enters the left atrium (see Fig. 8.1). It therefore has a moderate muscle layer.

● The left ventricle pumps blood throughout the body against a high resistance, the systemic arterial system being a high pressure system with a normal systolic pressure of about 120 mm Hg. The left ventricle therefore has the thickest myocardium (see Fig. 8.19c).

The outer surface of the myocardium beneath the pericardium is smooth, but the internal surface beneath the endocardium is raised into **trabeculations**, which are most marked in the ventricles. The trabeculations are covered by smooth endocardium and do not interfere with the smooth flow of the blood.

In both ventricles, raised mounds of cardiac muscle (**papillary muscles**) protrude into the ventricular lumina and point towards the atrioventricular valves. Papillary muscles are the site of attachment of **chordae tendinae**, which are narrow tendinous cords that tether the atrioventricular valve leaflets to the wall of the ventricle beneath them. Such tethering prevents eversion of the valve leaflets into the atrium during ventricular contraction.

Atrial natriuretic hormone

Atrial myocardial fibres are smaller than those of the ventricles and contain small neuroendocrine granules, which are usually sparse and located close to the nucleus; they are most numerous in the right atrium. These granules secrete **atrial natriuretic hormone** when the atrial fibres are excessively stretched.

Atrial natriuretic hormone increases the excretion of water, and sodium and potassium ions, by the distal convoluted tubule of the kidney. It also decreases blood pressure by inhibiting renin secretion by the kidneys and aldosterone secretion by the adrenals (see page 260).

Endocardium

The internal lining of all four heart chambers is the endocardium, which is composed of three layers.
• The layer in direct contact with the myocardium is composed of irregularly arranged collagen fibres, which merge with collagen surrounding adjacent cardiac muscle fibres. This layer may contain some **Purkinje fibres**, which are part of the impulse conducting system (see page 109).
• The middle layer is the thickest endocardial layer and is composed of more regularly arranged collagen fibres containing variable numbers of elastic fibres, which are compact and arranged in parallel in the deepest part of the layer. Occasional myofibroblasts are present.
• The innermost layer is composed of flat endothelial cells, which are continuous with the endothelial cells lining the vessels entering and emerging from the heart.

The endocardium is variable in thickness, being thickest in the atria and thinnest in the ventricles, particularly the left ventricle. The increased thickness is due almost entirely to a thicker fibroelastic middle layer (Fig. 8.4). Localized areas of endocardial thickening (jet lesions) are common, particularly in the atria, and result from turbulent blood flow within the chamber.

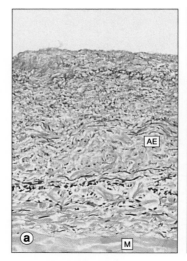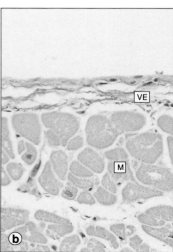

Fig. 8.4 Endocardium.
a Micrograph of elastic Van Gieson (EVG) stained right atrial endocardium (AE). The collagenous content stains red and elastic fibres stain black; myocardial muscle fibres (M) stain yellow. The nature of endocardial fibres is not apparent in a routine H&E stained section (see Fig. 8.25). The atrial endocardium is much thicker than that which covers the ventricles.
b Micrograph of EVG stained left ventricular endocardium (VE). It is a much thinner layer than in the atrium and contains much less elastic tissue; the muscle fibres (M) are large.

The inner mesothelial cell layer is always poorly preserved in post-mortem material, as here.

Valves

In the heart there are four valves, which permit blood flow in one direction only; in addition there is a small valve-like flap where the main vein from the lower part of the body (the **inferior vena cava**) enters the right atrium.

Anatomy

AORTIC AND PULMONARY (SEMILUNAR) VALVES
The outflow valves of the right and left ventricles, the **pulmonary** and **aortic valves**, are composed of three cup-like cusps that fit closely together when closed. Because of their shape they are sometimes called semilunar valves.

The base of each valve is attached to a fibrocollagenous valve ring (see page 104), and the junctions between one cusp and another are called **commissures** (Fig. 8.5).

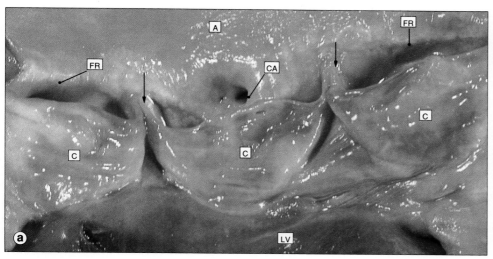 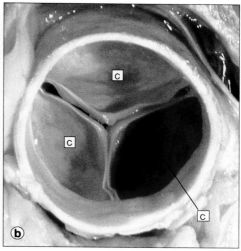

Fig. 8.5 Aortic valve.
a Photograph showing the opened aortic valve between the left ventricle (LV) and its large empyting artery, the aorta (A). The three cusps (C) of the valve, the commissures (arrows), the origin of one of the coronary arteries (CA) and the pale fibrocollagenous valve ring (FR) are clearly seen.
b Photograph of aortic valve viewed from above in the closed position. Note how closely the three cusps (C) fit together. The pressure of blood against the closed valve ensures coronary artery blood flow in diastole.

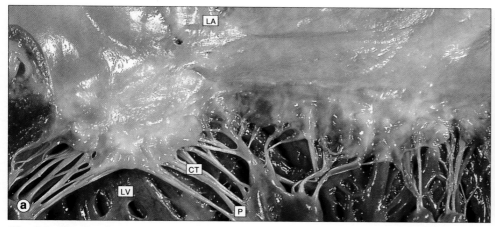 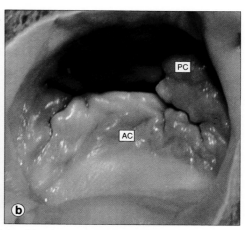

Fig. 8.6 Mitral valve.
a Photograph showing the opened left side of heart to demonstrate the mitral valve between the left atrium (LA) and the left ventricle (LV). It has two cusps, the free edges of which are tethered to the papillary muscles (P) by thin chordae tendinae (CT).
b Photograph of mitral valve viewed from above in the closed position. There are two cusps, one anterior (AC) and one posterior (PC).

MITRAL AND TRICUSPID (ATRIOVENTRICULAR) VALVES
The atrioventricular valves are thin flaps attached to their respective valve ring at their base, and tethered on their undersurface (ventricular surface) by numerous thin tendinous cords, the chordae tendinae. The chordae tendinae run from the valves to the tips of the papillary muscles in the ventricular wall (Fig. 8.6).

107

Histology

In general, each valve has a dense fibrocollagenous central plate (the **fibrosa**), which is an extension of the fibrocollagenous tissue of the central fibrous body and fibrocollagenous valve ring. The fibrosa is covered on both surfaces by a layer of fibroelastic tissue, and is covered by outer layers of flat endothelial cells. The thickness of the layers varies from valve to valve, and from site to site within the same valve, and with age (Fig. 8.7).

All four valves show localized areas of dense fibroelastic thickening at sites of apposition during valve closure.

ATRIOVENTRICULAR VALVES

In addition to the general histology described above, much of the lower ventricular surface of the atrioventricular valves is roughened, the roughening marking the points of insertion of the chordae tendinae. The chordae are not only inserted at the free edge of the leaflet, but some attach further back and a few small chordae insert near the base. The chordae fibres merge with the collagenous fibres of the central fibrosa of the valve leaflet.

The atrioventricular valves may also have a thin layer of muscle fibres, continuous with those of the atrial wall, on their upper surface.

AORTIC AND PULMONARY VALVES

In addition to the general histological structure of heart valves, the aortic valve shows prominent fibroelastic thickening at the sites of cusp apposition during valve closure, which is sometimes visible as white lines (**linea alba**) just below the free edge of the cusps, with a central nodule at the midpoint of each cusp (see Fig. 8.5). These are present but much less prominent on the pulmonary valve cusps because of the less forceful valve closure in the low pressure pulmonary system.

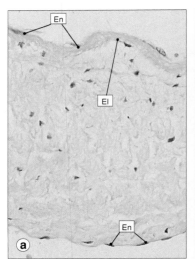
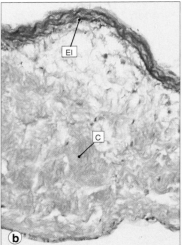
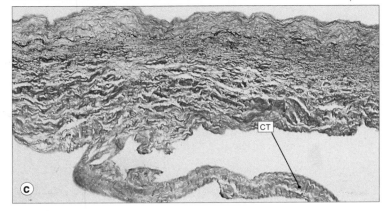

Fig. 8.7 Histology of heart valves.

a High magnification micrograph of H&E stained aortic valve. The bulk of the valve leaflet is composed of loose fibrocollagenous tissue with non-staining glycosaminoglycans between the collagen fibres. There is a dense area of elastic tissue (El) on the superior surface. The flat endocardial cells (En) can be clearly seen on both surfaces of the valve.

b High magnification micrograph of elastic Van Gieson (EVG) stained aortic valve. The dense elastic tissue (El) stains black and the collagen (C) stains red.

c Micrograph of EVG stained mitral valve close to its origin at the left atrioventricular valve ring. The leaflet is composed of red-staining collagen with some elastic fibres (black) running through it. The collagen is most thick, dense and irregular on its inferior (ventricular) surface where the chordae tendinae (CT) are attached. The chordae have a structure similar to that of tendon (see Fig. 14.10).

DISORDERS OF HEART VALVES

There are three important abnormalities of the heart valves, all most commonly affecting the valves of the left side of the heart.

Rheumatic valve disease

Heart valves are damaged during the acute stage of a childhood illness called rheumatic fever. Healing of such damage results in progressive scarring of the valve leaflets and their elastic content is replaced by irregular masses of collagen scar. The valves therefore become more rigid. The leaflets may also partially fuse, which limits their ability to open (**stenosis**) or close (**incompetence**).

Calcific valve disease

Calcific valve disease mainly affects the aortic valve, particularly if it is congenitally abnormal with only two cusps (i.e. **bicuspid**). The valves become thickened and distorted by fibrous scarring and deposition of calcium nodules (Fig. 8.8). This renders the valve leaflets immobile and impairs blood flow from the left ventricle during systole, leading to left heart failure (see page 113).

Infective valvitis

Heart valves may become infected by bacteria or fungi, most commonly when the valve has been previously damaged, for example, by rheumatic disease. The damaged endocardium is roughened, exposing collagen fibres, which act as a nidus for the formation of platelet aggregates, such aggregates eventually leading to the formation of thrombus (see page 116). Bacteria or fungi circulating in the blood stream can then settle in the thrombus and proliferate.

The effects of infective valvitis on the patient are two-fold.
• A fragment of infected thrombus may break off and enter the systemic circulation until it lodges in a small vessel. These small vessels are commonly arterioles in organs such as the brain, kidney or spleen. The resulting blockage of the arterial supply leads to ischaemic death (infarction) of the tissue cells supplied by the blocked vessels. This is called **embolization**.
• The proliferating bacteria may erode and destroy the tissues of the valve.

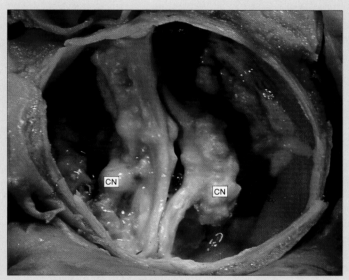

Fig. 8.8 Calcific valve disease.
Micrograph showing a bicuspid aortic valve that has become thickened and distorted by fibrous scarring and calcium nodule (CN) deposition. Compare with Fig. 8.5a.

Conducting system

The heart contracts independently of the will (i.e involuntarily), beating about 70/minute, any abnormality of the rhythm impairing the functioning of one or more chambers.

The rhythmic contractions of atria and ventricles do not depend on nerve stimulation, but result from impulses generated within the heart itself. This is fortunate since cardiac transplantation would otherwise be impossible as all of the nervous connections are severed during surgery. However, the autonomic nervous system can control the rate of the heartbeat; stimulation of the parasympathetic innervation (vagus) slows the heart rate, while sympathetic stimulation increases it.

The impulse for contraction is initiated at a small body called the **sinoatrial node**, which acts as a **pacemaker**, and stimulates atrial contraction. The impulse passes through the atrium and arrives at a further node, the atrioventricular node. This node initiates the marginally later contraction of the ventricles, the impulse passing down specialized bundles of cardiac muscle (**the main bundle**, **right and left bundle branches**, and so-called **Purkinje fibres**) to the furthest reaches of the bulky ventricular muscle (Fig. 8.9).

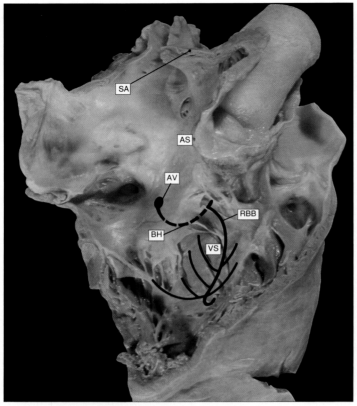

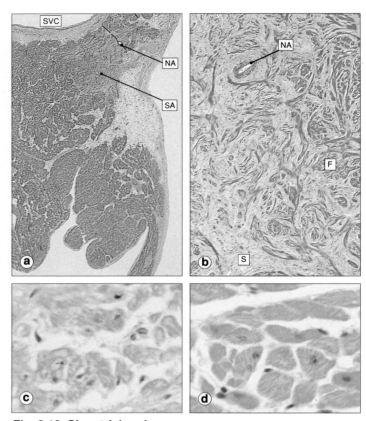

Fig. 8.9 Conducting system of the heart.
Photograph of opened right side of the heart trimmed to expose the septum between the two atria (AS) and the septum between the two ventricles (VS). The sinoatrial node (SA), atrioventricular node (AV), bundle of His (BH), and right bundle branch (RBB), are indicated; the left bundle branch runs down on the left ventricular side of the interventricular septum.

Fig. 8.10 Sinoatrial node.
a Micrograph showing the sinoatrial (SA) node situated in the atrial wall close to the entrance of the superior vena cava (SVC). The node is highlighted in this pentachrome stain by the prominent blue-staining fibrocollagenous support tissue in which the cardiac pacemaker cells are embedded. Note the nodal artery (NA).
b Medium power micrograph showing the irregular whorled network of small nodal fibres (F) embedded in the bulky fibrocollagenous stroma (S). A small nodal artery (NA) is present.
c High magnification view of the irregularly arranged small muscle fibres of the SA node.
d Normal atrial muscle fibres photographed at the same magnification as **c** for comparison.

Sinoatrial node

The sinoatrial (SA) node is located where the main vein from the upper part of the body (the **superior vena cava**) enters the right atrium (Fig. 8.10a&b). Its position is constant, but it is so small that it is not visible naked-eye, being a curved linear structure 1–1.5 cm long, but only 0.1–0.15 cm wide on the outer surface of the vena caval–atrial junction just beneath the pericardium.

The SA node is composed of an irregular meshwork of muscle fibres 3–4 μm in diameter, which are considerably smaller than normal atrial cardiac muscle fibres (Fig. 8.10c).

In contrast to normal cardiac muscle cells, SA muscle fibres do not have intercalated discs (see Fig. 5.8), but

connect with each other by desmosomes, contain few myofibrils and lack an organized striation pattern.

The cells of the SA node are embedded in a bulky fibrocollagenous support tissue containing numerous blood vessels, including a prominent central artery, the nodal artery. Numerous nerve fibres can be seen peripherally.

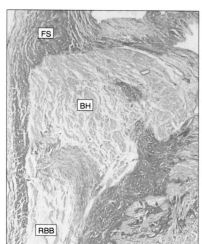

Fig. 8.11 Bundle of His and right bundle branch. Micrograph showing the bundle of His (BH) and origin of the right bundle branch (RBB). The His bundle is situated in the fibrous skeleton (FS), which appears red in this elastic Van Gieson stained section, the nodal and bundle branch fibres staining yellow.

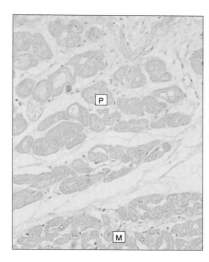

Fig. 8.12 Purkinje fibres. Micrograph showing the large pale-staining Purkinje fibres (P) in the endocardium lining the interventricular septum. Compare them with the normal myocardial fibres (M).

The impulse generated by the SA node passes quickly to the atrioventricular node, stimulating atrial contraction in the process.

The long-standing belief that the impulse travels to the atrioventricular node by diffuse radiation along all atrial muscle fibres is probably inaccurate, as specific bundles of atrial muscle (**internodal atrial muscle**), which preferentially conduct the impulse, have been identified. Three such specific bundles have so far been described, the **anterior**, **middle** and **posterior internodal tracts** and are histologically indistinguishable from other atrial fibres.

Atrioventricular node

The **atrioventricular (AV) node** is located beneath the endocardium of the medial wall of the right atrium just in front of the opening of the coronary sinus (see Fig. 8.24) and immediately above the tricuspid valve ring. It is thus situated at the base of the interatrial septum, at the junction between atria and ventricles, and between the central fibrous body and endocardium.

Histologically the AV node is composed of a network of small muscle fibres identical to those of the SA node, but less haphazardly arranged. Like the SA node, the fibres of the AV node are embedded in a fibrocollagenous stroma and have a rich blood and nerve supply.

Bundle of His, and right and left bundle branches

The small fibres at the anterior end of the AV node are more regularly arranged and eventually become a distinct bundle of parallel fibres, which forms the main bundle conducting the impulse from the AV node to the ventricles. This conducting bundle, the **bundle of His** (Fig. 8.11),

penetrates the collagen of the central fibrous body, and then runs anteriorly for a short distance along the upper border of the muscle of the interventricular septum before dividing into right and left bundle branches.

The **left bundle branch** arises fan-like over a broad area as individual fibres, which leave the bundle of His; the remaining fibres form a distinct **right bundle branch**.
• The left bundle branch fascicles run down beneath the endocardium of the left side of the interventricular septum in two main groups, a posterior group and a smaller anterior group.
• The right bundle branch runs down beneath the endocardium of the right side of the interventricular septum as a single bundle.

Purkinje fibres

The right and left bundle branches connect with a complex network of specialized conduction fibres, the **Purkinje fibres**, which are large fibres with vacuolated cytoplasm due to a high glycogen content, and scanty myofibrils. They lie in clusters of up to about 6 fibres (Fig. 8.12).

Arterial supply

Because of its constant contractile activity the heart has enormous energy demands and therefore a substantial arterial supply, the left ventricle having the greatest oxygen demand and consequently the best arterial supply. Thus, any interruption in the cardiac arterial supply particularly affects the structure and function of the left ventricle (see Fig. 8.13).

Coronary arteries

The heart is supplied by two **coronary arteries**, which arise as direct side-branches of the main artery leaving the left ventricle (the aorta), just above two of the cusps of the aortic valve.

LEFT CORONARY ARTERY
The left coronary artery divides into two main branches, the left anterior descending branch and the circumflex branch.

The left anterior descending branch passes down the front of the heart in the epicardium and is located approximately over the anterior part of the interventricular septum. It gives off numerous branches, which supply the anterior part of the left ventricle and anterior half of the interventricular septum.

The circumflex branch passes laterally in the groove between the left atrium and left ventricle before descending in the lateral wall of the left ventricle, which it supplies.

RIGHT CORONARY ARTERY
The right coronary artery passes to the right in the groove between the right atrium and right ventricle, running round to the posterior aspect of the heart.

The terminal branches of the right coronary artery supply the posterior wall of the left ventricle and the posterior half of the interventricular septum.

Venous drainage

Venous tributaries run with the major coronary arteries before draining into a large venous channel, the coronary sinus, which runs in the atrioventricular groove on the posterior aspect of the heart, before opening into the right atrium at the coronary sinus opening (see Fig. 8.24).

CORONARY ARTERY DISEASE

The most common and important disease of the heart is **atheroma** in the coronary arteries, which impairs the efficiency of the left ventricle because it reduces the blood and therefore oxygen supply. The coronary arteries are particularly prone to this common disease, the consequences on the left ventricle being severe and often fatal.

Angina

Slowly progressive reduction of coronary artery lumen by atheroma impairs oxygenation of the left ventricular muscle, leading to a characteristic pattern of chest pain (**angina**), which is usually brought on by exertion (i.e. when the left ventricular muscle is working harder).

Myocardial infarction

Complete obstruction of one of the coronary arteries or its branches (see Fig. 8.17) results in one area of the heart muscle receiving no blood or oxygen. Such affected heart muscle fibres die and cannot be replaced. This is called **myocardial infarction** (Fig. 8.13), which is colloquially known as a **heart attack**.

The heart can survive loss of part of its muscular wall, but pumping efficiency of the left ventricle is reduced, and may lead to **heart failure**, either sudden or slowly progressive.

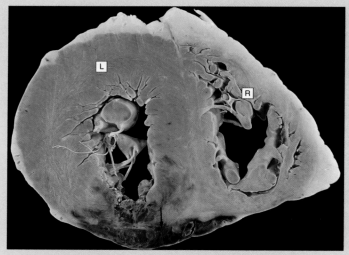

Fig. 8.13 Myocardial infarction.
Photograph showing a transverse slice across the left (L) and right (R) ventricles. The left ventricular myocardium is increased in thickness as a result of persistent high blood pressure (**hypertension**). Part of the left ventricular wall and septum shows reddish-black discoloration (arrow) due to infarction (i.e. death of tissue due to sudden cessation of its oxygenated blood supply) resulting from occlusion of a coronary artery. Blood has seeped into the dead myocardium and rupture of the heart is imminent.

HEART FAILURE

The term **heart failure** is imprecise since it is rare for all chambers of the heart to fail equally and at the same time.

A failing chamber is unable to empty itself of blood completely and this is most commonly due to:
- impaired contractile ability;
- blockage of its outflow tract, for example by a damaged heart valve (see Fig. 8.8).

Thus a failing atrium will fail to empty during diastole, and a failing ventricle will fail to empty during systole, and with each inefficient contraction, a little blood is left behind in the chamber. Progressive accumulations lead to distension of the chamber with blood, which increases the pressure in the chamber. Such increased pressure is commonly reflected back into the preceding chamber or blood vessel.

A failing heart chamber will attempt to overcome the resistance to emptying by increasing the thickness and work rate of the cardiac muscle in its wall. This is visible to the naked-eye as marked thickening of the chamber wall due to compensatory muscular hypertrophy; the chamber is also dilated because of its failure to empty.

Left heart failure

The most common type of heart failure affects the left side of the heart (**left heart failure**) and is usually due to incomplete emptying of the left ventricle with each systolic beat. Damage to the myocardium (see Fig. 8.13) is the most common cause, but it can also occur if the aortic valve is obstructed, for example by calcific aortic stenosis, (see Fig. 8.8).

Eventually a failing left ventricle is unable to accept the full load of blood from the left atrium during diastole, resulting in incomplete emptying of the left atrium. This emptying failure passes back along the pulmonary veins, which drain into the left atrium, so that the pulmonary capillaries and veins become distended with blood and their luminal pressure rises.

Right heart failure

Right heart failure may be due to:
- physical damage to the pulmonary capillary bed, as occurs in some chronic lung diseases;
- increasing pressure in the pulmonary capillary bed because of left heart failure.

Right heart failure resulting from left heart failure is often called **congestive cardiac failure**.

SYSTEMIC BLOOD VESSELS

The systemic circulation is an extensive high pressure system and the structure of its proximal vessels reflects the high pressures to which they are subjected. Furthermore, they are modified to smooth the flow of blood, since blood is impelled through them only during systole, and it is important to maintain an adequate pressure and flow during the diastolic intervals.

The structural modifications to handle the high systolic pressure and to maintain a respectable diastolic pressure are most refined in the large **elastic arteries**, which receive the output of the left ventricle (i.e. the aorta and its large branches such as the carotid, subclavian and renal arteries). Distal to these large elastic arteries, the artery walls gradually become more muscular (i.e. **muscular arteries**).

General structure

The walls of large and medium sized arteries have three identifiable layers. In veins these three layers are less clearly defined, and in small blood vessels (i.e. arterioles, capillaries and venules, see pages 116–118) they are so narrow that they are virtually indistinguishable.

The layers are the intima, media and adventitia.

Intima

The **intima** is the thin inner layer of a blood vessel wall. It is lined internally by flat **endothelial cells**, which normally provide a smooth, friction-free internal surface, permitting the free flow of blood. In certain vessels the endothelial cells may be more cuboidal.

Endothelial cells (see Fig. 8.20) contain occasional rounded membrane-bound bodies, which contain microtubules and are called **Weibel-Palade bodies**; their function is unknown.

The endothelial cells lie on a basement membrane, beneath which is a usually thin layer of collagen fibres and occasional elastic fibres. In large vessels, the elastic fibres may aggregate at the lower border of the intima to form a distinct **internal elastic lamina**, which is well-defined in muscular arteries, but indistinct in veins and elastic arteries.

Media

The **media** is the middle layer in a blood vessel wall and is particularly prominent in arteries, being indistinct in veins and virtually non-existent in very small vessels (e.g. capillaries). The composition of the media accounts for the main difference between elastic and muscular arteries (see below).

113

Adventitia

The **adventitia** is the outer layer of blood vessels, and is composed largely of collagen, but smooth muscle cells may be present, particularly in veins. In arteries it is demarcated from the media by a condensation of elastic fibres that forms a variably distinct **external elastic lamina**. The adventitia is the most prominent layer in the walls of the veins.

Within the adventitia of vessels with thick walls are small blood vessels, the **vasa vasorum**, which send penetrating branches into the media to supply it with blood. These are not seen in thinner vessels, which obtain their oxygen by diffusion from the lumen.

Elastic arteries

Elastic arteries are the largest arteries and receive the main output of the left ventricle, thus they need to withstand the high systolic pressure of 120–160 mm Hg and to maintain an adequate pressure during diastole.

Media. Elastic arteries have a thick, highly developed media in which elastic fibres are the main component, and are gathered together in sheets arranged in concentric layers throughout the thickness of the media. In the largest artery, the aorta, there are often 50 or more layers (Fig. 8.14).

The elastic fibres are arranged so that they run circumferentially rather than longitudinally in order to counteract the tendency for the vessel to over-distend during systole. Return of the elastic fibres from their stretched to unstretched state during diastole maintains a diastolic pressure within the aorta and large arteries of about 60–80 mm Hg. Interposed between the elastic layers are smooth muscle cells and some collagen.

Intima. The intima of elastic arteries bears the full force of the systolic output when the pressure is highest, and is therefore particularly prone to mechanical damage due to the shearing forces of the jets of blood.

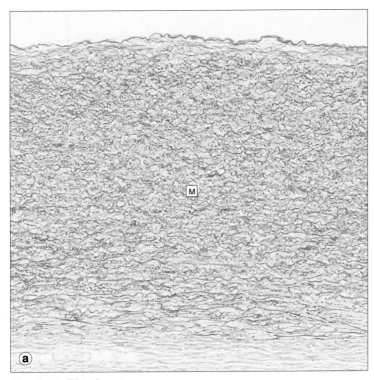

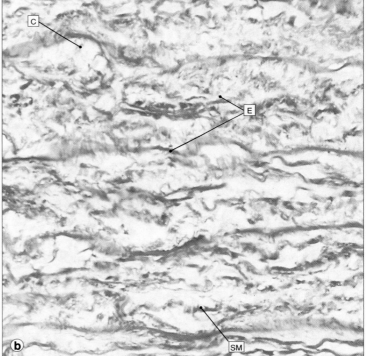

Fig. 8.14 Elastic artery
a Low power view of elastic van Gieson stained large elastic artery (aorta). The predominant layer is the media (M), which is composed of elastic fibres (black) arranged as concentric sheets and separated by smooth muscle fibres and collagen.
b High power view of the media to show the relationship between elastic fibres (E), smooth muscle (SM) and collagen (C).

Muscular arteries

The large elastic arteries gradually merge into muscular arteries by losing most of their medial elastic sheets, usually leaving only two layers, an internal elastic lamina and an external elastic lamina, at the junction of the media with the intima and adventitia, respectively.

Media. In a muscular artery the media is composed almost entirely of smooth muscle. These arteries are therefore highly contractile, their degree of contraction or relaxation being controlled by the autonomic nervous system. A few fine elastic fibres are scattered amongst the smooth muscle cells, but are not organized into sheets, and are most numerous in the large muscular arteries, which are a direct continuation of the distal end of the elastic arteries (Fig. 8.16).

Muscular arteries vary in size from about 1 cm in diameter shortly after their origin from the elastic arteries, to about 0.5 mm in diameter. In the larger arteries there may be 30 or more layers of smooth muscle cells, whereas in the smallest peripheral arteries, there are only 2 or 3 layers. The smooth muscle cells are usually arranged circumferentially at right angles to the long axis of the vessel.

The internal elastic lamina is commonly a distinct prominent layer, but the external elastic lamina is less well defined, and is often discontinuous.

ANEURYSM

With ageing, the elastic fibres in the media of the large elastic arteries degenerate and are replaced by inelastic collagen. As a result, the vessels lose their power of recoil after systole and tend to become permanently dilated over a period of years. They also fail to maintain the diastolic pressure effectively because of diminished elastic recoil, so diastolic pressure may fall.

When most of the elastic lamellae have become replaced by collagen, the artery may become so dilated that an aneurysm forms. An **aneurysm** (Fig. 8.15) is a permanently dilated thin-walled artery, which is prone to rupture, resulting in torrential and often fatal haemorrhage.

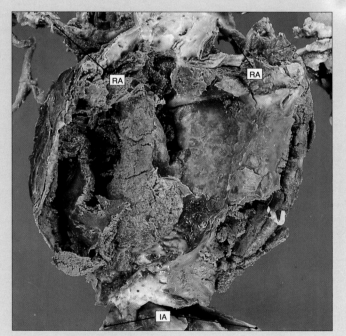

Fig. 8.15 Aneurysm.
Gross photograph of the abdominal aorta showing a ruptured aneurysm containing some red thrombus between the origins of the renal arteries (RA) and the bifurcation into two iliac arteries (IA).

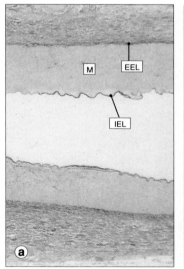 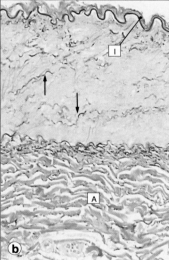

Fig. 8.16 Muscular artery.
a Elastic Van Gieson stained longitudinal section through a muscular artery. The intima is scarcely visible, the predominant layer being the muscular media (M) situated between an internal elastic lamina (IEL) and an external elastic lamina (EEL), which are composed of condensed sheets of elastic fibres (black). The outer adventitia stains red, being composed largely of collagen.
b Medium power view of the same artery showing the intima (I) and the fine black-staining elastic fibres running through the muscular media (arrows). In this large muscular artery the collagenous adventitia (A) is thick.

ATHEROMA

In elastic and proximal muscular arteries the intima is exposed to the full force of the high systolic pressure and, with the passage of time, becomes damaged, developing a disease called **atheroma.**

Atheroma is characterized by infiltration of the intima with fatty material, accompanied by increased deposition of collagen and elastic fibres, such intimal thickening forming a so-called **atheromatous plaque.**

The commonest consequences of atheroma are impaired blood flow, thrombus formation and aneurysm formation.

Impaired blood flow

In small bore arteries atheromatous change leads to reduction in the size of lumen of the vessel so that blood flow is decreased. This is particularly detrimental when it affects small muscular arteries supplying vital organs with a high blood and oxygen requirement, such as the heart. Partial occlusion of the coronary arteries may lead to the symptoms of **angina** (see page 112).

Thrombus formation

A further complication of atheroma is that it damages the smooth internal lining of endothelial cells, exposing the circulating blood to the underlying intimal collagen. This frequently triggers the formation of **thrombus** within the vessel, due initially to platelets aggregating over the damaged surface (see Fig. 6.17).

Thrombus further reduces the lumen of the vessel, and may block it completely (Fig. 8.17), resulting in **infarction** of the tissue supplied by the vessel. The myocardium of the left ventricle is particularly vulnerable to infarction (see Fig. 8.13), as is the brain (**stroke**) and the feet and toes (**gangrene**).

Aneurysm formation

Atheroma can also affect the media of the blood vessels, with loss of elastic in elastic arteries and of smooth muscle cells in muscular arteries, both these specialized components being replaced by non-contractile inelastic collagen. This predisposes to aneurysm formation (see Fig. 8.15).

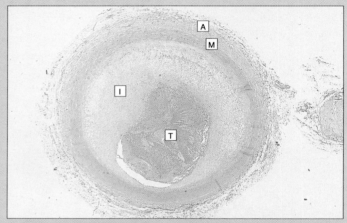

Fig. 8.17 Coronary atherosclerosis and thrombosis.
Micrograph showing a transverse section from the coronary artery supplying the area of dead muscle shown in Fig. 8.13. The lumen has been greatly reduced by thickening of the intimal layer (I). The media (M) and adventitia (A) are normal. The intimal thickening and irregularity has led to the formation of a thrombus (T), which further reduces the lumen and blood flow through it.

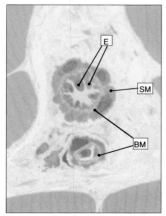

Fig. 8.18 Arteriole.
Micrograph of a thin epoxy resin toluidine blue stained section of two arterioles showing basement membrane (BM) as a pale-staining membrane surrounded by a number of smooth muscle cells (SM). The inner endothelial cells (E) in the larger vessel appear rather cuboidal because it has contracted during the biopsy process. Note that the two arterioles differ not only in size, but also with regard to the number of muscle cells.

Arterioles

The smallest terminal branches of the arterial system are called arterioles, and these vary in diameter ranging from 30 μm–400 μm (0.4 mm).

Intima. The intima of an arteriole is composed of endothelial cells lying on either a basement membrane (in the smallest arterioles), or an internal elastic lamina (in the larger arterioles).

Media. The arteriolar media is composed of one or two layers of smooth muscle cells (Fig. 8.18). As the arterioles get smaller, the continuous layers of smooth muscle become progressively discontinuous. In the smallest arterioles, the endothelial cells have basal processes, which pierce the basement membrane and make junctional contacts with the smooth muscle cells.

Adventitia. The adventitia of arterioles is insignificant.

Microvasculature

The arterioles represent the beginning of the **microvasculature** (Fig. 8.19), which is composed of small diameter blood vessels with partly permeable thin walls that permit the transfer of some blood components to the tissues and vice versa. Most of this exchange between blood and tissues occurs in the extensive capillary network, the smallest arterioles (**metarterioles**) emptying into the capillary system. The **capillary** networks drain into the first components of the venous system, the **venules** (see below).

Capillaries

Capillaries are the smallest vessels of the blood circulatory system, being 5–10 μm in diameter. They form a complex interlinking network.

Capillaries have the thinnest walls and are the major site of gaseous exchange, permitting the transfer of oxygen from the blood into the tissues, and carbon dioxide in the other direction. Fluids containing large molecules pass across the capillary wall in both directions.

The capillary wall (Fig. 8.20) is composed of endothelial cells, a basement membrane and occasional scattered contractile cells called **pericytes** (see page 66).

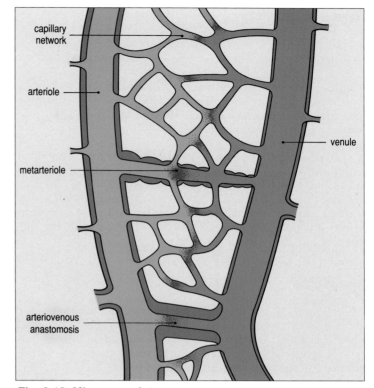

Fig. 8.19 Microvasculature.
Diagram showing the microvasculature. Blood flows from arteriolar to venular vessels through a complex network of capillaries, arising either directly from the arteriole or from the smaller metarteriole. Opening of the arteriovenous anastomosis directs blood flow out of the capillary network.

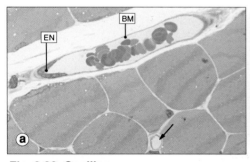
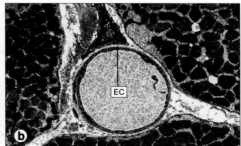
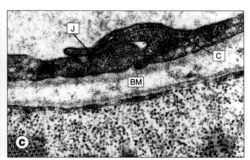

Fig. 8.20 Capillary.
a An epoxy resin section stained with toluidine blue of a capillary in longitudinal section. The wall is composed almost entirely of thin basement membrane (BM), the endothelial cytoplasm lining its internal surface not being visible at this magnification. An endothelial cell nucleus (EN) can be seen at one end. A similar but smaller capillary is seen in transverse section (arrow) between individual muscle fibres.

b Electronmicrograph of the capillary arrowed in **a**. At this low magnification the endothelial cytoplasm (EC) is just visible, but the basement membrane is indistinct.
c High power electronmicrograph of part of the capillary wall showing the basement membrane (BM), endothelial cytoplasm (C) and the anchoring junction (J) between the cytoplasm of adjacent endothelial cells.

117

Types of capillary

Capillaries are of two types according to their endothelial cell structure, which is either continuous or fenestrated.

Capillaries with continuous endothelium are the most common type, the endothelial cells forming a complete internal lining to the capillary without any intercellular or intracytoplasmic defects.

Capillaries with fenestrated endothelium are seen most commonly in the gastrointestinal mucosa, endocrine glands and renal glomeruli (see Figs 16.16 & 16.22). The endothelial cell cytoplasm is pierced by pores (**fenestrations**), which extend through its full-thickness. In some fenestrations there is a thin diaphragm, which is thinner than the cell membrane; its nature is uncertain.

Sinusoids

Highly specialized vascular channels called **sinusoids** are seen in some organs such as the liver (see Fig. 11.1) and spleen (see Fig. 7.18). They are endothelial-lined channels with a larger diameter than capillaries, and scanty, discontinuous or absent basement membrane.

The endothelial cells are commonly highly fenestrated, often with large pores, and there may be substantial gaps between the cells.

Venules

Post-capillary venules. Capillaries drain into post-capillary venules, which are the smallest venules, being 10–25 μm in diameter. They resemble capillaries in structure, but have more pericytes (Fig. 8.21).

Collecting venules. Post-capillary venules drain into larger collecting venules 20–50 μm in diameter in which the pericyte layer becomes continuous and surrounding collagen fibres appear.

Muscular venules. As the collecting venules become larger bore, the pericytes are progressively replaced by smooth muscle cells, which form a layer 1–2 cells thick, and a fibro-collagenous adventitia becomes identifiable; these are muscular venules and are 50–100 μm in diameter. Muscular venules drain into the smallest veins.

Veins

Veins vary in size from less than 1 mm–4 cm in diameter. In comparison with arteries of comparable external diameter, veins have a larger lumen and a relatively thinner wall, and are therefore commonly collapsed in histological sections unless inflation-fixed.

Although intimal, medial and adventitial layers are present in veins, they are less clearly demarcated than in arteries, and it is often difficult to identify where one layer

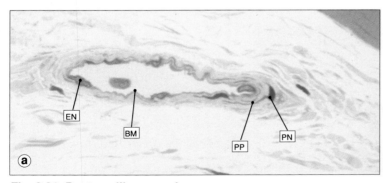

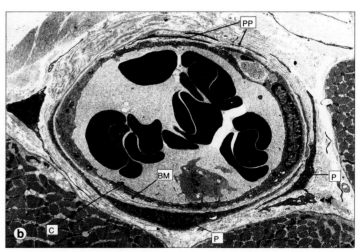

Fig. 8.21 Post-capillary venule.
a Toluidine blue stained epoxy resin section of a partly collapsed post-capillary venule. The endothelial cell nucleus (EN) and basement membrane (BM) can be identified. There are a few pericyte processes (PP) and a pericyte nucleus (PN) in the wall, but the details are not clearly visible.
b Electronmicrograph of a post-capillary venule showing the endothelial cell cytoplasm (C), basement membrane (BM) and pericytes (P) more clearly. Note that the finer pericyte processes (PP) apparently intervene between layers of the basement membrane (arrow).

ends and another begins. Furthermore, there is considerable variation in vein wall structure according to location. The following description of veins of different sizes is therefore a generalization.

Small veins, which are a continuation of the muscular venules and have a similar wall structure, but are larger, being up to 1 mm in diameter, with more clearly defined muscle cell and outer fibrocollagenous layers (Fig. 8.22a).

Medium sized veins are 1–10 mm in diameter. They have an inner layer of endothelial cells on a basement membrane, which is separated by a narrow zone of collagen fibres from an indistinct condensation of elastic fibres producing a poorly formed internal elastic lamina.

The inner layer is fairly consistent in structure, differing only in quantity of collagen and elastic fibres between the endothelium and the condensation of elastic fibres. However, the outer layers, still called the media and adventitia, but often arbitrarily and with little justification, vary considerably in thickness, proportions of collagen, elastic fibres and smooth muscle, and particularly in the orientation of the muscle fibres.

Large veins. The inner (intimal) layer of large veins resembles that of medium sized veins, but there are usually more collagen and elastic fibres between the endothelial basement membrane and the elastic lamina, which is often markedly fragmented. External to the elastic lamina there is a layer of smooth muscle embedded in collagen, and outside this a thick layer of collagen in which there are bundles of longitudinally orientated smooth muscle fibres. Some elastic fibres intermingle with the collagen (Fig. 8.22b).

Venous circulation and valves

Venous circulation of blood is maintained by contraction of venous smooth muscle, supplemented to varying degrees by external pressure from the contraction of surrounding skeletal muscle. Such assistance from skeletal muscle contraction is particularly important for the venous circulation of the arms and legs, most of which is surrounded by the skeletal muscles responsible for arm and leg movement.

As the veins in the arms and legs carry blood against gravity, they are equipped with valves to prevent blood flowing back down the vein. Such valves are thin flaps of intima that project into the lumen, the free edges of the valve flaps pointing towards the heart; thus they allow blood to flow towards the heart, but prevent backflow. Incompetence of the valves in the superficial veins of the legs causes varicose veins.

Valves are also present in other medium and large veins, their number depending on whether the vein is carrying blood against or with gravity.

Arteriovenous anastomoses

In addition to the microvasculature (i.e. arterioles emptying into a capillary network, which drains into a venular system), there are additional vessels that bypass the capillary bed, so that arterioles can communicate directly with venules; these are **arteriovenous anastomoses** (see Fig. 8.19).

At its arteriolar end, an arteriovenous anastomosis is thick-walled, mainly due to an abundant smooth muscle coat, which is richly innervated. Contraction of this thick

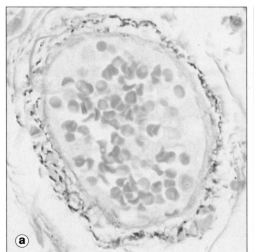

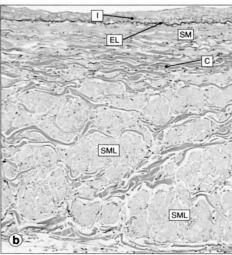

Fig. 8.22 Veins.
a Micrograph showing an elastic Van Gieson (EVG) stained small vein. The rather variable and irregular arrangement of smooth muscle (yellow), collagen (red) and elastic fibres (black) in its wall is evident.
b Micrograph showing the wall of the largest vein in the body, the inferior vena cava. There is a distinct intima (I) and internal elastic lamina (EL), a layer of smooth muscle (yellow, SM) and an irregular layer of thick collagen (red, C). This collagen indicates the approximate beginning of the adventitial layer, which is the thickest layer in large veins, being expanded by the presence of large bundles of longitudinally running smooth muscle (SML). (EVG stain).

smooth muscle layer closes off the lumen of the anastomosis at its origin and diverts blood into the capillary bed, whereas relaxation opens up the lumen allowing blood to flow directly into a venule, thus bypassing the capillary network.

Arteriovenous anastomoses are widespread, but are most common in certain regions of the skin such as the fingertips, lips, nose, ears and toes. They are thought to play an important role in the skin's thermoregulatory function (see Chapter 19), closure of the anastomosis diverting blood into the extensive dermal capillary system and permitting heat loss, while opening of the vessel closes down the capillary bed and conserves heat.

In the fingertips, there is a highly specialized type of arteriovenous anastomosis, the **glomus body,** which has a prominent arterial end (Sucquet-Hoyer canal) connecting directly to the venular end. The canal is surrounded by modified smooth muscle cells (glomus cells), which are richly innervated by the autonomic nervous system.

Innervation of blood vessels

Efferent innervation

Blood vessels that can significantly alter their lumen size by contraction and relaxation of their smooth muscle fibres have a major supply of adrenergic sympathetic fibres, stimulation of which causes muscle contraction and vasoconstriction.

Some blood vessels in skeletal muscles also have a cholinergic sympathetic innervation capable of producing vasodilation.

Afferent innervation

In certain areas blood vessels have an afferent innervation, which provides information about the luminal pressure (**baroreceptive information**) and blood gas (i.e. carbon dioxide and oxygen) levels (**chemoreceptive information**). These are mainly located in the carotid sinuses, and in the region of the aortic arch, pulmonary artery and large veins entering the heart.

Afferent fibres from the carotid sinus receptors travel in the glossopharyngeal nerve to the cardiorespiratory centres in the brain stem.

PULMONARY BLOOD VESSELS

The pulmonary vasculature is discussed in Chapter 9 (pages 124–142).

PORTAL BLOOD SYSTEMS

Portal circulations are venous channels that connect one capillary system with another and do not depend on the central pumping action of the heart.

The nature of portal connecting vessels varies from site to site; for example, the vessels of the hepatic portal system (see Fig. 11.2), which connects capillaries in the intestine to the capillary-like sinusoids in the liver, are venous in nature, being small venules adjacent to the capillary beds, and medium and large sized veins in between. In the other main portal system, between the hypothalamus and posterior pituitary (see Fig. 15.3) the connecting vessels are large capillaries and venules.

LYMPHATIC CIRCULATORY SYSTEM

The intercellular spaces of almost all tissues contain small endothelial-lined tubes, which are blind ending, but otherwise identical in structure to blood capillaries. These are **lymphatic capillaries** and are permeable to fluids and dissolved molecules in the interstitial fluid.

In some areas the lymphatic capillaries have a fenestrated endothelium and a discontinuous basement membrane, permitting the entry of larger molecules such as large molecular weight proteins, triglycerides, etc., and also some cells, particularly cells of the immune system.

The lymphatic capillary network acts as a drainage system, removing surplus fluid (**lymph**) from tissue spaces. Lymph is normally a clear colourless fluid, but lymph draining the intestine is often milky in appearance because of its high content of absorbed lipid and is called **chyle**.

The lymphatic capillaries merge to form thicker walled vessels, which resemble venules and medium sized veins.

Lymph moves sluggishly from the capillary network into the larger lymphatic vessels, backflow being prevented by numerous flap-like valves similar to those in veins (Fig. 8.23).

On its way to the larger vein-like lymphatics from the smaller lymphatics, lymph passes through one or more **lymph nodes**, entering the lymph node at its convex periphery, and leaving it through one or two lymphatic vessels at the concave hilum (see Fig. 7.8). During this passage, activated lymphocytes, which are important to immune defence, are added to the lymph.

The larger lymphatic vessels have muscular walls and pump the lymph into the following two main lymphatic vessels:
- the so-called **thoracic duct**, which empties lymph into the venous system at the junction of the left internal jugular and left subclavian veins;

- a more variable lymphatic vessel, the **right main lymphatic duct**, which empties into the junction between the right internal jugular and right subclavian veins.

These two main lymphatic vessels run alongside the lumbar and thoracic vertebrae in the posterior abdominal and posterior thoracic wall, receiving lymph from lymphatics as they progress towards the jugular veins.

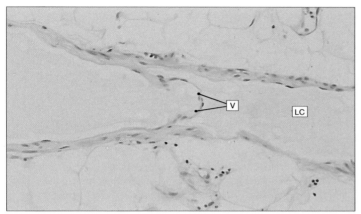

Fig. 8.23 Lymphatic capillary.
Micrograph showing a large lymphatic capillary (LC) containing pale pink-staining lymph. Note the delicate flap-like valves (V) controlling the direction of flow.

SPREAD OF CANCER BY LYMPHATICS

All lymphatic capillaries from a particular area drain their lymph into lymph nodes serving that area (**regional lymph nodes**). Such drainage is particularly important to the spread of cancer, since cancer cells can enter the lymphatic capillaries and be carried to other sites in lymph. Cancer cells may also be trapped in the regional lymph node, where they can multiply and produce secondary tumours at some distance from the site of the primary cancer (see Fig. 7.12).

For example most cancers that originate in the breast may travel in the lymph to the regional lymph nodes of the breast, most of which are in the subcutaneous tissue of the axilla. Careful palpation of the axillary lymph nodes is therefore a vital part of the physical examination of any patient with suspected breast cancer.

PRACTICAL HISTOLOGY

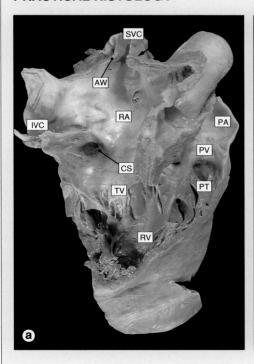

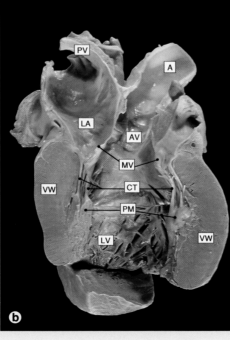

Fig. 8.24 Anatomy of the heart.
a Photograph of opened right side of the heart. In the right atrium (RA), note the opening of the superior vena cava (SVC), the inferior vena cava (IVC), the coronary sinus (CS), and the thin atrial wall (AW). The arrow marks the site of the sinoatrial node.

In the right ventricle (RV), note the flaps of the right atrioventricular (tricuspid) valve (TV) separating the ventricle from the atrium, the pulmonary outflow tract (PT) with the pulmonary valve (PV) between it and the pulmonary artery trunk (PA).
b Photograph of opened left side of the heart. Blood enters the left atrium (LA) through the pulmonary veins (PV), and leaves through the left atrioventricular (mitral, bicuspid) valve (MV) into the left ventricle (LV).

In the left ventricle, note the thick muscular wall (VW), the papillary muscles (PM) and the chordae tendinae (CT), which link them to the leaflets of the mitral valve. Blood leaves the left ventricle through the aortic outflow tract and the aortic valve (AV) and enters the aorta (A).

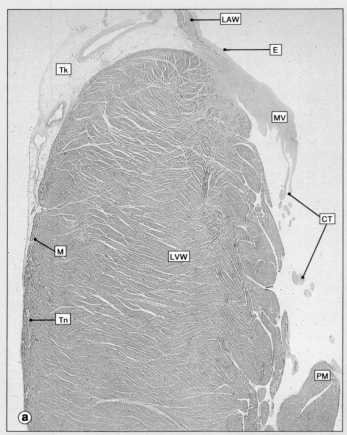

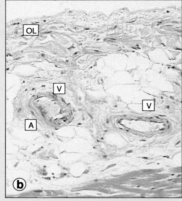

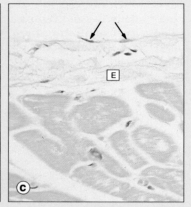

Fig. 8.25 Histology of the heart.

a Low power micrograph showing part of the wall of the left atrium (LAW) and left ventricle (LVW). Part of the mitral valve (MV), papillary muscles (PM) and chordae tendinae (CT) are also shown. Note that the left atrial wall has a relatively thick endocardium (E), whereas the thin endocardium of the left ventricle cannot be discerned at this magnification. Both thick (Tk), thin (Tn) and medium (M) pericardium can be seen on the outer surface of the heart.

b Medium power view of medium thickness pericardium from the area labelled M in **a**. The outer layer (OL) is mesothelial-covered collagenous and elastic tissue, beneath which is a narrow adipose tissue layer (A) containing blood vessels (V).

c High power view of the endocardium (E) lining the interior of the left ventricle, where it is normally a thin layer in which elastic and collagen fibres are difficult to identify. The nuclei of two flat endothelial cells on the surface are arrowed.

Fig. 8.26 Large blood vessels.

The structural details of large and medium-sized blood vessels are best seen in sections specifically stained to show their elastic and muscular components (see Figs 8.14, 8.16 & 8.22). The structural details of the microvasculature (i.e. arterioles, capillaries and venules) are only clearly seen by electron microscopy (see Figs 8.20b&c & 8.21b). It is important however to be able to identify the nature of a blood vessel in a routine H&E stained section, and the micrographs here and in Fig. 8.27 are shown to facilitate such recognition.

a Micrograph showing the H&E appearance of a typical large elastic artery in the systemic circulation, in this case the aorta. The media is a very thick layer with roughly alternating layers of smooth muscle fibres and laminae of intensely eosinophilic, slightly refractile, elastic tissue. Compare with Fig. 8.14.

b Micrograph showing a muscular artery in longitudinal section. The media (M) is composed almost entirely of smooth muscle fibres, and the elastic component is mainly concentrated as internal and external elastic laminae, which are not visible at this low magnification. Note the intimal (I) and adventitial (A) layers. Compare with Fig. 8.16.

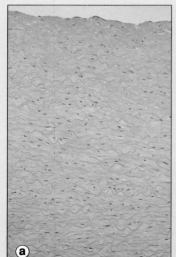

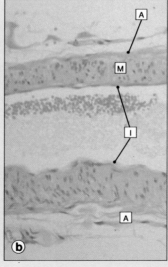

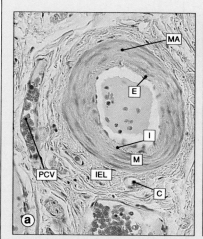

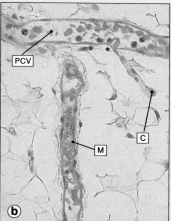

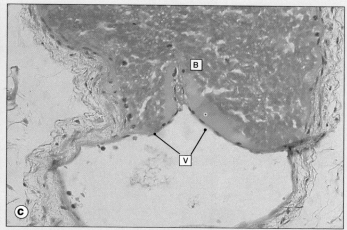

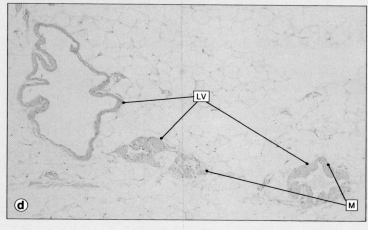

Fig. 8.27 Small blood and lymphatic vessels.

a In this high power micrograph of a small muscular artery (MA), seen here in transverse section, note the endothelial cell lining (E) and the just discernible internal elastic lamina (IEL) between the intima (I) and media (M). Also present are a small capillary (C) and a post-capillary venule (PCV).

b Micrograph of small vessels in adipose tissue, showing capillaries (C). One capillary is opening into a post-capillary venule (PCV), into which a direct metarteriole (M) is also opening.

c High power micrograph showing a thin-walled vein containing a column of blood (B), which is being held back by delicate flap-like valves (V).

d Three lymphatic vessels (LV), one of which is distended with lymph, stretching the muscle in its wall are shown in this micrograph. The less distended lymphatics show rather irregular smooth muscle (M) in their walls.

9. RESPIRATORY SYSTEM

The main function of the respiratory system is to permit oxygenation of the blood and removal from it of carbon dioxide.

In addition, the respiratory system is also involved in the perception of smell and flavour, and phonation (the production of speech).

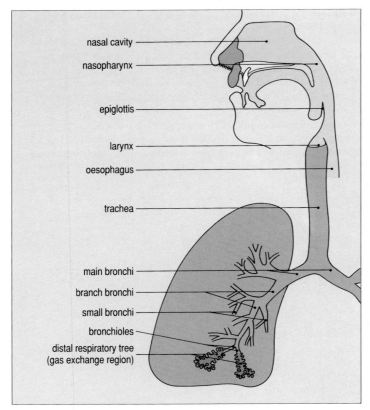

Fig. 9.1 Upper respiratory tract–transport passages.
Diagram to show the part of the respiratory tract that transports air from the atmosphere to the distal respiratory tract where gaseous exchange takes place.

UPPER RESPIRATORY TRACT

Air, from which oxygen is removed and to which carbon dioxide is added, enters and leaves the body through a series of passages known as the **upper respiratory tract** (Fig. 9.1).

On its way to the lungs, where gaseous exchange takes place, the air is cleaned (by removal of particulate matter), and moistened, and its temperature is approximately equated to that in the furthest reaches of the lung.

Nasal cavity and paranasal sinuses

Air enters the respiratory system through the **nostrils**, which are openings to the exterior at the front of the nasal cavity.

The external aspect of the nostrils is covered by keratinizing squamous epithelium, as is the face. This epithelium extends for a short distance into the openings of the nostril (the vestibule), but then becomes non-keratinizing.

Although occasional patches of stratified squamous epithelium persist, most of the epithelium then changes to a pseudostratified columnar pattern, many of the columnar cells bearing numerous cilia (Fig. 9.2). Scattered among these columnar cells are mucus-secreting (goblet) cells with microvilli on their luminal surface.

Beneath the nasal epithelium, the lamina propria contains many glands (Fig. 9.3) equipped with basal myoepithial cells (see page 66). Three main types of gland can be distinguished.
• Most are mucous glands, which secrete mucus to supplement that produced by the goblet cells in the lining epithelium.
• Some are serous cells containing basophilic granules (similar to those seen in the salivary glands, see page 152), which probably produce small amounts of amylase.
• Some are serous cells containing eosinophilic granules (similar to those seen in the lacrimal glands), which produce lysozyme.

Inspired air is moistened by the secretions of the serous components of the glands, while a sheet of mucus secreted by the goblet cells lies on the mucosal surface and traps any inhaled particulate contaminants. The mucus is then wafted backwards by cilia towards the pharynx, where it is swallowed or expectorated.

The lamina propria also contains variable numbers of immune cells (see Chapter 7), which are mainly lymphocytes, plasma cells and macrophages, together with a few neutrophils and eosinophils. Eosinophils are particularly numerous in people who suffer from allergic rhinitis (hay fever).

A characteristic feature of the lamina propria is the presence of many blood vessels, which form an interconnecting network, the vessels being surrounded by a supporting stroma in which smooth muscle is prominent. It is probable that this highly vascular submucosa makes a major contribution to the warming of inhaled air.

The **paranasal sinuses** (the **maxillary, ethmoid, frontal** and **sphenoid** sinuses, Fig. 9.4) are cavernous spaces in the maxillary, ethmoid, sphenoid and frontal bones of the face. Each sinus communicates with the main nasal cavity through a series of orifices, and is lined by epithelium similar to that of the main nasal cavity.

The architecture of the nasal cavity and sinuses provides a large surface area for warming and moistening inspired air, and for trapping particulate matter.

Nasopharynx

The nasopharynx is a posterior continuation of the nasal cavities and becomes the oropharynx at the level of the soft palate. The Eustachian tubes from the middle ear open into its lateral walls.

The nasopharynx is lined by columnar epithelium (like that of the nasal cavities) and stratified squamous epithelium, which becomes more prevalent as the oropharynx is approached; there are also areas of an intermediate epithelium resembling urothelium (see Chapter 16).

The stratified squamous epithelium is normally non-keratinizing and increases in amount with increasing age; keratinizing squamous epithelium is always abnormal and indicates disease.

Beneath the nasopharyngeal epithelium, abundant mucosa-associated lymphoid tissue (MALT) forms Waldeyer's ring. The most important component of this is the nasopharyngeal tonsil (**adenoids**), which is sited where the posterior wall of the nasopharynx joins its roof.

MALT samples inhaled antigenic material and prepares defence mechanisms against them (see page 99).

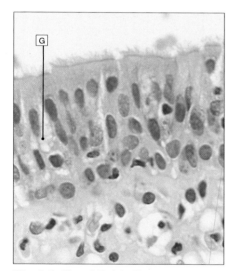

Fig. 9.2 Nasal Epithelium.
Micrograph showing the characteristic ciliated columnar epithelium lining the nasal cavity. There are occasional scattered mucus-secreting goblet cells (G). This pattern, with minor variations, is seen throughout most of the air-conducting part of the respiratory tract and is known as **respiratory-type epithelium**.

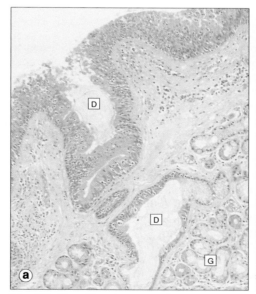
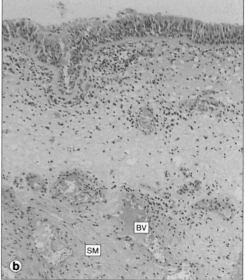

Fig. 9.3 Nasal lamina propria.
a Micrograph showing subepithelial tissue of the nose. Numerous seromucous glands (G) discharge their secretions onto the epithelial surface through wide ducts (D).
b Micrograph showing the prominent network of blood vessels (BV) in the lamina propria, which is supported by irregular bands of smooth muscle (SM) and resembles the vascular tissue of the corpora spongiosa and cavernosa of the penis (see Fig. 17.21), and the corpora of the clitoris (see Fig. 18.1). It is sometimes referred to as the 'erectile' tissue of the nose.

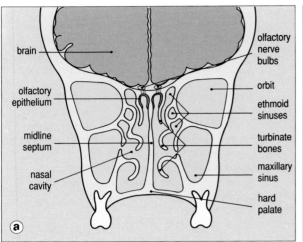

Fig. 9.4 Nasal cavity and paranasal sinuses.

a Coronal section showing the relationship between the nasal cavity and ethmoid and maxillary sinuses. The frontal (anterior) and sphenoid (posterior) sinuses are not shown in this plane of section.

The surface area of the respiratory mucosa is increased by long curved turbinate bones arising from the lateral walls of the nasal cavity, and by the paranasal sinus system. Note the olfactory

epithelium and its proximity to the olfactory nerves and bulbs.

b Sagittal section showing the relationship between the nasal cavity, the anterior nares (nostrils), vestibule, nasopharynx, and frontal and sphenoid sinuses. The opening of the frontal sinus is not shown in this plane of section. Note the openings beneath the two upper turbinates of the ethmoid and maxillary sinuses, and the opening in the nasopharyngeal fold of the Eustachian tube from the middle ear.

Olfactory mucosa

In the roof of the nasal cavity, and extending a short way down the septum and lateral wall is **olfactory mucosa**, which senses smell and the more sophisticated aspects of taste.

Olfactory mucosa has a pseudostratified columnar epithelium composed of olfactory receptor cells, supporting (sustentacular) cells and basal cells. The disposition of these cells results in the pseudostratified appearance since the nuclei of each type occupy different levels (Fig. 9.5a&b).

Basal cells. The nuclei closest to the basement membrane of olfactory epithelium belong to the small basal cells. These cells are not in contact with the lumen and form the stem cells from which new olfactory cells can develop. Olfactory cells normally survive for about one month and regenerate after damage, being the only neurone to do so.

Sustentacular cells. The nuclei closest to the lumen in olfactory epithelium belong to tall sustentacular cells, which have a narrow base in contact with the basement membrane, expanding to more bulky cytoplasm near the lumen.

The oval nuclei of sustentacular cells lie close to the lumen, and the perinuclear cytoplasm contains a moderate amount of rough endoplasmic reticulum and numerous mitochondria, implying a synthetic function. There are small cytoplasmic accumulations of yellow-brown pigment and numerous microvilli on the luminal surfaces.

Olfactory receptor cells. The olfactory receptor cells are bipolar neurones insinuated between the sustentacular and basal cells. They have a central bulge containing the nucleus and from this area extend two cytoplasmic processes, the dendritic and proximal processes.

• The **dendritic process** extends to the surface of the epithelium where its tip is expanded into a club-shaped prominence, the **olfactory vesicle**. This bears cilia, some of which protrude into the nasal cavity, while other lateral cilia insinuate between the microvilli of the sustentacular cells.

The cilia have the typical 9 + 2 arrangement (see Fig. 3.7) for some of their length, but there is a long distal portion, which contains only the 2 central fibres. The cilia are inserted into basal bodies in the olfactory vesicle.

• The **proximal process** is very narrow and passes down between the basal cells and basal portions of the sustentacular cells to penetrate the basement membrane. It then joins other non-myelinated processes to form the so-called **fila olfactoria**, which ultimately forms synaptic connections in the **olfactory bulb** (the first cranial nerve, Fig. 9.5c). The proximal processes are therefore regarded as axons.

Bowmans glands. Beneath the olfactory epithelium are small serous glands (of Bowman) with short ducts that penetrate the olfactory epithelium (Fig. 9.5d). Their secretion may act as the solvent in which odorous substances dissolve.

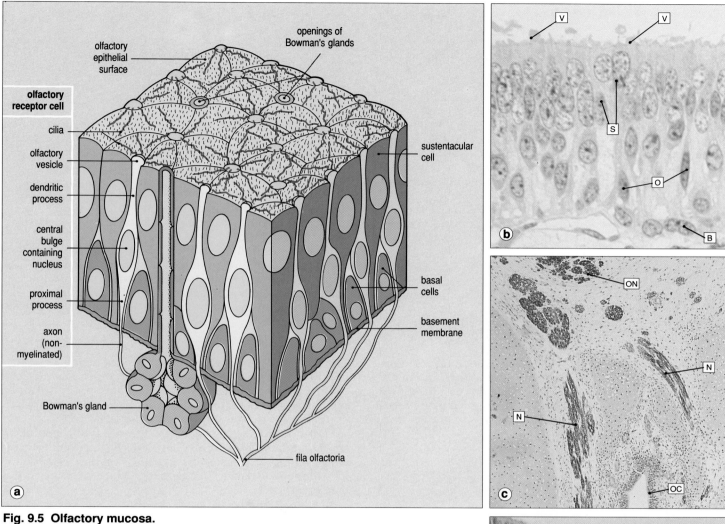

olfactory epithelial surface

openings of Bowman's glands

olfactory receptor cell

cilia

olfactory vesicle

dendritic process

central bulge containing nucleus

proximal process

axon (non-myelinated)

Bowman's gland

sustentacular cell

basal cells

basement membrane

fila olfactoria

a

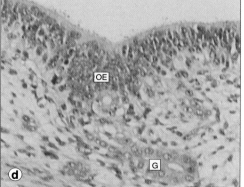

Fig. 9.5 Olfactory mucosa.

a A three-dimensional drawing showing the components of the olfactory mucosa, the Bowman's glands, and the nerves leaving the base of the olfactory epithelial cells on their way to the main olfactory nerve.

b Micrograph of a 0.5 μm acrylic resin section of human olfactory mucosa from an 18-week-old fetus before the associated bone plates have fully calcified. The nuclei of the basal (B), olfactory (O) and sustentacular (S) cells can be identified. The olfactory vesicles (V) on the luminal surface are just discernible. Compare with **a.**

c Micrograph showing the nerve twigs (N) from the olfactory receptor cells (OC) fusing before passing upwards through the cribiform plate of the skull to join the olfactory nerve (ON, first cranial nerve), demonstrated using an immunocytochemical method for neurofilament protein.

d Micrograph showing a small immature Bowman's gland (G). These open onto the luminal surface through narrow ducts, which run through the olfactory epithelium (OE).

Larynx and related structures

On its way to the trachea, air from the nasopharynx passes through the laryngeal region, which has a complex architecture in order to:
• prevent inspired air entering the oesophagus;
• prevent ingested food and fluid entering the trachea;
• permit the production of sounds.

Laryngeal architecture is maintained by a series of cartilaginous plates (mainly the thyroid, cricoid and arytenoid cartilages). These are joined together by densely collagenous ligaments, and are able to move by the action of small bands and sheets of striated muscle called the **intrinsic muscles of the larynx**.

The cartilages maintain openness and shape of the airway, and move to prevent food inhalation during swallowing, which is also partly the responsibility of the epiglottis.

Epiglottis

The epiglottis consists of a central sheet of elastic cartilage, covered by mucosa on both sides.
• The anterior (lingual) surface is covered by stratified squamous epithelium continuous with that of the dorsal surface of the posterior part of the tongue.
• The posterior surface, which faces the pharynx and larynx, is covered in its upper half by stratified squamous epithelium, and in its lower half by ciliated pseudostratified columnar epithelium. This lower half contains many seromucous glands, which penetrate deeply into the central elastic cartilage plate (Fig. 9.6).

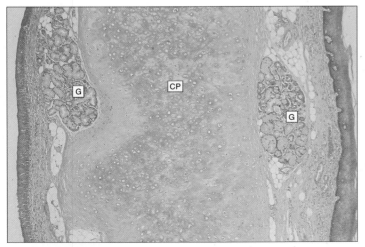

Fig. 9.6 Epiglottis.
Micrograph of epiglottis showing its central cartilaginous plate (CP), seromucous glands (G), some of which split the cartilage, and the two types of epithelium on its two faces.

Vocal cords

Below the epiglottis, the laryngeal mucosa is everted into the laryngeal lumen to form two pairs of folds, an upper pair of **false vocal cords**, and a lower pair of **true vocal cords**. Between these cords outpouching of laryngeal mucosa forms the ventricle and its upward extension, the **saccule** (Fig. 9.7).

The areas where the ends of the true cords are attached to the anterior and posterior walls of the larynx are called the **anterior** and **posterior commissures,** respectively.

FALSE CORDS
The false cords are covered by ciliated columnar epithelium, but islands of non-keratinizing stratified squamous epithelium are common in adults, becoming more extensive with increasing age.

Beneath the epithelium a loose fibrocollagenous supporting stroma contains numerous seromucinous glands and fibres of skeletal muscle from the thyroarytenoid muscle. Small islands of elastic cartilage and adipose tissue may also be found in adults, adipose tissue being most commonly seen in the elderly.

TRUE CORDS
The true cords are covered by stratified squamous epithelium, which shows a rete ridge formation (see Chapter 19) on its free edge and inferior surface, although its upper surface is flat. The epithelium contains occasional melanocytes, but no significant melanin is formed.

The immediate subepithelial support tissue (**Reinke's space**) contains loose fibrocollagenous tissue, which is virtually devoid of lymphatic vessels. This is an important factor in limiting or delaying the spread of cancers arising in the true vocal cords.

Beneath Reinke's space are the fibroelastic fibres of the vocal ligament, to which the skeletal muscle fibres of the vocalis part of the thyroarytenoid muscle are attached. There may be islands of elastic cartilage in the vocal ligament.

SACCULE AND VENTRICLE
The saccule and ventricle are covered largely by respiratory-type ciliated columnar epithelium, and contain seromucous glands in their subepithelial tissue. In children, lymphoid aggregates are common, some with germinal centres.

ANTERIOR AND POSTERIOR COMMISSURES
The anterior and posterior commissures are covered with ciliated columnar epithelium, and their subepithelial zone consists of dense fibrocollagenous tissue containing seromucous glands. Lymphatics and blood vessels are common in both regions and are an important factor in the further spread of cancers of the vocal cords that invade locally to the commissures.

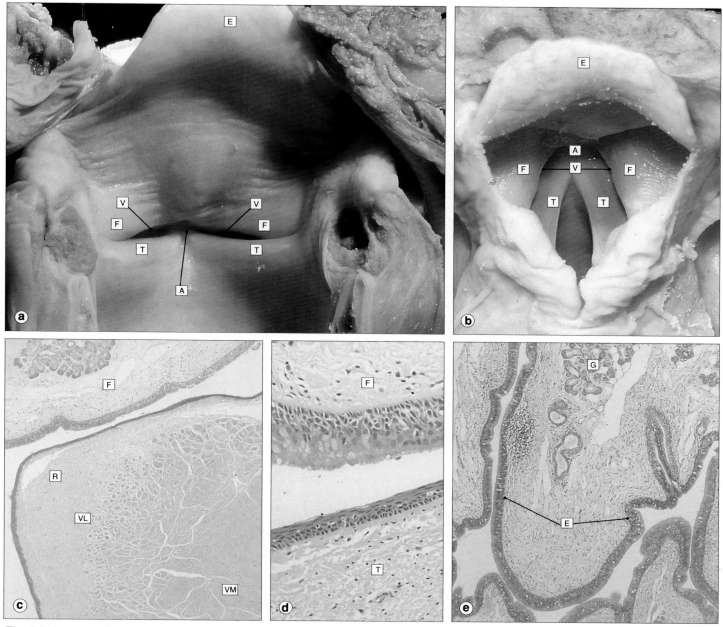

Fig. 9.7 Laryngeal region.

a Photograph of the laryngeal region opened in the midline posteriorly to show the epiglottis (E), the false cord (F), the true cord (T) and the openings of the ventricles (V) between them. This view also shows the anterior commissure (A).
b Photograph showing the vocal cords as seen from above when examined clinically with a laryngoscope. Note the epiglottis (E), false cords (F), true cords (T), the opening of the ventricles (V), and the anterior commissure (A) where the true vocal cords meet in the midline anteriorly.

c Micrograph showing the histology of the true and false cords at low magnification. The false cord (F) is covered by ciliated columnar epithelium and contains seromucous glands. The true cord is covered by non-keratinizing stratified squamous epithelium and contains Reinke's space (R), fibres of the vocal ligament (VL), and the skeletal muscle fibres of the vocalis muscle (VM).
d Micrograph showing the different epithelia of the false (F) and true (T) cords at higher magnification.
e Micrograph of the saccule, which is lined by ciliated columnar epithelium (E) and is rich in seromucous glands (G).

129

Trachea

Below the larynx, the airway continues as the trachea, which is a fairly rigid tubular structure about 10 cm long and 2–3 cm in diameter. The trachea runs down in the midline into the thoracic cavity, where it divides into two main bronchi, one to each lung.

The tracheal wall is rendered rigid and non-collapsible by a number, usually 15–20, of incomplete circular rings of cartilage, which occupy 70–80% of its circumference.

Only a narrow strip of the posterior tracheal wall is deficient in cartilage; here the gap between the ends of each cartilage ring is bridged by a dense fibro-collagenous ligament rich in elastic fibres and bundles of smooth muscle (**trachealis** muscle) which permit some constriction of the tracheal lumen. The ligament linking the two cartilage ends prevents dilation (Fig. 9.8a).

Mucosa

The trachea is lined by pseudostratified ciliated columnar epithelium containing scattered goblet cells. Subepithelial seromucous glands are particularly numerous in the posterior band devoid of cartilage (Fig. 9.8b).

Bronchi

The trachea bifurcates into two main bronchi. These are the largest bore tubes of the **bronchial tree**, which is an irregularly branching system of airways, the luminal diameter becoming smaller with each division.

The **main bronchi** are extrapulmonary and enter each lung with the pulmonary arteries at the lung hilum. They then divide into **lobar bronchi**, one of which supplies each lobe of the lung, two entering the lobes of the left lung (**left upper lobe bronchus** and **lower lobe bronchus**), and three entering the lobes of the right lung (**right upper lobe bronchus**, **middle lobe bronchus** and **lower lobe bronchus**).

Each of the five lobar bronchi divides into a variable number of **segmental bronchi** delivering air to one of the bronchopulmonary segments, where the bronchi divide for a further variable number of generations, eventually terminating in **bronchioles**.

Throughout their course, the bronchi have a similar structure to that of the trachea (Fig. 9.9), but there are variations. The basic structure comprises:
- a pseudostratified columnar ciliated epithelium;
- subepithelial fibrocollagenous tissue containing variable quantities of seromucous glands;

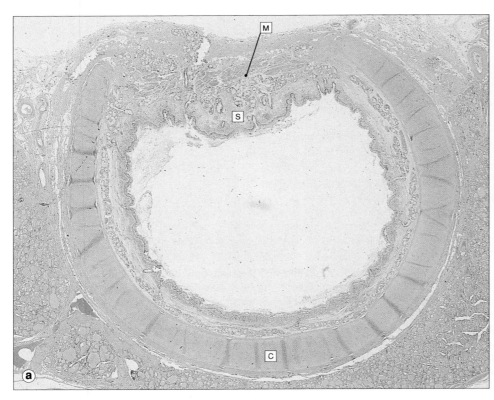

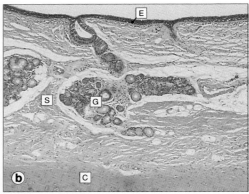

Fig. 9.8 Trachea.
a Micrograph showing a child's trachea with an incomplete cartilage hoop (C), the free ends of the cartilage being joined by a band of muscle (M). The submucosa (S) contains numerous seromucous glands, particularly where the cartilage is deficient.
b Micrograph showing tracheal mucosa with ciliated respiratory epithelium (E) on its surface, and seromucous glands (G) in the submucosa (S). The inner part of the tracheal cartilage ring (C) can be seen at the base of the micrograph.

- variable amounts of smooth muscle, with elastic fibres arranged in longitudinal bands;
- variable amounts of partial cartilaginous ring.

Epithelium

In health the bronchial tree is lined by a ciliated columnar epithelium, which is pseudostratified in the larger bronchi and becomes less complex in smaller peripheral branches. The epithelium contains basal cells, intermediate cells, mucus-secreting goblet cells and neuroendocrine cells (Fig. 9.10).

CILIATED CELLS
Ciliated cells are columnar in most of the bronchial tree, but are shorter and almost cuboidal in the most peripheral branches. They have a basal nucleus, and lysosomes and numerous mitochondria in their supranuclear cytoplasm. The luminal surface of each cell bears about 200 cilia and some microvilli, each cilium being about 6 μm long.

BASAL CELLS
Basal cells lie on the basement membrane and are small cells that are not in contact the lumen. They form a stem cell population from which the other cell types develop.

INTERMEDIATE CELLS
Intermediate cells are probably stem cells transforming into either a ciliated columnar cell or a mucus-secreting goblet cell.

GOBLET CELLS
Goblet cells are scattered between the ciliated cells and are most numerous in the main and lobar bronchi, becoming less common in the smaller branches. Their number increases in some chronic respiratory diseases.

NEUROENDOCRINE CELLS
Neuroendocrine cells are small round cells with dark staining nuclei and clear cytoplasm, similar to those seen in the alimentary tract (see Fig. 15.32), and are located on the basement membrane. They are scattered throughout the tracheobronchial tree, but are most numerous in the smaller bronchi.

Neuroendocrine cells possess cytoplasmic processes and contain characteristic neuroendocrine granules. They secrete hormones and active peptides, including bombesin and serotonin.

The neuroendocrine cells may be found in clusters (**neuroepithelial bodies**), particularly in the newborn and infants (see Fig. 9.11b).

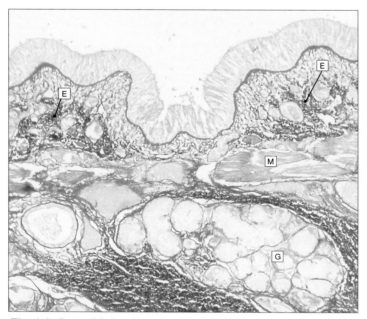

Fig. 9.9 Bronchial wall.
Micrograph showing part of the bronchial wall stained by a method to emphasize its longitudinal bands of elastic fibres (E), here cut in transverse section. The muscle (M) and glands (G) can also been seen.

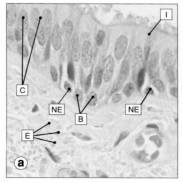
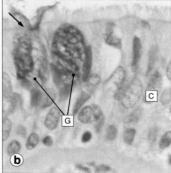

Fig. 9.10 Bronchial epithelium.
a High power micrograph of a thin acrylic resin section of the bronchial epithelium showing the various cell types present. Most of the cells are tall columnar ciliated cells (C), but scattered between them are occasional intermediate cells (I). Goblet cells are not seen in this section, but basal (B) and neuroendocrine (NE) cells are present on the basement membrane. Longitudinal elastic fibres (E) of the bronchial wall, here cut in transverse section, can also be seen.
b High power micrograph of bronchial epithelium stained with a mucin stain (PAS/alcian blue) to show the goblet cells (G) scattered amongst the ciliated columnar cells (C). The mucins are both acid mucins (blue) and neutral mucins (purple). One cell (arrow) has recently discharged its mucin onto the surface.

Submucosa

The submucosa of the bronchial tree contains variable amounts of both smooth muscle and seromucous glands in a loose fibrocollagenous stroma characterized by elastic fibres arranged in distinct longitudinal bands.

SMOOTH MUSCLE
In the main bronchi, the smooth muscle is largely confined posteriorly (as in the trachea), being attached to the ends of the incomplete cartilage rings.

In the intrapulmonary bronchi, the muscle is submucosal and arranged in an irregular spiral with two components, one spiralling to the left, the other to the right. It persists in the airway walls down to the smallest branches (bronchioles, see below), long after the cartilage component has disappeared.

Hypertrophy of the smooth muscle is an important component of some lung diseases.

BRONCHIAL GLANDS
The submucosal bronchial glands are seromucous glands, which empty into the lumen through short ducts. Other deeper glands with longer ducts are located between and beneath the cartilaginous plates. The serous component is thought to secrete lysozyme and glycoprotein.

Myoepithelial cells (see page 66) lie between the secretory and duct lining cells and their basement membrane, and some neuroendocrine cells are also present.

IMMUNE CELLS
Lymphocytes and IgA-secreting plasma cells are closely associated with the bronchial glands, and lymphoid aggregations are common, being most evident at bifurcations. The larger lymphoid aggregates occur in the proximal part of the bronchial tree and may have germinal centres.

CARTILAGE
Bronchi of all sizes contain some cartilage, the most distal branches of the bronchial tree, which lack cartilage, being called bronchioles (see below).

The main extrapulmonary bronchi have regular incomplete cartilage rings like the trachea, but the intrapulmonary bronchi have an irregular roughly circumferential arrangement of cartilage plates connected by dense fibrocollagenous bands.

As the bronchi branch and get smaller and more peripheral, the cartilage plates decrease in size and number, and are mainly concentrated at bifurcations.

Bronchioles

Bronchioles (Fig. 9.11) are defined as distal airways located between the cartilage-walled bronchi and the site where the ciliated epithelium ceases. Goblet cells persist, but bronchioles do not contain seromucous glands.

The bronchioles branch repeatedly, and thereby reduce their luminal size. With the absence of cartilage, smooth muscle becomes a major component of their wall.

EPITHELIUM
Bronchioles are lined by ciliated columnar epithelium without pseudostratification, and the cells become lower and near cuboidal in the small peripheral branches. Occasional goblet cells persist, and an additional cell type, the Clara cell is found.

The **Clara cell** is neither ciliated nor apparently mucus-producing. It contains numerous mitochondria and abundant smooth endoplasmic reticulum near the luminal surface, which bulges above the level of adjacent ciliated cells; small electron-dense granules are also seen in the apical cytoplasm.

The function of Clara cells is not known, but they are rich in oxidative enzymes and lipoprotein, suggesting a role in surfactant production.

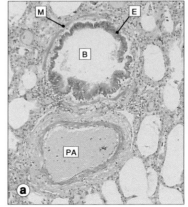
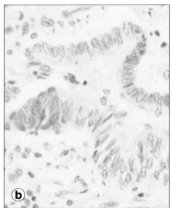

Fig. 9.11 Bronchiole.
a Micrograph of an H&E stained section showing a bronchiole (B) close to a pulmonary artery (PA) branch. The bronchiole does not contain cartilage in its wall, which is composed only of muscle (M). Its epithelium (E) is similar to bronchial epithelium.
b Micrograph showing part of a bronchiole wall from a newborn stained by an immunoperoxidase method for bombesin. This highlights in brown a cluster of neuroendocrine cells forming a so-called **neuroepithelial body**.

Terminal bronchioles

The final bifurcations of the bronchiolar tree produce **terminal bronchioles**, which are the smallest bronchioles concerned solely with air conduction.

DISTAL RESPIRATORY TRACT

The passages of the respiratory tract discussed above end in the terminal bronchiole and both transport and warm air from the outside environment. They also remove foreign particles (dust, bacteria, etc.) by a combination of mucus entrapment and ciliary action.

The terminal bronchiole leads into the distal respiratory tree, which is concerned with gaseous exchange. The first element of this system is the respiratory bronchiole.

Respiratory bronchioles

Respiratory bronchioles are lined by cuboidal ciliated epithelium, which merges with the flattened epithelium lining ill-defined conduits outlined by a spiral of smooth muscle (**alveolar ducts**). The walls of these ducts are composed largely of the openings of laterally disposed air sacs (**alveoli**). Each alveolar duct terminates in two or three **alveolar sacs** formed from the confluence of the openings of several alveoli (Fig. 9.12a).

Alveoli

Alveoli are air sacs and are the main site of gaseous exchange. They number 200–600 million in each normal healthy lung, and provide an enormous surface area (estimated at 70–80 m²) for gaseous exchange.

Each alveolus is a polygonal air space with a thin wall, which contains pulmonary capillaries and forms the air–blood barrier (see Fig. 9.14).

Most alveoli open into an alveolar sac, or into an alveolar duct, but a few open directly into a respiratory bronchiole. Pores (of Kohn) permit communication between adjacent alveoli.

The cellular components of the alveoli are type 1 and type 2 pneumocytes, which lie on the alveolar basement membrane, and alveolar macrophages (Fig.9.12b).

TYPE 1 PNEUMOCYTES
Type 1 pneumocytes represent about 40% of the alveolar cell population, but form most (i.e. 90%) of the lining to the alveolar sacs and alveoli.

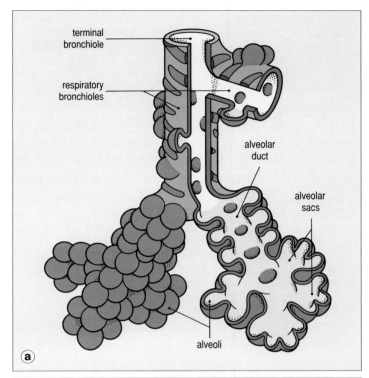

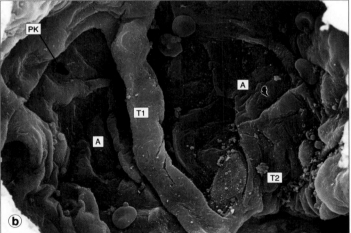

Fig. 9.12 Distal respiratory tree.
a Diagram showing the relationships between the terminal bronchiole, respiratory bronchiole, alevolar ducts, alveolar sacs and alveoli.
b Low power scanning electronmicrograph of an alveolar sac looking into two of the alveoli (A) that open into it. The two alveoli are separated by a wall, which is covered by type 1 pneumocyte cytoplasm (TI). On the left is a pore of Kohn (PK), and a round type 2 pneumocyte (T2) can be seen in the right alveolus.

Type 1 pneumocytes are attenuated flat cells with greatly flattened nuclei, and are joined together by tight junctions (see page 28). They contain scanty mitochondria and organelles, and their cytoplasm provides a very thin covering to the alveolar basement membrane, its thinness contributing to the efficiency of the air–blood barrier (see Fig. 9.14).

TYPE 2 PNEUMOCYTES

Type 2 pneumocytes represent 60% of the alveolar cell population numerically, but occupy very little (5–10%) of the alveolar surface, being larger rounded cells, which are commonly located in obtuse angles in the polygonal alveolus.

Type 2 pneumocyte nuclei are round and dark-staining, and their cytoplasm is rich in mitochondria, and both rough and smooth endoplasmic reticulum. They also contain electron-dense vesicles and large spherical bodies of lamellated material, which is composed of phospholipid, protein and glycosaminoglycans, and forms the basis of pulmonary surfactant. The granular surfactant material is extruded from their multilamellar bodies through their microvillar luminal surface (Fig. 9.13).

When the alveolar epithelium is exposed to certain toxic agents, particularly if there is extensive destruction of type 1 pneumocytes, type 2 pneumocytes increase in size and number; it is believed that some type 2 cells act as precursor stem cells for type 1 pneumocytes.

ALVEOLAR MACROPHAGES

Alveolar macrophages lie on top of the alveolar lining cells and may be seen apparently free in the alveolar space. They may contain phagocytosed material.

Alveolar macrophages patrol the alveolar air spaces and the interalveolar septa (interstitium, Fig. 9.14) passing freely between the two. They phagocytose inhaled debris (e.g. fine dust, including carbon) and bacteria, and are an important defence mechanism.

The macrophages then enter the respiratory and terminal bronchioles, where they either pass into lymphatic vessels and hence become transported to regional lymph nodes, or they adhere to the ciliated mucus-coated epithelium, which is the first step on the mucus/cilia escalator. This eventually carries them up to the trachea and main bronchi, from which they are cleared in the mucus by coughing. Alternatively the macrophages may remain in the interstitium.

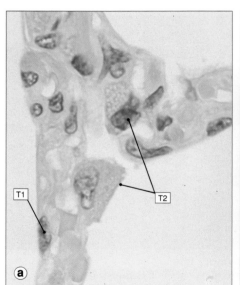
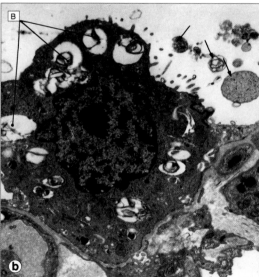
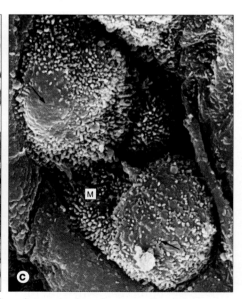

Fig. 9.13 Type 2 pneumocyte and surfactant.

a An H&E stained thin acrylic resin section showing the confluence of the alveolar walls of three adjacent alveoli. In the angles are rounded cells with vacuolated cytoplasm; these are type 2 pneumocytes (T2). The nucleus of a type 1 pneumocyte (T1) is also seen.

b Electronmicrograph showing an active type 2 pneumocyte. The cell is round, and has a convex luminal face, which is covered with microvilli. The most obvious intracytoplasmic organelles are large membrane-bound spherical bodies (B) containing lamellated lipoprotein material, which represents the surfactant substance. These can often be seen discharging their contents onto the luminal surface (arrows).

c Scanning electronmicrograph of two type 2 pneumocytes. Note the microvilli (M), and small amounts of granular material (arrow), which is recently disgorged surfactant.

Elastin

An important component of the alveolar wall is elastic tissue (see Fig. 4.8), which is present as coarse and fine fibres (see Fig. 9.14c).

Elastin has remarkable properties of stretch and recoil (see page 45), and has three important functions in the alveolar walls.

• It allows the lungs to stretch to accommodate the inhaled air.

• It allows air to be expelled from the alveoli by recoiling.

• It acts as a spring, tethering the soft-walled bronchioles, which contain no cartilage, to the lung parenchyma, and indirectly to the pleura, thus preventing bronchiolar and alveolar collapse during exhalation.

Gaseous exchange

Gaseous exchange occurs across the air–blood barrier, oxygen diffusing from the alveolar cavity into the blood to become linked to red cell haemoglobin, and carbon dioxide diffusing from the blood into the alveolar air.

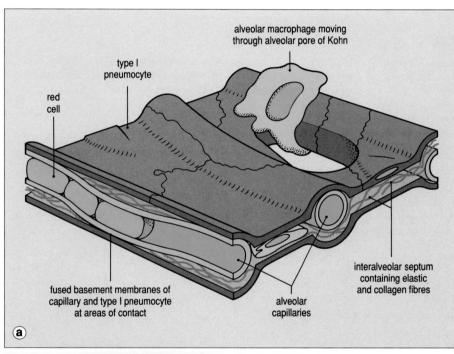

alveolar macrophage moving through alveolar pore of Kohn

type I pneumocyte

red cell

fused basement membranes of capillary and type I pneumocyte at areas of contact

alveolar capillaries

interalveolar septum containing elastic and collagen fibres

(a)

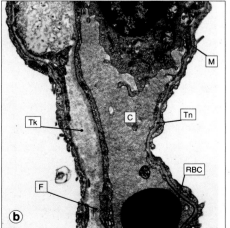

(b)

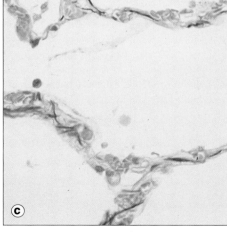

(c)

Fig. 9.14 Interalveolar septum and air–blood barrier.

a Diagram of the interalveolar septum showing the pulmonary capillaries (C) coursing through the alveolar wall, sometimes in close contact with one wall, then the other.

Each capillary is closely opposed to two alveolar cavities, and is therefore located in the interalveolar septum or interstitium. Where the capillary contacts the alveolar wall its basement membrane appears to fuse with that of the alveolar wall.

Parts of the interalveolar septum not occupied by the capillary contain fine collagen and elastic fibres, together with some fibroblasts and macrophages.

Thus, in some places the capillary is in direct contact with the alveolar wall (thin part), but in others is separated from it by cells and fibres (thick part). The thin part is the site of gas exchange and the thick part is where liquids can move between the air spaces and the interstitium.

Macrophages move freely from alveolus to alveolus through the pores of Kohn.

b Transmission electronmicrograph through the alveolar wall. It is largely occupied by a capillary (C) containing a red blood cell (RBC) and a monocyte (M). The monocyte will leave the capillary and ultimately enter the alveolar lumen to become an alveolar macrophage. Note the thin (Tn) and thick (Tk) parts of the alveolar wall.

Both sides of the alveolar wall are covered by a thin layer of type 1 pneumocyte cytoplasm. In the thick part, between type 1 pneumocyte cytoplasm and the capillary wall, there are collagen and elastic fibres (F).

c High magnification micrograph of elastic Van Gieson stained alveolar wall to show its dark elastic fibre content. Yellow staining red blood cells within alveolar capillaries are also evident.

INTERSTITIAL FIBROSIS

In some lung diseases, the fibroblasts in the interalveolar septum or interstitium increase in number and secrete excess collagen and elastin. This results in fibrocollagenous thickening of the septa (**interstital fibrosis**).

Interstitial fibrosis increases the rigidity of the lung and limits expansion, but most importantly impairs gaseous exchange because the presence of collagen fibres between the capillary and alveolar walls ruins their intimate contact.

CHRONIC OBSTRUCTIVE AIRWAYS DISEASE

The most common lung disease in the Western world is **chronic obstructive airways disease**, which is characterized by difficulty in getting air into and out of the distal respiratory tree.

There are three main disease processes causing chronic obstructive airways disease: **asthma**, **chronic bronchitis**, and **emphysema**. These conditions may be present alone or more commonly in combination.

Asthma

Asthma is caused by a combination of bronchoconstriction and excessive production of particularly viscid mucus, both of which obstruct the airways. Repeated attacks of asthma lead to permanent thickening of the muscle layers in the walls of the airways.

Chronic bronchitis

In chronic bronchitis, the bronchial walls are thickened by a combination of muscle layer thickening, inflammation and scarring of the submucosa, and increase in number and size of the mucous glands. These changes are the end result of repeated episodes of infection or inhaled toxins.

Emphysema

Emphysema is caused by destruction of the walls of the alveolar ducts, sacs and alveoli (Fig. 9.15).This leads to loss of the elastic

support for the bronchioles, and results in their collapse, particularly during exhalation, and air trapping, as air is unable to pass the obstructed lumen.

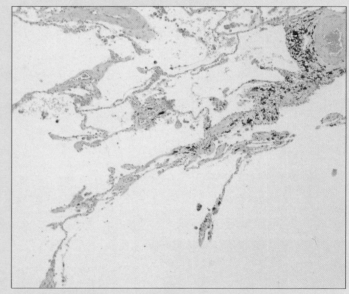

Fig 9.15 Emphysema.
Micrograph of lung from a patient with severe emphysema, showing extensive destruction of the alveolar walls. Compare with Fig. 9.14 c

PULMONARY VASCULATURE

The lungs have a dual blood supply and venous drainage, which is provided by the pulmonary and bronchial arteries and veins.

Pulmonary arteries

The pulmonary arteries supply the lung with relatively deoxygenated blood from the right side of the heart. Such blood has supplied the tissues with oxygen and received carbon dioxide (see Fig. 8.1).

The pulmonary arteries enter their respective lung at the hilum and closely follow the course of the adjacent bronchus and its branches, dividing more or less with the bronchi. Eventually the vessels culminate in the extensive intimate capillary network in the interalveolar septa (see Fig.9.14).

The capillary network empties its reoxygenated blood into pulmonary venules and veins, which eventually convey the blood to the left side of the heart for distribution to other organs.

As the pulmonary arterial and venous system is a low pressure system (i.e. pulmonary artery systolic pressure is 25 mm Hg, whereas systemic arterial systolic pressure is 110–135 mmg Hg), the structure of its vessels differ considerably from those of the systemic circulation (see page 113).

Microanatomy

ELASTIC ARTERIES
From their origin at the pulmonary valve ring to the intrapulmonary branches at the level where the bronchi lose their cartilage plates to become bronchioles, the pulmonary arteries are elastic arteries (see page 114), and are structured as outlined below (Fig. 9.16).
• A narrow intima is composed of a single layer of endothelium and lies almost directly on the innermost layer of the media, from which it is separated by scanty collagen fibrils and myofibroblasts.
• The media is composed of many layers of elastic fibres, which are irregular and fragmented in the pulmonary trunk and main pulmonary arteries, but more regular and intact in the peripheral branches. Between the elastic fibres are smooth muscle cells and some collagen.
• The elastic laminae are composed of longitudinally running fibres that form interlinked flat strands of varying

breadth. This particular orientation is probably an adaptation to counteract the stretching forces during lung expansion. In the aorta, which is exposed to circumferential stretch during systole, the elastic fibres are circumferential.

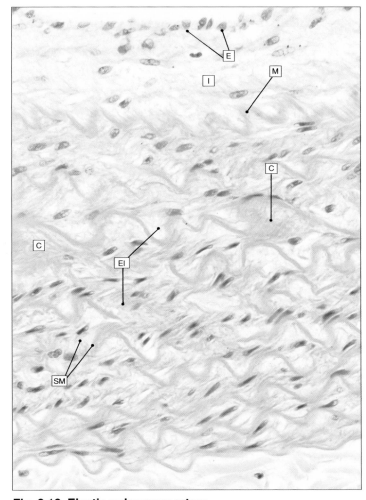

Fig. 9.16 Elastic pulmonary artery.
Micrograph of an elastic pulmonary artery from a child. Note the endothelium (E), the scanty myofibroblasts (M) in the narrow intima (I), the thick media composed of fairly regularly organized alternating lamellae of elastic fibres (El) and intervening smooth muscle cells (SM) and collagen (C). The elastic is easily seen in this H&E section because the lamellae are so thick.

MUSCULAR ARTERIES

At about the bronchial/bronchiolar junction, the medial elastic laminae largely disappear, and the arteries become muscular arteries (Fig. 9.17). These arteries continue to follow the bronchioles as far as the terminal and respiratory bronchioles, but also give off supernumerary arteries as side branches.

The media of the muscular pulmonary artery is composed largely of circularly orientated smooth muscle, and occasional collagen and elastic fibres. The organized laminated elastic tissue is confined to distinct internal and external elastic laminae (see page 115).

Continuous branching of the muscular pulmonary arteries produces progressively smaller vessels with narrower bores and thinner walls, because of diminishing smooth muscle in the media. The muscle layer becomes discontinuous, and finally disappears, the vessel then being called a **pulmonary arteriole**.

Arterioles are difficult to distinguish from venules. The alveolar capillaries are discussed in Fig. 9.14.

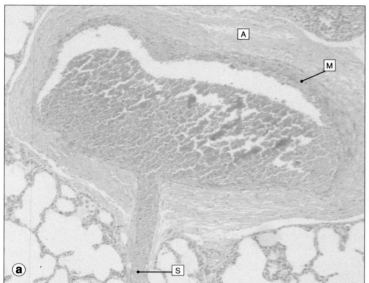

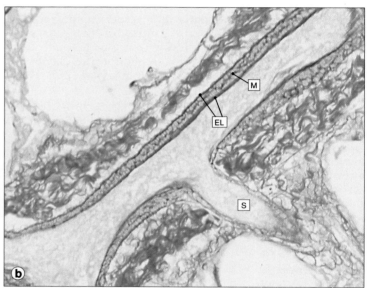

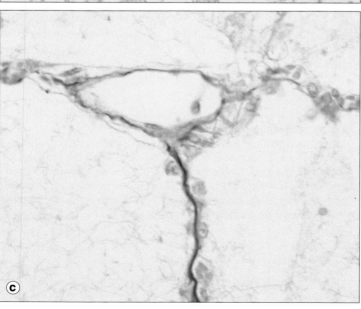

Fig. 9.17 Muscular pulmonary artery.
a Micrograph of muscular pulmonary artery stained with H&E. Note the media (M) and adventitia (A). A small supernumerary artery (S) arises as a direct side branch.
b Micrograph of a smaller muscular pulmonary artery stained by the elastic Van Gieson method to show the media (M) lying between two distinct dark-staining elastic laminae (EL). In addition to giving off a lateral supernumerary branch (S), this artery is bifurcating into two vessels with less well-formed arterial walls.
c Micrograph showing a small pulmonary arteriole. This is a thin walled vessel resembling a small pulmonary artery from which the muscular media between the two elastic laminae has disappeared. Transitional vessels with only an occasional remnant of the spirally arranged muscular media can sometimes be identified.

Pulmonary veins

Oxygenated blood from the alveolar capillaries enters small venules composed of a thin intima lying on a narrow zone of collagen and elastic fibres. These small tributaries fuse to form larger venules, which run in the fibrocollagenous septa and are associated with increasing numbers of myofibroblasts and smooth muscle cells in the media (Fig. 9.18).

Larger veins have a distinct media with a variably continuous internal elastic lamina and irregularly arranged smooth muscle fibres.

The largest veins have a media in which elastic fibres are irregularly interspersed with collagen and smooth muscle fibres, rather than confined to clearly defined elastic laminae.

Age-related variations in pulmonary vessels

Pulmonary vasculature varies considerably at the extremes of age.

Before birth, the pulmonary vasculature is barely perfused because of the bypass through the patent foramen ovale and ductus arteriosus. Thus, the muscular pulmonary arteries have a small lumen, large endothelial cells and a thick media. In addition there are small bundles of longitudinally running smooth muscle fibres in the intima.

These features change progressively to the adult pattern in the first few weeks of life, and new supernumerary arteries develop.

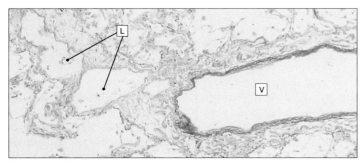

Fig. 9.18 Pulmonary vein.
Pulmonary veins (V) are thin-walled vessels, which run in the fibrocollagenous septa with pulmonary lymphatics (L). Small venules resemble pulmonary arterioles, but the larger veins contain collagen and elastic fibres, as well as smooth muscle, outside the basement membrane.

The smooth muscle cells and elastic fibres are haphazardly arranged, but in large pulmonary veins the elastic fibres may form an interrupted or continuous elastic lamina. There are no valves in pulmonary veins of any size.

In old age, the veins and muscular pulmonary arteries thicken as a result of irregular fibrocollagenous thickening of the intima.

Bronchial arteries

The bronchial arteries are direct lateral branches of the thoracic aorta, and perfuse the lung at systemic arterial pressure to provide it with oxygenated blood.

The bronchial arteries follow the course of the bronchial tree and its branches to the level of the respiratory bronchioles, where they anastomose with the pulmonary artery branches. They also communicate with the pulmonary artery system by capillary anastomoses in the bronchial submucosa.

Microanatomy

In children, the bronchial arteries are histologically similar to other systemic muscular arteries (see page 115). They have a muscular media and a distinct internal elastic lamina, but no cohesive external elastic lamina (Fig. 9.19a).

In adults, the bronchial arteries develop longitudinally running smooth muscle fibres arranged in small bundles in the intima. These are particularly prominent in some forms of chronic lung disease, but are found from about 20 years of age in normal healthy individuals (Fig. 9.19b).

Bronchial veins

There are numerous anastomoses between the bronchial and pulmonary veins, the bronchial veins running with the bronchial arteries in the adventitia of the airways. The bronchial veins drain into the azygos and hemiazygos veins.

Lymphatic drainage

There is no lymphatic drainage from the alveolar air sacs and interalveolar septa, any fluid in the air spaces being absorbed into the interstitium through the thick part of the alveolar wall. This fluid diffuses proximally in the interstitium until it enters small lymphatics at about the level of the respiratory bronchioles.

The small lymphatics merge to form larger vessels that follow the bronchial tree proximally as far as the lung hilum, draining into a series of peribronchial lymph nodes on the way.

Another system of lymphatics runs in the visceral pleura and fibrocollagenous septa that divide the lung parenchyma into discrete lobules; such peripheral pleural lymphatics drain directly into the pleural space.

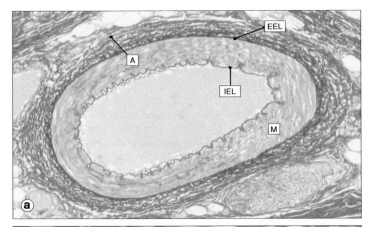

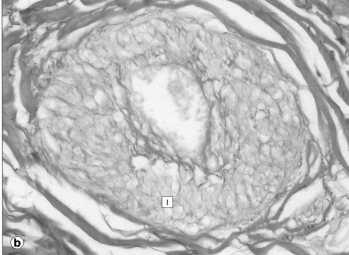

Fig. 9.19 Bronchial artery.
a Low magnification micrograph of a bronchial artery from a 2-year-old child stained by the elastic Van Gieson (EVG) method to show its muscular media (M) between the internal and external layers of elastic lamina (IEL and EEL). It is very similar to a normal systemic muscular artery and has a fibrocollagenous adventitial layer (A).
b High magnification micrograph of a bronchial artery from a healthy 50-year-old man stained by the EVG method. It shows marked hypertrophy of the intima (I) by longitudinal smooth muscle cells (yellow).

PLEURA

The lungs are contained within the thoracic cavity, which is capable of increasing and decreasing its size by intercostal muscle relaxation and contraction. The internal lining of the thoracic cavity and the outer surface of the contained lungs are smooth, low-friction surfaces bathed with a small amount of lubricant fluid. These surfaces are the pleurae.

Visceral pleura

The outer surface of the lungs is the visceral pleura, which is composed of the following five ill-defined layers.
• An outer layer of flat mesothelial cells.
• A narrow zone of loose fibrocollagenous tissue, with no identifiable basement membrane between this layer and the mesothelium.
• An irregular external elastic layer.
• An interstitial layer of loose fibrocollagenous stroma containing lymphatics, blood vessels and nerves, together with some smooth muscle fibres.
• An ill-defined internal elastic layer containing short lengths of elastic fibre, some of which merge with those of the interalveolar septa of the most peripheral alveolar groups.
These layers vary markedly from site to site (Fig. 9.20), and are particularly irregular in the region of a fibrocollagenous interlobular septum, the ill-defined elastic networks of the pleura often fusing into a single layer before extending partway into the septum.

Parietal pleura

Parietal pleura forms the internal lining of the thoracic cavity, and joins the visceral pleura at the hilum of each lung.
The structure of parietal pleura is similar to that of the visceral pleura, but simpler, with usually only one layer of elastic fibres.
Parietal pleura sits on a layer of adipose tissue beneath which is a layer of dense fibrocollagenous tissue. This fibrocollagenous tissue is continuous with the periosteum of the ribs and the perimysium of the intercostal muscles.

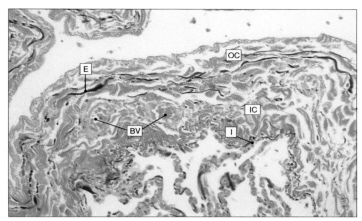

Fig. 9.20 Visceral pleura.
Visceral pleura stained by the elastic Van Gieson method to show its elastic (black) and collagen (red) content. The flat mesothelial cells on the surface cannot be identified, but the irregular external elastic layer (E) and ill-defined fragmented internal elastic layer (I) can be seen, as can the outer (OC) and interstitial (IC) collagenous layers, the latter containing blood vessels (BV).

PRACTICAL HISTOLOGY

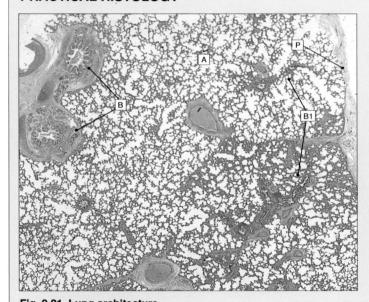

Fig. 9.21 Lung architecture.
Low power micrograph showing the general architecture of the lung of a child. Bronchi (B), bronchioles (B1), the alveolar network (A) and the outer covering of pleura (P) are indicated.

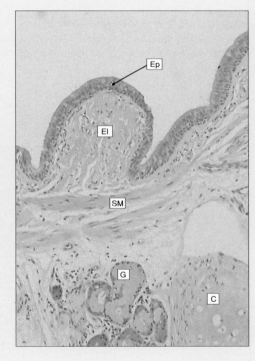

**Fig. 9.22
Bronchial wall.**
Medium power micrograph showing a segment of the bronchial wall. Note the pseudostratified ciliated columnar epithelium (Ep), longitudinally running bands of elastin (El), bands of smooth muscle (SM), seromucous glands (G) and an isolated island of cartilage (C).

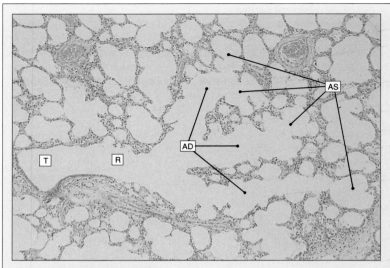

Fig. 9.23 Distal air passages.
Micrograph showing a terminal bronchiole (T) giving off a respiratory bronchiole (R), which has divided into three alveolar ducts (AD) with alveoli opening into them. They terminate in alveolar sacs (AS) into which a number of alveoli open directly.

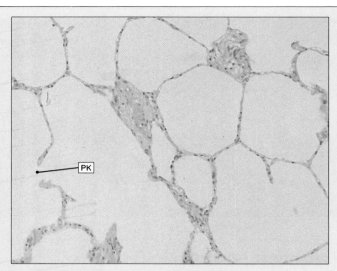

Fig. 9.24 Alveoli.
Micrograph showing the architecture of the alveolar sacs and alveoli. Note the pore of Kohn (PK), which is a communication between adjacent alveoli (see Fig. 9.14).

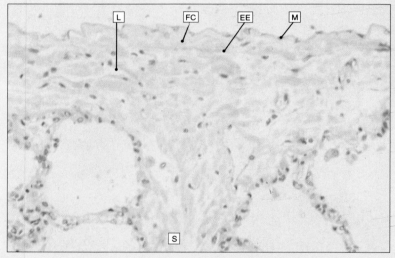

Fig. 9.25 Pleura.
Micrograph showing the visceral pleura. Its component layers described on page 140 are difficult to distinguish, but are more clearly seen if an elastic/collagen stain is used (see Fig. 9.20). Note the mesothelium (M), the narrow zone of fibrocollagenous tissue (FC), the irregular external elastic layer (EE), the lymphatic (L) and the fibrocollagenous interlobular septum (S).

10. ALIMENTARY TRACT

The alimentary tract is best considered as a muscular tube lined internally by an epithelium that varies in structure according to specialized functions required at particular sites along its length; with a few local variations, the structure of the musculature is similar throughout.

The function of the alimentary tract is to take in raw food material, and to fragment it into small portions. These are then acted upon by a series of secretions, mainly enzymes, which convert the large molecules into smaller molecules, thus permitting their absorption into the blood and lymph circulation.

The small molecules are mainly amino acids, small peptides, carbohydrates, sugars and lipids, which are transported by the blood and lymph, mainly to the liver, where they are used as the building blocks in the synthesis of essential proteins, carbohydrates and lipids.

The alimentary tract can be divided into three functional compartments.
• The **oral cavity and its contents** are responsible for ingestion and preliminary fragmentation of ingested food.
• **Simple passages** (i.e the oropharynx, oesophagus and anal canal) transport food or its residue from one part of the alimentary tract to another without significant metabolic activity.
• The **digestive tract** secretes enzymes and other substances involved in the breakdown of food, and absorbs the small molecules produced. It comprises the **stomach**, the **small intestine**, the **colon** and **rectum**.
    Secretory organs (i.e. the **liver**, **pancreas** and **salivary glands**) are glands located outside the alimentary tract, and disgorge their secretions into its lumen by long ducts. The liver performs numerous functions in addition to producing secretions to aid digestion and is discussed in detail in Chapter 11.

ORAL CAVITY AND ITS CONTENTS

The oral cavity communicates with the exterior at the oral orifice (the mouth). Here food enters the alimentary tract and undergoes preliminary fragmentation prior to its transmission to the first part of the digestive tract (i.e. the stomach).

In addition the food material is rendered moist by the secretion of the salivary glands, the moistening of the food facilitating fragmentation and subsequent swallowing.

General architecture

The wall of the oral cavity consists of three main layers.
• Stratified squamous epithelium, which is largely non-keratinizing, lines the cavity.
• A submucosa beneath the epithelium contains varying numbers of salivary glands, which can secrete both a serous and a mucus fluid
• Skeletal muscle fibres are common in the deeper layers and are responsible for altering the size and shape of the cavity, and for moving food.

One highly specialized area of the oral cavity is the **tongue**, which is a mobile muscular ingrowth from its floor. In addition to containing specialized taste receptors, it has a major function in the movement of food.

In some areas the deep tissues of the oral cavity consist of bone, either simple plates of bone (as in the **hard palate**), or modified bone (**teeth**). The immovable hard palate produces a rigid structure against which the tongue can move, while the teeth, which are embedded in bone supports (the **mandibles** and **maxillae**) are the main tools for fragmenting ingested food.

Fragmented food and secretions are propelled backwards from the oral cavity to the opening of the oesophagus, through which they are transmitted to the stomach.

Variations

There are variations to the general structure described above as follows.

ORAL ORIFICE
The oral orifice is lined by **lips**, the external aspects of which are covered by hair-bearing skin, with sebaceous glands and eccrine sweat ducts. Between the hair-bearing outer surface and the moist, fluid-bathed inner surface is a transitional zone known as the **vermilion** because of its pinkish-red appearance. Here the epithelium is non-keratinizing stratified squamous with a prominent rete ridge system (see Chapter 19), and the papillae between the epithelial downgrowths contain prominent blood vessels, which are responsible for the colour.

The inner surface of the lips is lined by a non-keratinizing stratified squamous epithelium with a less well developed rete ridge system, and small clumps of salivary tissue disgorge their secretions onto its surface through short ducts. In addition, occasional sebaceous glands (**Fordyce spots**), which are particularly common near the angles of the mouth, open directly onto the mucosal surface rather than into a hair follicle as in the skin.

In the deeper parts of the lips, bundles of striated muscle fibres (**orbicularis oris muscle**) are arranged mainly in a concentric manner around the oral orifice; this muscle is responsible, amongst other things, for opening and closing the oral orifice.

CHEEKS

Cheeks are lined by thick non-keratinizing squamous epithelium, the cells of which are often rich in glycogen. Areas of keratinization are common, usually as a result of chronic friction from ill-fitting dentures or from persistent cheek biting. The submucosa contains minor salivary glands (**buccal glands**), and occasional sebaceous glands (Fordyce spots), while the deep tissues contain the skeletal muscle fibres of the cheek muscles (**buccinator**).

HARD PALATE

The hard palate is covered by a keratinizing stratified squamous epithelium with a prominent rete ridge system, and a submucosa rich in salivary gland tissue (**palatine salivary glands**). Beneath the salivary gland tissue, the submucosa is firmly tethered to the periosteum of the palatal bone plate.

ORAL SURFACE OF SOFT PALATE

The oral surface of the soft palate is covered with non-keratinizing stratified squamous epithelium, which extends onto its free posterior edge where there is a transition to the ciliated columnar epithelium covering the nasal surface. There are numerous small salivary glands in the submucosa of the oral aspect.

FLOOR OF THE MOUTH

The floor of the mouth is covered by thin non-keratinized stratified squamous epithelium, which is continuous with that of the ventral surface of the tongue.

This region is rich in salivary gland tissue, with many minor salivary glands in the floor of the mouth (**minor sublingual glands**), and larger glands situated on either side of the midline frenulum of the ventral surface of the tongue (**major sublingual glands**).

Tongue

The tongue is a highly muscular organ protruding upwards and forwards into the oral cavity from its floor.

The ventral surface of the tongue is covered by thin non-keratinizing stratified squamous epithelium continuous with that of the floor of the mouth. In contrast, the dorsal surface, which is commonly in contact with the hard palate during feeding, talking and at rest, is covered with a thick keratinizing stratified squamous epithelium, which shows considerable specialization.

Dorsal surface

The dorsal surface of the tongue is divided into an anterior two-thirds and a posterior one-third by a V-shaped line of 6–10 dome-shaped protrusions, the **circumvallate papillae** (Fig. 10.1).

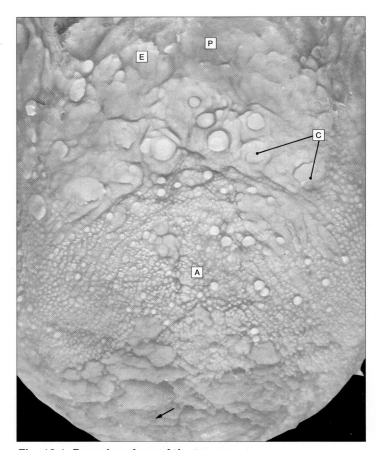

Fig. 10.1 Dorsal surface of the tongue.
The dorsal surface of the tongue can be divided into a posterior third (P) with smooth dome-shaped elevations (E), and an anterior two-thirds (A) by a V-shaped line of circumvallate papillae (C). The surface of the anterior two-thirds is roughened by the presence of small filiform and fungiform papillae and by a surface keratin layer. In places the surface keratin may become thick and stained by food (coated tongue, arrow), particularly in the elderly (as here), and contain numerous bacterial colonies.

NATURE OF THE IMMUNE RESPONSE

Antigen-presenting cells

Antigen-presenting cells (APCs) phagocytose antigenic material, process it, and present fragments to lymphocytes, and have several common attributes.

- They are monocyte-derived and express markers of white cell lineage (leukocyte common antigen).
- They have fine ramifying cytoplasmic processes, which increase the surface area of cell membrane interacting with other cells and antigen, and give rise to their descriptive name dendritic antigen-presenting cells (see Fig. 7.3).
- Although actively pinocytotic, they have low levels of lysosomal enzymes, unlike other monocyte-derived cells specialized for phagocytosis.
- They have high levels of class II MHC molecules (HLA-Dr), which is essential for presenting new antigen to T cells.

Cells that can be classified as dendritic APCs are:
- Langerhans' cells of the skin (see Fig. 19.9);
- dendritic reticulum cells of lymph nodes (see Fig. 7.3);
- interstitial dendritic cells, which form a population of dendritic cells in the support tissues of most organs;
- veiled cells of the blood, which are thought to be circulating forms of dendritic APCs in transit between tissues;
- microglia of the central nervous system (see Fig. 13.14).

Despite certain common attributes, each of these cell types is microenvironmentally specialized and each has slightly different cell surface receptors and proteins, which adapt them to antigen presentation in different sites.

In addition to this group of cells, which have a primary role in antigen presentation, several other cells can present antigen, particularly the nonspecific phagocytic macrophages.

NATURE OF THE IMMUNE RESPONSE

The production of an immune response depends on close interaction between the cells of the immune system. This preferentially takes place in specialized tissues and organs of the immune system, particularly lymph nodes and spleen, which contain structures to facilitate such interaction.

Activation of the immune system

An immune response is initiated when antigen interacts with lymphocytes; this usually involves antigen-presenting cells.

Processing by APC. Antigen is taken into an APC and partially fragmented. It is then bound to one of the class of histocompatability antigens termed an HLA protein, and transported to the cell surface. Here the HLA protein is incorporated into the cell membrane, so that a large part of the molecule, including the bound antigenic peptide, is exposed.

When the processed antigen meets a mature T cell bearing an appropriate receptor, it activates the T cell, the nature of the T cell response depending on whether the processed antigen is bound to HLA of class I or II. HLA class I proteins interact with CD8-bearing T cells, while HLA class II proteins interact with CD4-bearing T cells.

Thus antigenic peptides bound to class II HLA molecules produce a TH cell response, which is then available to help B cells respond to the same antigen.

The architecture of lymphoid tissues and the routes of circulation of T cells are designed to ensure that as many lymphocytes as possible come into contact with a potential antigen.

Direct interaction with B cells. Rarely, B cells may interact directly with a protein or polysaccharide antigen that has a repeating chemical structure (e.g. the polysaccharide coat of bacteria such as pneumococcus). There are however few antigens of this type.

Antigen synthesized within a cell. Antigen synthesized within a cell (e.g. tumour cell, cell infected by a virus) may be incorporated into the cell membrane bound to a class I HLA protein where it can be recognized by CD8-bearing T cells.

Immunological memory

When activated lymphocytes proliferate during an immune response, some of the cells mature to become memory T and B cells. These lymphocytes have a similar appearance to inactive naïve lymphocytes, but have already been adapted to recognize a specific antigen, and respond rapidly to the antigen by proliferation and activation on re-exposure.

B memory cells are known to have higher affinity receptors (surface immunoglobulin) for antigen than naïve B cells and produce IgG earlier in the response.

Memory cells circulate in the blood and lymphatics, and also reside in the specialized lymphoid organs.

Low smooth dome-shaped elevations of the covering epithelium of the posterior third of the tongue are due to lymphoid tissue (the **lingual tonsillar tissue**) in the submucosa (Fig. 10.2).

PAPILLAE

The surface epithelium of the anterior two-thirds of the tongue is raised in a series of elevations called papillae; the three types in man are circumvallate, filiform and fungiform.

Circumvallate papillae are the largest in size and smallest in number, and appear as flattened domes, the bases of which are depressed below the dorsal surface.

Each circumvallate papilla is surrounded by a narrow moat-like channel, in the epithelium of which are numerous taste buds. These taste buds are thought to detect bitter taste. Small salivary glands discharge their secretions into the channels (Fig. 10.3).

Filiform papillae are the most numerous papillae and are found all over the dorsum of the tongue. They are tall, narrow and pointed (Fig. 10.4) and are keratinized, particularly at their tips. Filiform papillae contain no identifiable taste buds.

Fungiform papillae (Fig. 10.4) are scattered apparently randomly among the filiform papillae on the dorsal surface of the tongue, and have a mushroom shape.

Taste buds are present in their covering epithelium, those at the anterior tip of the tongue detecting sweet taste, and those just behind the tip and partway along the lateral borders detecting salty taste.

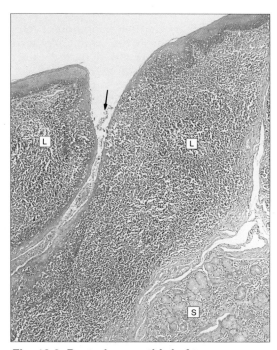

Fig. 10.2 Posterior one-third of tongue.
The posterior third of the tongue is characterized by the presence of lymphoid tissue (L), forming the lingual tonsillar tissue.

As in the palatine tonsils, it is penetrated by cleft-like downgrowths of the epithelium (arrow). Salivary glands (S) are numerous, particularly in the anterior portion near the line of circumvallate papillae.

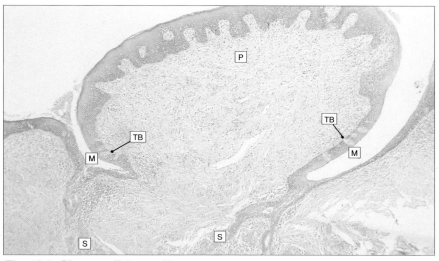

Fig. 10.3 Circumvallate papilla.
The circumvallate papilla (P) is surrounded by a moat (M) into the bottom of which empty prominent salivary glands (S). Taste buds (TB) are particularly numerous in the walls of the moat.

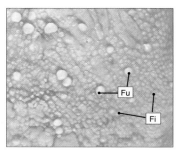

Fig. 10.4 Fungiform and filiform papillae.
Photograph of part of the dorsal surface of the anterior two-thirds of the tongue showing the gross appearance of the mushroom-like fungiform papillae (Fu) and the smaller filiform papillae (Fi).

TASTE BUDS

The taste buds of the dorsal tongue (Fig. 10.5) detect only acid, sweet, bitter, and salty, and provide early warning that food may be unpalatable. Appreciation of more subtle flavours depends on the smell receptors in the nose (see page 126).

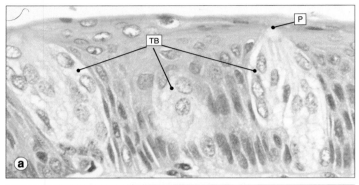

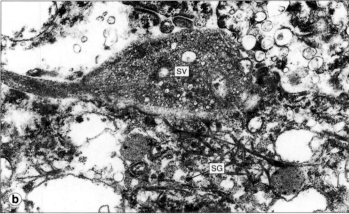

Fig. 10.5 Taste buds in circumvallate papilla.
a Each taste bud (TB) occupies the full-thickness of the epithelium and comprises pale staining spindle-shaped cells. The luminal surfaces of the cells open into a small defect in the epithelium, the taste pore (P), and each cell bears a number of microvilli.
b Ultrastructurally, some of the spindle-shaped cells have synaptic vesicles (SV) and are associated with small afferent nerve fibres, these are the taste receptor cells.

Other cells with more electron-dense cytoplasm and scanty secretory granules (SG) near the luminal surface are thought to act mainly as supporting sustentacular cells, but may also secrete glycosaminoglycans into the taste pore.

There are also cells resembling the taste receptor cells, but lacking the synaptic vesicles and afferent nerve connections. The turnover of these cells is rapid, (every 10–14 days), so there is a population of small rounded stem cells at the base of each taste bud, from which the other cell types derive.

Musculature

The musculature of the tongue comprises a complex pattern of skeletal muscle fibres running in bands longitudinally, vertically, transversely and obliquely, with a variable amount of adipose tissue in between (Fig. 10.6a).

This arrangement gives the tongue great mobility to manipulate food around the mouth for efficient fragmentation, and for moving fragmented food backwards prior to swallowing; it also provides the fine control of tongue movement that is essential for speech.

Abundant islands of salivary tissue are present in the submucosa between the muscular core of the tongue and the surface epithelium in the region of the junction between the posterior one-third and anterior two-thirds. Some of the deeper salivary gland collections extend down into the superficial parts of the muscular zone (Fig. 10.6b)

Teeth

The main task of the oral cavity, the fragmentation of large food masses, is performed by the teeth, which are hard, heavily mineralized structures embedded in the raised alveolar ridges of the maxilla and mandible.

Teeth are arranged so that the free surface of those embedded in the mandible (lower teeth) oppose and contact those in the maxilla (upper teeth), allowing food material to be trapped between them.

The anterior teeth (incisor and canine teeth) have narrow chisel-shaped or pointed free edges for chopping

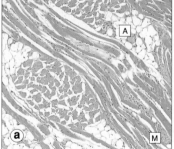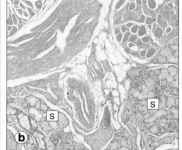

Fig. 10.6 Musculature of tongue.
a In the anterior two-thirds of the tongue the striated muscle bundles (M) are tightly packed with relatively little intervening adipose tissue (A). Note that the muscle bundles run in many directions. In the bulkier, less mobile posterior third, the adipose tissue is more abundant.
b Collections of salivary glands (S) are numerous in the submucosa and muscular core of the posterior tongue, particularly close to the junction between the posterior third and anterior two-thirds.

food into medium-sized pieces, whilst the posterior teeth (premolars and molars) have broader, flatter, free surfaces for grinding medium-sized food pieces into smaller fragments.

The mandible is joined to the body of the skull by the temporomandibular joint, which permits the mandible to slide backwards and forwards, and from side to side, thus aiding the grinding of food between the broad surfaces of the opposing molar teeth.

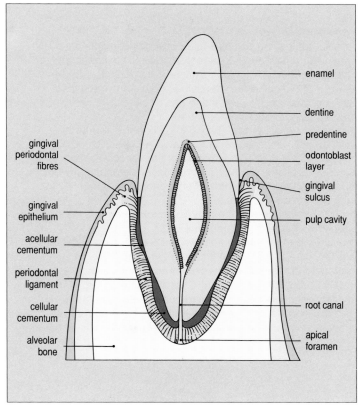

Fig. 10.7 Mature incisor tooth.
The central pulp cavity, the outer layer of which contains cells that produce the specialized extracellular matrix components of the teeth, is surrounded by dentine, a relatively acellular mineralized material forming the bulk of each tooth.

The dentine of the crown of the tooth is covered by enamel, a heavily mineralized material forming a resistant outer coat. At the neck of the tooth, enamel is continuous with cementum. This is a bone-like material forming an outer coat to the dentine in the root. Cementum is linked to the alveolar bone of the mandible or maxilla by the periodontal ligament, which is composed of tightly packed collagen fibres embedded at one end into the cementum of the tooth and at the other end into the bone forming the tooth socket.

Each tooth can be divided into two anatomical components, the crown and the root.
• The **crown** protrudes into the oral cavity.
• The **root** is embedded in the bone of the mandible or maxilla.

The junction between the crown and the root is called the **neck**. The mature tooth has five components: the central pulp cavity, dentine, enamel, cementum and periodontal ligament (Fig. 10.7).

Central pulp cavity

The **pulp cavity** is the soft central core of the tooth and approximates in shape to that of the tooth as a whole. It contains collagen and fibroblasts embedded in an acellular matrix composed of glycosaminoglycans.

Through the pulp cavity run the blood vessels that nourish the odontoblasts (see below) and the nerve twigs that provide dental sensation. These vessels and nerves enter and leave through a small apical foramen at the tip of the root.

The pulp cavity is narrow throughout most of the root (the root canal), but is expanded in the neck and crown (the pulp chamber). Its outer surface is lined by odontoblasts, which continually produce dentine. As dentine is progressively laid down, the pulp cavity diminishes in size.

Dentine

Dentine is a heavily calcified material composed of:
• inorganic calcium salts in the form of crystalline hydroxyapatite (about 70–80%);
• organic material in the form of the fine cytoplasmic processes of the odontoblasts, and the type 1 collagen fibres and glycosaminoglycans that they produce (about 20–30%).

Dentine is initally laid down as a glycosaminoglycan matrix in which collagen fibres are linearly arranged. This non-mineralized **predentine** is synthesized by odontoblasts located at the outer limits of the pulp cavity (Fig. 10.8).

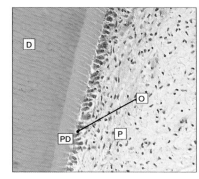

Fig. 10.8 Dentine, predentine and odontoblasts.
Micrograph showing pulp cavity (P) lined externally by a layer of odontoblasts (O), external to which is a pale staining band of predentine (PD). The outer layer is mineralized dentine (D), in which a pattern of dentinal tubules can be seen.

ODONTOBLASTS AND DENTINOGENESIS

Odontoblasts are tall columnar cells with nuclei arranged basally near the pulp cavity and their long cell bodies lying in neat palisades towards the forming predentine. Their cytoplasm is rich in rough endoplasmic reticulum and contains a prominent Golgi.

At the dentinal border, the odontoblasts terminate in long cytoplasmic processes, the odontoblast processes, which extend into the layers of predentine and dentine, running in parallel narrow channels, the **dentinal tubules.**

The dentinal tubules (and the odontoblast processes that they contain) are most broad near their origin at the odontoblast–predentine border, and become progressively narrower, terminating in fine branches near the junction between the dentine and enamel. The broad base of the odontoblast process contains secretory granules, vesicles and microfilaments.

Odontoblasts synthesize new predentine at the inner surface of the pulp cavity (Figs 10.9 & 10.10), and the cavity slowly decreases in size throughout life.

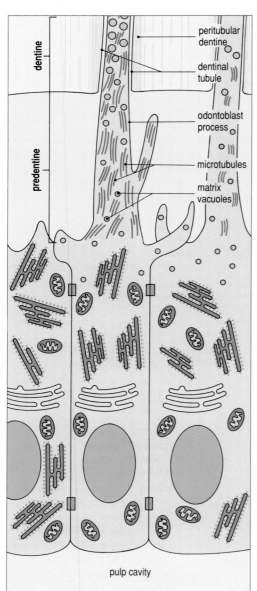

dentine

predentine

peritubular dentine

dentinal tubule

odontoblast process

microtubules

matrix vacuoles

pulp cavity

Fig. 10.9 Odontoblasts and dentinogenesis.
The functioning odontoblast is a tall narrow cell, the base of which contacts cells and fibres of the pulp cavity (mainly fibroblasts and collagen). Its nucleus is basal, and its cytoplasm is rich in mitochondria and rough endoplasmic reticulum. It has a large supranuclear Golgi. At the apex of the cell, the cytoplasm is drawn out into a long odontoblast process, which runs through the predentine and dentine layers in the dentinal tubule, while small side branches penetrate the predentine.

The cytoplasm of the odontoblast process and its branches contains numerous microtubules as well as small matrix vacuoles, which contain Ca^{2+} and PO_4^{2-} ions.

Dentinogenesis commences with the formation of predentine by odontoblasts. In predentine, randomly scattered collagen fibres (type 1 collagen) produced by the odontoblast are embedded in an extracellular matrix of phosphoprotein and glycosaminoglycans (mainly chondroitin-6-sulphate).

Mineralization is initiated by the discharge of the matrix vacuoles from the odontoblast process and its branches running through the predentine layer.

Some time after its formation, predentine becomes mineralized at its border with previously mineralized dentine; close to this predentine–dentine border the collagen fibres of predentine become more numerous and tightly packed. The dentine lining the dentinal tubules (peritubular dentine) is particularly compact and heavily mineralized.

In man, the odontoblast cytoplasmic processes extend only 25–50 % of the full length of the dentinal tubule, thus dentine close to the dentine–enamel border appears to contain empty tubules. In life these empty tubules may contain fluid, which is lost during tissue processing.

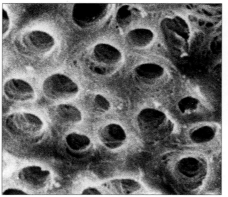

Fig. 10.10 Dentinal tubules.
Scanning electronmicrograph of dentine at a point well distant from the predentine layer. The mineral material contains regular empty dentinal tubules because the cytoplasmic processes of the odontoblasts extend only a short way into the tubules. Note the more compact dentine lining the tubules.

148

Enamel

Enamel is the hardest material in the body. It is composed almost entirely of the mineral hydroxyapatite ($Ca_{10}(PO_4)_6(OH)_2$), which is arranged in tightly packed hexagonal **enamel rods or prisms** (Fig. 10.11) about 4 μm in diameter, although some may measure up to 8 μm.

AMELOBLASTS AND ENAMEL FORMATION

Each enamel rod extends through the full thickness of the enamel. The small interstices between adjacent rods are occupied by hydroxyapatite crystals. A small amount of organic matrix (protein and polysaccharide) represents the remnants of the matrix synthesized and excreted by the enamel-producing cells, the **ameloblasts**, prior to mineralization of the enamel (Fig. 10.12).

Enamel is formed during tooth development by the ameloblasts, which degenerate when the tooth erupts, after which time the enamel cannot be replaced by new synthesis.

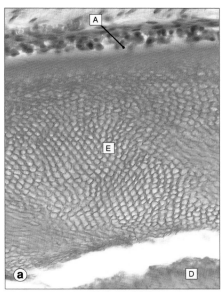

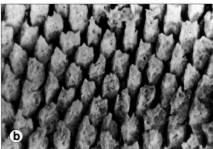

Fig. 10.11 Enamel.
a H&E stained section of early forming enamel (E), being produced by a layer of ameloblasts (A). The enamel shows a distinctive pattern due to the arrangement of enamel prisms, and abuts the dentine (D).
b Scanning electronmicrograph showing the characteristic arrangement of tightly packed enamel prisms or rods.

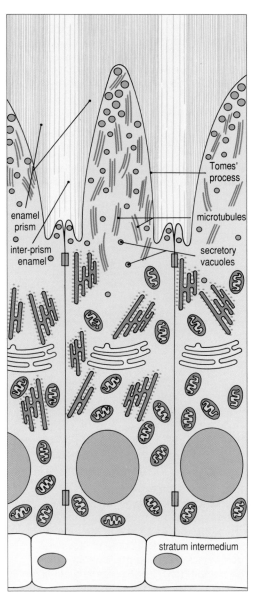

Fig. 10.12 Ameloblasts and enamel formation.
The functioning ameloblast is a tall narrow cell, with its base attached to the cells of the stratum intermedium. The nucleus is located basally and basal cytoplasm contains abundant mitochondria. The supranuclear cytoplasm contains a large, active Golgi and abundant rough endoplasmic reticulum, together with microtubules, which are predominantly longitudinally arranged, and secretory vacuoles which become larger and more numerous near the upper pole.

At the upper pole the cell elongates into a single large **Tomes' process**, and forms a fringe of smaller processes around its neck. The Tomes' process contains numerous microtubules, and large numbers of secretory vacuoles.

The rough endoplasmic reticulum synthesizes various proteins and glycoproteins (including amelogenin and enamelin), which form the organic matrix of enamel (**pre-enamel**), and are packaged by the Golgi into secretory vacuoles. These then move into the Tomes' process and the small neck processes, discharging their contents onto the surface.

Mineralization of the matrix proteins by hydroxyapatite occurs almost instantaneously producing small enamel crystallites, and with progressive mineralization, the enamel rods or prisms form.

The compact structured enamel prisms are probably derived from the surface of the main Tomes' process, while the small amount of less compact inter-prism enamel, which has a larger organic matrix component, is probably derived from the small neck processes.

Enamel covers the dentine (Fig. 10.13) only in the region of the exposed crown; in the root, the dentine is covered by cementum (see Figs 10.7 & 10.14).

Cementum

Cementum is a bone-like tissue; it is calcified and contains collagen.

A thin layer of cementum covers the root of the tooth, being thin, compact and acellular (**acellular cementum**) over the upper region, but thicker and containing lacunae and cementocytes (cellular cementum) lower down (Fig. 10.14).

CEMENTOCYTES, CEMENTOBLASTS AND CEMENTUM FORMATION
Cementocytes resemble osteocytes (see Chapter 14) and remain viable throughout life, being nourished through canaliculi, which link the lacunae. They can become activated to produce new cementum when required.

In addition to the cementocytes, which are scattered throughout the cellular cementum, there is a layer of cells called cementoblasts, which are similar to the actively synthetic osteoblasts of bone (see Fig. 14.15).

Cementoblasts lie against the surface of the periodontal ligament and probably produce most new cementum by appositional deposition.

Periodontal ligament

The **periodontal ligament** is a suspensory ligament tethering the tooth in the bony alveolar socket of the mandible or maxilla and permitting limited movement of the tooth within the rigid bony socket.

The periodontal ligament is composed of dense collagen and fibrocytes, with the fibres running across the gap between the cementum of the tooth and the bone of the alveolar socket (Fig. 10.15). As the collagen fibres are embedded in a ground substance, this ligament also acts as a shock absorber.

At its cemental and alveolar limits, some of the collagen fibres are inserted into the cementum and bone. The alveolar bone at the inner margin of the socket is composed of woven bone rather than compact lamellar bone. Above the upper limit of the alveolar bone, the fibres of the periodontal ligament become the gingival periodontal fibres and blend with the submucosa of the gingiva.

Tooth development

Teeth develop from both ectoderm and mesoderm:
- the ectodermal component produces the enamel;
- the mesodermal component produces the dental pulp, predentine and dentine (Fig. 10.16).

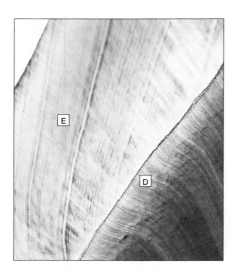

Fig. 10.13 Formed enamel.
Unstained ground section of a mature human tooth showing the characteristic patterns of enamel (E) and dentine (D); the tightly packed dentinal tubules are clearly seen.

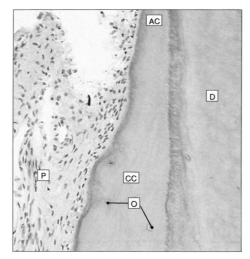

Fig. 10.14 Cementum.
Micrograph showing the dentine (D), cementum and fibrous periodontal ligament (P) of the root of a tooth at the junction between the narrow compact acellular cementum (AC) and the broader cellular cementum (CC) in which osteoblast-like nuclei can be seen (O).

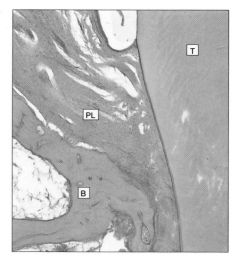

Fig. 10.15 Periodontal ligament.
H&E stained section showing the relationship between the tooth (T), bony socket (B) and the fibrous periodontal ligament (PL) at the neck of the tooth.

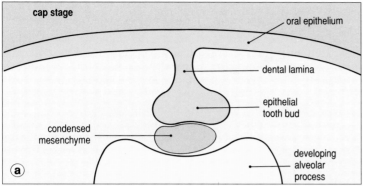

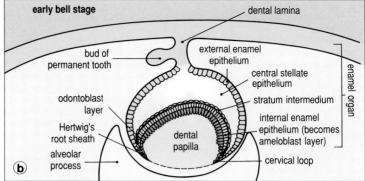

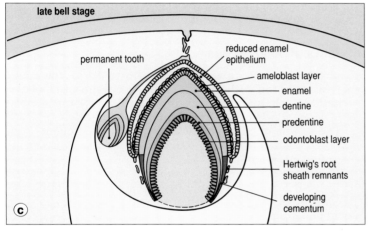

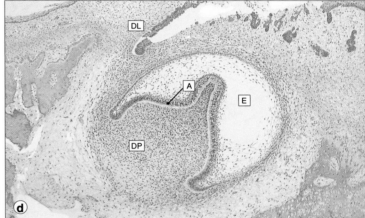

Fig. 10.16 Tooth development.

a Teeth develop from both ectoderm and mesenchyme of mesodermal origin, the ectodermal component being the enamel derived from the **enamel organ,** and the mesenchyme producing the rest of the tooth.

The enamel organ originates as a cellular downgrowth of the oral epithelium, initially in the form of a cap-shaped epithelial tooth bud, connected to the overlying oral epithelium by the dental lamina. Beneath the epithelial tooth bud, a condensation of mesenchyme contributes to the rest of the tooth.

b The cells of the epithelial tooth bud develop into the enamel organ by differentiating into a bell-shaped structure with a central core of loosely arranged stellate cells (**stellate epithelium**) and a peripheral layer of cuboidal or low columnar epithelium. The outer cell layer on the convex surface is the **external enamel epithelium**, and that of the concave surface the **internal enamel epithelium.**

The internal enamel epithelium differentiates into an outer layer of tall columnar **ameloblasts** (see Fig. 10.12) and a 2–3 cell thick inner layer called the **stratum intermedium.**

Where the external and internal enamel epithelium meet is called the **cervical loop.** An extension downwards of cells of the external enamel epithelium forms the so-called **Hertwig's root sheath** which defines the final size of the tooth root, being later replaced by the cementum.

In the concavity of the enamel organ, the mesenchyme continues to condense to form the **dental papilla,** and a row of odontoblasts develops at its junction with the enamel organ, in contact with the ameloblast layer.

In deciduous teeth, like the incisor shown here, the permanent tooth arises from a sidegrowth from the dental lamina.

c Odontoblasts begin to produce predentine, and this stimulates the production of enamel by the ameloblasts. Calcification of the predentine and pre-enamel begins almost immediately, and dentine and enamel continue to be laid down until the form of the tooth is complete. The dental papilla becomes enclosed by dentine to form the dental pulp.

The non-ameloblast components of the enamel organ become much reduced and eventually atrophy. When enamel formation is complete, the ameloblasts degenerate to form a thin layer of irregular cells, which ultimately disappear when the tooth errupts.

The cells of Hertwig's root sheath begin to degenerate as the cementum is deposited by cementoblasts on the surface of the dentine of the tooth root. Partial development of the permanent tooth continues alongside the deciduous tooth in the same manner.

d Micrograph of a resin section of a developing tooth at the bell stage, showing the enamel organ (E), including the ameloblast layer (A), the dental papilla (DP), and the degenerating dental lamina (DL).

151

Gingiva

The **gingiva** (gum) is the portion of oral mucosa covering the alveolar bone ridge surrounding the tooth; it is continuous with the alveolar mucosa covering the rest of the bone. A small sulcus lies between the tooth and the bulk of the gingiva.

The sulcal epithelium is thin stratified squamous, whereas that on the outer surface of the gingiva is thick and keratinized with prominent rete ridges.

The submucosa in the region of the gingival sulcus is commonly infiltrated by chronic inflammatory cells and also contains gingival periodontal fibres, which are an extension of the upper limit of the periodontal ligament.

DENTAL CARIES AND PERIODONTAL DISEASE

The most common disorders of teeth are:
- abnormal tooth eruption, leading to malalignment of teeth;
- dental caries;
- periodontal disease.

Dental caries result when weak acids in food and drink erode the calcified enamel, producing irregular holes and furrows. This erosion is augmented by acid produced by bacteria, which populate such holes. Such focal decalcification may progress until the erosion involves the deeper dentine, from where the acids and bacteria can advance more rapidly down the dentinal tubules to the pulp cavity, causing tooth pain.

Continued bacterial damage can produce a tooth abscess in the soft pulp.

Destruction of the pulp cavity and its contained blood vessels leads to death of the odontoblast layer and eventual death of the tooth.

Periodontal disease is caused by the accumulation of calcified food and bacterial debris in the gingival sulcus. This gradually forces the gingiva away from the tooth, widening and damaging the gingival sulcus and deep periodontal pockets form, in which food particles and bacteria become trapped. Bacterial proliferation then leads to inflammation of the gum (**gingivitis**) and the periodontal ligament (**periodontitis**).

Persistent periodontitis destroys the periodontal ligament, and the tooth becomes loose in its socket.

Salivary glands

The mouth receives secretions from salivary gland tissue located both inside and outside the mouth. These glands may contain mucus-secreting cells, serous cells or a mixture of both. The serous glands secrete a watery solution containing enzymes (e.g. amylase, lysozyme), IgA secretory piece and lactoferrin, an iron-binding compound.

The largest salivary glands are located outside the mouth and transfer their secretion into the oral cavity by long ducts; smaller glands, sited mainly in the submucosa of the oral lining, are less well-defined and empty their secretion into the mouth by short ducts.

The main salivary glands are the submandibular, the parotid and the large sublingual glands.

Submandibular glands

The **submandibular glands** are roughly ovoid in shape and are situated on either side of the neck just below the mandible. Their ducts open into the floor of the mouth, one on each side of the frenulum of the tongue.

The submandibular glands are typical mixed glands containing both serous and mucous elements, with serous elements predominating.

The secretory acini are composed mainly of epithelial cells, which are responsible for the serous secretion, and are plump cells filled with prominent purplish-staining zymogen granules.

The mucus-secreting cells are pale-staining with abundant clear cytoplasm, and often form blind-ending tubules, the blind end bearing a demilune or crescent of zymogen-rich serous cells (Fig. 10.17).

The secretory acini empty into **intercalated ducts**, which are lined by cuboidal or low columnar epithelium, and merge to form **intralobular ducts**. These are characterized by tall columnar epithelium, which stains pale pink and shows a characteristic striated pattern (see Fig. 3.23) of basal cytoplasm. Hence intralobular ducts are commonly called **striated ducts**.

Intralobular duct epithelium is biochemically active and modifies the concentration and content of the fluids produced by the secretory acini.

The intralobular striated ducts fuse to form larger **interlobular ducts**, which are lined by a non-striated, often pseudostratified, epithelium. Interlobular ducts then join to form the **major duct**s, some of which (particularly the main submandibular duct) may have a ciliated epithelium.

There is a network of myoepithelial cells between the epithelium and the basement membrane of the acini and much of the ductular system, contraction of the myoepithelial cells squeezing the secretion towards the major ducts.

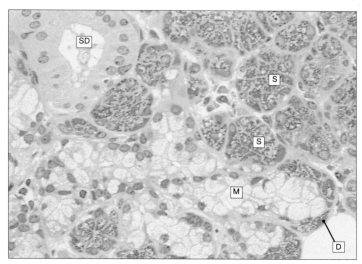

Fig. 10.17 Submandibular salivary gland.
The submandibular salivary gland has both a mucous and a serous component. The serous component (S) contains numerous large zymogen granules, while the mucous component (M) is often arranged in duct-like structures, the ends of which are capped by the so-called serous demilunes (D). A striated duct (SD) shows the characteristic features of an ion exchange epithelium.

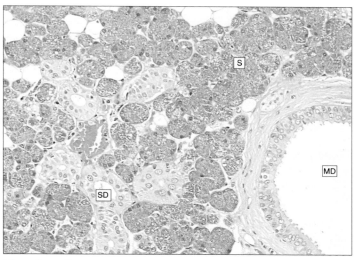

Fig. 10.18 Parotid salivary gland.
The parotid salivary gland is composed entirely of granular serous cells (S), with variable amounts of intervening adipose tissue. Note the cluster of small ducts (SD) and part of a major duct (MD).

Parotid glands

The **parotid glands** are situated below and in front of the pinna on each side of the face. They are flat and well encapsulated, and the facial nerve runs through them dividing them into superficial and deep portions. Their long ducts open into the oral cavity opposite the second upper molar tooth on each side.

The parotids are composed entirely of serous glands rich in zymogen granules, with a variable amount of adipose tissue in the interstitium between parotid lobules (Fig. 10.18).

Large sublingual glands

The large sublingual glands are located in the floor of the mouth, one on either side of the frenulum of the tongue, and their short ducts open into the mouth near to, or with, the submandibular ducts. These glands are composed predominantly of mucous cells.

Other salivary gland tissue

There are numerous smaller groups of salivary gland tissue, most of which have been mentioned on page 144. They include:
- **lingual glands** in the submucosa and muscle layers of the dorsal surface of the tongue (see Fig. 10.6);
- **minor sublingual glands** close to the larger major sublingual glands (other tongue glands are found on the inferior surface of the tip of the tongue and on its lateral borders);
- **labial glands** on the inner surface of the lips;
- **palatine glands** in the submucosa of the soft and hard palates;
- **tonsillar glands** in the mucosa associated with the palatine and pharyngeal tonsils;
- **buccal glands** in the submucosa lining the cheeks.

The labial, sublingual, minor lingual and buccal glands are composed predominantly of mucous cells, but some serous cells may be present. The palatine and lateral lingual glands are entirely mucus-secreting.

SIMPLE PASSAGES

The pharynx, oesophagus and anal canal are comparatively simple transport tubes through which ingested food is transmitted without undergoing significant metabolic change. They are muscular tubes lined internally by stratified squamous epithelium, and some mucous glands, which provide lubricating mucus.

Pharynx

The pharynx is located at the back of the mouth, and transfers partly fragmented food from the oral cavity into the upper end of the oesophagus. It also connects the nasal system of air chambers and the upper end of the trachea. The opening of the mouth into the pharynx is the **oropharynx**, while the nasal opening is the **nasopharynx**. The Eustachian tube from the middle ear (see Chapter 12) opens into the pharynx on each side.

The oropharynx and pharynx proper are lined by largely non-keratinizing stratified squamous epithelium. The nasopharynx is lined partly by stratified squamous epithelium, which changes to a ciliated columnar epithelium as the nasal cavities are approached.

The submucosa of the pharynx is well endowed with lymphoid tissue, with a particularly prominent aggregation in the nasopharynx forming the **pharyngeal tonsil** (**adenoids**). At the junction between the mouth and pharynx, in the oropharynx, are large lymphoid tonsillar masses in the gap between the glossopalatine and pharyngopalatine arches on each side. These are the **palatine tonsils**. The tonsils are discussed on page 100.

Oesophagus

The oesophagus lies between the pharynx and the stomach, and transports food in an undigested, but fragmented form to the stomach, where digestion begins.

The oesophagus is about 25 cm long, originating from the pharynx at the level of the cricoid cartilage, and extending down the posterior mediastinum in the midline to the level of the diaphragm; it penetrates the left crus before opening into the stomach.

Mucosa

The oesophageal mucosa is composed of non-keratinizing stratified squamous epithelium (except in the region of the oesophagogastric junction), with an associated lamina propria and muscularis mucosae (Fig. 10.19).

The basal zone of the epithelium may be several cell layers thick and consists of cuboidal or rectangular cells with dark nuclei and purple-staining cytoplasm in which there is no glycogen. Scattered in this layer are occasional melanocytes and neuroendocrine cells.

Above the basal zone the epithelial cells are larger and may be rich in glycogen, gradually becoming more flattened as the lumen is approached (Fig. 10.20).

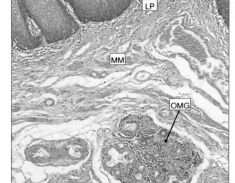

Fig. 10.19 Oesophageal mucosa and submucosa.
The oesophagus is lined by non-keratinizing stratified squamous epithelium (E), beneath which is a thick lamina propria (LP) and muscularis mucosae (MM). The submucosa contains abundant vessels and nerves together with oesophageal mucous glands (OMG), which are characteristically surrounded by lymphocytic infiltrate.

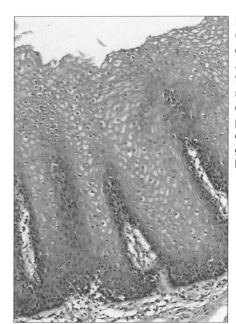

Fig. 10.20 Oesophageal epithelium.
At high magnification, the oesophageal squamous epithelium contains some pale-staining cells distended with glycogen, and its lower border is irregular.

The average epithelial thickness is 500–800 μm, but this is difficult to measure accurately because the lower border is irregular, and tongues of lamina propria extend up towards the luminal surface, giving an appearance similar to the rete ridge arrangement in the epidermis of the skin (see Chapter 19).

The oesophageal lamina propria consists of loosely arranged collagen fibres and fibroblasts embedded in an acellular glycosaminoglycan matrix, with a normal scattering of lymphocytes and eosinophils, as well as occasional mast cells and plasma cells.

The muscularis mucosae is of variable thickness, being particularly thick in the lower end of the oesophagus where it approaches the squamocolumnar junction. In the upper oesophagus the fibres appear to be arranged haphazardly, but in the lower third there are continuous sheets of longitudinal and circular fibres.

Submucosa

The submucosa of the oesophagus is broad and contains mucous glands (see Fig. 10.20), which secrete acid mucins.

Each gland has 2–5 lobes, which drain into a short duct lined by stratified columnar epithelium, the duct penetrating the muscularis mucosae, lamina propria and epithelial layer to open into the lumen. Lymphocytes, plasma cells and eosinophils are particularly common around the glands and their ducts (see Fig. 10.19). Aggregations of lymphoid cells forming small follicles are common in the oesophageal submucosa near the squamocolumnar junction.

Oesophageal submucosa is also particularly rich in blood vessels and lymphatics.

Musculature

The muscularis proper of the oesophagus varies along its length, although it is generally arranged in discrete circular and longitudinal layers.

In the upper third of the oesophagus the layers are composed almost entirely of striated muscle, but a gradual transition to smooth muscle occurs in the middle third where both striated and smooth muscle fibres are found together. The muscle layers in the lower third are composed entirely of smooth muscle, and are continuous with the smooth muscle layers of the stomach.

Oesophagogastric junction

Unlike the rest of the oesophagus, which is lined by stratified squamous epithelium, the short length (1–1.5 cm long) of oesophagus below the diaphragm, is lined by columnar epithelium similar to that of the cardiac region of the stomach; this is the **squamocolumnar (oesophagogastric) junction** (Fig. 10.21), and is an important site of pathological abnormality.

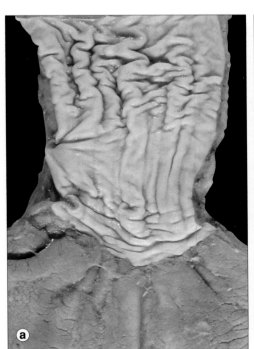

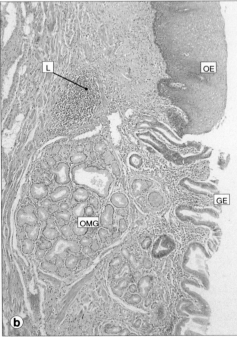

Fig. 10.21 Oesophagogastric junction.
a Macroscopic appearance of the junction between the oesophagus and stomach. Most of the oesophagus is lined by a stratified squamous epithelium (white) whilst the stomach epithelium appears brown.
b H&E section of the squamocolumnar junction in the region of the oesophagogastric junction showing the abrupt transition between oesophageal squamous epithelium (OE) and columnar gastric epithelium (GE). In the region of the junction, lymphoid aggregates (L) and oesophageal mucous glands (OMG) are particularly prominent.

OESOPHAGEAL ULCERATION AND BARRETT'S OESOPHAGUS

The squamous epithelium of the oesophagus is protected from exposure to gastric acid by:
- the anatomical arrangement of the oesophagogastric junction;
- the small oesophagogastric muscular sphincter, which in most cases prevents reflux of gastric contents into the lower oesophagus.

However the system is not foolproof, and ulceration of the oesophagus can occur as the result of reflux of gastric acid and digestive enzymes. This is most common in the junctional region of the lower oesophagus where the squamous epithelium changes to columnar epithelium.

Developmentally the oesophagus is lined initially by columnar epithelium with occasional cilia, the stratified squamous lining appearing later. Occasionally this change is not complete and islands of columnar epithelium persist in the oesophagus (**Barrett's oesophagus**).

The islands of columnar epithelium in Barrett's oesophagus are particularly prone to ulceration and inflammation (Fig. 10.22) when gastric acid refluxes into the oesophagus, and are also believed to be the site of development of one type of oesophageal cancer.

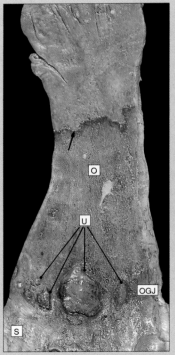

Fig. 10.22 Oesophageal ulceration and Barrett's oesophagus.
Photograph showing the lower half of the oesophagus (O) and the upper part of the stomach (S). Compare with Fig. 10.19a.

At the oesophagogastric junction (OGJ) are four ulcers (U), which lie in inflamed columnar mucosa that extends up as far as the arrow. Above the arrow there is normal oesophageal stratified squamous epithelium, which shows yellowish discoloration as a result of repeated vomiting.

Healing of such ulcers can lead to scarring of the lower end of the oesophagus, and thereby narrowing of its lumen, (i.e. an **oesophageal stricture**) so that swallowing becomes almost impossible.

Anal canal

The **anal canal** transports the residue of ingested food after it has been digested and most of its water content has been extracted (i.e. faeces) from the rectum to the exterior in the process known as defaecation.

Sphincters

Anatomically the anal canal is a tube 3–4 cm long (Fig. 10.23), the diameter of which is controlled by two sphincter systems.
- The **internal anal sphincter** is composed of smooth muscle, and is a localized thickening of the circular muscle of the lower rectum. It is under autonomic control and responds to distension of the rectal reservoir.
- The **external anal sphincter** is composed of skeletal striated muscle and is continuous with the fascia and muscles of pelvic floor. It is under voluntary control.

Mucosa

At its upper end the anal canal is lined by columnar epithelium identical to that of the rectum. This changes to a non-keratinizing stratified squamous type at the level of the **pectinate** (**or dentate**) **line**, which marks the site of the anal membrane of the fetus (i.e. the junction of gut endoderm and the ectodermal invagination of the proctodeal pit).

The pectinate line is a line of small crescentic valve-like mucosal extrusions, with small vertical folds, the **anal columns**, arising from their junctions.

Glands

Small branched tubular glands, the **anal glands**, open into the anal canal just above the pectinate line, while another set of glands, the prominent apocrine glands of the perianal skin (see Chapter 19), lie at the lower end of the anal canal (**circumanal glands**).

Venous plexuses

Two prominent venous plexuses are associated with the anal canal.
- The **internal haemorrhoidal plexus** lies in the submucosa of the upper end of the canal above the level of the pectinate line.
- The **external haemorrhoidal plexus** lies in the submucosa at the lower end in the region of the junction between anal canal and perianal skin.

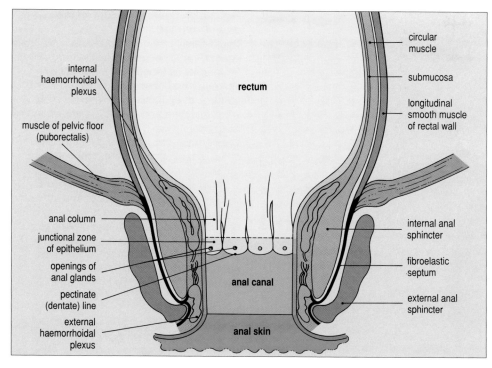

Fig. 10.23 Anal canal.
Diagram of the anal canal showing the epithelial linings of the rectum (columnar), anal canal (non-keratinizing stratified squamous), and anal skin (keratinizing epidermis rich in hair follicles, eccrine and apocrine glands). There is a variable junctional zone of epithelium at the pectinate line.

The internal sphincter is a continuation of the circular smooth muscle layer of the rectum, and the external sphincter is composed of skeletal muscle under voluntary control.

The rectal longitudinal muscle loses its fibres at the level of the puborectalis muscle of the pelvic floor and continues as a fibroelastic septum between the internal and external sphincter.

Note the position of the internal and external haemorrhoidal plexuses; haemorrhoids (piles) result from enlargement of the internal haemorrhoidal plexus.

DIGESTIVE TRACT

The digestive tract is the site of:
- major digestion of food material (some digestion begins in the mouth as a result of salivary secretion of diastase);
- absorption of the end products of digestion;
- absorption of ingested fluids and reabsorption of secreted fluids.

The digestive tract comprises the stomach, small intestine (i.e. duodenum, jejunum and ileum), and the large intestine (i.e. caecum, appendix, colon and rectum). Its basic structure is shown in Fig. 10.24.

Mucosa

The mucosa, which is composed of lining epithelium, lamina propria and muscularis mucosae, is the most variable component of the digestive tract and usually contains a mixture of epithelial cell types, both absorptive and secretory.

The efficiency of absorptive and secretory processes is improved by increasing the surface area of contact between the epithelial cells and the lumen. This is achieved by:
- intrusions or folding of the lining epithelium into the lumen (i.e. **villi** or **plicae**);
- inversions of the epithelium to form tubular structures, the lumina of which communicate with the main lumen;

- formation of complex glands within or exterior to the tract wall.

Examples of these structural modifications will be discussed in relation to specific areas of the digestive tract.

The epithelium is supported by a variable layer, the lamina propria, which is composed of supporting cells and their products (including collagen). Within the lamina propria are small blood vessels, lymphatics, nerve fibres and cells belonging to the immune and defence systems (see Chapter 7), particularly macrophages and lymphocytes.

The deep aspect of the lamina propria rests on a usually thin muscle layer, the muscularis mucosae.

Submucosa

The submucosa lies between the mucosa and the main muscle layer of the digestive tract wall. It is composed of fibroblasts, collagen and acellular matrix, and contains blood vessels, lymphatics and nerves, which supply or drain their smaller equivalents in the lamina propria of the mucosa.

In addition the submucosa contains clumps of ganglion cells associated with the autonomic nerve supply of the tract, and in some areas, contains lymphoid aggregates and follicles, which are part of the **gut-associated lymphoid tissue** (**GALT**) (see page 159).

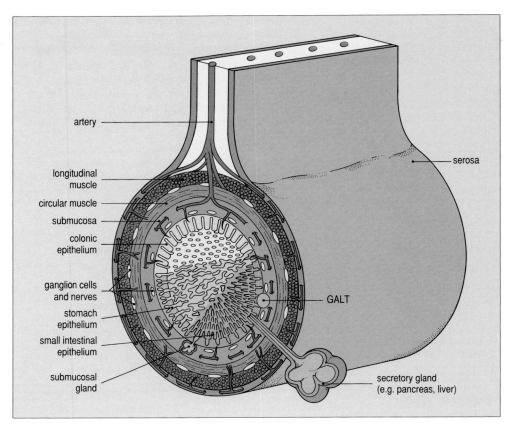

artery

longitudinal muscle

circular muscle

submucosa

colonic epithelium

ganglion cells and nerves

stomach epithelium

small intestinal epithelium

submucosal gland

serosa

GALT

secretory gland (e.g. pancreas, liver)

Fig. 10.24 Basic structure of the digestive tract.
The digestive tract is a muscular tube lined internally by specialized epithelium, which for most of its length has a combined secretory and absorptive function. Three patterns of epithelial structure (stomach, small intestine and colon) are shown in this diagram.

Externally, the tract has an outer layer of flat mesothelium where it runs through the peritoneal cavity.

Various secretory organs, which are derived embryologically as outgrowths of the putative alimentary tract, lie partly or completely outside it. These organs (e.g. pancreas and liver) produce secretions, which are vital for the tract to function normally and are transferred to the digestive tract lumen by one or more ducts.

Musculature

The musculature of the alimentary tract is responsible for moving the luminal contents along the tract caudally from mouth to anus, and therefore extends beyond the digestive part of the tract into the simple passages (i.e. the oropharynx, oesophagus and the anal canal).

The movement is achieved by **peristalsis**, whereby a wave of contraction moves distally, forcing the luminal contents onwards into the relaxed segment ahead.

There are two layers of smooth muscle throughout most of the digestive tract, and a third layer in the stomach (see below). Traditionally identified as an outer longitudinal layer and an inner circular layer, they are in fact arranged spirally, with the inner circular layer being a compact spiral, and the outer longitudinal layer being a more elongated helix (i.e. a similar arrangement to that of the smooth muscle of the ureter, see Fig. 16.40).

Between the two main smooth muscle layers of the digestive tract are small blood and lymphatic vessels, together with the nerves and ganglion cells of the autonomic nervous system.

The basic pattern of two muscle layers that extend into the simple passages of the alimentary tract, proximally into

the oesophagus and distally into the anal canal, is modified by the presence of some skeletal muscle.

In some areas, the basic muscle pattern is also modified by a localized increase in the circular muscle to act as a sphincter, which on contraction occludes the lumen, and thus prevents the passage of the luminal content.

The pyloric sphincter is the most important sphincter and is located at the junction between the stomach and duodenum. By contracting it delays stomach emptying, thereby permitting continued food breakdown in the stomach.

The oesophagogastric sphincter is located between the lower oesophagus and proximal stomach; it normally prevents reflux of gastric contents into the oesophagus.

The ileocaecal valve is situated between the terminal ileum and caecum, and delays discharge of ileal contents into the caecum.

The internal anal sphincter is sited at the upper end of the anal canal, and retains faecal waste material in the rectum until controlled defaecation.

Adventitia

Adventitia is the outer coat of the digestive tract and surrounds the external layer of muscle. It is composed of loosely arranged fibroblasts and collagen embedded in matrix, with variable numbers of adipocytes.

The adventitia contains large blood and lymphatic vessels, and nerves, the major arterial supply and venous drainage of the tract wall passing through it.

The digestive tract runs through the peritoneal cavity, and here the outer surface of the adventitia over much of its circumference is covered by a layer of flattened epithelium, the **mesothelium**. This is identical to and continuous with the mesothelium lining the peritoneal cavity internally and covering the mesenteric attachment of the alimentary tract to the posterior abdominal wall.

Adventitia covered by mesothelium (i.e. adventitia of stomach, most of small intestine and large intestine) is commonly called the **serosa**. Where adventitia is not covered by a mesothelium (i.e. adventitia of part of the duodenum and some of the colon), it merges with adjacent tissues.

Immune system (gut-associated lymphoid tissue)

Immunological defence against antigens ingested in the digestive tract is provided by the gut-associated lymphoid tissue (GALT).

Throughout the digestive tract, the lamina propria contains cells of the immune system (see Chapter 7), including lymphocytes, plasma cells and macrophages. In addition to these cells there are individual intraepithelial lymphocytes (see below).

The lymphoid cells are commonly arranged as large follicles, often with germinal centres, and are partly located in the mucosa and partly in submucosa, thus splitting the muscularis mucosae. In the ileum, the follicles aggregate to form substantial nodules called **Peyer's patches** (see page 100).

Although lymphoid follicles and Peyer's patches contain both B and T lymphocytes, the diffuse, non-follicular infiltrate in the lamina propria is composed largely of T lymphocytes.

The mucosal epithelial cells that overlie the lymphoid follicles and Peyer's patches differ from the usual epithelial cells in both structure and function, and are called **M cells** (Fig. 10.25). They are cuboidal or flat rather than tall columnar, and have luminal microfolds rather than tall microvilli.

M cells are believed to take up antigenic macromolecules from the intestinal lumen, incorporating them into endocytotic vesicles, and then transporting them to the lateral intercellular space in the region of an intraepithelial lymphocyte.

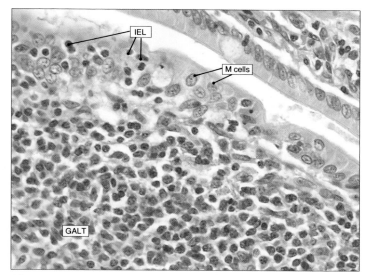

Fig. 10.25 Gut-associated lymphoid tissue (GALT).
Micrograph showing the typical arrangement of a nodule of gut-associated lymphoid tissue (GALT) in the lamina propria. The epithelial cells (M cells) closely associated with the lymphoid aggregate are cuboidal and show no cytoplasmic specialization such as mucin droplet formation. Note the intra-epithelial lymphocytes (IEL).

Innervation

The gut has both intrinsic and extrinsic innervations.

INTRINSIC
Collections of nerves and ganglion cells in the submucosa form an interconnected network called **Meissner's plexus** (Fig. 10.26a), while collections of nerves and ganglion cells between the inner circular and outer longitudinal components of the muscularis proper form a network called **Auerbach's plexus** (Fig. 10.26b).

EXTRINSIC
Autonomic input from parasympathetic (stimulatory) and sympathetic (inhibitory) abdominal plexuses modulate the activity of the intrinsic innervation of the gut. In addition sensory nerves derived from neurones in cranial and spinal nuclei terminate in the bowel as tendril-like sensory endings.

The afferent autonomic impulses mediate visceral reflexes and sensations such as hunger and rectal fullness.

The viscera are insensitive to pain, any painful sensations resulting from excessive contraction or distension of the bowel muscle.

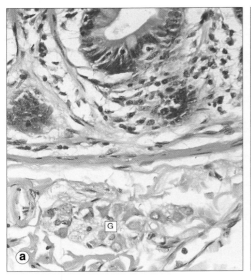
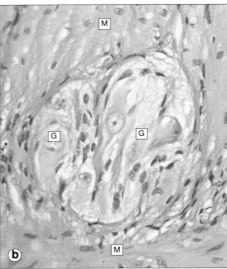

Fig. 10.26 Intrinsic innervation.
a High power micrograph showing a cluster of ganglion cells (G) in the small bowel submucosa (Meissner's plexus).
b High power micrograph showing clusters of ganglion cells (G) between the two muscle layers (M) of the muscularis proper (Auerbach's plexus).

Stomach

From the oesophagus, food enters the stomach, which is a dilated portion of the digestive tract where fragmented food is retained whilst it is macerated and partially digested. At the lower end of the stomach, the pyloric sphincter (see above) prevents the passage of food until it is converted into a thick semi-liquid paste or pulp (**chyme**).

The muscular wall of the stomach differs from the standard digestive tract pattern by the presence of a third layer of oblique muscle fibres internal to the circular layer to assist in the complex churning action necessary to thoroughly mix food with the secretions of the gastric mucosa.

The stomach muscle layers are thick. When contracted they decrease the stomach capacity and the mucosa is thrown up into longitudinal folds called **rugae**, which are most prominent on the convexity of the stomach (the **greater curve**). This is the state of the stomach when it is empty; when full the musculature relaxes and thins, and the rugae stretch flat as the stomach distends.

The stomach is ideally equipped for its role as a reservoir by its distensibility, the presence of the pyloric sphincter, and the mechanisms preventing reflux at its upper end.

Food is converted into chyme by the secretions of the gastric mucosa into the lumen. These are:
- a dilute solution of hydrochloric acid (approximately 0.16N);
- solutions of proteolytic enzymes, mainly pepsin;
- small amounts of other enzymes (e.g. rennin and gastric lipase);
- mucins, mainly in the form of neutral mucins.

Epithelium

The major functions of the gastric epithelium are the secretion of acid and digestive enzymes. It also secretes mucus to lubricate ingested food and to protect itself from the corrosive effects of the acid and enzymes. The surface area of the stomach is increased by downgrowths, which form glands.

The secretions are produced by three main cell types. In addition there is a population of endocrine cells and a population of stem cells from which the other cell types are derived. The cell types are **mucous cells**, **acid-producing cells** (**oxyntic** or **parietal cells**), **enzyme-producing cells** (**chief cells** or **peptic cells**), **stem cells**, and **enteroendocrine cells**.

MUCOUS CELLS
Gastric mucous cells are of two types: surface mucous cells and so-called neck mucous cells (Fig. 10.27), the latter occupying the necks of the gland.

Surface mucous cells are tall and columnar with basal nuclei and clear-staining luminal cytoplasm distended by numerous small mucin vacuoles, which are discharged into the stomach lumen by exocytosis. The cells also have prominent endoplasmic reticulum and the Golgi is located above the nucleus.

The luminal surface of surface mucous cells shows scanty short microvilli with a surface glycocalyx, and junctional complexes join adjacent cells near the luminal surface.

The lateral borders of the cells are often separated by a considerable intercellular gap, which is traversed by cytoplasmic protrusions of the lateral walls; this separation

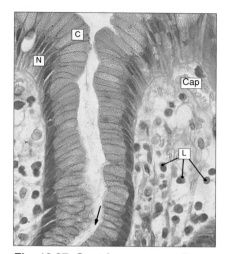

Fig. 10.27 Gastric mucous cells.
In this high power micrograph, the gastric surface mucous cells have basal nuclei (N) and bulky luminal cytoplasm (C) filled with pale-staining mucus. As the neck region is approached (arrow) the cells (neck mucous cells) are smaller and contain less mucus. Note the prominent capillaries (Cap) and lymphoid cells (L) in the lamina propria.

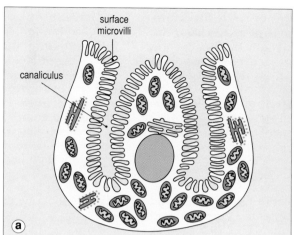

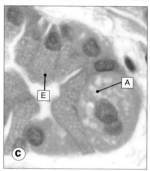

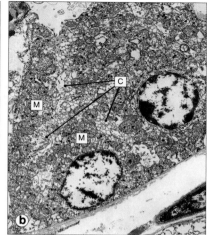

Fig. 10.28 Acid-producing cells.
a The acid-producing cell has an intricate system of invaginations lined by microvilli (canaliculi), which produce the perinuclear vacuolated appearance seen on light microscopy. The rest of the cytoplasm is packed with mitochondria, particularly at the cell periphery. A small Golgi and some rough endoplasmic reticulum are also present.
b Electronmicrograph showing the intricate canalicular system (C) of an acid-producing cell; the cytoplasm is largely occupied by tightly packed mitochondria (M).
c H&E appearance of an acid-producing cell (A) from the body of the stomach. Note the enzyme-producing cells (E, see Fig. 10.29).

disappears as the apical surface is neared where the binding of adjacent cells is very tight.

Surface mucous cells are also thought to produce blood group substances.

Neck mucous cells are smaller and less regular in shape than surface mucous cells, mainly because they are compressed and distorted by adjacent cells. They have a basal nucleus and finely granular cytoplasm due to the presence of small mucin vacuoles which are considerably smaller than those in the surface mucous cells.

The vacuoles are distributed throughout the cytoplasm and are not aggregated near the luminal surface as they are in the surface mucous cells. By light microscopy it is not always apparent that neck mucous cells contain mucin, and a PAS stain is often necessary to highlight it.

ACID-PRODUCING (OXYNTIC OR PARIETAL) CELLS
The acid-producing cells are large pyramidal cells with central nuclei and pale eosinophilic cytoplasm, which often appears vacuolated, particularly around the nucleus.

Their attachment to the basement membrane is broad, but their luminal aspect is narrow, being compressed between adjacent cells. Despite this these cells have a vast luminal surface area as a result of deep microvillar-lined invaginations producing so-called **canaliculi** (Fig. 10.28).

In the cytoplasm close to the canaliculi are clusters of round or oval vesicles, which have clear centres and distinct membrane borders, and are thought to be involved in the transfer of substances from the cytoplasm to the lumen of the canalicular system. The rest of the cytoplasm is packed with round or oval mitochondria with closely packed cristae. This high concentration of mitochondria is responsible for the eosinophilia of the cell cytoplasm, particularly at the periphery. A small Golgi and some rough endoplasmic reticulum is also present.

The acid-producing cells have abundant carbonic anhydrase, which is thought to play a vital role in generating H^+ ions for the production of hydrochloric acid (HCl). Carbon dioxide diffuses across the basement membrane from blood capillaries into the cell, where it links with water molecules (a reaction catalysed by carbonic anhydrase) to produce carbonic acid (H_2CO_3); this instantly dissociates into an H^+ ion and a HCO_3^- ion. The latter passes back into the blood, whilst the H^+ is pumped into the lumen of a canaliculus. Chloride ions (Cl^-) are actively transported across the cell into the canaliculus from the capillaries in the lamina propria.

Acid-producing cells are also believed to produce intrinsic factor, the glycoprotein that avidly binds to vitamin B_{12} to render it absorbable by the digestive tract. Its method of production is however not known.

ENZYME-PRODUCING (CHIEF OR PEPTIC) CELLS

The enzyme-producing cells have large basal nuclei, and contain eosinophilic refractile cytoplasmic granules, and a rich rough endoplasmic reticulum (Fig. 10.29); they therefore resemble the exocrine cells of the pancreas (see page 169).

The granules contain the inactive enzyme precursor, **pepsinogen**, which is disgorged into the gastric lumen where it is converted by gastric acid into the active proteolytic enzyme, **pepsin**.

Pepsin is a potent enzyme, breaking down large protein molecules into small peptides, and converting almost all of the structural proteins into soluble small molecular weight substances; it is largely responsible for the conversion of solid food particles to fluid chyme.

STEM CELLS

Stem cells are the precursor cells of all epithelial cells of the gastric mucosa. They are small cells with oval basal nuclei and show no cytoplasmic specialization when completely undifferentiated (Fig. 10.30), but are capable of differentiating into mucous, acid-producing, enzyme-producing or endocrine cells.

Normally present in very small numbers in humans, their number and activity are increased when the gastric epithelium is continually damaged, for example in chronic irritation of the gastric mucosa, (i.e. chronic gastritis). A surge of stem cell activity enables an ulcerated area of the stomach to be rapidly re-epithelialized. Such regeneration is an important final step in the healing of a stomach ulcer.

ENDOCRINE CELLS

Enteroendocrine cells (see Chapter 15) of the stomach are small and round, and are sited on the epithelial basement membrane. In H&E paraffin sections they have a round central dark-staining nucleus and a rim of clear cytoplasm (Fig. 10.31a).

Ultrastructurally the cytoplasm contains membrane-bound neurosecretory granules, the shape, size, number and electron density varying according to the substance secreted.

Immunocytochemical methods demonstrate that:

- endocrine cells storing and secreting serotonin, somatostatin (Fig. 10.31b) and a vasointestinal polypeptide (VIP)-like substance are present in the cardiac, body and antral regions;
- cells secreting gastrin and a bombesin-like peptide are concentrated in the pyloric mucosa, where gastrin-secreting cells are concentrated mainly in the neck region, with rare scattered cells in the depths of the glands.

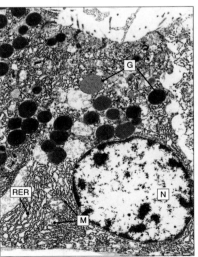

**Fig. 10.29
Enzyme-producing cells.**
Electronmicrograph of an enzyme-producing cell showing its large basal nucleus (N), abundant mitochondria (M), abundant rough endoplasmic reticulum (RER), and the grey-staining spherical granules (G), which contain pepsinogen and are responsible for the eosinophilic granular appearance of these cells in H&E stained sections (see Fig. 10.28b).

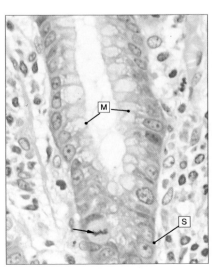

Fig. 10.30 Stem cells.
Micrograph from the neck region of the gastric body (see Fig. 10.32) showing a small population of uncommitted stem cells (S), one of which is in mitosis (arrow). Most of the stem cells are differentiating into mucous cells (M) and migrating upwards, but some will differentiate into enzyme-producing or acid-producing cells and migrate downwards.

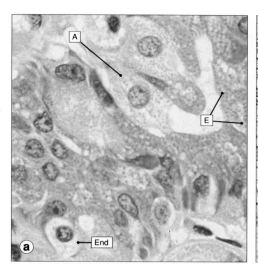
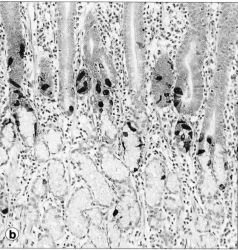

Fig. 10.31 Gastric endocrine cells.
a Micrograph of the base of glands in the body of the stomach showing the H&E appearance of gastric enteroendocrine cells (End). They are small with pale cytoplasm and a small dark-staining central nucleus. Acid-producing (A) and enzyme-producing (E) cells are also evident.
b Micrograph of an immunoperoxidase stained section of stomach showing the distribution of somatostatin-secreting endocrine cells in the pyloric gastric mucosa. The cells are numerous in the neck region, with a few scattered cells in the deep glands.

MUCOSAL ZONES

The gastric mucosa can be divided into three histological zones, a superficial zone, a neck zone and a deep zone.

- The **superficial zone** is composed of a layer of surface mucous cells with downgrowths, which are variously called **foveolae**, **pits** or **crypts**.

The mucous cells lining the pits are not so tall and columnar as those on the surface; in addition they contain less mucin.

The superficial zone is roughly constant in its content and structure throughout the stomach.

- The **neck zone** between the superficial and deep zones is narrow and composed largely of immature stem cells mixed with some neck mucous cells. The immature stem cells proliferate and migrate upwards to replenish the predominantly mucous cells of the superficial zone, and downwards to replenish the cell types in the glands of the deep zone.

- The **deep zone** is composed of glands, the bases of which lie close to or in the muscularis mucosae, while the upper ends open into the bases of the superficial zone pits.

The structure of the deep zone varies, there being three main histological patterns, which delineate three main areas of the stomach; these areas are the **cardia**, the **body** and the **pylorus** (Figs 10.32 & 10.33).

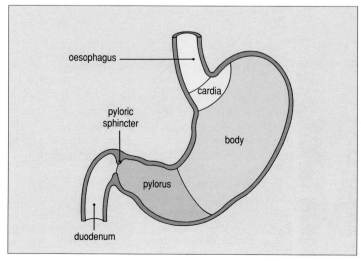

Fig. 10.32 Areas of the stomach.
Diagram of stomach showing the three histologically distinguishable areas.

The **cardia** extends from the squamocolumnar junction at the lower end of the oesophagus for a variable distance into the upper stomach, usually 2–3 cm down the lesser curve; cardiac mucosa may also extend part way into the fundus, which is an anatomical rather than a histological feature.

Pyloric mucosa lines a roughly conical area in the lower third of the stomach, starting about half-way down the lesser curve. The area is very variable and tends to begin higher on the lesser curve in women.

Body mucosa occupies the rest of the stomach, including most of the anatomical fundus. The transition between the various mucosal patterns is commonly gradual, with a narrow junctional zone showing features of both.

cardiac mucosa

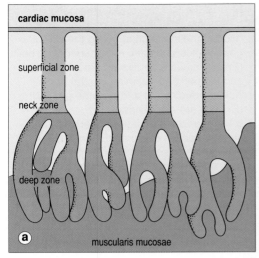

superficial zone

neck zone

deep zone

a

muscularis mucosae

body mucosa

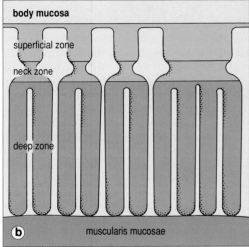

superficial zone

neck zone

deep zone

b

muscularis mucosae

pyloric mucosa

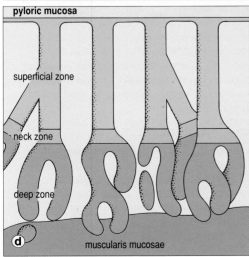

superficial zone

neck zone

deep zone

d

muscularis mucosae

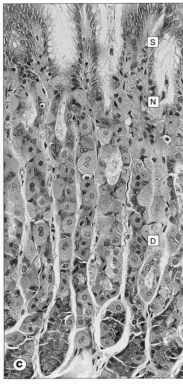

c

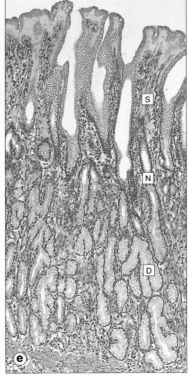

e

Fig. 10.33 Gastric mucosa.
a Cardiac mucosa. The superficial and deep zones of the cardiac mucosa are of about equal thickness. The surface and pit epithelium is composed of mucous cells, while the deep zone is composed of tubular and branched glands lined by mucous cells, with scattered endocrine and acid-producing cells becoming more numerous near the junction with the body mucosa. Some of the more complex glands are coiled.

The muscularis mucosae is thick and irregular, and often sends bundles of fibres towards the surface, interdigitating with the glands. The histological appearance of cardiac mucosa is shown in Fig. 10.21b.

b Body mucosa. The superficial zone of the body mucosa accounts for only 25 % or less of the mucosal thickness. Most pits open directly and singly onto the surface, but some fuse before opening, to form a wider crevice.

The deep zone is composed of tightly packed long straight tubular glands that end blindly at the muscularis mucosae. At their upper ends the glands open into the bases of the crypts through a variably constricted neck region. 1–4 gland opens into single crypts, and 2–8 into fused crypts.

The superficial zone is covered by surface mucous cells, with neck mucous cells covering the deeper parts of the pits. At the neck region, neck mucous cells are mixed with stem cells. The glands are composed of acid-producing cells, enzyme-producing cells, neck mucous cells and scattered endocrine cells.

c Body mucosa. H&E section of body mucosa showing the superficial zone (S) composed of mucus–secreting cells, a narrow neck zone (N) containing mainly stem cells and neck mucous cells, and the deep zone (D) largely composed of acid-producing and enzyme-producing cells.

d Pyloric mucosa. The superficial zone of the pyloric region occupies slightly more than 50 % of the mucosal thickness, and the crypts are often branched.

The deep zone is composed of tortuous single or branched glands extending down to the muscularis mucosae.

The cell content of the superficial and neck zones is the same as in the cardiac and body mucosa. The glands are lined by neck mucous cells, but scattered acid-producing cells and numerous endocrine cells are also present. Acid-producing cells become more numerous close to the pyloric sphincter.

e Pyloric mucosa. H&E section of pyloric mucosa showing the superficial zone (S) occupying about 50 % of the mucosal thickness. The narrow neck (N) and substantial deep (D) zones are composed of neck mucous cells, which form branching glands in the deep zone.

GASTRIC ULCER

The stomach normally contains an acid solution, but is protected from the damaging effects of the acid by various mechanisms, including the presence of a thin layer of mucus over the surface of the epithelial cells.

In some circumstances these protective mechanisms break down and the acidic gastric contents damage the mucosa. The resulting death of epithelial cells and lamina propria leads to the formation of a shallow ulcer. Continued exposure of such an unprotected area leads to the formation of a deep ulcer (**chronic gastric ulcer**), which can extend through the submucosa and the muscle layers (Fig. 10.34), and takes a long time to heal.

If an ulcer penetrates the full thickness of the stomach wall, the wall may perforate and the gastric contents can then pour into the peritoneal cavity, causing peritonitis and often death.

Treatment of gastric ulcer is based on removing or decreasing the levels of gastric acid either by neutralizing them (e.g. with oral alkalies), or by decreasing the amount of gastric acid produced by blocking its secretion by the acid-producing cells (e.g. using H1 antagonists or by surgically cutting the vagus nerve). If severe, the entire acid-producing part of the stomach can be surgically removed.

As gastric acid also enters the first part of the duodenum, this area may also be subject to ulceration (**duodenal ulcer**), as may the lower oesophagus if gastric acid refluxes (see Fig. 10.22)

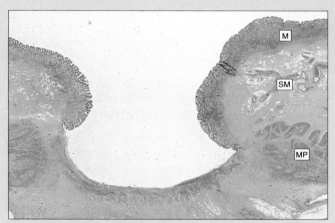

Fig. 10.34 Chronic gastric ulcer.
Micrograph of an H&E section through a chronic gastric ulcer, which has extended through the mucosa (M), submucosa (SM) and muscularis proper (MP).

Small intestine

When the pyloric sphincter (see page 158) opens, partially digested food (chyme) empties from the stomach into the small intestine, which is the main site for the absorption of amino acids, sugars, fats, and some larger molecules produced by digestion of food. The small intestine also secretes enzymes to complete the digestive processes begun in the stomach.

As the major absorptive site, the small intestine shows a number of architectural modifications to its mucosa and submucosa to increase its surface area.
• The mucosa and submucosa are thrown up into a large number of folds or **plicae** arranged circularly around the lumen. These are most prominent in the jejunum (Fig. 10.35a), and are absent from the distal end of the small intestine.
• The surface of the plicae is further arranged into villi, which protrude into the intestinal lumen (Figs 10.35b&c and 10.36).
• Tubular glands or crypts extend down from the base of the villi to the muscularis mucosae.

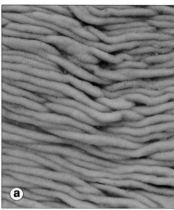
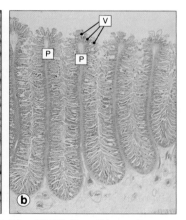
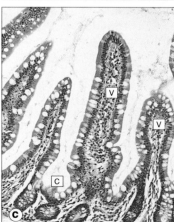

Fig. 10.35 Small intestine – general architecture.
a Macroscopic view of small intestinal mucosal surface showing tightly packed circumferential mucosal folds or plicae.
b Low power micrograph of the plicae (P) showing their complex mucosal surface, which is composed of large numbers of villi (V).
c Micrograph showing the villi (V) protruding into the small intestinal lumen; note the crypts (C) between their bases.

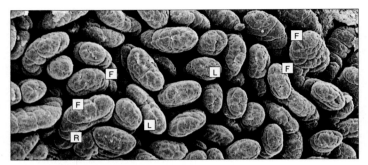

Fig. 10.36 Villi.
In two dimensions, the villi appear to have the same structure, but in three dimensions their structure can be seen to correspond to one of three main patterns; they are either finger-like (F), leaf-like (L), or ridge-like (R), as shown in this scanning electron micrograph. There are also occasional intermediate forms. The proportions of these patterns vary from site to site and also with age.

In adults most villi are finger-like, but leaf-like and ridge-like forms are also found, particularly in the duodenum; leaf-like forms may be dominant in the proximal duodenum resulting in the histological appearance of shorter and broader villi.

In babies and young children, the villi of the duodenum and proximal jejunum are almost entirely leaf-like and ridge-like, and occasionally ridge-like villi are the only type found. Finger-like forms appear progressively with growth and by 10–15 years of age, the adult pattern is acquired.

The small intestine has the standard arrangement of musculature (i.e. an external layer of longitudinal muscle and an inner circular layer), and a substantial submucosa in which GALT (see page 159) is particularly prominent.

The small intestine begins at the pylorus, the distal limit of the stomach, and ends at the ileocaecal valve, the proximal limit of the large intestine. At autopsy, when the longitudinal muscle is relaxed, the small intestine usually measures about 6 m, but in life it measures only about 3 m long. It is divided into three sections (**duodenum, jejunum, and ileum**), although the transitions from one to the other are not precise.

Duodenum is the proximal 20–25 cm of small intestine and is entirely retroperitoneal. It has the shape of a letter C, with the head of the pancreas fitting into its concave edge. The bile and pancreatic ducts open into the duodenum in this concavity.

Jejunum begins where the duodenum emerges from behind the peritoneum and extends to an ill-defined junction with the ileum.

Ileum extends from the jejunum to the ileocaecal valve.

GLUTEN ENTEROPATHY (COELIAC DISEASE)

The absorptive function of the jejunum depends on the integrity of the villi, and if enough villi are damaged, food material can not be absorbed, leading to weight loss, diarrhoea, etc.

One important cause of extensive loss of villi is coeliac disease, due to sensitivity to the wheat protein, **gluten**. This leads to flattening of the jejunal surface with extensive loss of the villi (Fig. 10.37).

Gluten enteropathy commonly presents in babies and young children with failure to thrive and to gain normal height and weight for their age.

The villi usually assume their normal structure when wheat and its products are excluded from the diet (i.e. a gluten-free diet), and the malabsorptive state subsequently improves.

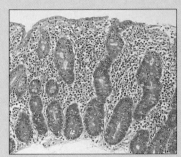

Fig. 10.37 Gluten enteropathy (coeliac disease).
Micrograph of villous damage resulting from gluten sensitivity. The jejunal mucosal surface is flattened due to extensive loss of villi. Compare with Fig. 10.35c.

Epithelium

Three zones of small intestinal epithelium can be identifed; these are the villi, the crypts, and the neck zone where villi and crypts merge.

The cells of the epithelium are **enterocytes**, **mucous cells**, **Paneth cells**, **endocrine cells** and **stem cells**, and their numbers and distribution vary in the different zones of the epithelium.

ENTEROCYTES
Enterocytes are the main absorptive cell of the villi (Fig. 10.38), being absorptive in function. They are tall columnar cells with round or oval nuclei in the lower third of the cell.

The luminal surface of enterocytes is highly specialized; each cell bears 2–3000 tightly packed tall microvilli, which are coated by a glycoprotein, the **glycocalyx** (see Fig. 10.38d). This is composed of fine filamentous extensions of the microvillar cell membrane.

The glycocalyx contains a number of enzymes (**brush border enzymes** e.g. lactase, sucrase, peptidases, lipases and alkaline phospatase), which are important in digestion and transport (see Fig. 10.38f).

Beneath the microvillar surface, the enterocyte cytoplasm contains lysosomes and smooth endoplasmic reticulum, and paired centrioles in the terminal web region (see Fig. 3.15). Nearer the nucleus the cell is rich in rough endoplasmic reticulum and mitochondria, and there is a prominent Golgi. Between the nucleus and the basement membrane are mitochondria, and many ribosomes and polyribosomes. The lateral walls of enterocytes show complex interdigitations, and are the sites of Na$^+$ and K$^+$

ATPase activity. The lateral walls are separated from the microvillar surface by desmosomes and tight junctions (see Fig. 3.7).

The ultrastructural features of the enterocyte are linked to its absorptive function, and therefore many of the features and mechanisms are common to other active absorptive cells, such as those of the proximal convoluted tubule cell of the kidney. These absorptive mechanisms are illustrated and discussed in Chapter 16.

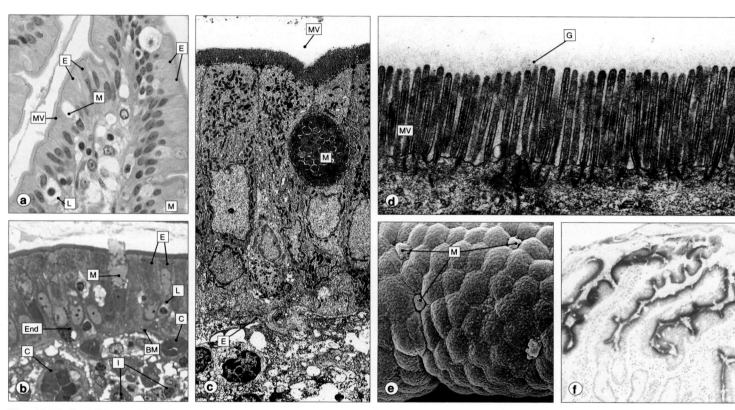

Fig. 10.38 Small intestine villus.

a Thin acrylic resin section stained with H&E showing a single villus, which is covered by tall enterocytes (E) bearing a prominent microvillar brush border (MV). Scattered among the enterocytes are occasional mucous cells (M) and intraepithelial lymphocytes (L). The stromal core contains small capillaries and lymphatics (not shown), and a number of lymphocytes, plasma cells and macrophages.

b An epoxy resin section stained with toluidine blue, showing enterocytes (E). A mucous cell can be seen discharging its contents onto the surface (M), and there are a number of small lymphocytes (L) in the epithelium, as well as a small endocrine cell (End) with basal granules. Basement membrane (BM) between the epithelium and the supporting stroma is also evident as are the immune cell population (I) in the stroma, and small capillaries (C) close to the base of the enterocytes.

c Electronmicrograph prepared from an area similar to that shown in **b**. Note the microvillar border (MV), part of a mucous cell (M) and the endocrine cell with basal granules (E).

d Electronmicrograph of microvillar brush border (MV) at high magnification. The glycocalyx (G) can be seen as a faint greyish haze on the surface of the microvilli.

e Scanning electronmicrograph of part of a villus surface. Note the tightly packed enterocytes, the microvilli of which are partly obscured by the layer of glycocalyx. Mucous cells discharging their mucus (M) are clearly seen.

f Histochemical preparation of small intestine showing the distribution of the enzyme lactase (blue staining), which is localized to the luminal surface of the enterocytes. Like many other cell-bound enzymes responsible for food breakdown in the small intestine, the enzyme molecules reside in the glycocalyx.

MUCOUS (GOBLET) CELLS

Mucous cells are found mainly in the upper two-thirds of the crypts, but occasional cells are scattered among the enterocytes of the villi (see Figs 10.38a,b&c).

Mucous cells contain globules of mucin in their luminal cytoplasm, the mucin being discharged onto the surface when the cytoplasm is fully expanded by mucin granules (see Figs 10.38b&e). The scanty basal cytoplasm is rich in rough endoplasmic reticulum.

Mucous cells are least frequent in the duodenum, and increase in number in the jejunum and ileum, being most numerous in the terminal ileum close to the caecum.

PANETH CELLS

Paneth cells are found in the lower third of the crypts.

Paneth cells have basal nuclei and prominent large eosinophilic granules in their luminal cytoplasm (Fig. 10.39). Ultrastructurally these granules are spherical and electron-dense, the remaining cytoplasm being rich in rough endoplasmic reticulum; these are features of a protein-secreting cell (see Fig. 3.20).

The antibacterial enzyme, lysozyme, is abundant in Paneth cells, suggesting a possible role in controlling the bacterial flora of the small intestine.

ENDOCRINE CELLS

Endocrine cells are located mainly in the lower third of the crypts, but are also seen higher up in the villi. They resemble those seen in the stomach (see Fig. 10.31), being roughly triangular in shape, the broad base being in contact with the basement membrane, the narrow apex reaching the lumen. Their nuclei are spherical and their cytoplasm pale staining (Fig. 10.40).

Ulstructurally, the cytoplasm contains neuroendocrine granules, and the luminal surface bears microvilli.

Small intestinal endocrine cells secrete a number of hormones and peptides, including serotonin (5HT), enteroglucagon, somatostatin, secretin, gastrin, motilin and vasoactive intestinal peptide (VIP).

STEM CELLS

Stem cells are found in the lower third of the crypts, and their replication replenishes the stock of the other cells, including the Paneth and endocrine cells. Most replication is to replace the mucous cells and enterocytes of the villi since these cells have a rapid turnover, being shed from the tips of the villi about 5 days after production.

Before developing into the mature form of the two cell types, the stem cells differentiate into **intermediate cells**, which show some features of both mucous cells and enterocytes. These cells occupy much of the upper two-thirds of the crypts.

Stem cells and intermediate cells are particularly numerous when there is increased cell loss from the villi,

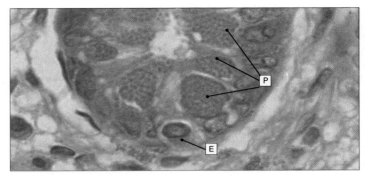

Fig. 10.39 Paneth cells.
Micrograph of the base of a small intestinal crypt from a paraffin section showing numerous Paneth cells (P) containing large numbers of bright red granules. A small endocrine cell (E) with ill-defined fine basal eosinophilic granules can also be seen.

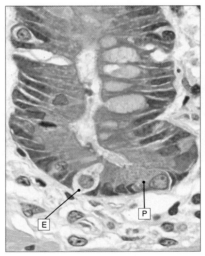

Fig. 10.40 Endocrine cell.
Micrograph of the base of a small intestinal crypt showing a typical pale-staining enteroendocrine cell (E). In this thin acrylic resin section the Paneth cell (P) granules are difficult to see.

which is a common feature of many diseases affecting the small intestine; the crypts increase in length and show increased numbers of cells in mitosis (i.e. **crypt** or **gland hyperplasia**).

Lamina propria

The lamina propria of the small intestine is most clearly seen in the core of the villi, but also surrounds and supports the glands. It is composed of collagen, reticulin fibres, fibroblasts and glycosaminoglycan matrix, through which run blood capillaries, lymphatics and nerves. It contains some smooth muscle fibres.

The blood vessels and lymphatics are particularly prominent in the villi, a central lymphatic (**lacteal**) running vertically down the centre of the core of each villus.

The lamina propria also contains lymphocytes, plasma cells, eosinophils, macrophages and mast cells.

Lymphocytes and plasma cells (GALT). The lymphocytes are largely T lymphocytes (approximately 70% T-helper and 30% T-suppressor, see Chapter 7); most of the plasma cells are IgA-producers. Lymphocytes are also present in the villous epithelium, usually in a basal position between the lateral intercellular spaces and like those in the lamina propria, they are also T lymphocytes, but the subset pattern is different, about 80% being T-suppressor, the rest being T-helper types.

Eosinophils are common in the lamina propria throughout the digestive tract.

Macrophages are found mainly beneath the basement membrane in the upper reaches of the villi. They are thought to engulf particulate antigens and to ingest soluble antigens before presenting them to T lymphocytes.

Mast cells are seen mainly in the crypt region.

Submucosa

The small intestinal submucosa contains lymphatics, blood vessels and the submucosal plexus of nerves and ganglion cells (see Fig. 10.26a). In addition it contains part of the larger lymphoid aggregates of the gut-associated lymphoid tissue, which cross the muscularis mucosae.

In the duodenum the submucosa contains mucus-secreting Brunner's glands.

Regional differences

DUODENUM
The duodenum differs from the rest of the small intestine as follows.
• It is entirely retroperitoneal.
• Its villous pattern contains a high proportion of leaf and ridge forms (see Fig. 10.36).
• It contains prominent mucus-secreting submucosal glands (**Brunner's glands**, Fig. 10.41), which penetrate and split the muscularis mucosae so that some acini are located within the lamina propria of the mucosa.
• It receives secretions of glands located outside the digestive tract through long ducts; these glands are the liver (see Chapter 11) and the exocrine component of the pancreas.

Brunner's glands are similar to the submucosal glands of the pyloric region of the stomach, being composed of mucous cells lining short ducts, which open into the bases or sides of the crypts of the mucosa. Brunner's glands secrete an alkaline mucoid material (pH 8.0–9.5), which

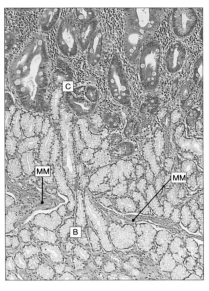

Fig. 10.41 Brunner's glands.
The first part of the duodenum is characterized by the presence of large fluid-secreting mucous glands, called Brunner's glands (B), which empty their secretions into the neck of the crypts (C). The Brunner's glands are partly located in the lower mucosa, but pass through the muscularis mucosae (MM) into the submucosa.

may protect the duodenal mucosa from the acid chyme, bringing its pH towards the level at which the pancreatic enzymes are most effective (see below).

Brunner's glands are also thought to secrete **urogastrone**, a peptide that inhibits acid secretion by the stomach. Endocrine cells can be demonstrated in these glands immunocytochemically.

Exocrine pancreas. The exocrine component of the pancreas forms a distinct organ, separate from the wall of the digestive tract in birds and mammals, but in lower animals it forms part of the cellular component of the digestive tract wall of the liver.

In man, the pancreas can be divided into four sections; these are the **head**, **neck**, **body** and **tail**. It is a long organ extending from its head, which occupies the space formed by the concavity of the duodenum, to its tail, which is situated in the left hypochondrium and terminates near the hilum of the spleen.

The pancreas has a thin ill-defined fibrocollagenous capsule from which narrow irregular septa penetrate it, dividing it into lobules. Each lobule is composed of roughly spherical clusters (**acini**) of secretory exocrine cells (Fig. 10.42). Each acinus has an individual **intra-acinar duct**, which drains into progressively larger ducts.

The pancreatic acinar cells produce and secrete the precursors of a wide range of enzymes involved in the breakdown of food in the lumen of the duodenum, including those of proteolytic enzymes (particularly trypsinogen, chymotrypsinogen, procarboxypeptidases A & B and proelastase) and lipolytic enzymes (prophospholipase and prolipase). The pancreas also secretes amylase, cholesterol esterase and ribonucleases.

Activation of the proenzymes occurs only in the duodenal cavity with the conversion of trypsinogen to active trypsin by an enterokinase located in the duodenal brush border, triggering a cascade of reactions in which the inactive precursors are converted to active enzymes.

Pancreatic secretion is alkaline due to the selective secretion of bicarbonate ions, which is thought to be performed by the ductular system rather than by the acinar cells.

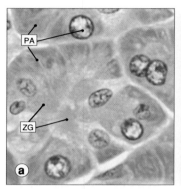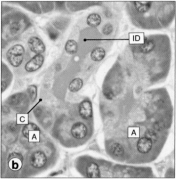

Fig. 10.42 Exocrine pancreas.
a The **acini** are composed of protein-secreting cells (pancreatic acinar cells, PA) which have a broad base and narrow apical surface covered by a few short microvilli.

The cells are rich in rough endoplasmic reticulum, which is concentrated mainly in the lower half of the cell, and is responsible for their cytoplasmic basophilia. The upper half of the cell, close to the lumen, contains variable numbers of eosinophilic **zymogen granules** (ZG), which contain the pre-enzymes synthesized by the cell. Some cells contain large numbers of these granules, while others, which contain few or none, are thought to have recently disgorged their granules by exocytosis into the acinar lumen. It is thought that the pre-enzymes are synthesized by the rough endoplasmic reticulum, and then transferred to the Golgi, which packages them into granules.
b The pancreatic ductal system begins in the acinus (A). Pale-staining cells, the **centroacinar cells** (C) represent the intra-acinar component of the **intercalated duct** (ID). In a fortuitous section, pale centroacinar cells can be seen leaving the acinus as the intercalated duct. These ducts are lined by a simple monolayer of cuboidal epithelium and form a complex network.

The intercalated ducts from individual acini fuse to form larger **interlobular ducts**, which run in the fibrocollagenous septa between the ill-defined pancreatic lobules and are lined by columnar epithelium.

Interlobular ducts join the **main pancreatic ducts**, which run longitudinally from the tail of the pancreas to its head and empty into the duodenal lumen at the **ampulla of Vater**. The main pancreatic ducts are lined by tall columnar epithelium containing a number of mucin-secreting goblet cells.

The control of pancreatic secretions is mainly mediated through hormones, the most important being secretin and **cholecystokinin** (**pancreozymin**).
• Secretin stimulates the formation of the bicarbonate-rich fluid.
• Cholecystokinin is thought to stimulate the acinar cells to release their enzymes.

Secretin and cholecystokinin are produced by the endocrine cells of the digestive tract mucosa, in response to the entry of acidic gastric contents into the duodenum.

The main pancreatic duct joins the distal end of the bile duct to open into the concavity of the duodenum at a small raised mound, the **ampulla of Vater**.

JEJUNUM
The jejunum is the main absorptive site of the digestive tract, and shows not only the greatest development of plical folds (see Fig. 10.35a), but also the most complex villous system, with finger-like villi being predominant.

ILEUM
The ileum is characterized by the greatest development of GALT. The lymphoid cells aggregate into large nodules (**Peyer's patches**), which expand the lamina propria of the mucosa, split the muscularis mucosae and extend into the submucosa. The mucosal epithelial cells overlying these lymphoid aggregates are modified in structure and function (see page 100).

Large intestine

The **large intestine** comprises:
• **caecum**;
• **ascending**, **transverse** and **descending colon**;
• **sigmoid colon**;
• **rectum**.

The structure of the large intestine is fairly constant throughout, although there are regional variations, particularly between the caecum and the rectum.

The main function of the large intestine is to convert the liquid small intestinal contents to solid indigestible waste material, **faeces**. This is achieved by extensive reabsorption of water and soluble salts from the bowel content, until it is semi-solid. With increasing solidity, mucin is required to lubricate its passage along the bowel. The **appendix** is a small appendage arising from the caecum.

Epithelium

The epithelial component of the mucosa of the large bowel is a mixture of absorptive cells and mucous cells, which are arranged as simple straight unbranching tubular downgrowths extending from the surface to the muscularis mucosae. The cell types present are columnar cells, mucous cells, stem cells and endocrine cells (see Fig. 10.43).

Other epithelial cells are found adjacent to the lymphoid aggregates in the lamina propria and are tightly packed cuboidal or columnar epithelial cells, which have a relatively high nucleus:cytoplasm ratio, and do not contain mucin. These cells are similar to the M cells associated with the lymphoid tissue in the small intestine.

COLUMNAR CELLS

Columnar cells (Figs 10.43b&c) are the most numerous type of epithelial cell in the large intestine. They are narrow slender cells and appear to be in a minority because they are compressed between the much larger mucous (goblet) cells. Their luminal surfaces have a microvillar brush border, and there is evidence that they can produce and secrete a neutral polysaccharide, possibly glycocalyx material.

Columnar cells are thought to carry out the salt and water absorptive function of the colon. They lack brush border enzymes and so play no part in digestive breakdown, but have prominent lateral intercellular spaces, which suggests active fluid transport. Furthermore they are well-equipped with Na^+ and K^+-ATPases in their lateral cell membranes.

MUCOUS (GOBLET) CELLS

Mucous cells (Figs 10. 43 b&c) possess large numbers of mucin granules, which produce the bulging rounded cytoplasm responsible for their synonym **goblet cells**.

The mucin vacuoles are larger in the sigmoid colon and rectum than in the caecum and ascending colon, and there appears to be a difference in the type of mucin secreted. Mucin from the colon and rectum is highly sulphated, and that from the caecum and ascending colon is less sulphated, and contains sialic acid radicals.

As the goblet cells approach the surface of the large intestine, they begin to discharge their mucus, and continue to migrate upwards to form part of the surface epithelium, which is mainly composed of columnar cells.

STEM CELLS

Stem cells (Fig. 10.43d) are the precursor cell of other cell types and are located at the bases of the tubular downgrowths. They develop into either mucous or columnar cells or into large intestinal endocrine cells.

ENDOCRINE CELLS

Endocrine cells (Fig. 10.43d) are comparatively few in number in the large bowel and are scattered amongst the other cells, mainly in the lower half of each tubular downgrowth; they have a broad base, narrowing to a small luminal surface covered with microvilli. Their neuroendocrine granules are situated basal to the nucleus and can sometimes be seen as small eosinophilic dots in H&E paraffin sections.

Immunocytochemical methods have shown that these cells contain a number of substances, including chromogranin, substance P, somatostatin, and glucagon.

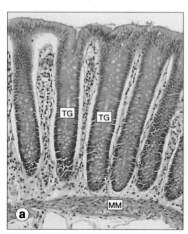 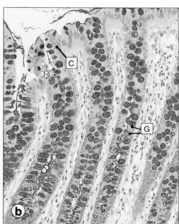 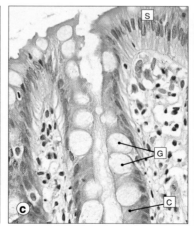 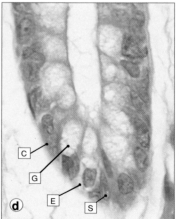
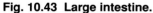

Fig. 10.43 Large intestine.
a Micrograph showing large intestine mucosa. The surface is flat, and simple straight tubular glands (TG) extend down to the muscularis mucosae (MM).
b The glands are lined by two populations of cells, the most numerous but less obvious being compressed tall columnar cells (C). The more easily seen cells are the mucous cells (mucus-secreting goblet cells, G), here stained blue by alcian blue .
c High power micrograph showing both columnar cells (C) and goblet cells (G) in the upper part of the tubular gland, while the surface cells (S) are mainly columnar and contain little mucin.
d At the bases of the glands the cell population is a combination of uncommitted stem cells (S), goblet cells (G), columnar cells (C), and occasional small pale-staining endocrine cells (E).

Lamina propria

The large intestinal lamina propria consists of collagen, reticulin, and fibroblasts, embedded in a glycosaminoglycan matrix.

There is a layer of compact collagen immediately beneath the basement membrane of the surface epithelium, and thin smooth muscle fibres from the muscularis mucosae insert into it.

The cell content of the lamina propria includes lymphocytes and scattered eosinophils, the lymphocytes being mainly T cells. Also present are small lymphoid follicles (part of the GALT, see page 159), the larger of which breach the muscularis mucosae and extend into the submucosa. Cells containing PAS positive granules, known as **muciphages** are a common finding, particularly in the rectum.

Muscularis mucosae

The muscularis mucosae consists of a two-layered smooth muscle arrangement, with an inner circular and an outer longitudinal layer, but this distinction is usually only clear in abnormally thickened muscle layers. Elastic fibres are also present.

The muscularis mucosae is penetrated by fine nerve twigs from the submucosal plexus, the fine nerves continuing vertically into the lamina propria. The innervation of the colon is particularly important in the diagnosis of Hirschsprung's disease (see Fig. 10.46).

Muscularis proper

The muscularis proper of the large intestine consists of an inner circular muscle layer and an outer longitudinal layer, which is not continuous, being concentrated into three bands, the **taeniae coli**.

Appendix

The appendix is a small blind-ending tubular diverticulum arising from the caecum. It is normally 5–10 cm long and about 0.8 cm in diameter. Both measurements vary from person to person, but its diameter decreases with increasing age, being at its greatest at 7–20 years of age.

The wall of the appendix is composed of a muscularis proper, which has an outer longitudinal and an inner circular component like the rest of the digestive tract. The submucosa contains blood vessels, nerves and variable amounts of lymphoid tissue.

The mucosal epithelium is colonic in nature, with straight tubular glands containing tall columnar absorptive cells, mucin-secreting goblet cells and some enteroendocrine cells, which are mainly found in the bases of the glands. Enteroendocrine cells are also found in the submucosa, closely related to nerves and ganglion cells, particularly near the closed tip of the appendix.

In children, the lamina propria and the submucosa contain abundant lymphoid tissue with prominent follicle formation (Fig. 10.44a). This is not present at birth, but progressively populates the appendix over the first 10 years of life, thereafter progressively disappearing, so that the normal adult appendix shows only traces of this tissue (Fig. 10.44b).

As the lymphoid tissue atrophies in the adult, the submucosa becomes progressively more collagenous, and in the elderly the mucosa itself may become fibrotic, particularly near the tip.

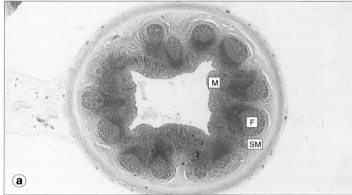

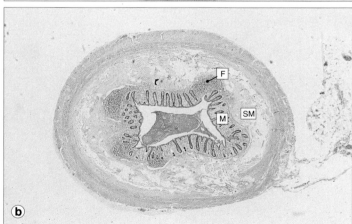

Fig. 10.44 Appendix.
a Transverse section of appendix from a 10-year-old child. It is lined by large bowel type mucosa (M) in which there are large lymphoid follicles (F) extending into the submucosa (SM).
b Transverse section of appendix from a 36-year-old man at the same magnification as **a**. Note the relative reduction in size and the virtual disappearance of the lymphoid follicles (F).

Low fibra, high fat

DISORDERS OF THE LARGE BOWEL

The colon and rectum are subject to a number of disorders, many of which are transient, and the result of dietary indiscretion, for example diarrhoea following the ingestion of large volumes of beer. The three most important diseases of long duration in adults are:

- **cancer** of the large bowel epithelium;
- **diverticular disease,** in which increased pressure in the bowel lumen forces mucosa to balloon through the muscle layers;
- **ulcerative colitis**, which is a severe ulcerating disease of the colonic mucosa.

Ulcerative colitis

The cause of ulcerative colitis is not known, but large bowel mucosa is lost over an extensive area, with ulceration and destruction of the absorptive epithelium (Fig. 10.45).

This mucosal damage impairs water resorption from the colonic contents, and thus the normal solid faeces are replaced by large quantities of watery diarrhoea, which is similar in content and texture to the contents of the ileum. Destruction of the mucosa also leads to bleeding, so the watery diarrhoea is often mixed with blood.

Hirschsprung's disease

In infants and children the most important disease of the large bowel is **Hirschsprung's disease**, in which defaecation is not possible because a segment of the lower rectum is completely devoid of ganglion cells in the submucosa and muscularis layers. Normal innervation has been described on page 159 and illustrated in Fig. 10.26.

The affected segment of bowel remains closed and the child's abdomen distends with unpassed faeces, fatal perforation occurring if it is not treated.

Although the abnormality primarily affects the lower rectum, the aganglionic segment may be extensive, involving much of the distal colon.

Diagnosis is established by rectal biopsy in which submucosal ganglion cells are absent. A characteristic feature is hypertrophy of nerve twigs in the muscularis mucosae, submucosa and lamina propria (Fig. 10.46).

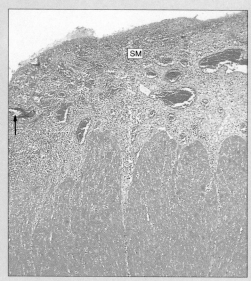

Fig. 10.45 Ulcerative colitis. Micrograph of wall of sigmoid colon from a patient with ulcerative colitis. Note the complete destruction of the mucosa and some submucosa (SM); only a few scattered remnants of absorptive and mucus-secreting epithelium remain (arrow).

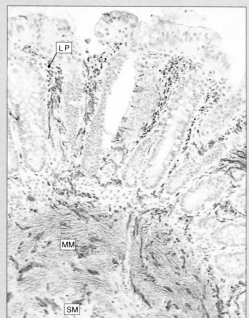

Fig. 10.46 Hirschsprung's disease. Micrograph showing prominent nerve twigs in the lamina propria (LP), muscularis mucosae (MM) and submucosa (SM). This rectal biopsy from a child with Hirschsprung's disease, has been stained by the cholinesterase enzyme histochemical technique.

173

PRACTICAL HISTOLOGY

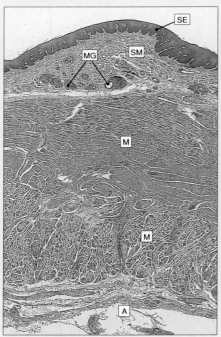

Fig. 10.47 Oesophagus.
This low power micrograph shows the squamous epithelium (SE) of the lower third of the oesophagus, and the submucosa (SM) containing oesophageal mucous glands (MG) surrounded by a prominent lymphocytic infiltrate.

At this level of the oesophagus the muscle layers (M) are composed entirely of smooth muscle. Higher in the oesophagus there is a moderate amount of skeletal muscle.

The outer adventitial layer (A) contains adipose tissue, and a number of nerves and blood vessels.

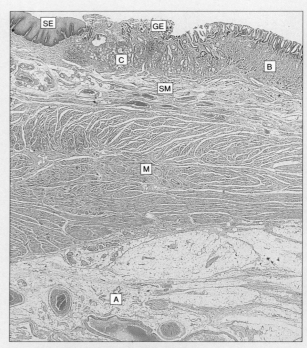

Fig. 10.48 Oesophagogastric junction.
This micrograph shows the junction between the squamous epithelium (SE) of the lower oesophagus and the glandular epithelium (GE) of the stomach.

Two patterns of gastric mucosa can be seen, that closest to the oesophageal squamous epithelium being cardiac-type (C, see Fig. 10.33), which in this case forms a narrow zone before gastric mucosa of body-type (B, see Fig. 10.33).

In this region, the submucosa (SM) is highly vascular, as is the adventitial layer (A).

The distinction of the muscle layers (M) into circular and longitudinal layers becomes indistinct in this oesophagogastric area.

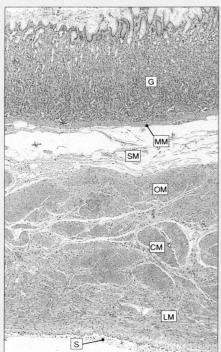

Fig. 10.49 Stomach wall.
Micrograph showing the stomach wall in the body region. The body mucosa is thick and composed largely of glands (G, see Figs 10.21 & 10.33). The distinct muscularis mucosae (MM) can be seen separating the epithelium from a loose textured submucosa (SM).

The three muscle layers frequently seen in the stomach are evident. There is an inner oblique (OM) layer, a middle circular (CM) layer and an outer longitudinal (LM) layer.

The stomach lies within the peritoneal cavity and its outer coat is therefore a serosal (S) layer covered by mesothelial cells.

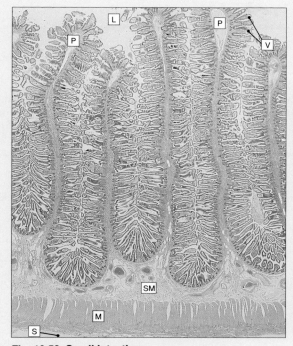

Fig. 10.50 Small intestine.
This low power micrograph from the first part of the jejunum shows the characteristic structure of the small intestinal wall.

The mucosal layer is thrown up into high folds (plicae P, see also Fig. 10.35), the surfaces of which are modified to form numerous villi (V, see Fig. 10.36). This modification enormously increases the surface area of epithelium exposed to small intestinal contents in the lumen (L).

The submucosa (SM) is highly vascular and the double muscle layer (M) can be seen. The outer surface is covered by serosa (S).

The pattern of extensive plication becomes progressively less marked in the lower reaches of the small intestine.

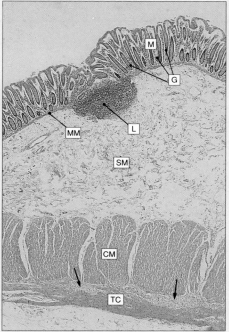

Fig. 10.51 Colon.
Micrograph showing the colon with its flat surfaced mucosa (M) composed of simple tubular glands (G, see Fig. 10.43). There is a distinct muscularis mucosae (MM), which in this micrograph is breached in one area by a lymphoid aggregate (L) that lies partly in the mucosa and partly in the submucosa. This lymphoid aggregate is part of the GALT.

The submucosa (SM) is loose and fibrocollagenous, allowing movement of the mucosa on the muscle layer.

The muscle layer is composed mainly of circular muscle (CM), but there is a narrow discontinuous longitudinal muscle forming the taenia coli (TC). There is a prominent collection of ganglia and nerves between the two muscle layers (arrows, see Fig. 10.26).

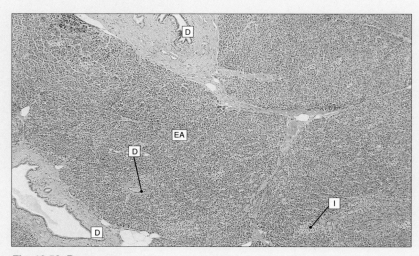

Fig. 10.52 Pancreas.
Low power micrograph showing the pancreas with its duct systems (D), which drain the secretions of the exocrine acini (EA, see Fig. 10.42) into the main pancreatic duct prior to discharge into the duodenum.

Most of the pancreatic tissue shown here is composed of tightly packed exocrine acini, the details of which are not visible at this low magnification. A small islet of Langerhan's (I), the endocrine component of the pancreas (see Chapter 15) is also present in this field.

11. HEPATOBILIARY SYSTEM

LIVER

The liver acts as a vast chemical factory, synthesizing large complex molecules from low molecular weight substances brought to it in the blood, particularly substances recently absorbed by the intestine and transported by a **portal** blood system. The liver also breaks down toxic substances brought to it by the **hepatic artery**, and synthesizes **bile**, which is transferred by a system of ducts (the **biliary system**) to the duodenum.

All of the biochemical functions of the liver are carried out by the epithelial parenchymal cell of the liver, the **hepatocyte** and are dependent on complex interrelationships between:
- the **vasculature** (hepatic artery and portal vein branches, sinusoids and central veins);
- the **hepatocytes**;
- the **bile drainage systems** (bile canaliculi and intrahepatic bile ducts, Fig. 11.1).

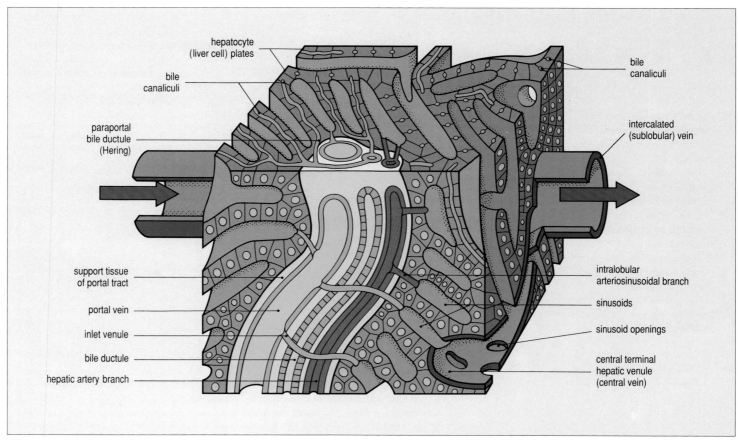

Fig. 11.1 Architecture of the liver.
Hepatocytes (liver cells) are arranged as interconnecting flat plates, between which are sinusoids containing blood supplied by small side branches of the hepatic artery and portal vein. Sinusoidal blood drains into a central terminal hepatic venule, each of which empties into an intercalated (sublobular) vein. Bile produced by hepatocytes enters narrow canaliculi, which drain into small bile ducts running with the hepatic artery and portal vein branches.

Afferent vasculature

The liver receives blood from two sources, the hepatic artery and the hepatic portal vein .

The hepatic artery perfuses the liver with oxygenated flood from the coeliac axis branches of the aorta. On entering the liver it divides into increasingly smaller branches.

The hepatic portal vein carries blood from the digestive tract and spleen to the liver, the blood from the digestive tract being rich in amino acids, lipids and carbohydrates absorbed from the bowel, and that from the spleen being rich in haemoglobin breakdown products.

After entering the liver at the porta hepatis, the portal vein divides into smaller distributing veins, which then branch further, eventually forming **terminal portal venules**.

Microvasculature

In the liver, the two input circulations (hepatic artery and hepatic portal vein) discharge their blood into a common system of small vascular channels, the **sinusoids** (Fig. 11.2), which are in intimate contact with the hepatocytes.

The hepatic artery carries oxygenated blood containing metabolites for reprocessing and toxins for detoxification by hepatocytes. It divides into successively smaller branches, the terminal elements running with the terminal branches of the hepatic portal vein before emptying into the hepatic sinusoids by short side branches (the **arteriosinusoidal branches**). A peribiliary plexus of small arterial branches supplies oxygenated blood to the large intrahepatic bile ducts before draining into the sinusoids.

The hepatic portal vein carries poorly oxygenated blood, which is rich in carbohydrates, lipids and amino acids absorbed from the gut, and haemoglobin-breakdown

products from the spleen. It divides within the liver into successive generations of progressively smaller branches (interlobar, segmental and interlobular branches), culminating in terminal portal venules, which run with the terminal branches of the hepatic artery.

Lateral side branches (**inlet venules**) of the terminal portal venules empty blood into the sinusoids where it blends with blood from the terminal hepatic artery branches. The terminal parts of the hepatic portal and arterial systems run together in the **portal tracts**, which also contain bile ductules.

Hepatic sinusoids

Hepatic sinusoids are vascular channels about 10–30 μm in diameter, lined by a thin discontinuous highly fenestrated endothelium, which does not rest on a basement membrane. Instead it is closely related externally to plates and cords of hepatocytes (Fig. 11.3), though separated from them by a space. This **perisinusoidal space of Disse** is the main site where material is transferred between the blood-filled sinusoids and hepatocytes in both directions.

The hepatic sinusoids are partly lined by a scattering of phagocytic cells (**Kupffer cells**), which are derived from circulating blood monocytes.

Sinusoids receive blood from the terminal portal venules and terminal branches of the hepatic artery, and empty blood, which has undergone considerable modification of its contents, into **terminal hepatic venules**.

Efferent vasculature

Blood which has passed through the functioning liver parenchyma enters terminal hepatic venules (**central veins** of the lobules, see Fig. 11.7), which in turn unite to form **intercalated veins**; these then fuse to form larger **hepatic vein** branches. Hepatic veins are devoid of valves, and open separately into the inferior vena cava as it passes through the liver on its way to the right atrium.

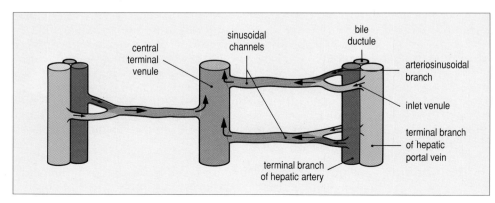

Fig. 11.2 Hepatic microcirculation.
Diagram of the hepatic microcirculation. Blood from the terminal branches of the hepatic artery and the portal vein enters the sinusoidal system via small side branches, the arteriosinusoidal branch and inlet venule, respectively. It then passes along the sinusoid lumina towards the terminal hepatic venule (central vein). The sinusoidal system is an interconnecting system of capillary-like channels in close contact with the functioning liver cells (hepatocytes); it is not a system of simple tubes as shown here.

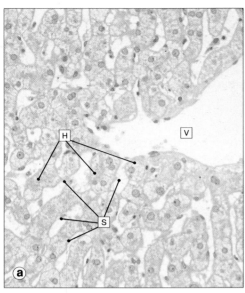

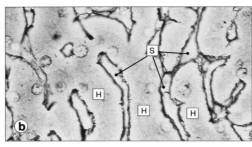

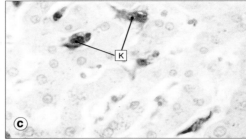

Fig. 11.3. Hepatic sinusoids
a High power micrograph showing the relationship between the sinusoidal channels (S) and the cuboidal hepatocytes (H). Note the terminal hepatic venule.
b Micrograph of liver stained to demonstrate reticulin fibres (black), which run in the space of Disse between the hepatocyte surface and the endothelial cells lining the sinusoid (see Fig.11.4c&d). This method delineates the outline of the sinusoid (S) and the hepatocyte columns (H) and is used in the histological diagnosis of liver disease on small cores of liver tissue obtained by needle biopsy (see Fig. 1.1).
c Immunoperoxidase preparation (showing lysozyme) identifying scattered phagocytic Kupffer cells (K) in the sinusoid lining.

Hepatocytes (liver cells)

Intimately associated with the skeleton of blood vessels (sinusoids) are the parenchymal cells of the liver, the hepatocytes.

Hepatocytes are polarized polyhedral cells with three identifiable types of surface (see below). As would be expected in cells that are so metabolically active, their cytoplasm is packed with a wide range of organelles.
• The nuclei are large, spherical and central, and contain scattered clumps of chromatin and prominent nucleoli. Many cells are binucleate, and nuclei are frequently polyploid; progressively more tetraploid nuclei develop with age.
• The Golgi is large and active, or small and multiple, and is mainly seen near the nucleus, with an extension lying close to the canalicular surface (see below).
• The vesicles and tubules of the abundant smooth and rough endoplasmic reticulum are continuous with the Golgi. There are numerous free ribosomes in the cytosol, as well as large glycogen deposits and some lipid droplets, the glycogen often being closely related to the smooth endoplasmic reticulum.
• Lysosomes (see page 17) of various sizes are numerous, some containing lipofuscin and lamellated lipoprotein. They are particularly large and numerous near the canalicular surface.
• Peroxisomes (see page 19) usually number 200–300/cell.
• Mitochondria are also abundant, numbering more than 1000 / cell and are randomly scattered. This vast mitochondrial component gives the hepatocyte cytoplasm its eosinophilic granular appearance in H&E stained paraffin sections.

Hepatocyte surfaces

The hepatocyte surfaces are important because they are involved in the transfer of substances between the hepatocyte, blood vessels and bile canaliculi.

The three types of surface are sinusoidal, canalicular and intercellular (Fig. 11.4).

SINUSOIDAL SURFACES
Sinusoidal surfaces are separated from the sinusoidal vessel by the space of Disse, and account for approximately 70% of hepatocyte surface. They are covered by short microvilli, which protrude into the space of Disse. Between the bases of the microvilli are coated pits (see Fig. 2.5), which are involved in endocytosis.

The sinusoidal surface is the site where material is transferred between the sinusoids and the hepatocyte.

CANALICULAR SURFACES
Canalicular surfaces are the surfaces across which bile drains from the hepatocytes into the canaliculi. They account for approximately 15% of the hepatocyte surface, and are closely apposed except at the site of a canaliculus, which is a tube formed by the exact opposition of two shallow gutters on the surface of adjacent hepatocytes.

Canaliculi are about 0.5–2.5 μm in diameter, being smaller close to the terminal hepatic venule, and are lined by irregular microvilli arising from the canalicular surfaces of the hepatocytes.

Hepatocyte cytoplasm close to the canaliculi is rich in actin filaments, which are possibly capable of influencing the diameter of the canaliculus and thus the rate of flow.

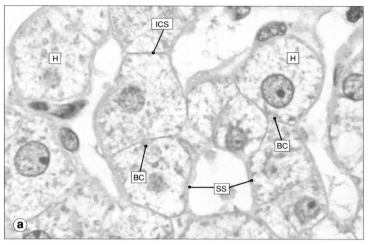

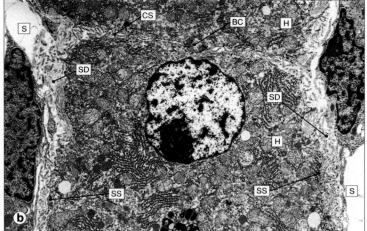

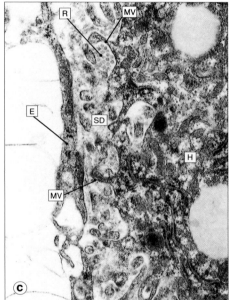

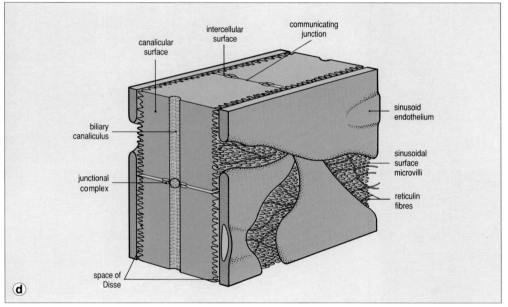

Fig. 11.4 Hepatocyte.

a Micrograph of a thin acrylic resin H&E stained section of hepatocytes (H), which are roughly cuboidal and have a pale granular eosinophilic cytoplasm, much of the pallor being due to the presence of glycogen. The nuclei are central with a distinct nuclear membrane and prominent nucleoli.

Some of the hepatocyte surface lines the sinusoidal channel (i.e. sinusoidal surface, SS), whilst other surfaces are in contact with adjacent hepatocyte (i.e. intercelluar surfaces, ICS), some of the adjacent hepatocyte surfaces having bile canaliculi (BC) running between them. Details of the canaliculi cannot be distinguished by light microscopy.

b Low power electronmicrograph showing some of the cytoplasm of two adjacent hepatocytes (H), joined by their canalicular surfaces (CS) in which a bile canaliculus (BC) can be seen.

The other surfaces of the hepatocyte are the sinusoidal surfaces (SS) bordering the sinusoid lumen (S). The space between the hepatocyte surface and the sinusoid is the space of Disse (SD).

c Medium power electronmicrograph showing the space of Disse (SD) between the sinusoidal surface of the hepatocyte (H) and the endothelial cell (E) lining the sinusoid. A number of irregular microvilli (MV) protrude into the space of Disse from the hepatocyte surface. The microvilli are much less regular in humans than in rodents. Some of the support fibres of the reticulin network (R) can be seen.

d Diagram showing the space of Disse lying between the hepatocyte and the discontinuous endothelium lining the sinusoid. The space contains microvillar processes from the hepatocyte surface and collagenous reticulin fibres, which form a supportive mesh.

179

The cell membrane around the canalicular lumen is rich in alkaline phosphatase and adenosine triphosphatase, and the canalicular lumen is isolated from the rest of the canalicular surface by junctional complexes (Fig. 11.5).

INTERCELLULAR SURFACES

The intercellular surfaces are the surfaces between adjacent hepatocytes that are not in contact with sinusoids or canaliculi. They account for about 15% of the hepatocyte surface.

These intercellular surfaces are comparatively simple, but specialized for cell attachment and cell to cell communication via communicating junctions (see Fig. 3.14).

INTRAHEPATIC BILIARY TREE

Bile produced by hepatocytes passes into bile canaliculi and flows towards the portal tracts (i.e. in the opposite direction to the blood).

As the canaliculi approach the **bile ductules** (Fig. 11.6a) in the portal tracts, they open into short passages lined by small cuboidal cells (the **canals of Hering**). From here, bile flows into the bile ductules in the portal tract.

Bile ductules anastomose freely, fuse and increase in size to form larger ducts, the **trabecular ducts** (Fig. 11.6b).

Many of these ducts fuse to form large **intrahepatic ducts**, which converge near the liver hilum into the **main hepatic ducts** (see page 184).

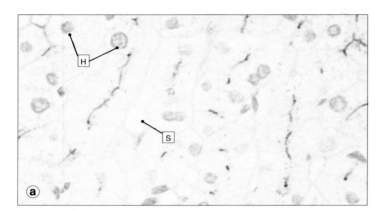

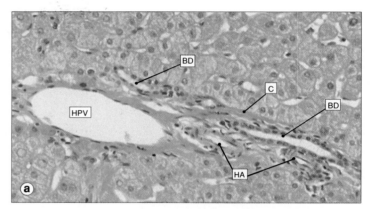

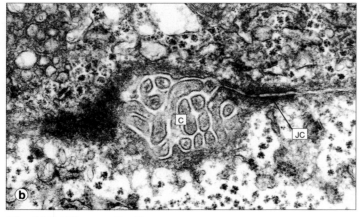

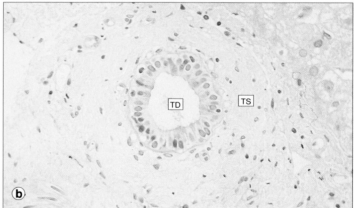

Fig. 11.5 Bile canaliculi.

a Micrograph showing bile canaliculi highlighted by an immunoperoxidase method for CEA, which shows the canaliculi as brown lines or dots depending on whether they have been sectioned longitudinally or transversely. The nuclei and outlines of hepatocytes (H) can be seen as can an occasional sinusoid (S).
b Electronmicrograph of the canalicular surface of two apposed hepatocytes showing the structure of the bile canaliculi. Note the canaliculus (C) and the junctional complexes (JC) separating the canalicular lumen from the rest of the apposed hepatocyte.

Fig. 11.6 Intrahepatic bile ducts.

a Micrograph showing a small bile ductule (BD) in the portal tract. It has a simple structure with low cuboidal epithelium, and a narrow surrounding zone of collagen (C) and some smooth muscle fibres. A terminal branch of the hepatic portal vein (HPV) and hepatic artery (HA) are also present in the tract.
b Micrograph of a transverse section of a trabecular duct (TD), which is larger than a bile ductule, with a larger lumen, and a well-formed wall. It is surrounded by dense fibrocollagenous tissue of the trabecular septum (TS) in which it runs.

Hepatic lobule *vs* acinus controversy

Historically, the arrangement of the components of the liver has been described as having a lobular pattern, and a vocabulary has arisen which enables normal histological features and abnormal pathological changes to be described in relation to the lobule unit. This device has stood the test of time. Recently however, it has been proposed that the structure of the liver should be considered in terms of another structural unit, the acinus (Fig. 11.7).

Lobule concept

The components of the liver (i.e. the hepatocytes, terminal hepatic venules, portal triads and sinusoids) are arranged in a fairly constant pattern, which has been described as lobular, the classical lobule being composed of:
- a central terminal hepatic venule, into which drains a converging series of sinusoidal channels like the spokes of a cycle wheel;
- interconnecting plates of hepatocytes, which surround each sinusoidal channel and run between the central terminal hepatic venule and the periphery of the lobule;
- peripherally arranged portal tracts, each containing terminal branches of the hepatic artery and portal vein, and a small tributary of the bile duct.

Thus a ring of portal tracts forms the outer limit of each classical lobule.

The channels within each portal tract are surrounded by a small amount of fibrocollagenous tissue, and in some animals, particularly the pig, fibrocollagenous septa extend from one portal triad to another, clearly outlining the limits of each lobule. In humans, however these fibrous septa are absent, and so the lobule is less clearly defined.

In the lobule, various zones of hepatocytes can be identified. These are the centrilobular, periportal and mid zones.

The centrilobular zone is composed of hepatocytes surrounding the central terminal hepatic venule, and is the zone most distant from the oxygenated arterial blood supply.

The periportal zone at the periphery of the lobule is closely related to the portal tracts. The outermost layer of periportal hepatocytes immediately adjacent to the portal tract is called the **limiting plate**, and is the first group of hepatocytes to be damaged in liver disorders that primarily involve the portal tracts.

As the cells of the limiting plate are exposed to hepatic artery and portal venous blood before other hepatocytes, they receive maximum exposure to any toxins in the systemic blood or absorbed by the digestive tract.

The mid zone is the zone of hepatocytes between the centrilobular and periportal zones.

Acinus concept

Another way of describing the architecture of the liver is the acinus concept. This views the blood supply as the focal point, the periphery of one segment of the lobule being its short axis.

Lobular or acinar

The architectural arrangement of the liver remains immutable, the lobular and acinar concepts are simply two different ways of looking at the structure. In man, neither lobules nor acini have a clearly visible outline, but most of the nomenclature used in the descriptions of disease processes (e.g. centrilobular necrosis, limiting plate inflammation) is based on the lobular concept.

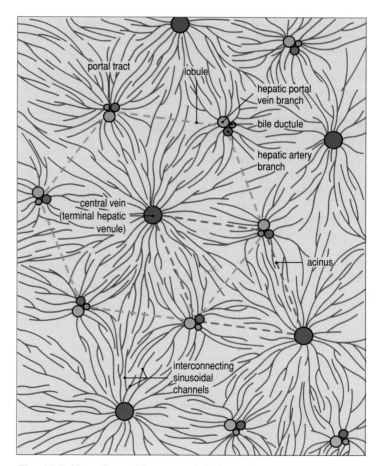

Fig. 11.7 Hepatic architecture–lobule and acinus.
Diagram showing the architecture of the liver and the relationship between the vessels and ducts in the portal tract, the sinusoidal system and the central veins. The lobular and acinar concepts (see Fig. 11.12) are overdrawn.

Liver function

The liver has a wide range of functions, which account for its complex structure.

Bile synthesis and secretion. The liver produces bile, which is an alkaline secretion containing water, ions, phospholipids, bile pigments (mainly bilirubin glucuronide) and bile acids (glycocholic and taurocholic acid).

Bile is transported in the bile ducts from the liver to the gallbladder, where it is stored and concentrated, prior to excretion into the duodenum via distal bile ducts.

Bile neutralizes the acid chyme, which enters the duodenum from the stomach, and bile acids in the bile emulsify fat globules in the chyme, thereby facilitating lipid digestion by lipases.

Most of the bile acids in the bile are reabsorbed in the ileum and recirculate to the liver, but about 10–15% is broken down in the intestine or lost in the faeces. Liver cells synthesize replacement bile acids.

Excretion of bilirubin. Bilirubin is produced in the spleen from the breakdown of the haem component of haemoglobin. In the liver the bilirubin is conjugated with glucuronic acid, and the conjugate (bilirubin glucuronide) is excreted in the bile and thence in the faeces.

Protein synthesis. The liver synthesizes many proteins including albumen, and blood clotting factors such as fibrinogen and prothrombin.

Gluconeogenesis. Lipids and amino acids are converted into glucose in the liver by gluconeogenesis.

Storage. Triglycerides, glycogen and some vitamins are stored in the liver.

Deamination of amino acids. In the liver amino acids are deaminated to produce urea, which is excreted by the kidney.

Conjugation and chemical breakdown of toxins. The smooth endoplasmic reticulum of the liver possesses large numbers of enzymes that break down or conjugate toxic substances (e.g. alcohol, barbiturates, etc.) to convert them into harmless products.

LIVER FAILURE

Liver disease can affect any of its functions, though when large numbers of hepatocytes are damaged, all of the functions tend to be disturbed.

Failure of synthetic functions. The liver fails to produce important proteins such as albumen and the various protein clotting factors.
- The reduced synthesis of albumen leads to a reduced oncotic pressure of the blood, which results in **oedema** and accumulation of watery fluid in the peritoneal cavity (**ascites**).
- Failure of clotting factor synthesis leads to spontaneous bleeding.

Failure of detoxification functions. The liver fails to convert metabolic waste products into innocuous substances. Toxic substances therefore circulate in the blood and cause a number of symptoms including confusion, altered consciousness and eventually coma (**hepatic coma**), which is rapidly fatal.

Failure of adequate bile secretion into the alimentary tract leads to retention of bile in the liver, with some of the components of the retained bile entering the blood and producing yellowish discoloration of the blood plasma and tissues (i.e. **jaundice**).

Chronic hepatic failure

If hepatocyte damage is slowly progressive the abnormalities outlined above develop insidiously over a period of years. This is called **chronic hepatic failure**, and is most commonly associated with the disease called cirrhosis (see Fig. 11.8).

Acute hepatic failure

If the liver disease is severe and of sudden onset, the metabolic abnormalities appear suddenly. This is **acute hepatic failure**, and is most commonly associated with some acute virus infections (e.g. hepatitis B virus infection) or exposure to liver toxins (e.g. paracetamol). In both cases acute hepatic failure is the result of widespread death of most liver cells.

CIRRHOSIS

Many slowly progressive diseases destroy hepatocytes and lead to distortion of liver architecture, particularly the relationships between the sinusoids, the portal venous system and the bile ducts.

Death of hepatocytes is followed by scarring, and although hepatocytes can regenerate and produce a new population of cells, their connections with the portal system and the biliary drainage are destroyed. This pattern of liver disorder is known as **cirrhosis** (Fig. 11.8), and is a common cause of chronic liver failure.

Cirrhosis is characterized by:
- continuing death of hepatocytes;
- collapse of normal architecture;
- increased production of fibrocollagenous tissue, leading to irregular scarring;
- attempted regeneration of surviving hepatocytes, which form irregular nodules, and have abnormal relationships with the microvasculature and bile drainage system.

Regenerating hepatocytes are able to continue some synthetic functions, but eventually fail to keep pace with normal demands, and the symptoms of liver failure begin to manifest themselves.

Cirrhosis produces chronic liver failure, and symptoms appear progressively over a period of some years, usually culminating fatally in coma or as a result of the complications of portal hypertension.

Portal hypertension

In cirrhosis, the sinusoidal connections between the portal venous system and the draining central terminal hepatic venules and hepatic veins are destroyed.

Portal venous blood cannot therefore escape through its normal channels (i.e. through sinusoids into central terminal hepatic venules). Thus, the blood pressure in the portal venous system increases considerably and causes **portal hypertension**.

One escape route for portal venous blood is via anastomoses with the systemic venous system; these are normally closed when portal pressure is low, but open when portal pressure rises.

When these anastomotic channels are distended with blood, they are called **varices.**

One of the sites of such an anastomosis is at the lower end of the oesophagus, which is unfortunate since the distended submucosal blood vessels (**oesophageal varices**) bulge into the lumen of the oesophagus and are easily eroded by gastric acid, resulting in torrential haemorrhage.

Bleeding from oesophageal varices is a severe complication of portal hypertension and cirrhosis, and may be fatal.

Cirrhosis and portal hypertension most commonly follow persisting hepatocyte destruction due to alcohol toxicity, some forms of viral infection, and autoimmune liver disease.

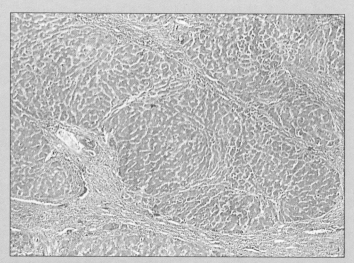

Fig. 11.8 Cirrhosis.
Micrograph of liver from a patient with cirrhosis. Compare with Fig. 11.12 and note the fibrous scarring (blue), which has distorted the normal architecture. There are nodules of regenerating liver cells but their connections with the vascular supply and bile drainage system are destroyed. Masson trichrome stain.

EXTRAHEPATIC BILE DUCTS

The small tributaries of the intrahepatic biliary tree fuse to become increasingly larger channels, eventually fusing to become two large ducts, the **right** and **left lobar bile ducts**. These join at the hilum of the liver to form the **common hepatic duct**, which is the first part of the extrahepatic bile duct system (Fig. 11.9).

About 3–4 cm after leaving the liver, the common hepatic duct receives the **cystic duct** (a small duct from the gallbladder) and becomes the **common bile duct**.

The common bile duct is about 6–7 cm long and opens into the duodenum at the **ampulla of Vater**, having passed through the head of the pancreas and combined with the pancreatic duct.

GALLBLADDER

The gallbladder is an ovoid sac with a muscular wall, and is capable of moderate distension. It concentrates and stores bile, receiving dilute watery bile from the common hepatic duct, and emptying thick concentrated, variably mucoid, bile into the common bile duct.

Bile is transported in and out of the gallbladder through a short duct, the **cystic duct.** This duct contains a spirally arranged outgrowth of mucosa, which forms the **spiral valve of Heister**.

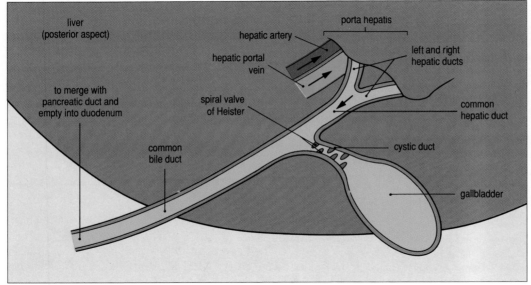

Fig. 11.9 Extrahepatic biliary tree.
Diagram of the drainage system whereby bile leaves the liver, is stored and concentrated in the gallbladder, and eventually enters the duodenum.

The right and left hepatic ducts emerge from the posterior aspect of the liver at the porta hepatis and join to form the common hepatic duct. A side branch of this duct (the cystic duct) conducts bile into and out of the gallbladder.

The common hepatic duct then continues as the common bile duct, passing through the head of the pancreas, where it merges with the pancreatic duct before entering the duodenum.

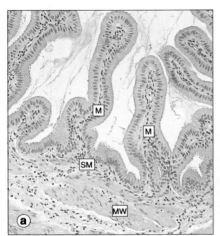
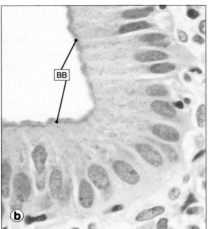

Fig. 11.10 Gallbladder.
a Low power micrograph of the gallbladder showing the mucosa (M) with its ridged mucosal folds, the submucosa (SM) and the muscular wall (MW).
b High power micrograph of gallbladder epithelium. The cells are tall and columnar with basal nuclei, and a luminal surface bearing microvilli. The microvilli are discernible as a faint brush border (BB).

Mucosa

The gallbladder mucosa is covered by tall columnar epithelial cells with numerous microvilli on their luminal surfaces, and complex interdigitations of their lateral walls (Fig. 11.10); these differently specialized surfaces are separated by junctional complexes (see Fig. 3.13).

Gallbladder epithelial cells are adapted for salt and water absorption, and have abundant basal and apical mitochondria, and Na^+ and K^+ transport ATPases in their lateral walls.

Na^+ and Cl^- ions are actively pumped out of the cell cytoplasm into the lateral intercellular space to produce an osmotic gradient between it and the gallbladder lumen. Water is therefore drawn into the space from the lumen, and then enters the abundant capillary network in the lamina propria.

This mechanism is similar to that employed by the proximal convoluted tubule epithelial cell in the kidney to absorb water and ions (see Chapter 16).

Gallbladder epithelium is thrown up into folds or plicae, which flatten when the gallbladder is distended.

GALLSTONES

Gallstones (i.e. stones or calculi in the gallbladder or biliary tree) form when solid concretions of bile act as a nidus for calcium salt deposition. Small gallstones are asymptomatic; larger gallstones can cause obstructive jaundice or cholecystitis.

Obstructive jaundice

Obstructive jaundice results from the blockage of a bile duct, for example by a gallstone that has passed out of the gallbladder and become impacted in the common bile duct on its way to the duodenum.

Blockage of the bile duct impedes the flow of bile into the duodenum. This results in:

- damming of bile in the proximal biliary tree, intrahepatic bile ducts and eventually bile canaliculi;
- passage of retained canalicular bile into the hepatic sinusoids and thence into the blood stream, producing **jaundice**;
- impaired intestinal breakdown of fat due to lack of the emulsifying bile acids normally present in bile;
- pale faeces, normal faecal colour being due to the presence of bile and its breakdown products.

Cholecystitis

Gallstones may become impacted in the cystic duct (Fig. 11.11a) and obstruct the flow of bile at this point. This has the following consequences, which are the basic features of so-called **chronic cholecystitis** (Fig. 11.11b).

- The gallbladder contracts more strongly to try to overcome the obstruction, and consequently its musculature thickens.
- Resulting high pressure within the gallbladder lumen pushes pouches of mucosa into the muscle layers (**Aschoff-Rokitansky sinuses**).
- Stasis of bile within the gallbladder predisposes to infection, and episodes of pain and fever are common.

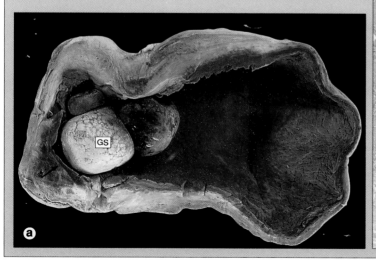

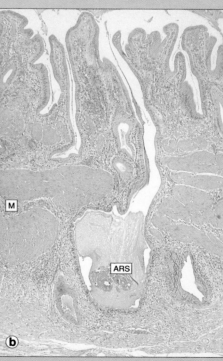

Fig. 11.11 Obstructive biliary disease.
a Photograph of a greatly enlarged gallbladder with a gallstone (GS) impacted in its neck, close to the cystic duct. Obstruction of bile drainage has led to bile stasis and consequent infection, producing red inflamed mucosa (arrow). **b** Micrograph of a chronically obstructed gallbladder. The muscle layer (M) is thickened by hypertrophy, and a pouch of epithelial-lined mucosa (Aschoff-Rokitansky sinus, ARS) has bulged through it. Compare with Fig. 11.10a.

PRACTICAL HISTOLOGY

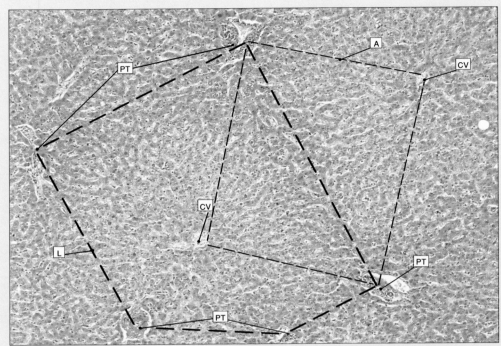

Fig. 11.12 Liver architecture.
Low power micrograph showing the general liver architecture. Note the central terminal hepatic venules (CV), portal tracts (PT), and the interconnecting cords of hepatocytes.

The concepts of the hepatic lobule (L) and hepatic acinus (A) are overdrawn (see Fig. 11.7).

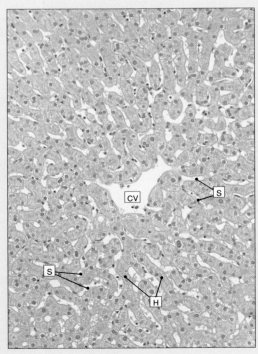

Fig. 11.13 Liver sinusoids and hepatocytes.
Micrograph showing sinusoidal channels (S) passing between the interconnecting columns of hepatocytes (H) on their way to the central terminal hepatic venule (CV).

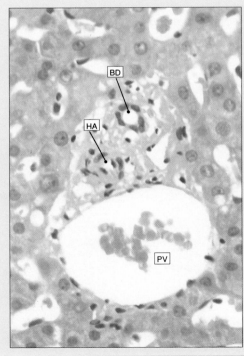

Fig. 11.14 Portal tract.
Portal tracts contain a small bile ductule (BD), a terminal branch of the hepatic artery (HA), and a component of the distal part of the hepatic portal venous system (PV). All are contained within a fibrocollagenous supporting stroma.

12. SPECIAL SENSES

Sensory information is derived from a variety of specialized sensory nerve endings, which include:
- sensory endings in the skin to detect touch (fine touch, pressure), pain and temperature (see Chapter 19);
- tendon endings and muscle spindles to detect movement and position of the limbs (see page 230);
- chemoreceptive organs such as the carotid body (see page 268);
- sensory endings on the tongue to detect taste (see page 146);
- sensory endings in the olfactory mucosa to detect smell (see page 126).

In addition, there are the specialized sensory organs, the eye and the ear; the ear and the vestibular system detects sound, acceleration and position, and the eye perceives light.

EAR

The ear is composed of external ear, middle ear and inner ear (Fig. 12.1).

External ear

The external ear comprises the **pinna** and **external auditory canal**.
- The pinna is composed of elastic cartilage (see page 53) covered by hair-bearing skin.
- The external auditory canal is lined by hair-bearing skin, and within its subcutaneous tissues are wax-secreting **ceruminous glands**, which are modified sebaceous glands. The outer two-thirds of the canal is surrounded by elastic cartilage in continuity with the pinna; the inner third is surrounded by the temporal bone of the skull.

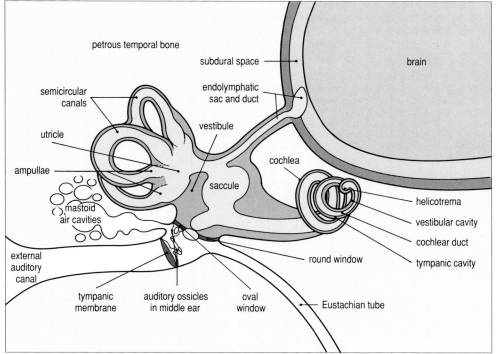

Fig. 12.1 Anatomy of the ear.
The ear consists of external ear, middle ear and inner ear. The inner third of the external auditory canal of the external ear is surrounded by the temporal bone, while the middle ear and inner ear are contained within cavities in the temporal bone.

The middle ear is an air-filled cavity containing the auditory ossicles. It is connected to the naspharynx by the Eustachian tube and is in direct continuity with the mastoid air cells.

The inner ear is a fluid-filled cavity divided into three main spaces (semicircular canal space, vestibule and cochlea).

Within the inner ear are a series of interconnecting fluid-filled membranous sacs (semicircular canals, utricle, saccule and cochlear duct).

The endolymphatic duct runs from the membranous sacs to the subdural space around the brain.

Middle ear

The tympanic membrane marks the boundary between the external auditory canal and the cavity of the middle ear, which is also termed the **tympanic cavity**.

Tympanic membrane

The tympanic membrane is a three layered structure.
• On the outer aspect it is covered by stratified squamous epithelium.
• The central portion is composed of fibrocollagenous support tissue containing numerous elastic fibres to provide mechanical strength.
• The inner portion is lined by a low cuboidal epithelium, which is continuous with that lining the rest of the middle ear.

Middle ear cavity

The middle ear cavity contains three auditory ossicles, the **incus**, **malleus** and **stapes**, which are:
• composed of compact bone;
• articulate by synovial joints (see page 246);
• covered externally by the same low cuboidal epithelium that lines the inner ear.
Two small skeletal muscles, the **stapedius** and the **tensor tympani** are associated with the ossicles and dampen motion between the bones, which occurs in response to loud noise.
The middle ear cavity communicates directly with air-filled spaces in the mastoid bone (**mastoid sinuses**), which are lined by low cuboidal or flattened squamous epithelium.

Eustachian tube

The **auditory (Eustachian) tube** extends from the middle ear cavity to the nasopharynx and is lined by ciliated epithelium similar to that of the respiratory tract. Its function is to equilibrate pressure between the middle ear cavity and the atmosphere.
Normally the Eustachian tube is collapsed, but is opened by movement of muscles in the nasopharynx such as occurs with swallowing or yawning.

Inner ear

The inner ear consists of fluid-filled sacs (**membranous labyrinth**) lying within cavities in the temporal bone of the skull (**bony or osseous labyrinth**).
• The membranous labyrinth comprises the **cochlear duct**, the **saccule**, the **utricle** and **semicircular canals,** and the **endolymphatic sac** and **duct**, the walls of which are composed of sheets of fibrocollagenous support tissue lined by a flat epithelium. These sacs are filled with a fluid called **endolymph**, and have epithelial and sensory specializations to detect position and sound.
• The osseous labyrinth is composed of three cavities, the **vestibule**, the **semicircular canals** and the **cochlea**, which are lined by periosteum and filled with fluid called **perilymph**.

Mechanoreceptors

The special receptors in the inner ear that sense movement (**mechanoreceptors**) are **hair cells**. These are specialized epithelial cells bearing a highly organized system of microvilli (**stereocilia**) on their apical surface.
Deflection of the microvilli causes electrical depolarization of the hair cell membrane, which is transmitted to the central nervous system by the connecting axons of sensory nerve cells (Fig. 12.2).
Patches of hair cells are located:
• within the vestibular apparatus in the ampullae of the semicircular canals to detect acceleration;
• within the macula of the utricle and saccule to perceive the direction of gravity and static position;
• within the organ of Corti of the cochlea to detect sound vibration.
At each site the hair cell microvilli are embedded in a gelatinous matrix, which moves according to the stimulus it is detecting. Movement of the microvilli towards the tallest row excites (depolarizes) the hair cell membrane, while movement towards the shortest row inhibits (hyperpolarizes) it.
Hair cells are arranged in different parts of the membranous labyrinth (Fig. 12.3) in order to sense movement generated by different causes.
Support cells surround the hair cells and are anchored to them at their apex by occluding junctions. These junctions maintain ionic gradients (see Fig. 3.7) between the endolymph and the extracellular fluid around the cells, the gradients being reversed on depolarization.

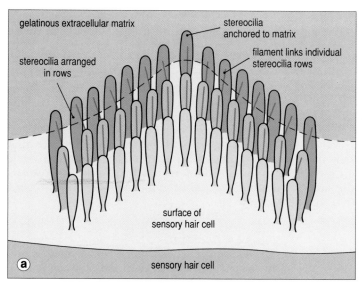

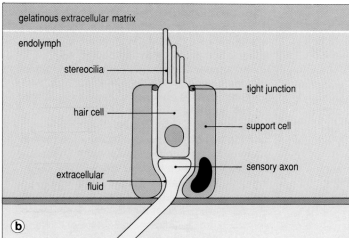

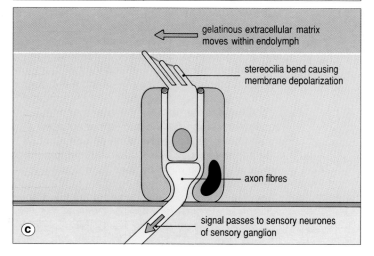

Fig. 12.2 Hair cell microvilli.

a The apical surface of each hair cell bears a highly organized system of microvilli (stereocilia), which are arranged as three parallel rows in a V or W-shaped pattern.

The height of the microvilli progressively decreases from the back to the front of the hair cell to form a so-called 'organ pipe' arrangement.

Fine filaments link individual microvilli from each row, with the tips of the shorter microvilli being coupled to the shafts of the taller microvilli behind.

While the hair cell is rigidly fixed in place by support cells, the tips of the tallest row of microvilli are embedded in a gelatinous extracellular matrix, which is free to move within the fluid cavities of the inner ear or vestibular system.

b Hair cells are supported by adjacent cells and are in contact with the axon of a sensory nerve. The support cells are anchored to the hair cells by occluding junctions. The stereocillia are embedded in a gelatinous matrix.

c Movement of the gelatinous matrix deflects the stereocilia causing membrane depolarization of the hair cell, which is relayed to the central nervous system via the axon of a sensory nerve.

Hair cells are arranged in different patterns in the cochlea and vestibular apparatus to detect acceleration (movement), gravity (position), or sound (hearing).

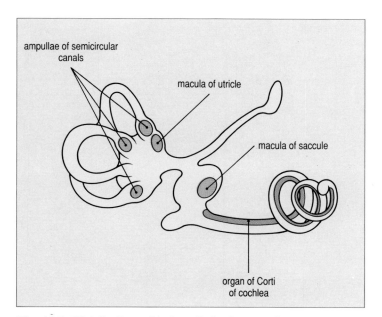

Fig. 12.3 Distribution of hair cells in the membranous labyrinth.

The hair cells are arranged in patches in the ampullae of the semicircular canals to detect acceleration, in the maculae of the utricle and saccule to perceive gravity direction and static position, and in the organ of Corti of the cochlea to detect sound vibration.

189

DETECTION OF SOUND

The **cochlear duct** is a blind-ended tubular diverticulum filled with endolymph. It makes 2 ³/₄ turns within the spiral-shaped bony cochlea in the temporal bone, and is compressed between two other tubular spaces, the **vestibular** and **tympanic cavities**, which are filled with **perilymph** (Fig. 12.4).

Within the cochlear duct is the **organ of Corti**, which is a special adaptation of the epithelial cells lining the cochlear ducts and detects sound vibration (Fig. 12.5).

Mechanism. Sound waves cause vibration of the tympanic membrane, which is then transmitted to the oval window membrane via the auditory ossicles.

Pressure waves are thence transmitted to the perilymph of the vestibular cavity causing the vestibular and basilar membranes to bow inwards towards the tympanic cavity, and to the round window, which bows outwards.

Because the tectorial membrane remains relatively rigid, bowing of the vestibular and basilar membranes causes relative movement of the hair cell sterocilia, which results in membrane depolarization.

This signal is transmitted to the sensory nerves of the spiral ganglion, and thence through the cochlear cranial nerve to the brain, where it is perceived as sound.

Low frequency sound is detected by stereocilia towards the apex of the cochlea, while high frequency sounds are detected at the base.

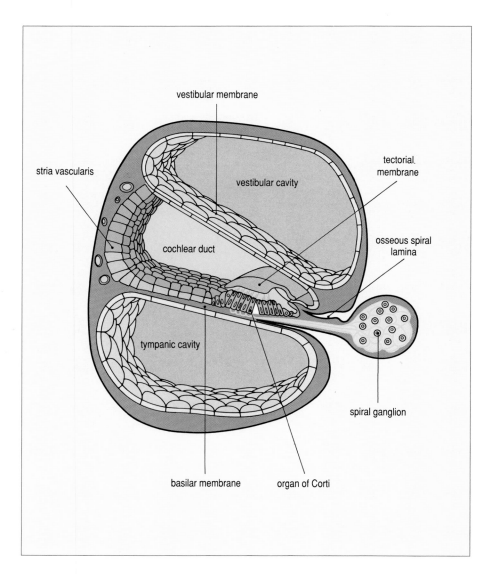

Fig. 12.4 Cochlea.
The cochlea of the osseous labyrinth contains three spaces, the vestibular cavity, the cochlear duct, and the tympanic cavity.

The vestibular cavity and the tympanic cavity contain perilymph continuous with that in the vestibule (see Fig. 12.1), while the cochlear duct, which is continuous with and part of the membranous labyrinth, is filled with endolymph.

At the apex of the cochlea the vestibular and tympanic cavities connect at an opening termed the **helicotrema**.

The **vestibular membrane (Reissner's membrane)** consists of two layers of flattened epithelium separated by a basement membrane, one cell layer being in continuity with the cells lining the vestibular cavity and the other in continuity with the cells lining the cochlear duct. The cells are held together by well developed occluding junctions to maintain different electrolyte concentrations (see Fig. 3.7) between the endolymph and perilymph.

The s**tria vascularis** is a specialized area of epithelium with a rich vascular supply in the lateral wall of the cochlear duct. Many of the cells in this area have ultrastructural features indicating an ion transport function (see page 37) and it is thought that they secrete endolymph.

The **basilar membrane** is thicker than the vestibular membrane and consists of collagen fibres as well as a basement membrane. On one side it is covered by cells lining the tympanic cavity, and on the other by specialized cells lining the cochlear duct.

Medially, the basilar membrane is continuous with the organ of Corti, which is a specialized area of support cells and sensory hair cells subserving hearing (see Fig. 12.5).

Labels in figure: vestibular membrane, stria vascularis, vestibular cavity, tectorial membrane, cochlear duct, osseous spiral lamina, tympanic cavity, spiral ganglion, basilar membrane, organ of Corti

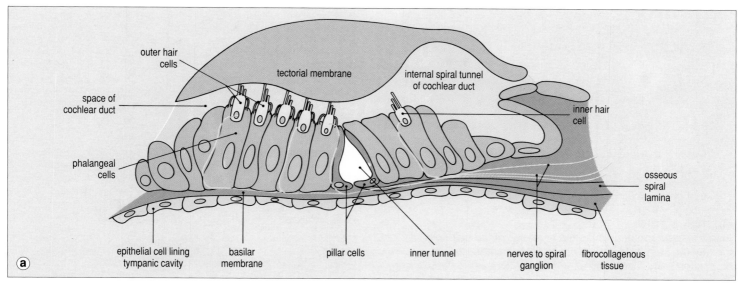

outer hair cells

tectorial membrane

internal spiral tunnel of cochlear duct

space of cochlear duct

inner hair cell

phalangeal cells

osseous spiral lamina

(a)

epithelial cell lining tympanic cavity

basilar membrane

pillar cells

inner tunnel

nerves to spiral ganglion

fibrocollagenous tissue

Fig. 12.5 Organ of Corti.

The organ of Corti is composed of epithelial support cells and sensory hair cells. Medially it rests on the rigid bony osseous spiral lamina, while laterally it is located on the deformable basilar membrane.

There are two groups of hair cells, an **inner group** and an **outer group**, which are separated by a small opening at the end of the osseous spiral lamina termed the **inner tunnel** (**tunnel of Corti**). The inner group are smaller and rounder than the outer group and arranged as a single row along the cochlea. The outer group are tall and thin and arranged as five parallel rows.

The hair cells are surrounded by epithelial support cells, the inner hair cells being completely surrounded, while the outer hair cells are enclosed only at their extreme apex and basal portions leaving a bare mid-zone in contact with extracellular fluid.

The microvilli of the outer hair cells are attached to a sheet of gelatinous extracellular matrix braced by filamentous proteins (**tectorial membrane**), while those of the inner hair cells are free. Axons make synaptic contact with the hair cells and run to the spiral ganglion. The tectorial membrane is secreted by epithelial cells (**interdental cells**).

There are several classes of support cell in the organ of Corti. **Pillar cells** contain abundant scaffolding microtubules, and

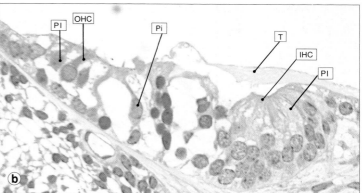

surround and support the triangular cavity (inner tunnel) at the level of the lip of the osseous spiral lamina. In contrast, **phalangeal cells** support the hair cells and are attached to them by occluding junctions at their apices, thus isolating the basal membrane of hair cells from the endolymph and maintaining electrochemical gradients.

b Micrograph of the organ of Corti. Note the tectorial membrane (T), the inner hair cells (IHC), the phalangeal cells (Pl), the pillar cells (Pi) and the outer hair cells (OHC).

DETECTION OF GRAVITY AND STATIC POSITION

Two areas of hair cells have a primary role in detecting the direction of gravity and thereby the static position of the head; they are located in the **macula of the utricle** and the **macula of the saccule** (see Fig. 12.3).

The macula of the utricle lies in the horizontal plane, while the macula of the saccule lies in the vertical plane at right angles to the macula of the utricle.

Each macula is histologically identical, and is composed of the following three cell types (Fig. 12.6):

- support cells (sustentacular cells), which are columnar cells with short apical microvilli;
- type I hair cells, which are polygonal in shape and surrounded by a network of afferent and efferent nerve endings;

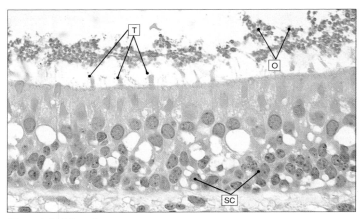

Fig. 12.6 Macula.
In this micrograph of macula, the sterocilia of the hair cells of the macula are embedded in the otolithic membrane. The otoconia (O) are visible as numerous purple-stained particles. The sterocilia appear as pink tufts (T) arising from the cell surface, but neither individual microvilli nor type of hair cell can be identified at this magnification. The support cells (SC) appear as an epithelial sheet.

- type II hair cells, which are cylindrical in shape, with basal synaptic afferent and efferent nerve endings.

In addition to an organ-pipe arrangement of tall microvilli stereocilia on their apical surface (see Fig. 12.2), these hair cells possess a single true cilium termed a **kinocilium**, which is located just behind the tallest row of sterocilia.

The stereocilia and kinocilium of each hair cell are embedded in a gelatinous plaque of extracellular matrix called the **otolithic membrane**, which is suspended in the endolymph. This membrane is covered by numerous small particles composed of protein and calcium carbonate, the **otoconia (otoliths)**.

Mechanism. The macula can detect the direction of gravity by sensing the direction of pull of the otolithic membrane and otoconia on the mass of hair cells that results from head movement either backwards and forwards (macula of utricle) or from side to side (macula of saccule).

DETECTION OF ACCELERATION AND MOTION
Hair cells that detect direction and magnitude of acceleration and motion are located in the ampullae at the end of the three semicircular canals, which assume posterior, superior, and horizontal positions.

Each ampulla is a 1 mm long dilated region of the membranous labyrinth and contains a patch of hair cells arranged in a tall, finger-like structure (an **ampullary**

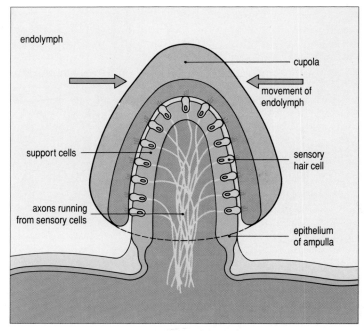

Fig. 12.7 Ampullary region of semicircular canal.
Within the ampullae of the semicircular canals, hair cells are arranged over a finger-like protrusion of the lining called the ampullary crista. The hair cells are both type I and type II and are associated with adjacent support cells.

The axons innervating the cells emerge from the base of the ampullary crista, being derived from sensory nerve cells in the ganglion of the vestibular nerve (Scarpa's ganglion), which connect with the vestibular nucleus in the brain stem.

The hair cell stereocilia and kinocilium are embedded in the gelatinous matrix of the cupola which, unlike the tectorial membrane of the maculae, does not contain otoconia.

crista). The sterocilia of the sensory hair cells are attached to a dome-shaped gelatinous matrix termed a **cupola** (Fig. 12.7).

Mechanism. With rotary motion of the head endolymph moves within the membranous labyrinth because of the static inertia of the fluid relative to the rest of the vestibular apparatus. Such movement causes displacement of the cupola, and the direction of this displacement is detected by the hair cells.

When integrated, perception from the three semicircular canals arranged in planes perpendicular to each other provides information on the direction and rate of acceleration of head movement.

EYE

The eye is designed to focus light onto specialized receptors that respond to light, and is composed of sclera, cornea, uvea and retina arranged around three chambers (Fig. 12.8).

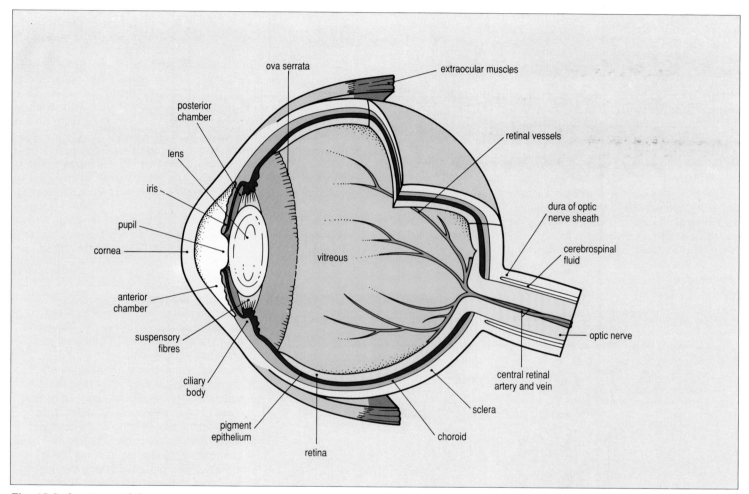

Fig. 12.8 Anatomy of the eye.

The eye is a spherical structure with a translucent disc-shaped area (cornea) on its anterior surface. This merges at its margins with a tough fibrocollagenous outer coat (sclera), which surrounds the globe of the eye and is attached to a series of skeletal muscles (extraocular muscles) responsible for eye movement.

The choroid is composed of blood vessels and support cells posteriorly and is continuous with the ciliary body and iris anteriorly, the iris being a disc-shaped membrane containing smooth muscle with a central aperture (the pupil) to allow the passage of light.

A special epithelial layer (pigment epithelium) lies inside the choroid and inside this is the receptor and nerve cell layer of the eye (retina). The ora serrata marks the end of the specialized sensory layer of the retina anteriorly.

Nerves from the retina emerge from the posterior aspect of the globe in the optic nerve, which is surrounded by a covering layer of fibrocollagenous tissue and cerebrospinal fluid, in continuity with that surrounding the brain.

Blood is supplied to the retina by the central artery of the retina, which runs with the optic nerve.

The transparent biconvex lens is suspended by a series of fine filaments from the ciliary body. The ciliary body contains smooth muscle and its contraction regulates the lens shape.

The globe is divided into three chambers; the anterior chamber in front of the iris, the posterior chamber behind the iris, and the vitreous behind the lens. The anterior and posterior chambers contain a clear fluid called the aqueous. The vitreous is a gelatinous transparent extracellular matrix material.

Sclera

The sclera proper is the outer fibrocollagenous coat of the globe of the eye. It varies in thickness from 1 mm posteriorly to 0.5 mm anteriorly, and is composed of flat plates of collagen orientated in different directions, but parallel to the surface.

The sclera is composed of three layers:
• The **episclera** is an external layer of loose fibrocollagenous tissue running adjacent to the periorbital fat.
• The **stroma** is the middle layer and is composed of thicker bundles of collagen than those of the episclera. These bundles run in sweeping branching patterns mainly looping from front to back, within the stroma.
• The inner part of the sclera, adjacent to the choroid layer, is the **lamina fusca** and contains small numbers of elastic fibres.

The blood vessels and nerve (including the optic nerve) running to and from the eye pass through the periscleral and scleral layers, but the scleral stroma itself is avascular. Anteriorly, the sclera blends with the cornea in a transition zone (the **limbus**), which is 1 mm wide.

Cornea

The cornea is the transparent disc-like anterior portion of the globe, and in the adult typically measures 10.5 mm from top to bottom and 11.5 mm from side to side. It is more curved than the globe and protrudes anteriorly.

The cornea has five layers; these are epithelium, Bowman's membrane, stroma, Descemet's membrane and endothelium (Fig. 12.9).
• **Corneal epithelium** is non-keratinizing squamous epithelium with a basal cell layer giving rise to 5–6 superficial layers with a total thickness of about 50 μm. Numerous free nerve endings terminate in this epithelium, and are the afferent part of the blink (ciliary) reflex, which is mediated through the sensory part of the fifth cranial nerve.
• **Bowman's membrane** is composed of fine collagen fibrils embedded in extracellular matrix, and is 8–10 μm thick. It is limited anteriorly by the basement membrane of the corneal epithelium, and blends posteriorly with the cornea stroma.
• **Corneal stroma** is the main layer of the cornea and is composed of 60–70 broad sheets of tightly bound, parallel collagen fibres (**corneal lamellae**) embedded in an

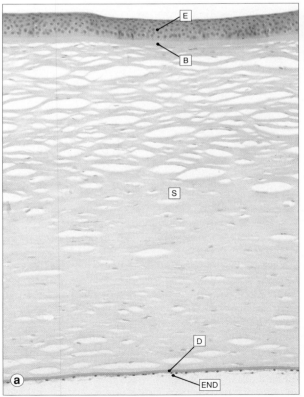

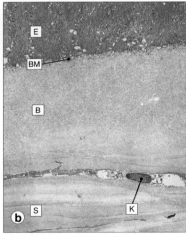

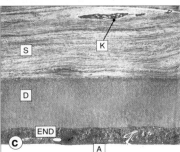

Fig. 12.9 Cornea.
a Micrograph of the five layers of the cornea showing epithelium (E), Bowman's membrane (B), stroma (S), Descemet's membrane (D), endothelium (End). Bowman's membrane and Descemet's membrane appear as homogeneous hyaline layers, which stain bright pink with H&E. In paraffin processed material, as here, artefactual splitting of the collagen plates forming the corneal stroma is common and gives rise to small spaces.
b Electronmicrograph showing the base of a corneal epithelial basal cell (E) and its basement membrane (BM) resting on Bowman's membrane (B), in which a felt-like arrangement of fine collagen fibrils can just be discerned. Beneath this are the collagen lamellae of the corneal stroma (S) and a corneal fibrocyte (keratocye, K).
c Electronmicrograph showing endothelium (End) resting on Descemet's membrane (D). Above are the collagen lamellae of the corneal stroma (S) and a corneal fibrocyte (keratocyte, K). Below is the anterior chamber (A).

extracellular matrix composed mainly of sulphated gly-cosaminoglycans (see page 42). To provide maximum mechanical strength the direction of the collagen fibres differs in each layer.

Between the lamellae are sparse inactive spindle-shaped fibrocytes, (**keratocytes**).

As there are no blood vessels in the cornea, the regular parallel arrangement of the collagen and the paucity of cells renders the cornea translucent and allows it to transmit light.

• **Descemet's membrane** is 7–10 μm thick and is a hyaline layer on the posterior aspect of the corneal stroma. It is produced by the corneal endothelial cells and is a true basement membrane.

• **Corneal endothelium** is a single layer of polygonal, plate-like cells, which line the inner surface of the cornea. They are adapted for ion-pumping and therefore possess numerous mitochondria, and are linked together by both desmosomal and occluding junctions (see Fig. 3.6 & 3.11).

The corneal endothelial cells pump fluid from the corneal stroma, and thereby prevent excessive hydration of the extracellular matrix, which would result in opacification of the cornea.

Uvea

The uvea is an intermediate layer in the eye between the dense support tissue of the sclera and the functional neural tissue of the retina. It contains blood vessels, nerves, support cells, contractile cells and melanocytes, and is divided into three specialized areas, these are the choroid, ciliary body and iris.

Choroid

The choroid extends from the ora serrata to the optic nerve, and contains the blood vessels and lymphatics supporting the retina. (Fig. 12.10). It is a dark brown sheet and blends with the lamina fusca of the sclera in its outer portion, while in its inner portion it is attached to the retina. It is composed of three main layers:

• the **choroidal stroma**, which is a loose fibrocollagenous support tissue interspersed with melanocytes, lymphocytes and mast cells, and through which the main arteries and veins run;

• the **choriocapillary layer**, which is a capillary layer supporting the deep layers of the retina, arises from the larger vessels in the stroma;

• Bruch's membrane.

BRUCH'S MEMBRANE
Bruch's membrane consists of:

• the basement membrane of the choriocapillary endothelial cells;

• an outer collagen fibre layer 0.5 μm thick;

• an elastic fibre layer 2 μm thick;

• an inner collagen fibre layer;

• the basement membrane of the retinal pigment epithelium (part of the retina).

CORNEAL DISEASE

The cornea contributes to the refraction of light into the eye, and damage resulting in corneal opacity may impair vision.

Although loss of corneal epithelium (**corneal abrasion**) is exquisitely painful, it is soon repaired by regeneration of new cells. Damage to Bowman's membrane, however, results in the formation of an opaque corneal scar because it is repaired by the haphazard deposition of collagen. If such scarring occurs in the visual axis, it causes loss of visual acuity.

The corneal endothelial cells are not replaced during life, and in some instances become depleted with age. They may also be damaged by disease processes in the anterior chamber of the eye. When the corneal endothelial cells are sufficiently depleted, fluid accumulates in the corneal stroma, which then becomes less transparent. Such waterlogging of the corneal stroma (corneal oedema) may cause the overlying epithelium to separate and this is intensely painful.

Diseases of the cornea, including endothelial failure, may be treated by corneal transplantation.

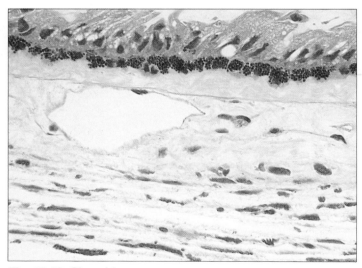

Fig. 12.10 Choroid.
Micrograph showing the vascular choroid layer posterior to the retinal pigment epithelium.

Iris

The **iris** is a sheet-like diaphragm located in front of the lens and delineates the anterior and posterior chambers of the eye. It has a circular aperture (**pupil**), which can be opened and closed by the action of groups of smooth muscle.

Contraction of the pupil reduces the amount of light entering the eye and thereby reduces glare from light scattered from the periphery of the lens.

The iris contains pigmented cells and muscle and is composed of four layers. These are the anterior limiting membrane, the stroma, the dilator muscle layer and the posterior epithelium (Fig. 12.11).

• The **anterior limiting layer** is an incomplete, fenestrated layer formed from stellate fibroblastic cells and stellate melanoctyes.

• The **stroma** is a loose fibrocollagenous support tissue associated with spindle-shaped fibroblasts (**stromal cell**s), blood vessels, nerves and macrophages containing phagocytosed melanin pigment; at the pupil margin is the circumferentially arranged smooth muscle of the sphincter muscle of the pupil.

The blood vessels of the iris generally run in a radial direction with frequent anastomotic channels forming circumferential vascular plexuses.

• The **dilator muscle layer** is composed of the contractile processes of the myoepithelial cells of the inner layer of the posterior epithelium; it extends from the base of the iris to the sphincter muscle.

• The **posterior epithelium** is composed of two layers of cells, which are densely pigmented with melanin. The inner layer of cells are more correctly myoepithelial in type with a basal zone around the nucleus containing melanin

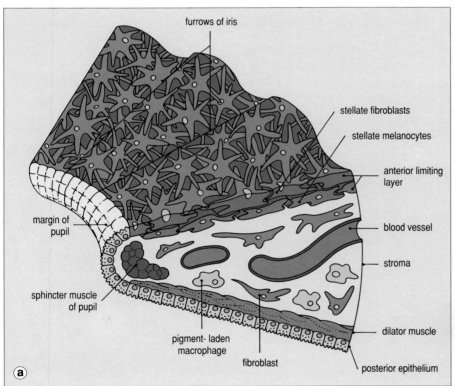

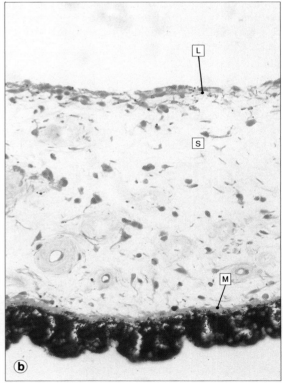

Fig. 12.11 Iris.

a Diagram of the free margin of the iris at the pupil showing its four consituent layers. An incomplete and fenestrated anterior limiting layer containing stellate fibroblasts and melanocytes lies on a loose fibrocollagenous stroma containing the sphincter muscle of the pupil, as well as radially orientated collagen fibres, which give the iris its ribbed and trabeculated surface. Behind the stroma is the dilator muscle, which is backed posteriorly by two layers of melanin-pigmented cells.

b Micrograph showing the histological appearance of the iris. The four layers are not well defined. The anterior limiting layer (L), merges with the stroma (S). The pigmented posterior epithelium cannot be resolved into two layers because of the density of melanin pigment. The dilator muscle (M) is visible as a pink band.

granules, and an apical portion which is melanin free, constituting the dilator muscle layer. This inner layer is bound by desmosomal junctions to the outer layer cells, which contain numerous melanin granules and are continuous with the retinal pigment epithelial layer.

The pigmented cells eliminate light from the eye and reduce glare.

Eye colour is determined by the relative number of melanocytes in the stroma; few cells give a blue colour, while many melanin-containing cells produce a dark brown colour; grey and green are the intermediate colours.

Ciliary body

The **ciliary body** extends from the base of the iris to the ora serrata where it is continuous with the choroid (see Fig. 12.7). In section (Fig. 12.12) the ciliary body is roughly triangular in shape and is composed of a vascular stroma, smooth muscle, and covering epithelium; it has two anatomically recognizable regions, the pars plica and pars plana.

The ciliary body contains the **ciliary muscle**, which is a form of smooth muscle. Contraction of the ciliary muscle lessens tension on the suspensory fibres of the lens and allows the lens to assume a more spherical shape.

• **The pars plica** contains the ciliary processes, which are ridges or folds 2 mm long, each with a core of stroma and blood vessels and covered by two layers of columnar epithelium. The outer layer of epithelium is pigmented, but the inner layer, which is in contact with the aqueous is not.

The non-pigmented epithelial cells in the grooves between the ciliary processes give rise to the suspensory fibres of the lens which are composed mainly of the protein **fibrillin** (see page 45). The ultrastructural features of these non-pigmented cells are those of ion-pumping cells (see page 37); they secrete the aqueous.

• **The pars plana** is a posterior flat area, which is 4 mm long. Its stroma is continuous with the choroid, while the outer pigmented epithelium of the ciliary body is continuous with that of the retina at the ora serrata.

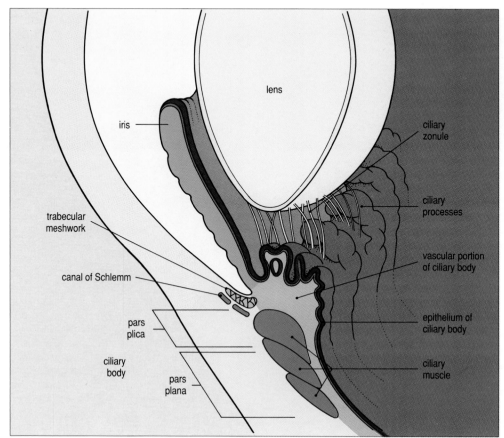

Fig. 12.12 Ciliary body.
The ciliary body is continuous with the base of iris and is divided anatomically into the pars plica and pars plana. The ciliary processes give rise to the suspensory fibres of the lens (**ciliary zonule**), while the ciliary muscle controls the tension on the suspensory fibres, and thereby controls the shape of the lens. The epithelium of the pars plana secretes the aqueous.

lens

iris

trabecular meshwork

canal of Schlemm

pars plica

ciliary body

pars plana

ciliary zonule

ciliary processes

vascular portion of ciliary body

epithelium of ciliary body

ciliary muscle

Retina

The retina is the innermost layer of the eye and is derived embryologically from an outgrowth of the developing brain (the **optic cup**).

It is composed of pigment epithelial cells, photoreceptor cells, retinal support cells and nerve cells.

Pigment epithelial cells

The retinal pigment epithelium is a single layer of melanin-containing polygonal cells, extending from the optic nerve to the ora serrata. Internally it lies adjacent to the photoreceptor layer of the retina, and externally its basement membrane is a component of Bruch's membrane.

The apical surfaces of the pigmented epithelial cells are covered with large microvilli, which extend upwards and surround the photoreceptors of the retina: Retinal pigment epithelial cells phagocytose worn-out components of the photoreceptor cells.

Photoreceptor cells (rods and cones)

The two types of photoreceptor are rods and cones, which have a similar basic structure (Fig. 12.13).

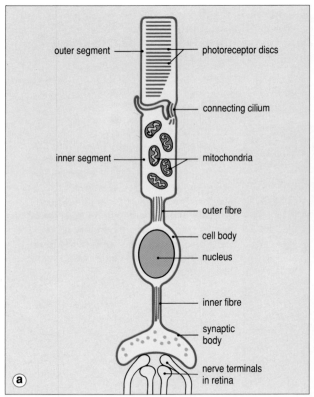

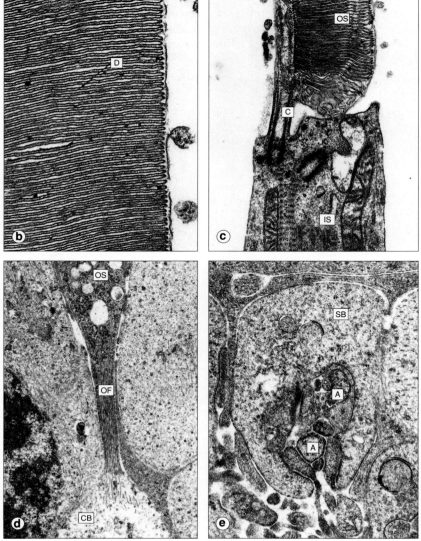

Fig. 12.13 (a–e) Photoreceptors.
Diagram and ultrastructural details of a photoreceptor cell. Light is detected by its outer segment (OS), which contains flat plates of membrane (photoreceptor discs, D).

The outer segment is connected to the inner segment (IS) by a connecting cilium (C). The inner segment contains numerous mitochondria.

The cell body (CB) connects to the outer segment by a microtubule-rich outer fibre (OF).

The synaptic body (SB) is cup-shaped and connects to axons (A) from other retinal neurones.

The light sensitive structures (**photoreceptor discs**) in the photoreceptor cell, form huge stacks 600–1000 deep in the outer segment of the cell and originate as deep infolds of the cell membrane.

In rods photoreceptor discs are formed constantly and pinch off to form free discs, which are shed from the cell when old (Fig. 12.14). In cones, however photoreceptor discs remain as deep infolds of cell membrane, and do not form free discs. The turnover of cone photoreceptor discs is not clear, but it does not appear to be the same relentless turnover characteristic of rods

Rods are about 2 μm thick and average 50 μm in length, possessing a roughly cylindrical outer segment. The tips of these cells are embedded in the microvilli of pigment epithelial cells, which phagocytose the old photoreceptor discs.

Cones are thicker and slightly shorter than rods being 3–5 μm thick, and about 40 μm long; their outer segment is conical in shape. Like rods, cones are also located close to the microvilli of the retinal pigment epithelial cells.

The distribution of rods and cones varies within the retina.
• Cones, which perceive colour, are concentrated in the optical centre of the retina in a small pit (the **fovea**).
• Rods, which perceive light intensity, but not colour, are concentrated at the periphery of the retina.

Between the fovea and the periphery of the retina there is a mixture of rods and cones (Fig. 12.15).

MECHANISM OF LIGHT DETECTION

In the dark, the photoreceptor cell is strongly depolarized and this holds voltage-gated Ca^{2+} ion channels open in the synaptic region, resulting in a constant release of an inhibitory transmitter substance at the synaptic terminal. This inhibitor prevents firing of nerve cells connected to the photoreceptor.

When stimulated by light, the photoreceptor becomes hyperpolarized and release of the inhibitory transmitter substance at the synaptic terminal is reduced. This reduction allows the axons of nerve cells connected to the photoreceptors to fire.

Photoreceptor cells detect light through its interaction with **rhodopsin** molecules. These are membrane-associated glycoproteins in the photoreceptor discs, and are composed of a protein (opsin) and a light sensitive group (cis-retinal).

When cis-retinal interacts with a photon it undergoes a conformational change to the trans form, which causes a fall in the concentration of a secondary messenger (cyclic GMP) within the cytosol of the photoreceptor. This results in closure of sodium channels in the cell membrane and hence hyperpolarization.

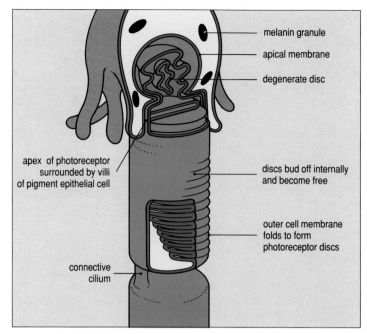

melanin granule

apical membrane

degenerate disc

apex of photoreceptor surrounded by villi of pigment epithelial cell

discs bud off internally and become free

outer cell membrane folds to form photoreceptor discs

connective cilium

Fig. 12.14 Turnover of photoreceptor discs in rods.
In the rod photoreceptor cell, photoreceptor discs originate at the cilial pole of the outer segment as deep infoldings of the cell membrane. These migrate up through the cell and eventually bud off internally to form free discs within the outer segment.

At the rod apex, effete and aged discs are eliminated and extruded into the extracellular space where they are phagocytosed by the retinal pigment epithelial cell, into which the rod outer segment is buried. Thus is a constant flow of new photoreceptor discs along the rod outer segment.

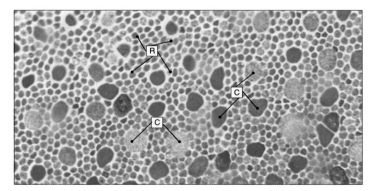

Fig. 12.15 Rods and cones.
Micrograph of a resin section taken tangentially through the retina at the level of the inner segment of the photoreceptors. Rods (R) are identified as thin circular profiles, while cones (C) are larger. There is a mosaic of rods and cones in this retinal area 6 mm temporal to the fovea.

Retinal support cells

The two types of retinal support cell are Müller's cells and astrocytes.
- **Müller's cells** are tall retinal support cells. They extend from the base of the inner segment of the photoreceptor cells, where they link to each other by adherent junctions (see Fig. 3.9) to form the structure known as the **outer limiting membrane**, up to the retinal surface, where they rest on the **internal limiting membrane**.
- **Astrocytes** (see page 213) act as support cells to the nerve cells throughout the retina and are characterized by long dendritic processes, which form a scaffold for the delicate processes of nerve cells.

Nerve cells of the retina

The retina contains several classes of nerve cell, which connect to photoreceptors and form interconnections between different parts of the retina. These include bipolar cells, ganglion cells, horizontal cells, amacrine cells and interplexiform cells.
- **Bipolar cells** connect with the synaptic end of the photoreceptor cells and transmit signals to ganglion cells.
- **Ganglion cells** send axons from the eye to the brain in the optic nerve.
- **Horizontal cells, amacrine cells**, and **interplexiform cells** are neurones that act as 'gates' to modulate the passage of impulses from the photoreceptors to the ganglion cells. Their processes interpose the connections between bipolar cells and photoreceptors, and between bipolar cells and ganglion cells. This group of gate cells allows integration of signals from adjacent groups of photoreceptors.

Retinal structure

The sensory retina is composed of nine layers (Fig. 12.16).
- The **photoreceptor layer** of rods and cones extends from the retinal pigment epithelium and consists of outer and inner segments of the photoreceptor cells.
- The **external limiting membrane** is not a true membrane, but a line marking the zone of adherent junctions between Müller cells.
- The **outer nuclear layer** consists of the nuclei and cell bodies of the photoreceptor cells, which form 8–9 rows of nuclei. The nuclei of rods are small and densely stained, while those of cones are larger and pale stained.
- The **outer plexiform layer** contains the cell processes and synaptic connections between the photoreceptor cells, bipolar neurones, and horizontal cells. The synaptic connections to rods are termed **spherals** while those to cones are termed **pedicles**. For both cell types the terminal of a horizontal cell is interposed between the photoreceptor and the bipolar cell to form a structure termed a **triad**. The horizontal cell can therefore modulate the impulse from the photoreceptors to the bipolar cells and allows integration of signals from adjacent photoreceptors.
- The **inner nuclear layer** is composed of the nuclei and cells bodies of bipolar cells, horizontal cells, interplexiform cells and amacrine cells, as well as the nuclei of the Müller cells.
- The **inner plexiform layer** contains the cell processes and synapses of bipolar cells, amacrine cells, interplexiform cells and ganglion cells. The amacrine cells interpose processes between the processes of bipolar cells and ganglion cells and thereby modify the transmission of impulses from the bipolar cells. The interplexiform cells are similar to amacrine cells but also send a process to synapse in the outer plexiform layer.
- The **ganglion cell layer** consists of a row of ganglion cells which have large nuclei with visible nucleoli, and prominent rough endoplasmic reticulum visible as Nissl substance. The ganglion cells are separated by the cytoplasm of Müller cells.
- The **nerve fibre layer** is composed of the axons of the ganglion cells *en route* to the central nervous system via the optic nerve with supporting astrocytic cells.
- The **internal limiting membrane** is a barely visible basement membrane at the interface between the vitreous and the retina.

REGIONAL RETINAL VARIATIONS

Optic disc. The axons of the nerve fibre layer converge at the optic disc, which is visible in the retina and gives rise to the optic nerve. This area is devoid of photoreceptors and therefore produces a blind spot in the visual field.

Macula. The macula is a small yellow area located 2.5 mm lateral (temporal) to the optic disc. At its centre there is a thin zone of retina composed exclusively of cones (the **fovea**), each cone synapsing with a single bipolar cell and thence linking with a single ganglion cell, thus producing a high degree of resolution. This area is at the centre of the visual axis and provides high detail colour vision.

The yellow colour of the surrounding macula is due to the presence of yellow xanthophil pigment in ganglion cells from the fovea, which are displaced laterally so that light can impinge on the cones of the fovea without being dispersed by an overlying neural layer.

Peripheral retina. In the peripheral retina, many photoreceptors are mapped onto one ganglion cell and form a receptive field with low visual resolution. Electrophysiology has shown that these receptive fields are triggered by different visual stimuli for example some ganglion cells only fire in response to a bright light, while others only respond to a moving edge.

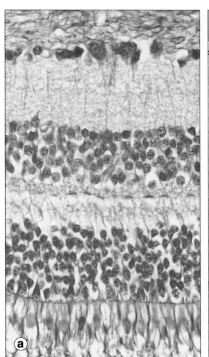

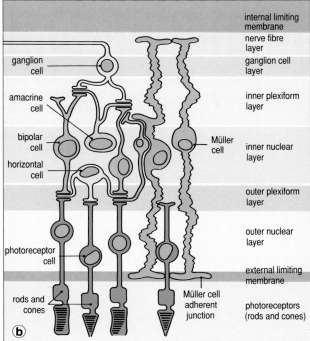

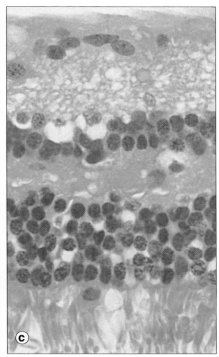

Fig. 12.16 Sensory retina.

a Micrograph of silver stained sensory retina showing its nine constituent layers.

b Diagram of the sensory retina showing its nine layers.

c Micrograph of H&E stained sensory retina.

Vasculature

The central artery and vein of the retina enter the back of the eye in the optic nerve and branch in the plane between the vitreous and the inner limiting membrane.

The capillaries, which form a dense plexus within the retina and supply all cells apart from the rods and cones, are characterized by tight junctions between their constituent endothelial cells to prevent diffusion of substances into the neural retina (i.e. they form a **blood–retinal barrier**). The rods and cones are supplied by choroidal vessels.

The retinal vessels are visible by ophthalmoscopic examination and may be damaged in disease, for example high blood pressure (hypertension) causes visible thickening of the arterial walls.

DIABETIC RETINOPATHY

Ophthalmoscopic examination of the retina (**fundoscopy**) is an important part of a general medical examination because it provides a direct view of blood vessels in a critical area of the circulation; retinal blood vessels are frequently affected in disease, particularly diabetes mellitus.

In diabetes mellitus, the basement membrane of small blood vessels in the retina thickens and the vessels show dilatations termed microaneurysms.

The abnormal vessels become leaky and exude fluid into the retina, which is visible as white spots. Haemorrhages may also occur. This particularly affects the macula leading to loss of visual activity.

If these changes become severe the blood supply to the retina is reduced (i.e. ischaemia) and this stimulates abnormal growth of new retinal blood vessels (**proliferative retinopathy**). The newly formed vessels may bleed and also result in retinal detachment.

The severity of diabetic retinopathy, which is the most common cause of blindness, is greatly reduced by the careful control of blood sugar levels. Laser coagulation of leaking vessels delays or prevents development of severe visual loss.

Optic nerve

The optic nerve contains the axons from the retinal ganglion cells *en route* to the central nervous system, as well as the central artery and vein of the retina.

The optic nerve leaves the retina at the optic disc and penetrates the collagen of the sclera through a sieve-like plate of channels in an area termed the **lamina cribosa**. Within the orbit the optic nerve is surrounded by a sheath of dura and an extension of the subarachnoid space (Fig. 12.17).

The optic nerve is invested in the pia arachnoid layers (see page 305) and septa from this layer enter the optic nerve and divide the axons into fascicles.

PAPILLOEDEMA

If pressure of the CSF within the skull increases (i.e. raised intracranial pressure), pressure of the CSF around the optic nerve increases. Initially this impairs cytoplasmic flow along the optic nerve axons, which swell and cause engorgement of the central artery and vein.

Ophthalmoscopic examination of a normal optic disc reveals that it is a cup-shaped depression, but in cases of raised intracranial pressure, the disc is swollen (**papilloedema**) with loss of the cup-shaped depression.

Papilloedema is an important physical sign and usually denotes abnormal brain swelling caused by disease.

Lens

The lens is a soft transparent biconvex structure and in the adult is 9 mm in diameter and 3.5 mm thick. It has
- an outer capsule 10–20 μm thick of hyaline material containing type IV collagen;
- a layer of large cuboidal epithelial cells, (the **lens epithelium**) beneath the capsule;
- a centre composed of tightly packed cells, which have lost their nuclei and become packed by special transparent proteins (**crystallins**) to form so-called **lens fibres** (Fig. 12.18).

New lens cells are added to the margin of the lens throughout life from the lens epithelium, but the cells at the centre of the lens do not undergo turnover or replacement and are therefore the oldest cells in the body of an adult.

The lens is avascular and is nourished by diffusion from the aqueous and vitreous (see below).

The lens is suspended by suspensory fibres to the ciliary body, the radial arrangement of suspensory fibres being termed the **ciliary zonule**. These fibres are composed mainly of the fibrillar protein **fibrillin** (see page 45).

Chambers of the eye

The three chambers of the eye are the vitreous body, and the anterior and posterior aqueous chambers.

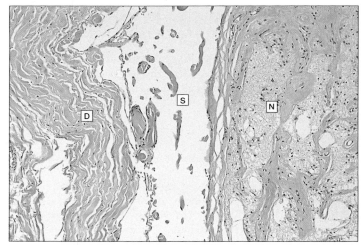

Fig. 12.17 Optic nerve and sheath.
Micrograph showing the optic nerve (N) in longitudinal section. The central artery and vein of the retina run along its centre. Around the optic nerve is the optic nerve sheath, which is composed of an extension of the dura (D) and subarachnoid space (S) and is filled with cerebrospinal fluid.

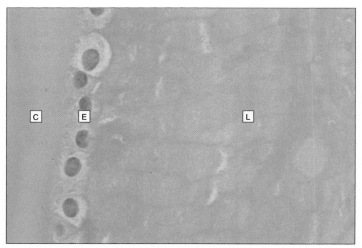

Fig. 12.18 Lens.
Micrograph showing the lens capsule (C) as a pink-staining hyaline layer, and the subcapsular lens epithelium (E). The centre of the lens (L) is composed of cells devoid of organelles (lens fibres) packed with crystalline proteins.

Vitreous

The vitreous body is a transparent gelatinous structure located behind the lens and occupying the space bounded by the inner surface of the retina.

The vitreous has a volume of 4 ml and is a specialized support tissue, being composed of a few scattered spindle-shaped cells (**hyalocytes**), fine highly dispersed collagen fibres, and an abundant extracellular matrix rich in hyaluronic acid.

Aqueous chambers

The **anterior** and **posterior** chambers lie anterior to the lens, are delineated by the iris and communicate with each other via the aperture of the pupil (see Fig. 12.8).

The **aqueous humor** is a watery fluid resembling cerebrospinal fluid and is secreted at a rate of about 2 μl/minute by the epithelial cells of the ciliary body in the posterior chamber. It provides nutrients to the structures it bathes and flows from the posterior chamber, through the pupil into the anterior chamber.

The aqueous then filters through a network of spaces lined by endothelium, the **trabecular meshwork** (see Fig. 12.12),

which runs around the circumference of the root of the iris, at the periphery of the anterior chamber, and enters the **canal of Schlemm** (Fig. 12.19). This canal runs around the whole circumference of the limbus within the sclera. From the canal of Schlemm, the aqueous enters venous vessels.

The angle between the margin of the cornea and the iris root where the trabecular meshwork lies is the **irido-corneal drainage angle**.

There is a normal resistance to the flow of aqueous at the level of the trabecular meshwork such that continued secretion and resorption of the aqueous results in a normal intrinsic resting pressure within the globe (intraocular pressure) of 10–22 mm Hg.

GLAUCOMA

Abnormalities in the drainage pathway of aqueous humor result in a rise in the intraocular pressure (**glaucoma**), which if untreated damages the nerve cells of the retina and causes blindness.

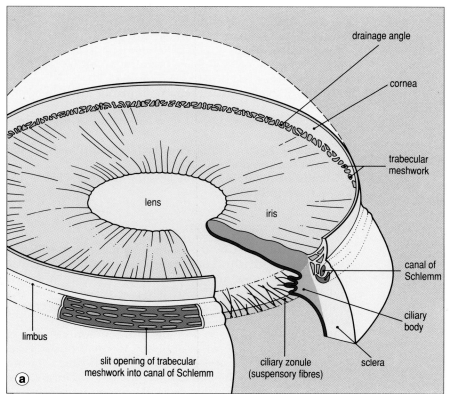

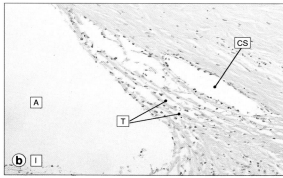

Fig. 12.19 Canal of Schlemm and trabecular meshwork.

a The canal of Schlemm runs around the circumference of the cornea at the limbus and communicates with the trabecular meshwork, which runs around the circumference of the root of the iris. The aqueous from the anterior chamber of the eye filters through the trabecular meshwork into the canal of Schlemm, and thence drains into venous vessels.
b Micrograph showing the trabecular meshwork (T) as an area of slit-like spaces with the canal of Schlemm (CS) within the sclera. The aqueous filters from the anterior chamber (A) just above the iris (I).

RETINAL DETACHMENT

The term **retinal detachment** is used to describe splitting of the retina through the photoreceptor layer to leave the attached pigment epithelium.

Retinal detachment usually follows a tear in the retina caused either by retinal degeneration or by traction by the vitreous.

The vitreous is normally in contact with the whole of the retina and rotational shearing forces generated by pulling of the extraocular muscles are transmitted uniformly to the whole globe. If the vitreous becomes detached from the retina posteriorly, rotational shearing forces are focally concentrated and cause tearing of the retina.

If the retina does not re-attach, the cell bodies of the rods and cones in the detached area degenerate, with loss of visual function.

Accessory components of the eye

The conjunctiva, eyelids and lacrimal drainage system are the accessory components of the eye.

Conjunctiva

The normal conjunctiva is a translucent membrane that lines the inner surface of the eyelids (**palpebral conjunctiva**) and reflects onto the globe (**bulbar conjunctiva**) to cover its anterior surface up to the margin of the cornea (**limbus**).

The conjunctiva is covered by two layers of stratified columnar epithelium, which give way to a flattened squamous epithelium towards the limbus. Goblet cells (see page 37) are present in this epithelium but mainly in the medial portion, being scarce in the temporal bulbar conjunctiva (Fig. 12.20).

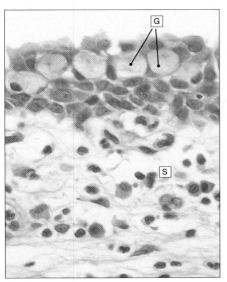

Fig. 12.20 Conjunctiva.
Micrograph showing conjunctival epithelium with goblet cells (G) containing mucin overlying the subepithelial support tissues (S), which contain vessels and lymphoid cells.

Beneath the epithelium the conjunctival stroma is composed of loose fibrocollagenous support tissue with small blood vessels and lymphatics running through it. With ageing, there is loss of collagen in this tissue.

Eyelids

The structure of both upper and lower eyelids is similar and comprises the following four layers:
- skin;
- orbicularis muscle (a layer of skeletal muscle);
- tarsal plate (a plate of dense fibroelastic tissue);
- conjunctiva.

Within these layers are various types of glands (Fig. 12.21).
- **Meibomian glands** are sebaceous in type and secret a lipid-rich substance that delays evaporation of the tear film, which lubricates and protects the cornea.
- **Glands of Zeis** are small sebaceous glands associated with the eyelashes.
- **Glands of Moll** are apocrine sweat glands at the margin of the eyelid.
- **Glands of Krause** are accessory lacrimal glands in the fornix of the conjunctiva.
- **Glands of Wolfring** are accessory lacrimal glands just above the tarsal plate.

Lacrimal drainage system

Tears are produced by the main lacrimal gland, which is located beneath the conjunctiva on the upper lateral margin of the orbit, and by the accessory glands of Krause and Wolfring (see Fig. 12.21). The glands secrete a serous fluid and have a complex branched structure with secretory acini and ducts (see Fig. 3.25).

The main lacrimal gland drains into the upper fornix of the conjunctiva via a series of about 10 small ducts. Tears then wash over the surface of the eye and drain via two ducts located at the medial end of the eyelids. These ducts, the **superior** and **inferior lacrimal ducts**, merge into a

common lacrimal duct and drain into the **lacrimal sac**; this empties, via the **nasolacrimal duct**, into the nasal cavity through an opening beneath the inferior turbinate bone (see page 126).

The superior and inferior lacrimal ducts are lined by stratified squamous epithelium, whereas the lacrimal sac and nasolacrimal duct are lined by respiratory-type pseudostratified ciliated columnar epithelium.

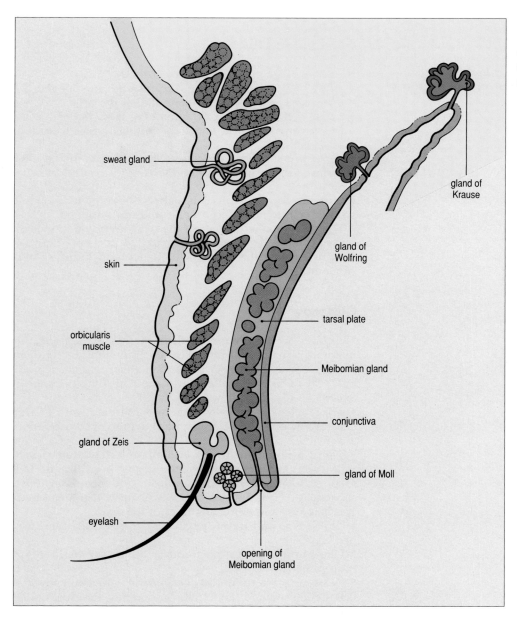

Fig. 12.21 Structure of the eyelid.
Diagram of eyelid, which is composed of skin, orbicularis muscle, tarsal plate and conjunctiva and contains various types of glands.

sweat gland

gland of Krause

gland of Wolfring

skin

tarsal plate

orbicularis muscle

Meibomian gland

conjunctiva

gland of Zeis

gland of Moll

eyelash

opening of Meibomian gland

13. NERVOUS SYSTEM

The nervous system allows rapid and specific communication between widely spaced areas of the body by the action of specialized **nerve cells** (**neurones**), which gather and process information and generate appropriate response signals.

NERVE CELLS (NEURONES)

Neurones form a network of highly specific connections between cells in order to:
● gather information from sensory receptors;
● process information and provide a memory;
● generate appropriate signals to effector cells.

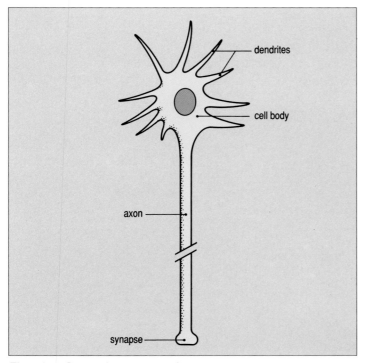

Fig. 13.1 General structure of a neurone.
Neurones consist of a cell body, axon and dendrites, the axon carrying pulses to its terminal, the **synaptic bouton**, which makes contact with another cell. The dendrites connect with synaptic boutons from other neurones.

General structure

Neurones (Fig. 13.1) are characterized by:
● a cell body containing the nucleus and most of the cell organelles responsible for maintaining the cell;
● a long cell process (**axon**) stretching from the cell, often over a long distance, and transmitting signals from it to other cells;
● numerous short cell processes (**dendrites**) to increase the surface area available for connecting with axons of other neurones;
● specialized cell junctions (**synapses**) between its axon and other cells to allow direct cell communication.

The functional attributes of the nervous system are determined mainly by the network of connections between neurones rather than on specific structural features of individual neurones.

Cytology

Neurones are highly metabolically active as they not only maintain a massive surface area of cell membrane, but also constantly require energy to develop electrochemical gradients. This activity is reflected in their histological appearance (Fig. 13.2) as follows.
● The nucleus is typically large and rounded, with a large central nucleolus, reflecting a high degree of transcriptional activity.
● There is abundant rough endoplasmic reticulum, which synthesizes the necessary proteins, and is visible in H&E sections as purple-stained granules in the cytoplasm (**Nissl substance**). The Nissl substance is present in the cell body (**perikaryon**) and dendrites, but not the axon.
● There is a well developed Golgi to produce secretory products.
● Large numbers of mitochondria supply the high energy requirements.
● Lysosomes are numerous because of a high turnover of cell membrane and other cell components. Residual bodies containing lipofuscin are often prominent, particularly in the elderly.

The cytoskeleton of neurones is highly organized to maintain the unique shape of these cells, and particularly their long axons which may be up to 1 m long.

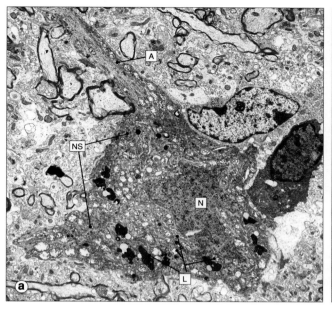

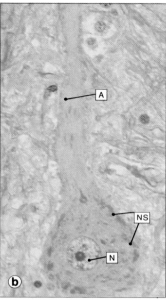

Fig. 13.2 Neurone.
a Electronmicrograph of a neurone showing the axon (A) containing mitochondria and cytoskeletal filaments, and the cell body containing a nucleus (N), dark staining lysosomal bodies (L), and abundant rough endoplasmic reticulum (Nissl substance, NS).
b Micrograph showing a neurone with a large nucleus (N) containing a prominent nucleolus. Within the cell body purple-staining Nissl substance (NS) composed of rough endoplasmic reticulum can be seen. The axon (A) stretches away from the cell body.

Neurofilament protein, the intermediate filament of nerve cells, is thought to act as an internal scaffold to maintain the shape of the axon and cell body, and in the axon, certain membrane proteins are anchored in place in an organized pattern by attachment to cellular neurofilaments.

There is also a highly organized network of microtubules, which transport substances and organelles up and down the axon.

Architecture

Different types of neurone have different shapes, which reflect their function (Fig. 13.3).
• **Motor neurones** have a large cell body to provide metabolic support for the large axon. They also have many dendritic processes and are therefore classed as a **multipolar neurone**.
• **Sensory neurones** are commonly **unipolar** cells, which are characterized by the possession of one major process. This divides into two branches, one running to the central nervous system and one to a sensory area of the body.
• **Interneurones** are generally small simple cells with short processes that provide local connections within the central nervous system. Many such cells are **bipolar** in type, having two main processes of equivalent size: one dendritic, and one axonal.

In addition to these general types of neurone, there are many types of neurone that are unique to a particular part of the brain, for example the **Purkinje cells**, which are large multi-processed cells in the cerebellum (see Fig. 13.25).

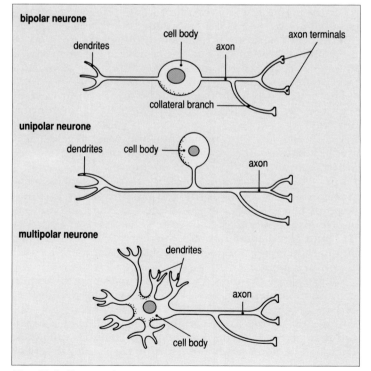

Fig. 13.3 Types of neurone.
There are many different types of neurone, which are shaped according to their function. Bipolar cells are commonly interneurones, while unipolar cells tend to be sensory neurones and multipolar cells are often motor neurones.

Axonal transport

The metabolic maintenance of the long cell process of the axon requires a transport system for organelles, enzymes, and metabolites from the cell body.

• Enzymes and elements of the cytoskeleton are transported down the axon at a speed of 1–5 mm/day by an unknown mechanism (**slow axonal transport**).

• Membrane-bound organelles, such as neurosecretory vesicles are transported at speeds of 400 mm/day (**antero-grade fast axonal transport**). This method is mediated by microtubular transport mechanisms using the molecule **kinesin** as a molecular motor.

• The return of effete organelles as well as recycled membrane from the synaptic ending back to the neuronal cell body for processing occurs at a rate of 300 mm/day (**retrograde rapid transport**). This is mediated by micro-tubular transport mechanisms, using the molecule **dynein** as a molecular motor.

Electrophysiology of neuronal signalling

Neurone signalling is controlled by the electrical (ionic) gradient across their cell membranes.

Firing of a neurone is associated with depolarization of the cell membrane, which is propagated along the axon of the cell at up to 100 m/sec. In a resting axon, the membrane potential is negative (-70 mV).

The cell membrane of neurones is divided into several regions, each containing highly specialized membrane proteins.

• Membrane ion pumps maintain the baseline electrical gradient between the outside and inside of the cell and are widely distributed in the cell membrane.

• Ion channel proteins modify the electrochemical gradient across the neurone cell membrane by forming pores or gates, which can switch their permeability to ions in response to specific signals (**gated channels**).

Ligand-gated channels close or open in response to binding to chemical transmitter substances and are located mainly in synapses.

Voltage-gated channels are involved mainly in the explo-sive and rapid depolarization that occurs as nerve cells fire, and are widely distributed in the cell membrane.

If an area of the axon membrane is locally depolarized and the current is small, then no gated channels will open. The current flows down the axon by **passive local spread** for a small distance before dissipating because of leakage from the membrane.

In this situation the axon behaves like an electrical cable, simply conducting a current along its surface with the speed of conduction related to the resistance and capaci-tance of the axon.

If an area of axon membrane is depolarized and the current is large, Na^+ and K^+ gated channels open and lead to an explosive change in the membrane potential, termed an **action potential**.

The opening of voltage-gated channels to produce an action potential can be considered as a local amplification system for membrane depolarization; the current does not now dissipate over a small length of the axon, but propa-gates to the end of the axon by causing a chain reaction triggering of gated ion channels along the way.

Action potentials propagate along an axon at the speed of passive local spread, which is determined by the resis-tance and capacitance of the axon; the larger the diameter of the axon the greater the speed of propagation.

SYNAPSE

A synapse is a special cell junction that allows direct com-munication between cells; a transmitter substance is secreted in a highly localized fashion by one cell and received uniquely by the other.

Structure

The terminal end of an axon is swollen to form a **synaptic bouton**, which is closely applied to the surface of a target cell, leaving a small gap 20 nm wide (the **synaptic cleft**). The cell membrane on each side of the synaptic cleft contains special membrane proteins and receptors involved in neurotransmission.

Ultrastructurally the cell membrane on each side of the synaptic cleft is slightly thickened and the synaptic bouton contains mitochondria, microtubules, and neurofilaments, as well as membrane-bound vesicles 40–65 nm in diameter (**neurosecretory vesicles** or **granules**, Fig. 13.4). The ap-pearance of these vesicles is variable; most are small and round with a clear centre, others are elliptical. Certain neu-rosecretory granules (dense-core granules) have an electron-dense core with a pale 'halo' beneath the membrane.

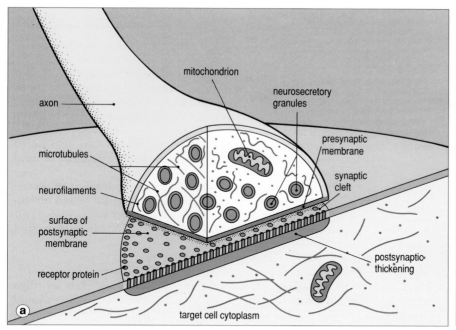

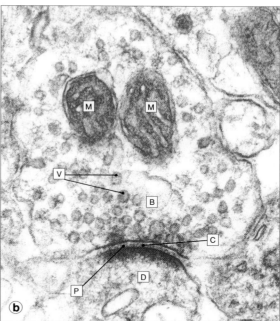

Fig. 13.4 Synapse.

a Diagram showing an axon terminating as a synaptic bouton on the surface of a neurone. The postsynaptic membrane bears arrays of receptors for the neurotransmitter contained in the axonal vesicles, and is released into the synaptic cleft by exocytosis.

b Electronmicrograph showing a synaptic bouton (B) making contact with a dendrite (D). The bouton contains small vesicles (V), mitochondria (M), and cytoskeletal filaments. The synaptic cleft (C) contains faint granular material above the thickened postsynaptic membrane (P).

In tissue sections it is possible to detect transmitter substances in neurones and their terminals by immuno-chemistry using antibodies specific for the transmitter.

Neurosecretory granules also contain unique non-transmitter proteins. Again, these may be detected by immunochemistry, for example, **synaptophysin,** which is a glycoprotein in the membrane of neurosecretory granules, and **chromogranins,** which are proteins involved in the packaging of transmitter into the vesicles.

Function

When a wave of depolarization reaches the synaptic bouton, it triggers the release of the transmitter substance from the neurosecretory granules by exocytosis (see Fig. 2.4). The transmitter substance then diffuses across the synaptic cleft and is able to interact with receptors in the postsynaptic membrane of the target neurone.

The three possible effects of transmitter release on the target (postsynaptic) cell are depolarization, hyperpolariza-tion and altered cell sensitivity.

DEPOLARIZATION

The target cell depolarizes if the transmitter substance binds to a ligand-gated receptor (i.e. Na^+ ion channel protein) and causes it to open allowing ions to diffuse into the neurone.

If many receptors are activated at the same time, the al-teration in membrane potential causes activation of voltage-gated ion channels, leading to an action potential.

Only a small group of transmitter substances act in this way, which generally results in rapid neural transmission. These include **acetylcholine,** which is the major transmitter in this group, and glutamate.

In any given nerve terminal more than one transmitter substance may operate.

HYPERPOLARIZATION

The target cell hyperpolarizes if the transmitter substance binds to a ligand-gated receptor that admits small negative ions into the cell. Hyperpolarization inhibits depolariza-tion.

The main transmitter substances causing hyperpolariza-tion are γ-**aminobutyric** acid and **glycine**.

ALTERED CELL SENSITIVITY

The overall sensitivity of a cell to stimulation is altered if the transmitter substance binds to one of the class of non-channel linked receptors. These receptors generate secondary messengers (e.g. cAMP) within the target neurone to modify the overall sensitivity of the cell to depolarization mediated by the ligand-gated receptors; such behaviour is called **neuromodulation**.

Many of the transmitters causing altered cell sensitivity are monoamines (e.g. **dopamine**, **5-hydroxytryptamine**), but some are small neuropeptides.

Patterns of synapse

Within the central nervous system, synapses form in a diversity of combinations between axons and dendrites, axons and cell bodies, axons and other axons (Fig. 13.5).

Because axons may be excitatory, inhibitory, or modulatory, certain synapses are formed from the coincidence of many axons from different neurones onto one part of a target neurone. The target neurone can then integrate the overall input into an appropriate output. Such functional clusters of synapses are commonly isolated from the adjacent nervous system by support cells of the brain such as astrocytes.

The neuromuscular junction (see page 229) is a specialized form of synapse between a motor nerve axon and skeletal muscle.

MYELIN

The speed of conduction along nerves is limited by the electrical capacitance and resistance of the axon.

Because wide axons have a lower capacitance than narrow ones, increasing the diameter of axons is a useful means of increasing the speed of nerve conduction. This is, however, inefficient, as giant axons require a high metabolic upkeep.

The speed of conduction along axons can also be increased if leakage of current from the membrane is minimized by insulation.

The two functions of insulation and reduction of electrical capacitance are performed by a substance called **myelin**, which is produced by specialized support cells. These cells wrap layers of cell membrane around axons to form a lipid-rich insulating layer, and are:

- oligodendrocytes in the central nervous system;
- Schwann cells in the peripheral nervous system.

A **Schwann cell** myelinates only one axon, but an **oligodendrocyte** may myelinate several adjacent axons. Although largely identical in structure, there are minor differences in the composition of myelin formed by these two cell types.

Myelin can be stained by histological methods with affinity for the lipid or protein components of the myelin sheath, and such methods highlight the structural difference in the central nervous system between neurone-rich areas low in myelin (**grey matter**) and tracts of axons with abundant myelin (**white matter**).

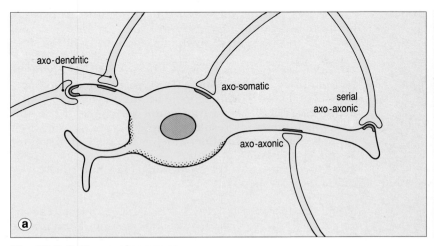

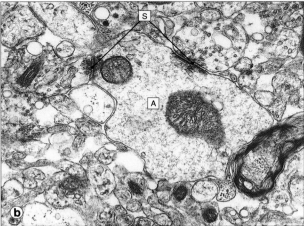

Fig. 13.5 Patterns of synapse.

a Diagram to illustrate the combinations of synapse. Synapses can form between axons and dendrites, axons and cell bodies, axons and other axons.

b Electronmicrograph showing two axo-axonic synapses (S) onto the same axon (A). Firing of A will depend on the integration of these separate inputs.

Structure

The myelin sheath is formed by the oligodendrocytes or Schwann cells wrapping spiral layers of cell membrane around the axon.

Myelination begins with the invagination of a single axon into the support cell, which brings its outer cell membranes into close apposition and seals them together to form a sheet of internal membrane (the **mesaxon**, Fig. 13.6). The line of fusion is between the outer surfaces of the cell membrane, and ultrastructurally forms a line (the **intraperiod line**). Myelination then proceeds as the support cell wraps numerous layers of the mesaxon around the axon. A tight spiral composed of double-thickness cell membrane fused together forms because the cytoplasm of the support cell is excluded from most of the space between the membrane layers.

The inner surfaces of the cell membranes also fuse and form a dense line, the **major dense line**.

The thickness of the myelin sheath depends on the number of layers (lamellae) wrapped around the axon.

The cell membrane of the support cells that form myelin contains special lipids and proteins, for example, the glycolipid **galactocerebroside,** which is abundant in myelin.

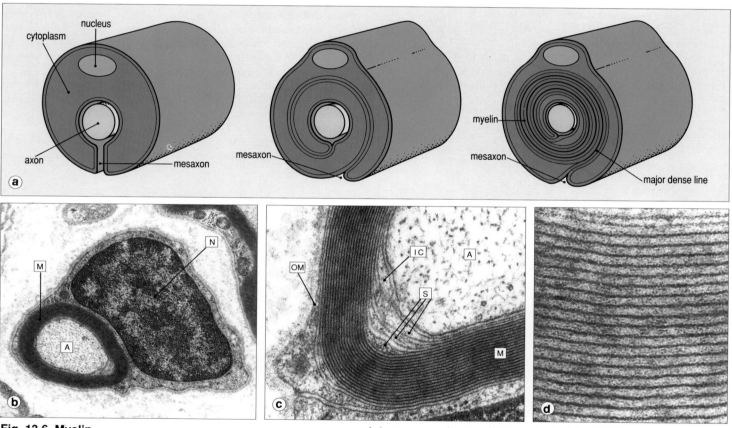

Fig. 13.6 Myelin.

a Diagram to show myelin formation. First an axon invaginates a myelin-forming cell and the outer leaflets of the myelin-forming cell's membrane fuse to form the mesaxon.

The myelin-forming cell then wraps layers of the mesaxon around the axon; the inner cytoplasm is lost when the inner leaflet of the cell membrane fuses to form the major dense line. Myelin forms into numerous lamellae of fused membrane, the lamellae being separated by alternating major dense lines and mesaxon (intraperiod line).

b Low power electronmicrograph showing an axon (A) surrounded by myelin (M) and the nucleus (N) of a Schwann cell.

c Medium power electronmicrograph showing the fine structure of myelin. The axon (A) is surrounded by myelin lamellae (M). Note the outer mesaxon (OM). The areas of cytoplasm in the myelin represent Schmidt-Lantermann incisures (S, see Fig. 13.7), and the inner collar of cytoplasm (IC).

d High power electronmicrograph showing the fine detail of myelin lamellae; the dark lines are the major dense lines while the intraperiod lines are barely visible in between.

Myelination of an axon is not continuous along its length, but occurs in small units 1–2 mm long, each unit being formed by an individual support cell. The small space between each unit of myelin is the **node of Ranvier** and has an important physiological role in increasing the efficiency of nerve conduction.

The cytoplasm of the myelin-forming support cell remains in the myelin sheath at three sites to maintain the cell membrane. These sites are located:

- adjacent to the axon (**inner collar**);
- between the internodal myelin lamellae of peripheral nervous system myelin formed by Schwann cells (**Schmidt-Lantermann incisures**);
- at each end of the myelin segment adjacent to the nodes of Ranvier (**paranodal area**, see below);
- adjacent to the cell body on the outer aspect of the myelin (**outer collar**).

The cytoplasm in all these areas is in continuity with that of the cell body of the support cells so that the membrane forming the myelin can be maintained (Fig. 13.7).

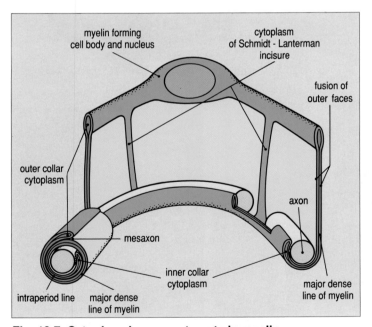

Fig. 13.7 Cytoplasmic compartments in myelin.
If the myelin around an axon is theoretically unwrapped, the relationships between the cytoplasmic compartments become evident.

The inner collar and outer collar run along and parallel to the axon, while the cytoplasm of the Schmidt-Lantermann incisures is wrapped around the axon in between myelin lamellae. These zones of cytoplasm are continuous with the cell body of the myelin-forming cell and serve to maintain the membrane forming the myelin.

NODES OF RANVIER

The myelin insulation is not continuous along the axon, but occurs in small segments about 1–2 mm long. Between each segment there is a bare area of the axon in a region termed the node of Ranvier (Fig. 13.8).

At the node of Ranvier the myelinating cells form paranodal loops of cytoplasm in continuity with the cell body.

In the central nervous system the axons in the nodes of Ranvier are bare, while those in the peripheral nervous system are partly covered by tongues of cytoplasm from adjacent Schwann cells.

The axon at the node of Ranvier is slightly thicker than in the internodal regions and contains most of the Na^+ gated channels of the axonal cell membrane, which is reflected ultrastructurally as a fuzzy thickening of the membrane. These gated channels are anchored via the link protein ankyrin to the cytoskeleton. There are no gated channels in the internodal region beneath the myelin sheath.

Depolarization at a node of Ranvier is followed by rapid passive spread of the depolarization current along the axon beneath the myelin to the next node because leakage of current is minimized by the insulation.

As the membrane capacitance is low, which is also the result of the myelin, only a small charge is required to cause a significant voltage difference.

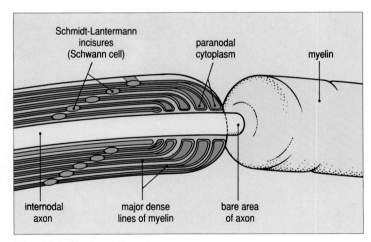

Fig. 13.8 Node of Ranvier.
Diagram of a node of Ranvier in longitudinal section. At the end of a myelin segment the myelin lamellae give way to a series of paranodal loops containing cytoplasm. The adjacent bare area of axon is generally slightly wider than the internodal axon and is the region containing the voltage-gated Na^+ channels, which are necessary for the formation of action potential. Compare the Schmidt-Lantermann incisures in this plane with those in Fig. 13.7.

When such passively spread conduction encounters the zone of highly concentrated gated channels in the next node of Ranvier along the axon, there is further local depolarization. Thus the depolarization progresses in a series of jumps, with passive spread of charge in between.

Depolarization in a myelinated nerve is much more efficient metabolically than in a non-myelinated nerve, because the restricted entry of Na^+ ions to small areas, instead of to the whole axonal surface, reduces the demand for energy to pump the ions back out again.

CENTRAL NERVOUS SYSTEM

The central nervous system comprises the brain and spinal cord. These contain nerve cells and their processes together with a series of specialized support cells.

Support cells

The central nervous system (CNS) contains numerous non-neural support cells. These are astrocytes oligodendrocytes, ependyma, and microglial cells (Fig. 13.9), which are collectively called **the glia**.

Astrocytes

Astrocytes are large, multi-processed cells with several functions.
• In embryological development, they form a structural framework to guide the migration of developing nerve cells.
• In the developed brain, they form a structural scaffolding for the more specialized neural elements.
• Certain astrocytes transport fluid and ions from the extracellular space around neurones to blood vessels.

Astrocytes are characterized by oval or slightly irregular nucei with an open chromatin pattern, and a spectacular stellate morphology with numerous fine processes radiating in all directions. These processes contain a specific form of cytoskeletal intermediate filament (see page 21) called **glial fibrillary acidic protein (GFAP)**.

The stellate morphology is not evident in conventional H&E section because the processes merge with the processes of other cells, but is seen with special staining methods (Fig. 13.10).

Two types of astrocyte have been identified.
• **Fibrous astrocytes** are most evident in the white matter and have long cell processes, which are rich in bundles of GFAP.
• **Protoplasmic astrocytes** are most evident in the grey matter of the brain and have long thin processes containing few bundles of GFAP.

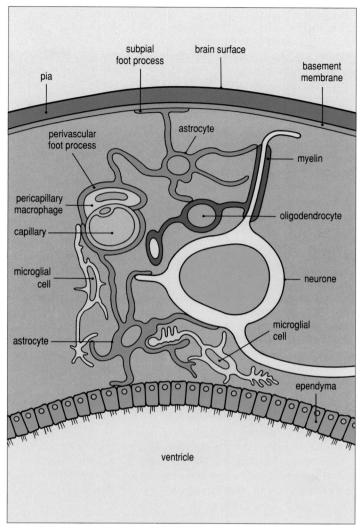

Fig. 13.9 Support cells of the CNS.
The support cells of the CNS are called glia and have several roles.

Astrocytes not only form a scaffolding for the other cells, but also extend foot processes around capillaries to maintain a blood–brain barrier. At the surface of the brain, astrocytes line a basement membrane and form the **glia limitans**, which surrounds the whole CNS.

Oligodendrocytes myelinate the axons of the nerve cells, while a vast network of antigen-sensing microglial cells is present throughout the CNS. Phagocytic macrophages, which also have an immune defence role, reside in the perivascular space, outside the CNS substance.

The ependymal cells form an epithelial sheet, which unlike other epithelia, does not lie on a basement membrane. This sheet lines the fluid-filled ventricular cavities of the brain, and the central canal of the spinal cord.

213

One important structural adaptation of astrocytes is seen in their interaction with the blood vessels of the brain, which they surround by forming flat plates termed **end feet** (see Fig. 13.9). The interaction induces changes in the structure of the cerebral vascular endothelium, rendering it highly impermeable, so that it acts as a barrier to diffusion between the blood and brain.

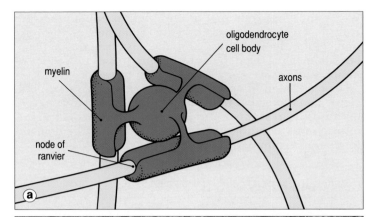

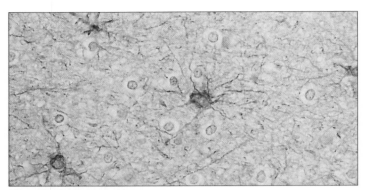

Fig. 13.10 Astrocytes.
Micrograph stained by an immunoperoxidase method to show glial fibrillary acidic protein (GFAP), the intermediate filament of astrocytes. The astrocyte is stained brown and shows the characteristic stellate morphology.

GLIOSIS

When neurones die, the dead cells are removed by macrophages by phagocytosis. The damaged area is then repaired by proliferation of astrocytic cells, which fill the defect and form an astrocytic scar in a process termed **gliosis**.

Oligodendrocytes

Oligodendrocytes produce myelin within the CNS. One oligodendrocyte sends out several cell processes and myelinates several nearby axons (Fig. 13.11).

In routine histological preparations of oligodendrocytes their branching morphology is not seen, but they do show a rounded nucleus with moderately dense-staining chromatin and, in most preparations, a cytoplasm containing a clear 'halo' around the nucleus. Such a halo is an artefact of preparation because oligodendrocytes are fragile and contain few cytoskeletal elements.

Immunohistochemical staining for myelin-related proteins, for example myelin basic protein, can be used to specifically identify oligodendrocytes (Fig. 13.11c).

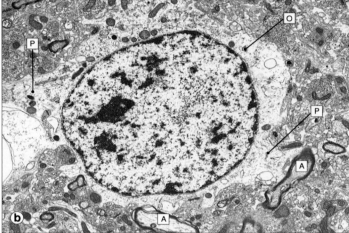

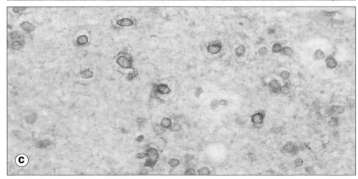

Fig. 13.11 Oligodendrocytes.
a Oligodendrocytes myelinate several adjacent axons within the CNS.
b Ultrastructurally, the oligodendrocyte (O) has abundant mitochondria and Golgi, but few cytoskeletal elements.
Note processes (P) myelinating nearby axons (A).
c Oligodendrocytes can be identified by immunochemical staining for specific proteins; in this instance highlighting oligodendrocytes (brown), but not other cells such as microglia or astrocytes.

214

DEMYELINATION

Multiple sclerosis

The myelin of the CNS is the target for attack by the immune system in **multiple sclerosis** (Fig. 13.12), which is of unknown cause.

Myelin is vital for the CNS to function effectively and its destruction in multiple sclerosis results in severe functional deficits, such as paralysis, loss of sensation and/or loss of co-ordination. The nature of the deficit depends on the area of the CNS affected.

Leukodystrophies

Several inherited diseases of metabolism result in defective production of myelin within the nervous system. Such disorders are called **leukodystrophies**. Affected children have severe neurological deficits and impaired neural development.

One of the most common leukodystrophies is due to a metabolic defect in peroxisomal function (see page 19), which causes adrenoleukodystrophy. In this disorder, there is widespread degeneration and loss of myelin in the cerebral hemispheres.

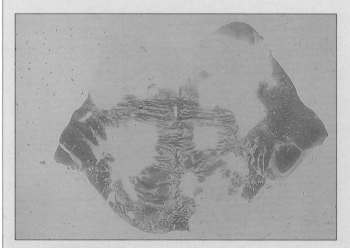

Fig. 13.12 Multiple sclerosis.
Low power micrograph of the pons region of brain, which has been stained by a method that stains myelin blue. Large patches of myelin have been destroyed, leaving a pale-stained space and only a little blue-stained myelin remains.

Ependyma

Ependymal cells are epithelial in type and line the cavities in the brain (**ventricles**) and the **central canal** of the spinal cord, forming a sheet of cuboidal cells in contact with the cerebrospinal fluid.

Each ependymal cell has a small oval basal nucleus with dense chromatin, and many are ciliated (Fig. 13.13).

Ultrastructurally the cells are bound to each other by prominent desmosomal junctions and have apical microvilli in addition to cilia.

Unlike other epithelial cells, the ependymal cells do not lie on a basement membrane, but have tapering processes, which merge with the processes of underlying astrocytic cells.

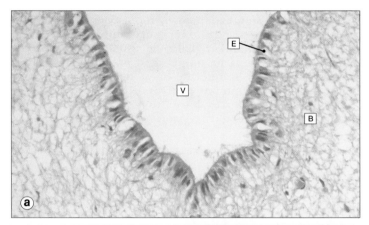

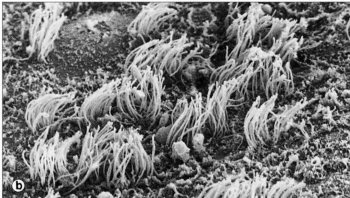

Fig. 13.13 Ependyma.
a Micrograph showing ependymal cells (E) lining the lateral ventricle (V) of the brain. They are cuboidal epithelial cells and rest on underlying glial processes in the brain (B).
b Scanning electronmicrograph showing that many of the ependymal cells bear tufts of surface cilia.

215

Microglia and immune cells

The CNS has its own unique set of immune cells, the main type being the **microglial cells**, which are specialized macrophages.

In conventional H&E preparations microglial cells are not easily seen, appearing only as rod-shaped nuclei with no discernible cytoplasmic borders. Immunohistochemical staining (Fig. 13.14), however, shows that they have extensive fine ramifying processes and form a widespread network of cells throughout the brain.

The phenotype of microglia suggests that they are dendritic antigen-presenting cells (see page 83), having a low level of phagocytic activity, and expressing class II major histocompatibility molecules.

In disease states microglial cells become activated and increase in size and number. Under these circumstances they are usually supplemented by monocytes, which enter the brain from the blood and form macrophagic cells.

In addition to the microglial cells, which are intrinsic to the brain there are large numbers of macrophages in the perivascular spaces outside the brain substance, and these cells can also act as immune effector cells.

The brain appears to have no significant traffic of lymphoid cells in the normal state.

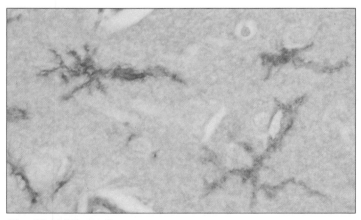

Fig. 13.14 Microglia.
Micrograph of brain stained by a lectin technique using ricinus communis agglutinin, which binds to a sugar on the surface of microglial cells and endothelial cells in the brain.

Microglial cells (brown) have a rod-shaped or elliptical dark-staining nucleus and a fine ramified dendritic morphology consisting of numerous extremely fine cell processes.

Microglial cells can also be immunostained by antisera to leukocyte common antigen (CD45) and HLADr (class II MHC antigen). The level of HLADr expression increases in disease states with an immune basis, for example multiple sclerosis (see page 215).

Meninges

The CNS is invested by three protective coats, the **meninges**, which are composed of fibrocollagenous support tissue and epithelial cells (Fig. 13.15). There are three meningeal layers: the dura, the arachnoid and the pia.

The dura is a tough fibrocollagenous layer, which forms the outer coat of the CNS. It blends with the periosteum of the skull and is attached to the periosteum of the vertebral canal by the dentinate ligaments. It is covered on its internal surface by an incomplete layer of flat epithelial cells.

The dura is reflected down from the skull to form sheets of tissue, the tentorium cerebelli and the falx cerebri, which separate the structures of the brain. The venous sinuses of the brain run at the base of these sheets by dura.

The arachnoid is a layer of fibrocollagenous tissue covered by inconspicuous flat epithelial, cells and is located beneath, but not anchored to, the dura. Web-like strands of fibrocollagenous tissue extend down from the arachnoid into the subarachnoid space, which contains the cerbrospinal fluid.

The main arteries and veins to and from the brain run in the subarachnoid space.

The pia is a delicate layer of epithelial cells associated with loose fibrocollagenous tissue. It lies external to a basement membrane, which completely invests the CNS. This basement membrane is formed by a special set of astrocytes, termed the **limiting glia (glia limitans)**.

MENINGEAL SPACES IN DISEASE

There are several spaces defined by the meninges of clinical importance. These are the subdural space, the subarachnoid space and the extradural space.

Extradural haematoma. Fracture of the skull causes an accumulation of blood outside the dura in the **extradural space**.

Subdural haematoma. Following trauma bleeding may occur into the space between the dura and the arachnoid (**subdural space**) from venous channels.

Subarachnoid haemorrhage. Rupture of arteries running outside the brain causes bleeding into the subarachnoid space between the arachnoid and pia.

Meningitis. The cerebrospinal fluid in the subarachnoid space is the site of infection in meningitis.

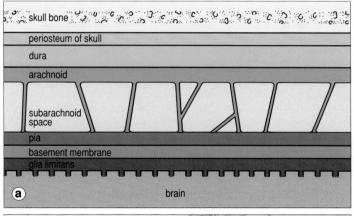

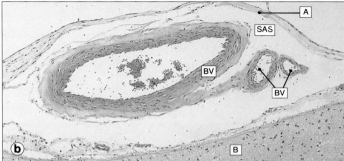

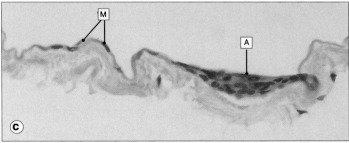

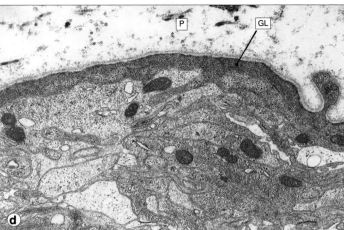

Fig. 13.15 Meninges and glia limitans.

a The meninges cover the CNS and are divided into three layers, dura, arachnoid, and pia. Below the pia there is a basement membrane giving rise to a set of astrocytic cells, which form a barrier around the CNS termed the glia limitans. The subarachnoid space contains the cerebrospinal fluid.

b Micrograph showing the arachnoid (A), subarachnoid space (SAS) and underlying brain (B). Blood vessels (BV) run in the subarachnoid space.

c Meningothelial cells are normally flat, inconspicuous cells, which line the dura, arachnoid and pia, but with age some of these cells become histologically prominent; in this micrograph from the arachnoid of a 60-year-old man, the meningothelial cells (M) form a small aggregate (A).

d Electronmicrograph showing the glia limitans (GL) , which forms an outer barrier investing the whole of the CNS. It is composed of a basement membrane, which is seen just beneath the pia collagen (P), and is produced by a sheet of closely adherent foot processes from astrocytic cells in the underlying brain.

MENINGIOMA

The epithelial cells of the meninges (meningothelial cells) may form tumours termed **meningiomas.** These tumours are:

- most common in women;
- increase in frequency after 45 years of age;
- one of the commonest tumours involving the CNS;
- mostly benign and slow growing.

Meningiomas are most common around the falx cerebri and appear macroscopically as rounded nodules, typically 3–4 cm in size, but can be much larger.

Symptoms are caused by compression of the underlying brain, which may result in paralysis, epileptic fits, or swelling of the brain.

Histologically meningiomas are made up of sheets of meningothelial cells, which characteristically form spherical whorls. Ultrastructurally the epithelial characteristics of desmosomal junctions are usually prominent.

Meningiomas can usually be successfully treated by surgical removal.

Choroid plexus

The choroid plexuses are located in the ventricular system of the brain and produce cerebrospinal fluid. Each choroid plexus consists of a vascular stroma covered by columnar epithelial cells, which form large frond-like masses (Fig. 13.16). The epithelial cells are anchored by junctional complexes, rest on a basement membrane, have apical microvilli, and are adapted for secretion (see page 35).

The cerebrospinal fluid produced in the ventricles flows out through exit foramina at the base of the brain, and circulates in the subarachnoid space. It is reabsorbed by the venous sinuses in the dura.

Vasculature

The brain is supplied with blood from major arteries that form an anastomotic link around the base of the brain. From this region, the arteries run in the subarachnoid space before turning and dipping down into the brain.

Around the large vessels within the brain is a perivascular space, called eponymously the **Virchow-Robin space**. In man this space is sealed from the subarachnoid space by reflections of the pia onto the blood vessels as they enter the brain (Fig. 13.17), and is therefore continuous with the potential subpial space.

The perivascular space is bounded externally by the basement membrane of the glia limitans (see Fig. 13.15d) as far as the capillaries, where the vascular and glial basement membranes fuse.

The endothelial cells of brain capillaries are joined by occluding junctions and are not fenestrated, thus they form a barrier to the diffusion of substances from the blood to the brain (i.e. a **blood–brain barrier**).

The brain endothelial cells have systems for active transport of substances such as glucose into the brain.

External to the capillary endothelium is a basement membrane and external to this are the foot processes of astrocytes (see Fig. 13.9), which are responsible for induction of the special properties of the endothelial cells (see page 214).

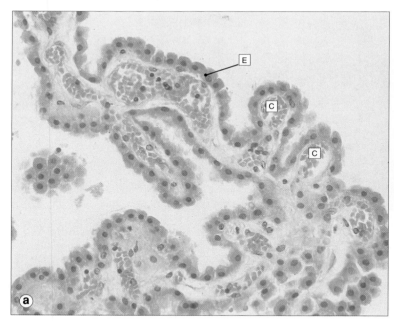

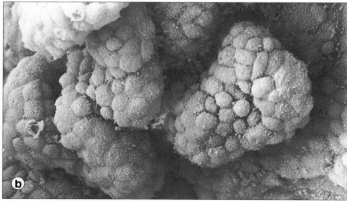

Fig. 13.16 Choroid plexus.
a Micrograph showing a portion of choroid plexus covered with a columnar epithelium (E), which is arranged as papillae over vascular stromal cores (C).
b Scanning electronmicrograph showing the convoluted surface of the choroid plexus, which is thrown into deep folds, and the fine microvilli on the apical surface of the covering epithelium.

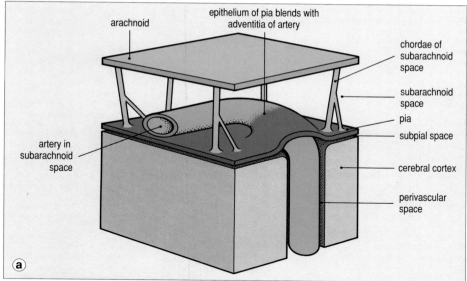

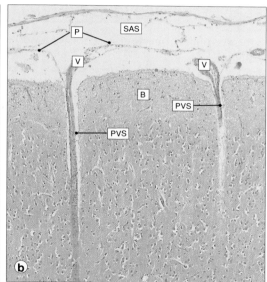

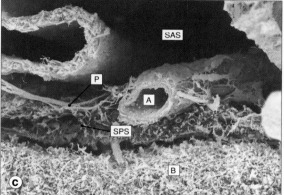

Fig. 13.17 Vascular arrangement in the brain.
a Arteries running in the subarachnoid space penetrate the pia, which is reflected up onto the wall of the vessel, thus isolating the perivascular space from the subarachnoid space. The layer of pia reflected onto the vessel is composed of a single layer of flat meningothelial cells anchored by junctional complexes. The perivascular space is continuous with the potential subpial space.
b Micrograph showing vessels (V) penetrating the surface of the brain (B) from the subarachnoid space (SAS). The pia (P) is reflected onto the vessel wall and separates the subarachnoid space from the perivascular space (PVS).
c Scanning electronmicrograph showing the subarachnoid space (SAS) with an artery (A) becoming invested by pia (P). Note the underlying subpial space (SPS) and brain (B).

TUMOURS OF THE NERVOUS SYSTEM

Gliomas

Primary brain tumours are most commonly derived from the glial cells and are collectively termed **gliomas**.

The most common glioma is derived from astrocytes (**astrocytoma**), and varies from a slow-growing lesion, which diffusely infiltrates the brain over many years, to a rapidly growing lesion that soon compresses vital structures.

Ependymomas commonly arise in the region of the ventricles and are recognized histologically by their epithelial characteristics. **Oligodendrogliomas** are most common in the temporal lobe, when they may be a cause of temporal lobe epilepsy.

Certain tumours of the CNS resemble the primitive embryonic cells of the developing brain and are grouped together as Primitive Neuroectodermal Tumours (PNET). These are commonest in childhood and may show differentiation towards neuronal, astrocytic, or ependymal cells.

Confirming the diagnosis

The diagnosis of CNS tumours must be confirmed by histology of tumour biopsies, and immunohistochemistry is used increasingly in the laboratory to identify cell types within a tumour. Finding glial fibrillary acidic protein (GFAP) is a strong indication that a tumour is of glial origin.

PERIPHERAL NERVOUS SYSTEM

The peripheral nervous system is composed of nerves and ganglia.
- A **nerve** is a collection of axons, linked together by support tissue into an anatomically defined trunk. The axons may be either motor or sensory, myelinated or non-myelinated.
- A **ganglion** is a peripheral collection of nerve cell bodies together with efferent and afferent axons, and support cells. Ganglia may be sensory (e.g. spinal sensory ganglia), or contain the cell bodies of autonomic nerves (i.e. sympathetic or parasympathetic ganglia).

Peripheral nerve

A peripheral nerve is composed of:
- axons;
- Schwann cells, which make myelin;
- spindle-shaped fibroblast support cells, which produce fibrocollagenous tissue;
- blood vessels.

Support tissue

There are three types of support tissue in a nerve trunk the endoneurium, perineurium and epineurium (Fig. 13.18).

Endoneurium is composed of longitudinally orientated collagen fibres, extracellular matrix material rich in glycosaminoglycans, and sparse fibroblasts. It surrounds the individual axons and their associated Schwann cells, as well as capillary blood vessels.

Perineurium surrounds groups of axons and endoneurium to form small bundles (**fascicles**). It is composed of 7–8 concentric layers of flattened cells separated by layers of collagen. The cells are joined by junctional complexes and each layer of cells is surrounded by an external lamina.

Epineurium is an outer sheath of loose fibrocollagenous tissue, which binds individual nerve fascicles into a nerve trunk. The epineurium may also include adipose tissue, as well as a main muscular artery supplying the nerve trunk.

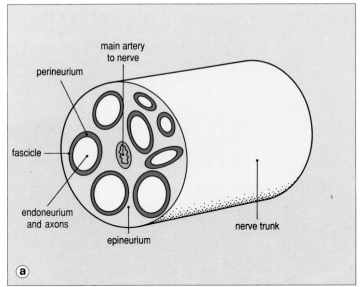

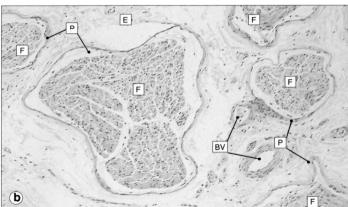

Fig. 13.18 Support tissue of peripheral nerve.
a Diagram showing the arrangement of support tissue in a peripheral nerve. Individual axons and their associated Schwann cells are sheathed by epineurium, and bound into fascicles by perineurium. The epineurium binds individual fascicles into a nerve trunk, and may contain the main muscular artery supplying the nerve trunk.
b Micrograph showing nerve fascicles (F) surrounded by perineurium (P) and grouped into a nerve trunk by epineurium (E). Note blood vessels (BV).

Myelinated and non-myelinated axons

Within a peripheral nerve there are both myelinated and non-myelinated axons.

In addition to producing the myelin of peripheral nerves, Schwann cells support non-myelinated axons, which bury themselves into the Schwann cell cytoplasm (Fig. 13.19).

Each Schwann cell has a well-defined external lamina which separates the cell from the endoneurium.

Variations

Nerves vary in their relative composition of myelinated and non-myelinated fibres from one anatomical site to another.

Myelinated fibres in a typical peripheral nerve in the lower limb of an adult vary in diameter from 2–17 μm (including myelin), there being a bimodal distribution with peaks around 5 μm and 13 μm.

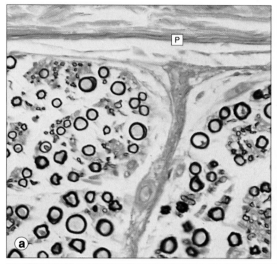

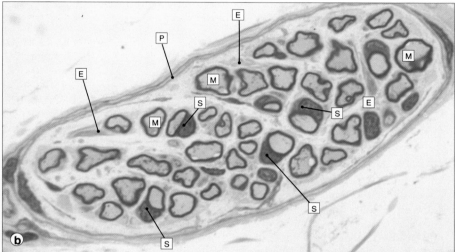

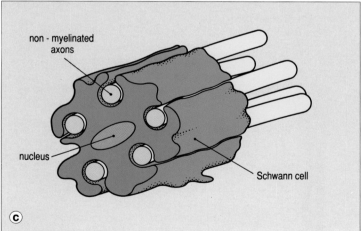

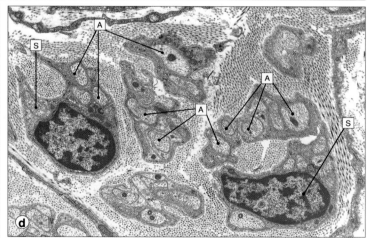

Fig. 13.19 Peripheral nerve.

a Micrograph of the edge of a single fascicle from a peripheral nerve stained with osmium, which stains myelin black. The perineurium (P) surrounds the fascicle. The myelinated axons appear as circular profiles with the central non-staining area occupied by axon. Non-myelinated fibres are not visible.

b Micrograph of a small nerve fascicle embedded in resin and stained with toluidine blue. The increased resolution allows myelinated axons (M) to be seen with associated Schwann cell nuclei (S) and endoneurial support tissue (E). The perineurium (P) is visible as 2–3 thin cell and collagen layers.

c Non-myelinated fibres are buried into and thereby supported by the cytoplasm of Schwann cells.

d Electronmicrograph showing non-myelinated axons (A) of a peripheral nerve embedded in the cytoplasm of a Schwann cell (S).

Ganglia

A ganglion is composed of
- neurone cell bodies;
- support cells (satellite cells and Schwann cells);
- axons;
- loose fibrocollagenous support tissue (Fig. 13.20).

The neurone cell bodies are large; they have abundant cytoplasm containing Nissl substance and large nuclei with prominent nucleoli.

Satellite cells are small support cells resembling Schwann cells, which surround the neurone cell bodies.

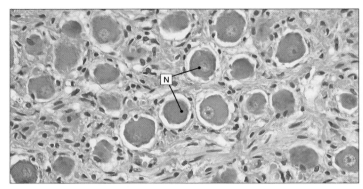

Fig. 13.20 Ganglion.

Micrograph showing a peripheral sensory ganglion containing neurones (N) with large nuclei and prominent nucleoli, surrounded by small darkly-stained satellite support cells. Axons running to and from the ganglion are supported by Schwann cells and a loose fibrocollagenous stroma.

REPAIR IN THE PERIPHERAL NERVOUS SYSTEM

The axons of neurones can regenerate following damage if the cell body remains alive.

Following section of a nerve supplying a muscle, the axons and myelin beyond the area of damage degenerate and are removed by Schwann cell lysosomes and by macrophages, which migrate into the nerve. The neurone cell body accumulates large amounts of neurofilaments, and the Nissl substance and nucleus migrate peripherally, so that it appears pale and swollen with an eccentric nucleus (**chromatolysis**).

The Schwann cells proliferate and form longitudinal columns of cells in the distal damaged nerve. At the proximal end the damaged axons re-grow by sprouting, the sprouts growing down the cords of Schwann cells at 2–5 mm/day. One fibre eventually connects with the muscle, becomes remyelinated and reestablishes innervation (Fig. 13.21). The cell body then resumes a normal appearance.

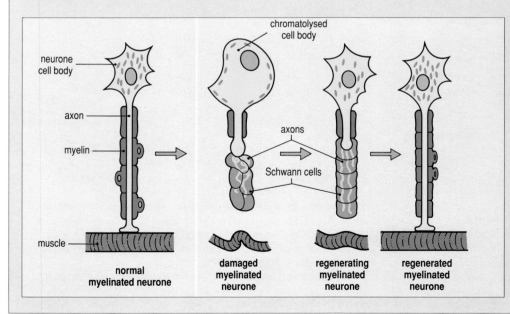

Fig. 13.21 Repair in the peripheral nervous system.

Following damage to a myelinated neurone innervating a muscle fibre, the distal axon and myelin are phagocytosed by proliferating Schwann cells.

The muscle fibre, devoid of innervation undergoes wasting, while the cell body of the neurone undergoes chromatolysis, with swelling, lateral migration of the nucleus, and loss of Nissl substance.

Axons then sprout from the damaged end of the nerve and grow down the column of Schwann cells, eventually restoring innervation of the muscle.

The Schwann cells remyelinate the axon, but the myelin segments are much shorter than before damage.

PRACTICAL HISTOLOGY

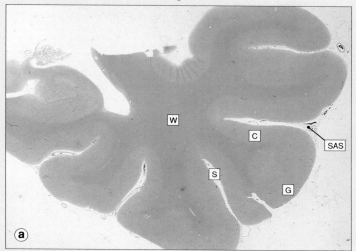

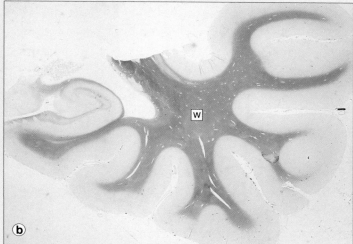

Fig. 13.22 Cerebral hemispheres.
a Micrograph of a section through the temporal lobe of the brain at low magnification. The cerebral hemisphere is thrown into a series of convolutions, **the gyri** (G), which are separated by intervening **sulci** (S).

The arachnoid covers the brain and is just visible at this magnification over the subarachnoid space (SAS). The white matter (W) contains the axons of nerve cells, which run to and from the cortex (C). The cortex is composed of nerve cells and does not contain myelin.

In H&E preparations the white matter stains more intensely with eosin (pink) than the cortex.
b Micrograph of the same section shown in **a** after staining with a dye with an affinity for myelin. Such a dye delineates the white matter (W) but does not stain the cortex (grey matter).

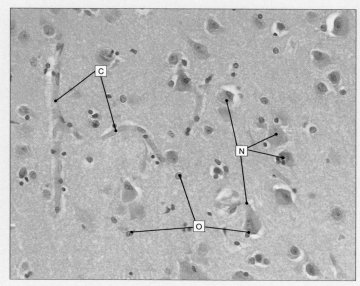

Fig. 13.23 Cerebral cortex
High power micrograph of cerebral cortex. Neurones (N) vary in size and shape according to their function, which is specific for different levels in the cortex, and in most of the cerebral cortex there are six distinct layers of different neuronal types. Capillary vessels (C) are plentiful.

The small densely stained nuclei belong to a mixture of glial cells, of which oligondendrocytes (O) are most prominent. Cortical oligodendrocytes do not make myelin, but act as support cells for axons and neurones. The oligodendrocytes adjacent to neurones are called satellite cells.

The pink stained background is a mat of neuronal and glial cell processes (neuropil).

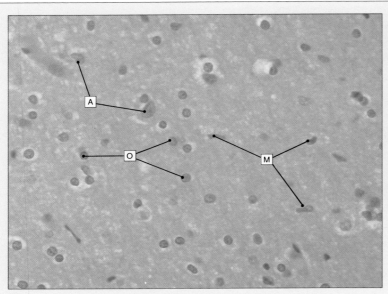

Fig. 13.24 White matter.

High power micrograph of white matter, in which it is generally not possible to perceive individual nerve fibres or cell processes because they merge into the pink-staining background of the neuropil.

The nuclei of glial cells are prominent but again details of the cytoplasm merge into the neuropil. Different glial types can be distinguished by the character of their nuclei. Oligodendrocytes (O) are most numerous and have rounded nuclei, which are often surrounded by an ill-defined clear perinuclear halo. Astrocytes (A) are fewer in number and are characterized by larger polygonal nuclei, which commonly contain central nucleoli. The nuclei of microglial cells (M) are frequently rod-shaped or comma shaped and stain more densely than those of the other glia.

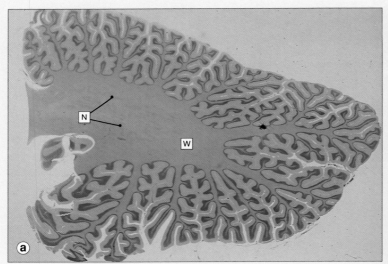

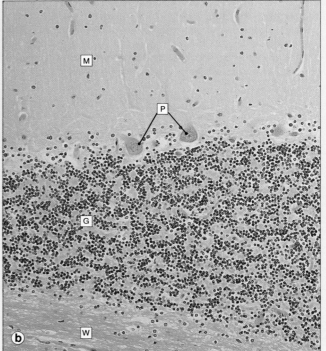

Fig. 13.25 Cerebellum.

a Micrograph of cerebellum, which is a distinct part of the brain and is characterized by complex folding of cerebellar cortex, generating a pattern of pleats (**cerebellar folia**). The folia contain the nuclei of nerve cells, which produce a purple staining ribbon at this low magnification. The centre of the cerebellum is composed of white matter (W) in which a serpiginous aggregate of nerve cells, termed a **nucleus** (N) is seen.

b Higher power micrograph of cerebellum showing that the outer part of the cerebellar cortex is composed of nerve cell processes with scanty glial cells (**the molecular layer M**), while the bulk of the purple staining ribbon is formed by a band of small nerve cells with dark-staining rounded nuclei (the **granular layer, G**). Below the granular layer is the white matter (W), which contains myelinated fibres. At the junction of the molecular layer with the granular layer is a row of large nerve cells (**Purkinje cells**, P), which are characterized by a vast branching pattern of dendrites in the molecular layer, but this is only visible by special staining methods.

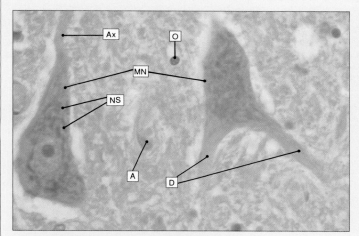

Fig. 13.26 Motor neurones of spinal cord.
Micrograph of spinal motor neurones (MN), which send axons (A) out to supply voluntary muscles and lie in the anterior part of the spinal cord. These neurones are large because they maintain an axon that may be up to 1 m long. The nucleus is large with a prominent nucleolus and the cytoplasm is packed with purple staining Nissl substance (NS).

Motor neurones make multiple connections with the axons of other neurones via large dendrites (D). The axon (Ax) of a motor neurone passes out through the spinal nerve roots and eventually forms part of a peripheral nerve.

The background in this micrograph is composed of a neuropil of nerve cell and glial processes and cannot be resolved with this type of preparation. The nuclei of oligodendrocytes (O) and astrocytes (A) are visible.

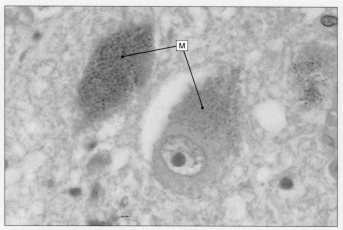

Fig. 13.27 Melanin-containing neurones.
Micrograph of neurones containing brown melanin pigment (M). Such cells are part of the substantia nigra, so-named because of its black colour imparted by the melanin and contain transmitter substance dopamine, which is responsible for coordination and fluidity of movement.

Destruction of these neurones results in Parkinson's disease, which is characterized by rigid, slow movement and a tremor.

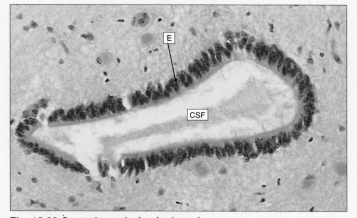

Fig. 13.28 Central canal of spinal cord.
Micrograph showing the central canal of the spinal cord. It is lined by ependymal cells (E) and contains cerebrospinal fluid (CSF).

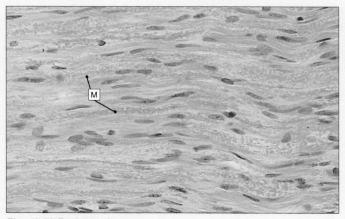

Fig. 13.29 Peripheral nerve.
In this micrograph of a longitudinally sectioned peripheral nerve, myelin (M) is just visible as long tapering profiles with a granular or foamy texture. The nuclei of the Schwann cells, which make the myelin, are the most conspicuous feature, and are typically long and tapering.

14. MUSCULOSKELETAL SYSTEM

The musculoskeletal system provides mechanical support and permits movement, and is composed of:
- skeletal muscle;
- tendons;
- bones;
- joints and ligaments.

Skeletal muscles act as contractile levers, which are inserted into bone via tendons, while bones act as rigid levers, which can articulate with other bones through joints.

A special characteristic of muscle, tendons and joints is the possesion of a rich sensory nerve supply, which detects position and velocity of movement. The integration of this sensory information by the central nervous system is vital for the musculoskeletal system to function normally.

The main functional attribute of bone is its specialized extracellular matrix, which is hardened by the deposition of calcium so that it can function as a rigid lever.

The rigid, hard character of bone belies its importance as a metabolic reservoir of mineral salts and that it is in a constant state of dynamic remodelling.

SKELETAL MUSCLE

The histological characteristics of skeletal muscle cells and the structural basis of muscle contraction are described on pages 57–61.

To generate movement through contraction, individual muscle cells are arranged into large groups to form anatomically distinct **muscles**, which are characterized by:
- an orderly alignment of the constituent cells to generate a directional force following contraction;
- anchorage to other structures by highly organized fibro-collagenous support tissues;
- a rich blood supply reflecting their high metabolic demands;
- innervation and control by specialized neurones (**motor neurones**), which terminate on muscle cells at specialized nerve endings (**motor end plates**);
- incorporation of specially adapted skeletal muscle cells into structures called **spindles**, to act as sensors of muscle stretch.

Structure

Embryologically, muscle fibres develop from mesenchymal tissues (Fig. 14.1).

Each skeletal muscle cell is typically extremely long (up to 10 cm in length), and it is therefore more usual to use the term skeletal muscle fibre rather than cell.

A muscle fibre is composed of large numbers of **myofibrils** bounded by a cell membrane termed the **sarcolemma** (see Fig. 5.2 & Fig. 14.2). Many muscle fibres are arranged together to form a muscle (Fig. 14.3).

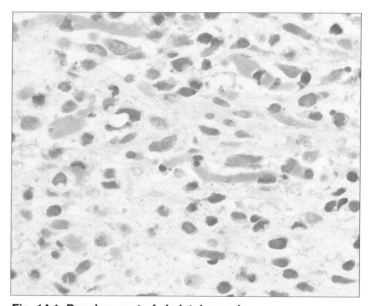

Fig. 14.1 Development of skeletal muscle.
In embryogenesis, skeletal muscle develops from mesenchymal tissues with the formation of small spindle-shaped mononuclear cells (rhabdomyoblasts). Multinucleate muscle fibres then form from the fusion of numerous individual rhabdomyoblasts, and enlarge in size following connection to the nervous system.

Residual cells with the function of rhabdomyoblasts persist in adult skeletal muscle as satellite cells. Following damage, these cells proliferate and can produce new muscle cells in adult life.

In order to transmit mechanically the force of contraction, the cell surface at the end of the muscle fibres is adapted for attachment to highly organized fibrocollagenous support tissues, which anchor the muscle to other structures.

Such anchorage may be provided by anatomically distinct tendons, broad areas of anchorage to a bony surface, or broad areas of anchorage to sheets of fibrocollagenous support tissue (**fascia**), which run between muscles.

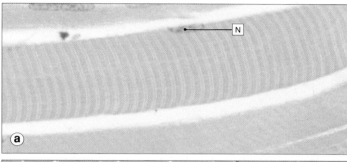

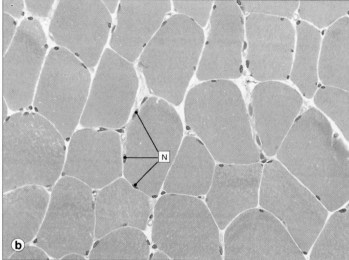

Fig. 14.2 Skeletal muscle fibres.
a Micrograph of skeletal muscle fibres in a longitudinal frozen section showing prominent cross striations. The dark bands are termed **A bands** (anisotropic, i.e. birefringent in polarized light), while the light bands are termed I bands (isotropic, i.e. no interference with polarized light). These bands correspond to the arrangement of thick and thin filaments in myofibrils (see Fig. 5.2). Nuclei (N) appear as elongated structures just beneath the cell membrane and each fibre contains by many nuclei.
b Micrograph of skeletal muscle fibres in a transverse frozen section showing roughly hexagonal profiles with flattened sides where they are compressed by adjacent fibres. Nuclei (N) appear as small circular profiles at the periphery of each fibre. Individual myofibrils are generally not identifiable by light microscopy.

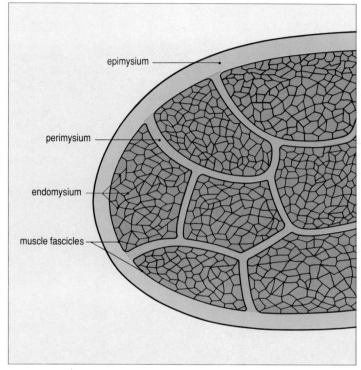

Fig. 14.3 Organization of muscle fibres into muscle.
Individual muscle fibres (see Fig. 5.2) are surrounded by **endomysium** which is composed of sheets of external lamina identical to basement membrane (see page 49).

Endomysium anchors the muscle fibres to each other and contains both capillary blood vessels, and individual nerve axons (see page 206).

Clusters of muscle fibres are held together by fine sheets of fibrocollagenous support tissue (**perimysium**) to form **fascicles**. Blood vessels, lymphatic vessels and nerves run in the endomysial support tissues.

An anatomically defined muscle is composed of many fascicles, which are surrounded externally by a thick layer of fibrocollagenous support tissue, the **epimysium**.

Although elongated cells, individual muscle cells do not extend for the full length of a muscle, but are arranged in overlapping bundles, the force of contraction being transmitted through the arrangement of the support tissues.

Muscle fibre types

Different muscles are characterized by different physiological and metabolic properties, which are determined by differences in the structure of their constituent muscle fibres.

In both animals and man it has been possible to define several subtypes of muscle fibre by macroscopic, physiological, biochemical and histochemical criteria, but there are marked interspecies variations.

Histochemical staining for specific enzymes (see glossary) delineates several types of fibre and is a useful method for analysing muscle. Two main types of fibre are identified (**type 1** and **2**), and the type 2 fibres can be subdivided into types **2A**, **2B** and **2C** (Fig. 14.4). Such histochemical staining is used routinely in the study of muscle pathology and allows the histological diagnosis of certain muscle diseases.

Histochemical staining can also be correlated with other functional and biochemical attributes of muscle (Fig. 14.4c).

Not all muscles have the same proportions of type 1 and type 2 fibres. In general, muscles with a role in maintaining posture (e.g. calf muscles) have a high proportion of type 1 fibres, while muscles used for short bursts of power have a high proportion of type 2 fibres.

Different individuals are genetically endowed with variable proportions of muscle fibre types in defined muscles, and this may limit athletic prowess at a particular sport; training does not affect the proportion of muscle fibres in any given muscle, but does alter their size.

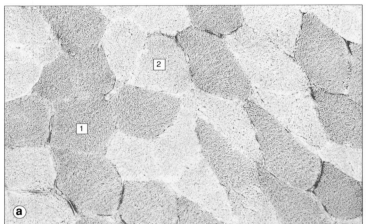

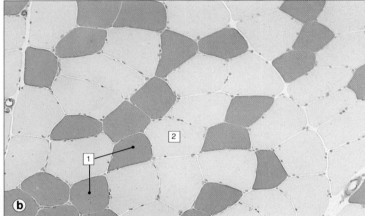

fibre type	colour	metabolism	contractile behaviour
1	intermediate	oxidative	slow twitch
2A	red	oxidative and glycolytic	fast twitch, fatigue resistant
2B	white	glycolytic	fast twitch, fatigue sensitive

Fig. 14.4 Fibre types.
a Micrograph of a transverse frozen section of muscle stained by an enzyme histochemical method to demonstrate NADH transferase which indicates oxidative capacity. Two different subtypes of fibre are evident. Type 1 fibres (1) show a high level of activity and stain darkly, while type 2 fibres (2) are paler because of their lower level of activity.
b Micrograph of muscle stained for one form of myofibrillar ATPase at pH 4.2. This technique also delineates two fibre types. Type 1 fibres stain darkly having a high level of activity, while type 2 fibres have a low level of activity and stain lightly. Note that the type 1 and 2 fibres are arranged in a haphazard or checkerboard pattern.
c Table detailing the physiological features of different fibre types.

DISEASES OF MUSCLE

Several diseases of muscle have been attributed to specific metabolic or structural abnormalities (Fig. 14.5a).

Duchenne muscular dystrophy is the most common inherited muscle disease and characteristically affects male children. Such individuals become unable to stand unaided in early childhood and develop progressive muscle weakness, becoming wheelchair-bound by their mid teens and typically dying in early adult life.

The abnormality in Duchenne muscular dystrophy is due to a defect in the gene coding for a protein termed **dystrophin** (Fig. 14.5b). Although the function of this protein is at present unknown, its absence leads to abnormal muscle fibre fragility, and the muscle fibres are ultimately replaced by fibrous tissue.

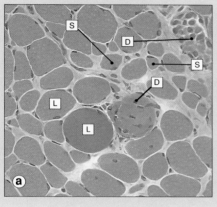
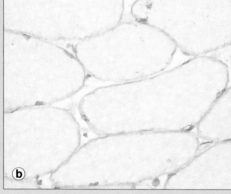

Fig. 14.5 Diseases of muscle.
a Micrograph of frozen section of skeletal muscle from a child showing the typical appearance of dystrophy, which is a congenital primary disorder of muscle. There is marked variation in fibre size, with some large fibres (L) and some abnormally small fibres (S). Some fibres are dead (D) and are being removed by phagocytic cells (see page 73).
b Micrograph of normal skeletal muscle stained by an immunocytochemical method for dystrophin (which stains brown), showing its localization in the sarcolemma. In Duchenne muscular dystrophy this protein is absent.

Vascular supply

Muscle is characterized by a rich blood supply because of the high energy demands of contraction.

Large arteries penetrate the epimysium and divide into small branches, which run in the perimysial support tissues, forming perimysial arteries and veins. These branches terminate in a vast capillary network, which runs in the endomysium. Each muscle fibre is associated with several capillary vessels.

Satellite cells

Normal adult skeletal muscle cells do not undergo cell division. Any increased demands placed on a muscle, for example by weight training, result in increased muscle size because the muscle cells themselves increase in size (i.e. hypertrophy).

It is possible, however, for skeletal muscle cells to re-grow because a pool of inactive stem cells in adult muscle called **satellite cells** can be stimulated to divide following damage. These cells are not discernible by light microscopy, but may be seen ultrastructurally (Fig. 14.6). They are infrequent and appear as small spindle-shaped cells lying just beneath the external lamina of a muscle fibre.

Fibres that have regenerated in adult life following damage to a muscle can be detected histologically because they commonly contain centrally placed nuclei rather that the peripheral nuclei typical of normal fibres.

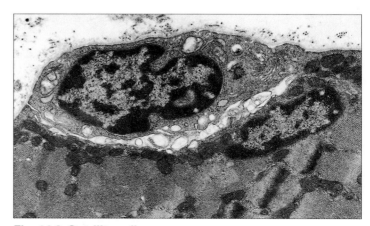

Fig. 14.6 Satellite cells.
Electronmicrograph showing a satellite cell. These cells are small spindle-shaped cells lying immediately beneath the external lamina of a muscle fibre and act as stem cells in adult muscle.

Sensory innervation of muscle

Although there are no pain receptors in skeletal muscle, there are receptors sensitive to stretch, which function as part of a feedback system to maintain normal muscle tone (i.e. the spinal stretch reflex arc).

Sensory fibres that provide information on the tension of skeletal muscle arise from two sources:

- encapsulated nerve endings responding to stretch in the tendon of muscle;
- spiral nerve endings (**sensory afferent fibres**) sensing stretch and tension of specialized muscle fibres contained in a special sense organ in muscle called the **muscle spindle** (Fig. 14.7).

The muscle spindle sensory mechanism maintains normal tone and muscle coordination.

Motor innervation of muscle

Large nerves, containing both motor and sensory axons, enter muscles by penetrating the epimysium and branch to form small nerves, which run in the perimysium.

Perimysial nerves contain axons to provide both motor and sensory functions. The motor axons destined to innervate skeletal muscle (α **efferent fibres**) enter the endomysium as nerve twigs and branch to innervate several fibres.

At the end of each twig each axon becomes modified to form a **motor end plate**, which controls skeletal muscle contraction (Fig. 14.8).

Activation of the motor axon causes the release of acetylcholine from its storage granules by exocytosis. Acetylcholine then diffuses across the gap between the axon and muscle fibre, and interacts with specific membrane receptors to cause depolarization of the muscle fibre; this initiates contraction as described on page 60.

The activity of secreted acetylcholine is rapidly curtailed by the activity of an enzyme called acetylcholinesterase, which is bound to the basement membrane investing the junctional folds.

In addition to nerve fibres controlling voluntary movements, specialized motor axons (γ **efferent fibres**) innervate muscle fibres in the muscle spindle.

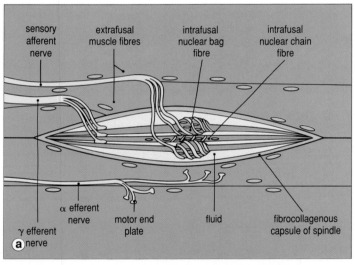

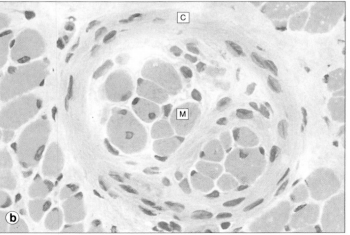

Fig. 14.7 Sensory innervation of skeletal muscle.

a Diagram illustrating the sensory innervation of muscle, which arises from two sources: encapsulated nerve endings in the tendons respond to stretch, and spiral nerve endings in muscle spindles sense stretch and tension.

The muscle spindle is composed of a fusiform capsule of fibrocollagenous tissue (continuous with the perimysium) surrounding a group of 8–15 thin muscle fibres. These fibres are termed **intrafusal fibres** to distinguish them from normal skeletal muscle fibres (i.e. **extrafusal fibres**).

Two types of intrafusal fibre can be distinguished; those with a fusiform shape and central aggregate of nuclei (**nuclear bag fibres**), and those of uniform width with dispersed nuclei (**nuclear chain fibres**).

Specialized motor nerve fibres (γ efferent fibres) innervate the intrafusal fibres and adjust their length according to the state of stretch of the muscle, which is detected by spiral nerve endings. The spiral nerve endings are wrapped around the intrafusal fibres and form special **sensory afferent fibres** running back to the spinal cord.

b Micrograph of frozen section from a child's muscle showing a muscle spindle, identified by its circular fibrocollagenous capsule (C) and its content of intrafusal muscle fibres (M).

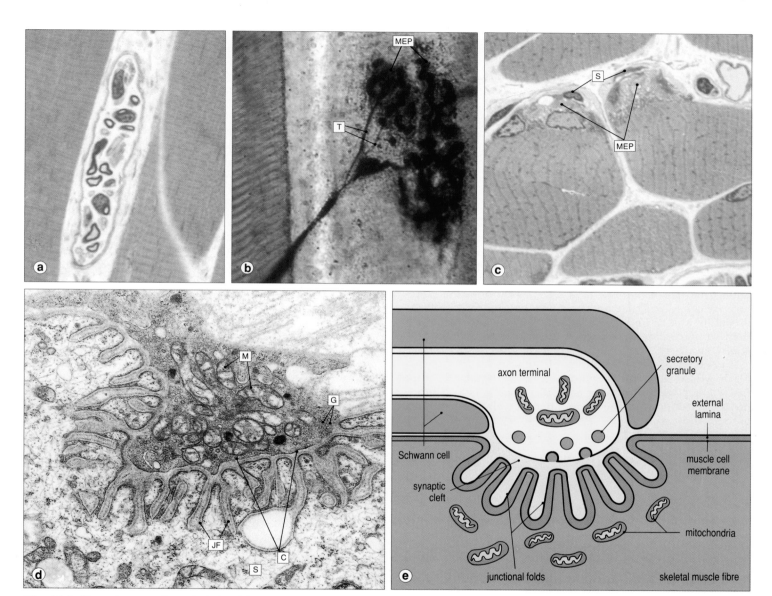

Fig. 14.8 Motor innervation of skeletal muscle.

a A thin resin section of skeletal muscle stained with toluidine blue showing a small perimysial nerve, which contains both motor (efferent) and sensory (afferent) fibres.

b A methylene blue stained teased preparation of muscle showing several nerve twigs (T) branching from a single axon to innervate muscle fibres. There is a bulbous swelling (the motor end plate, MEP) at the end of each twig at the site of connection with the muscle. The group of fibres innervated by a single axon is a motor unit.

c Micrograph of a thin resin section of skeletal muscle stained with toluidine blue to show the motor end plate (MEP). The axon terminates in a dome-shaped swelling of the nerve terminal in direct apposition to the cell membrane of the muscle fibre, to form

the MEP. This is invested by a layer of Schwann cell cytoplasm (S).

d Electronmicrograph of a motor end plate showing the cell membrane of the muscle fibre thrown into a series of deep folds (junctional folds, JF) beneath which the sarcoplasm (S) contains numerous mitochondria (M). In the terminal swelling of the motor axon neurosecretory granules (G) containing the transmitter substance, acetylcholine, and mitochondria are abundant.

The terminal swelling of the axon is separated from the muscle cell membrane by a gap of 30–50 nm (the synaptic cleft, C), which includes the external lamina of the muscle.

e Diagram of motor end plate. The sarcoplasmic membrane in the region of the motor end plate contains specialized receptors for acetylcholine, which when activated by acetylcholine cause muscle cell membrane depolarization.

MYAESTHENIA GRAVIS

Myaesthenia gravis is a disease caused by antibodies to the acetylcholine receptor on the sarcolemma in the junctional folds of the motor end plates. The antibodies bind to the acetylcholine receptors and thereby prevent released acetylcholine from interacting with the receptors and causing depolarization.

Affected individuals develop tremendous muscle weakness manifest by fatiguability, inability to lift the arms, inability to maintain an upright posture of the head, and drooping of the eyelids.

Treatment is by the administration of drugs (anticholinesterases), which inhibit acetylcholinesterase. This potentiates the action of released acetylcholine and allows it to bind to receptors not blocked by antibody.

Myaesthenia gravis is an **autoimmune disease** because the body generates an antibody to a normal consitituent.

TENDONS

Tendons are the means by which many muscles are attached to bone. They are long cylindrical structures of tightly packed longitudinally running collagen fibres, with the nuclei and scanty cytoplasm of fibrocytes compressed almost flat between them (Fig. 14.9). Tendons are therefore relatively acellular and have low oxygen and nutrient demands; this is important because in order to maximize their strength they are relatively avascular, and contain only scanty capillaries.

Many tendons lie within fibrocollagenous sheaths, particularly where they rub over bone, and are separated from their sheath by a thin layer of fluid, which acts as a lubricant. The tendons of the fingers have a well-developed set of tendon sheaths.

The collagen fibres of tendons are firmly tethered to the muscle fibres in specialized areas called **myotendinous insertions** (Fig. 14.10), while at the bone end, the collagen fibres of the tendon merge with the collagen of the periosteum.

The original tendon collagen is probably incorporated into bone when the periosteum makes new bone, as it does with bone growth during childhood (see page 245); such intraosseous tendon collagen fibres are called **Sharpey's fibres**.

Maintenance of the tendon at the site of bony attachment is the responsibility of the spindle cells of the periosteum (see page 44), which also have the capacity to convert into chondroprogenitor cells (i.e. produce cartilage) or osteoprogenitor cells (i.e. produce bone, see Fig. 14.13). For this reason, the tendon close to its attachment to the bone may contain small islands of cartilage or bone.

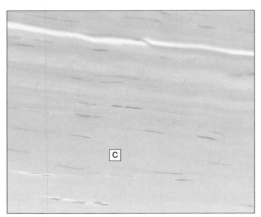

Fig. 14.9 Tendon.
Micrograph of tendon showing highly organized regular bundles of collagen (C) with a few interspersed fibrocytes.

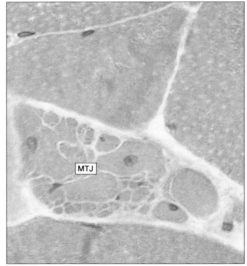

Fig. 14.10 Myotendinous junction.
At the point where skeletal muscle is attached to a tendon or fascia individual skeletal muscle fibres develop a complex interdigitating surface, which is tightly anchored to the support tissues.

This micrograph of a myotendinous junction (MTJ) shows apparent splitting of the rounded contour of a muscle fibre to form several small rounded structures separated by fibrocollagenous tissue. Such splitting of the terminal portion of the fibre increases the surface area available for anchorage to support tissues and thus contributes to the mechanical strength of insertion.

BONE

Bone is a highly specialized support tissue, which is characterized by its rigidity and hardness. Its four main functions are:
- to provide mechanical support (e.g. ribs);
- to permit locomotion (e.g. long bones);
- to provide protection (e.g. skull);
- to act as a metabolic reservoir of mineral salts.
  Bone is composed of:
- support cells (**oesteoblasts** and **osteocytes**);
- a non-mineral matrix of collagen and glycosaminoglycans (**osteoid**),
- inorganic mineral salts deposited within the matrix;
- remodelling cells (**osteoclasts**).

Osteoblasts and osteocytes secrete and nourish the osteoid, into which inorganic mineral salts are deposited to make it rigid and hard. Osteoclasts constantly reshape the deposited bone (i.e. the mineralized osteoid).

Bone is a dynamic tissue, being formed and destroyed continually under the control of hormonal and physical factors. This constant activity permits the process of modelling (i.e. modification of the bone architecture to meet physical stresses).

Bone turnover is normally low in mature adults, but in babies and children it is high to allow the growth and active remodelling required to cope with new demands, for example with the onset of walking.

In the adult, bone turnover can increase from its normal basal level to meet any increased demand, for example to repair a fracture (see below). In addition, increased bone turnover can be caused by pathological processes and lead to disease of the bone.

Osteoid is a collagenous support tissue of type 1 collagen embedded in a glycosaminoglycan gel containing specific glycoproteins (e.g. osteocalcin), which strongly bind calcium. Deposition of mineral salts in the osteoid gives bone its characteristic rigidity and mechanical strength.

Lamellar and woven bone

Two types of bone can be identified according to the pattern of collagen forming the osteoid.
- **Woven bone** is characterized by haphazard organization of collagen fibres and is mechanically weak.
- **Lamellar bone** is characterized by a regular parallel alignment of collagen into sheets (lamellae), and is mechanically strong (Fig. 14.11).

Woven bone is produced when osteoblasts produce osteoid rapidly; the collagen fibres are deposited in an irregular, loosely intertwined pattern. This occurs initially in all fetal bones (see Fig. 14.22), but the resulting woven bone is gradually replaced by remodelling and the deposition of more resilient lamellar bone.

In adults, woven bone is formed when there is very rapid new bone formation, as occurs in the repair of a fracture or Paget's disease (see Fig. 14.21). Following a fracture woven bone is remodelled and lamellar bone is deposited, but in Paget's disease the woven bone persists and leads to mechanical weakness and bone deformity. Virtually all bone in the healthy mature adult is lamellar bone.

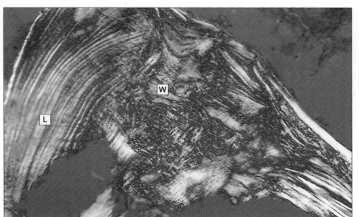

Fig. 14.11 Woven and lamellar bone.
Polarizing micrograph of repairing bone showing both recently formed woven bone (W) at the centre, and original lamellar bone (L) on either side. Note the haphazard arrangement of the collagen fibres in the woven bone, and the regular parallel arrangement in the lamellar bone.

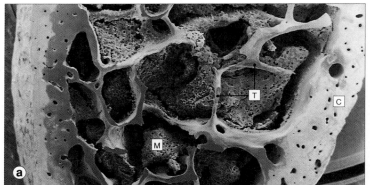

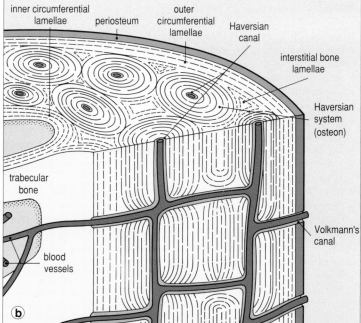

Fig. 14.12 Bone architecture–cortical and trabecular bone.

a Low power scanning electronmicrograph showing the architecture of bone (cortical and trabecular) and its relationship to bone marrow (see page 67). The cortical bone (C) is dense and forms a compact outer shell, which is bridged by interconnecting narrow and delicate plates of trabecular bone (T). The spaces between the trabecular bone are occupied by yellow marrow (adipose tissue) or haemopoietic red marrow. In this micrograph the marrow (M) has retracted from the bone during tissue preparation.

b Diagram of cortical bone. There is a network of vertically running **Haversian canals**, which are linked by transverse **Volkmann's canals**. The canals contain blood vessels and some nerves. Each vertical Haversian canal is surrounded by concentric layers of lamellar bone. The concentric bone layers contain concentrically arranged rings of osteocytes, each lying in its small lacuna, and communicating with osteocytes in its own layer and adjacent layers through cytoplasmic processes lying in narrow canaliculi.

The Haversian canal and its concentric bone and osteocyte system is called an **Haversian system** or **osteon**. Each Haversian canal is lined internally by flat osteoprogenitor cells or inactive osteoblasts, as is the internal surface of the cortical bone plate, and the outer surfaces of the bone trabeculae. This layer is called the **endosteum**, and provides a source for new osteoblasts necessary for new bone formation if remodelling is needed. Cortical remodelling in the Haversian canals is common.

The Haversian canal system occupies the bulk of the cortex, but there are irregularly arranged **interstitial bone lamellae** acting as packing between them; the **inner** and **outer circumferential bone lamellae** separate the collection of Haversian systems from the endosteum and the outer surface of the bone, the fibrocollagenous **periosteum** respectively.

c Polarizing micrograph of a single osteon (Haversian system). A central Haversian canal (H) is surrounded by concentric layers of lamellar bone, which contains a number of non-polarizing spaces marking the sites of osteocytes (O). Outside the Haversian system are less regularly arranged interstital bone lamellae (I), which act as packing between adjacent Haversian systems

d Medium power scanning electronmicrograph showing more detail of cortical (C) and trabecular bone (T). The outlines of a number of Haversian systems (H) of various sizes, each with a central canal, can be seen.

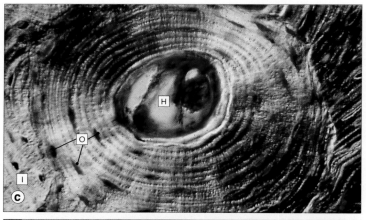

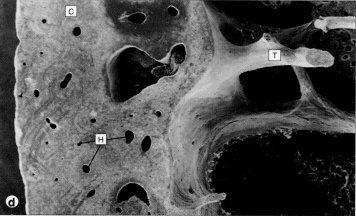

234

Architecture

Most bones have a basic structure composed of:
- an outer **cortical** or **compact** zone;
- an inner **trabecular** or **spongy** zone.

Cortical bone forms a rigid outer shell, which resists deformation, while the inner trabecular meshwork provides strength by acting as a complex system of internal struts. The spaces between the trabecular meshwork are occupied by bone marrow (see page 67).

In bones with a substantial weight-bearing function, the trabecular pattern is arranged to provide maximum resistance to the physical stress to which that bone is normally subjected.

The specialized support cells of the bone reside either on the surfaces of the bone or within small spaces in formed bone termed **lacunae** (Fig. 14.12).

ABORMALITIES OF BONE ARCHITECTURE

Abnormal bone architecture may result from:
- damage to both cortical and trabecular bone due to fracture;
- decreased cortical and trabecular bone due to osteoporosis;
- destruction of trabecular bone due to cancer;
- maldevelopment of bone.

Osteoporosis. In old age both cortical and trabecular bone become thinned (osteoporosis, see Fig. 14.21) and are therefore more fragile and more prone to fracture. Fracture of the neck of the femur is common in the elderly.

Osteoporosis may also develop following disuse, for example in the leg bones of a wheelchair-bound person.

There is some evidence that hormonal disturbances may induce osteoporosis in women around and after the menopause.

Bone involvement in cancer. The bone marrow is a common site of spread of some forms of cancer, particularly cancers that originate in the breast (see Fig. 19.30), bronchus, thyroid and kidney. Growth of the tumour cells frequently destroys the trabecular bone, and thus leads to an increased tendency to bone fracture (**pathological fracture**), which is an important complication of widespread cancer.

Maldevelopment. There are a number of diseases in which bone formation is impaired in embryological development. Many of these are incompatible with survival and such children commonly die *in utero* or shortly after birth.

The most common maldevelopment of bone that is compatible with life is achondroplasia, which produces a form of dwarfism characterized by a normal sized trunk but short limb bones.

Bone cells

Cells concerned with the production, maintenance and modelling of the osteoid are:
- osteoprogenitor cells;
- osteoblasts;
- osteocytes;
- osteoclasts.

Osteoprogenitor cells

Osteoprogenitor cells are derived from primitive mesenchymal cells and form a population of stem cells that can differentiate into the more specialized bone-forming cells (i.e. osteoblasts and osteocytes).

In mature bone in a low turnover phase, osteoprogenitor cells are insignificant spindle cells, which resemble fibroblasts and are closely applied to the bone surface.

In actively growing bone, however, for example in fetal bone or in a period of high turnover in adult bone, these cells are much larger and more numerous, containing plump oval nuclei and more abundant spindle-shaped cytoplasm (Fig. 14.13).

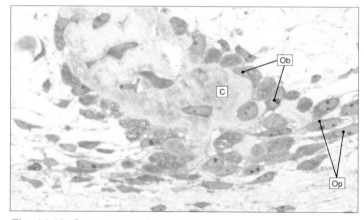

Fig. 14.13 Osteoprogenitor cells.
Micrograph of toluidine blue-stained acrylic resin section showing numerous plump spindle-shaped osteoprogenitor (Op) cells in the developing skull bone of a 15-week-old human fetus. Derived from primitive mesenchymal cells, they are transforming into osteoblasts (Ob), which are larger and more cuboidal. The osteoblasts have begun to deposit osteoid collagen (C).

In mature bone in which there is no active new bone formation or remodelling, the osteoprogenitor cells become flattened spindle cells closely applied to the bone surface, when they are sometimes called inactive osteoblasts. If there is a stimulus to new bone formation, these cells enlarge and convert to active osteoblasts.

Osteoblasts

Osteoblasts are derived from osteoprogenitor cells and synthesize the organic component of the bone matrix (osteoid), which consists of type 1 collagen, glycosaminoglycans and proteoglycans.

When fully active, osteoblasts are cuboidal or polygonal cells, with basophilic cytoplasm, which reflects the abundance of rough endoplasmic reticulum in their cytoplasm resulting from their role as active protein synthesizing and secreting cells (Fig. 14.14).

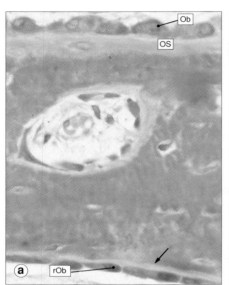

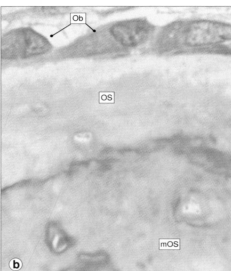

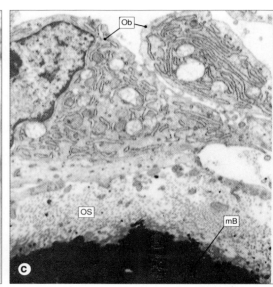

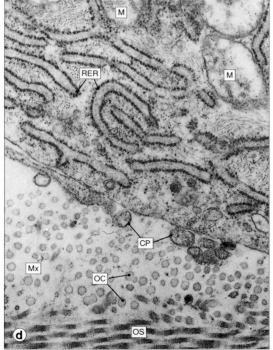

Fig. 14.14 Osteoblasts.

a Micrograph of an acrylic resin section of actively growing fetal bone stained by Goldner's method, which distinguishes mineralized bone (green) from unmineralized osteoid. Note the zone of unmineralized newly formed osteoid (OS) adjacent to the row of actively synthesizing osteoblasts (Ob) on one side of the trabeculum. On the other side, a layer of now flattened osteoblasts have entered an inactive resting phase (rOb) and its recently formed osteoid is now almost fully mineralized (arrow).

b Micrograph of a toluidine blue stained thin epoxy resin section of actively growing bone, with a row of cuboidal osteoblasts (Ob) actively synthesizing and secreting organic matrix (osteoid, OS); the cells have bulky basophilic cytoplasm due to their protein-synthesizing rough endoplasmic reticulum. Some of the osteoid is lightly mineralized (mOS).

c Low power electronmicrograph showing an osteoblast (Ob) at the face of newly forming bone. Note the zone of unmineralized osteoid (OS), which has recently formed between the active osteoblast and the older mineralized bone (mB).

d High power electronmicrograph showing the characteristic cytoplasmic features of an active osteoblast. The cytoplasm is rich in rough endoplasmic reticulum (RER) and there are prominent mitochondria (M); the collagenic protein precursors and glycosaminoglycans are synthesized in the RER and then packaged in the Golgi prior to transfer to the cell surface in secretory vesicles

The cell surface shows numerous cytoplasmic processes (CP), particularly on the face in contact with existing osteoid (OS). The secretory vesicles discharge their contents from this surface to form identifiable osteoid collagen fibres (OC) embedded in an electron-lucent matrix (Mx) of glycosaminoglycans and proteoglycans.

The formation and secretion of collagen is described on page 43.

Osteocytes

When osteoblasts have completed a burst of osteoid-producing activity, most return to an inactive state, becoming flattened and spindle-shaped and closely applied to the now inactive bone surface. Some osteoblasts however become surrounded by mineralizing bone matrix and lie within small cavities (**lacunae**) in the bone. When this happens the cell is called an **osteocyte** (Fig. 14.15).

Adjacent osteocytes can communicate with each other by long cytoplasmic processes, which lie in narrow channels called **canaliculi**. Usually they are arranged haphazardly,

but in cortical bone they assume a regular pattern (see page 234).

The function of osteocytes is not known, but each osteocyte in its lacuna maintains a narrow zone of osteoid around it and retains the prominent Golgi and a fraction of the rough endoplasmic reticulum of its parent osteoblast. This suggests that it may be able to maintain the organic matrix.

Through their interconnecting cytoplasmic processes, osteocytes receive enough nutrient to survive. They may also resorb formed bone matrix to release calcium (a process called osteocytic osteolysis), though the evidence for this is poor.

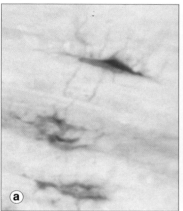

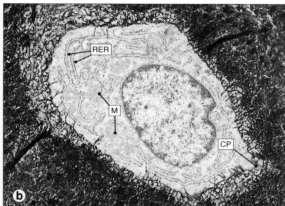

Fig. 14.15 Osteocytes.
a Micrograph of a toluidine blue stained acrylic resin section of bone showing osteocytes trapped within mineralized bone matrix. Note their fine cytoplasmic processes, which lie in narrow canalicular channels within the mineralized bone and link one osteocyte with another.
b Electronmicrograph of a recently entrapped osteocyte. It shows some of the cytoplasmic rough endoplasmic reticulum (RER) and mitochondria (M) of the osteoblast from which it is derived. Note the origin of one of its cytoplasmic processes (CP), the rest being out of the plane of section.

TUMOURS OF OSTEOBLASTS AND OSTEOCYTES

Osteosarcoma

The most important tumour derived from bone cells is **osteosarcoma** which is a malignant tumour of osteoblasts. It is most common in children, and usually involves the bones around the knee joint, either the lower end of the femur or the upper end of the tibia.

The tumour cells resemble osteoblasts in structure and in function, in that they synthesize osteoid; however, the production of osteoid is scanty, haphazard and irregular, and it does not mineralize normally.

The malignant osteoblasts in osteosarcoma are largely primitive, and more closely resemble the immature osteoprogenitor cells than the mature osteoblasts.

Osteosarcoma spreads extensively through the blood, often producing secondary (metastatic) tumours in the lungs.

Osteoid osteoma

Benign tumours of osteoblasts produce localized swellings in bone. Again the tumour cells produce osteoid, but in contrast to osteosarcoma, there is more osteoid formation and a greater degree of mineralization.

In one form of **osteoma**, the cells produce large amounts of regular osteoid, which becomes fully mineralized, producing a dense hard bony nodule; this is **ivory osteoma** and may be derived from osteocytes.

Benign osteomas remain at their site of origin and do not spread.

Osteoclasts

Osteoclasts are large cells with multiple nuclei and abundant cytoplasm (Fig. 14.16) and are thought to be derived from blood monocytes. It is not known whether they form from fusion of a number of monocytes, or from repeated monocyte nuclear division not associated with cytoplasmic splitting.

Osteoclasts are found attached to the bone surface at sites of active bone resorption, often in depressions, where they have eroded into the bone. These depressions are called **resorption bays** or **Howship's lacunae**.

Mineralization of osteoid

The hardness and rigidity of bone is due to the presence of mineral salt in the osteoid matrix. This salt is a crystalline complex of calcium and phosphate hydroxides called **hydroxyapatite** $(Ca_{10}(PO_4)_6(OH)_2)$.

For mineralization to occur, the combined local concentrations of Ca^{2+} ions and PO_4^{2-} ions must be above a threshold valve and a number of factors operate to bring this about.

• A glycoprotein (osteocalcin) in osteoid binds extracellular Ca^{2+} ions, leading to a high local concentration.

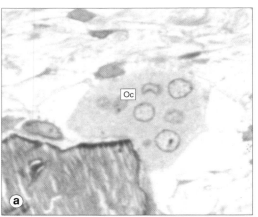

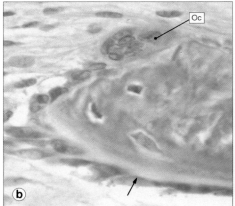

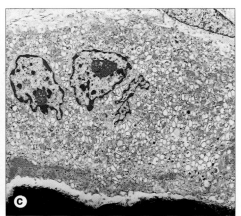

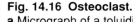

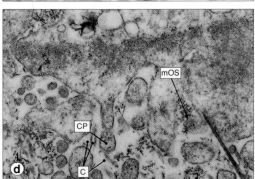

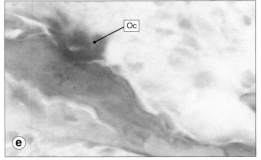

Fig. 14.16 Osteoclast.

a Micrograph of a toluidine blue stained epoxy resin section showing a single osteoclast (Oc), which has alighted on an irregular spur of bone prior to reabsorption. At a later stage the spur of bone will have been eroded and levelled as a result of osteoclast activity.

b Micrograph of Goldner stained acrylic resin section of bone showing active resorption of bone on one face, with a multinucleate osteoclast (Oc) lying in a Howship's lacuna. There is active osteoblast deposition of new osteoid on the other face (arrow), in a bone which is undergoing active modelling (see Fig. 14.19).

c Electronmicrograph of an osteoclast, showing that ultrastructurally it is rich in Golgi, lysosomes, and secretory vesicles, and has abundant mitochrondria. At its interface with the bone is a ruffled border, which is produced by highly complex cytoplasmic protrusions from the osteoclast surface.

d High power electronmicrograph of the ruffled border region where numerous fine cytoplasmic processes (CP) extend from the surface of the osteoclast, and some interdigitate with the collagenic fibres (C) of the osteoid. Fragments of mineralized osteoid (mOS) can be seen between the cytoplasmic processes.

e Micrograph of a frozen section of bone demonstrating abundant acid phosphatase activity (red) in an osteoclast (Oc), which is actively eroding the bone surface.

- The enzyme alkaline phosphatase, which is abundant in osteoblasts, increases local Ca^{2+} and PO_4^{2-} ion concentrations.
- Osteoblasts produce **matrix vesicles**, which can accumulate Ca^{2+} and PO_4^{2-} ions, and are rich in the enzymes alkaline phosphatase and pyrophosphatase, both of which can cleave PO_4^{2-} ions from larger molecules. Matrix vesicles are round membrane-bound vesicles, which are probably derived from the cell membrane. During osteoid formation they bud off from the osteoblast into the matrix and form the nidus for the initial precipitation of hydroxyapatite.

It is currently believed that osteoblast-derived matrix vesicles are the most important factor controlling the initial site of mineral deposition in osteoid, and that once the first few crystals of hyoxyapatite have precipitated out, they grow rapidly by accretion until they join foci growing from other matrix vesicles. In this way, a wave of mineralization sweeps through new osteoid (Fig. 14.17).

Other cells that produce matrix vesicles are the ameloblasts and odontoblasts of the developing tooth (see page 149), and chondrocytes; hence the frequent mineralization of cartilage.

If the local concentrations of Ca^{2+} and PO_4^{2-} ions are normal, then mineralization occurs shortly after the new osteoid has been formed. However, when there is a state of high turnover, the osteoblasts produce large amounts of osteoid in a short time, and mineralization lags behind, catching up only when the rate of new osteoid production falls.

During a lag phase, distinct layers of unmineralized osteoid can be seen between the layer of active osteoblasts and the previously mineralized bone. This is evident in the phases of rapid bone growth in fetal life, and also in adult life during periods of active remodelling of bone such as following fracture, or as part of some disease processes.

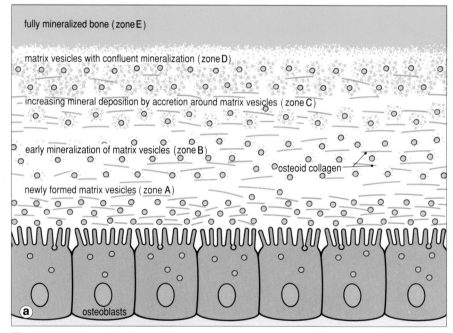

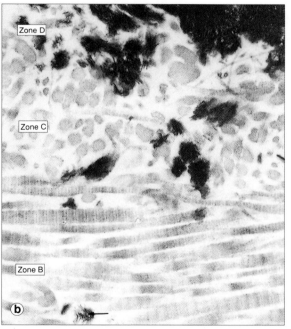

Fig. 14.17 Mineralization of bone.

a Diagram of the events believed to occur in newly formed osteoid. Immediately adjacent to the irregular osteoblast surface is a zone (A) of freshly deposited osteoid collagen and glycosaminoglycan, containing newly formed matrix vesicles.

Next is a zone (B), in which early crystals of hydroxyapatite are being deposited in slightly older matrix vesicles, and beyond it a zone (C) in which the foci of mineralization rapidly enlarge by accretion of mineral salts.

In zone D the individual foci of mineralization, each centred on a matrix vesicle remnant, have become almost completely confluent.

In zone E mineralization is complete, and the underlying osteoid collagen is obscured.

The junction betwen zones C and D is the so-called calcification front, but as this term is used inaccurately in an entirely different context in pathological studies of bone disease it is best avoided unless carefully defined.

b High power electronmicrograph showing early mineral deposition in a zone of recently formed osteoid from fetal bone. Note the early crystalline pattern of mineralization of a matrix vesicle (arrow) in zone B, enlargement of foci of mineralization in zone C, becoming confluent in zone D. Zones A and E are not shown.

OSTEOMALACIA (FAILURE OF MINERALIZATION)

Mineralization of osteoid can take place only if there are sufficient Ca^{2+} and PO_4^{2-} ions.

If the blood level of Ca^{2+} ions is low (due to, for example, inadequate dietary intake by vegans, or malabsorption resulting from small intestinal disease), or if PO_4^{2-} ion levels are low (which is uncommon, and usually due to excessive PO_4^{2-} ion loss in the urine), then mineralization is impaired.

This leads to the disease known as **osteomalacia** (Fig. 14.18).

Patients with osteomalacia develop softening of the bone, which results in an increased tendency to bone fracture, either major fractures or a series of smaller microfractures producing bone pain.

Osteomalacia in the growing bones of children leads to the disease called **rickets**, and produces permanent deformity of the soft, poorly mineralized bones.

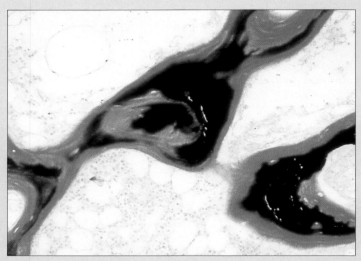

Fig. 14.18 Osteomalacia.
Micrograph of iliac crest bone embedded in acrylic resin without prior decalcification from a patient with osteomalacia. Note the broad zone of unmineralized osteoid (red) and the central zone of mineralized bone (black), in this section stained black by the Von Kossa silver technique.

Bone modelling

In rapid bone growth in fetal development and childhood, large quantities of bone are produced by osteoblastic synthesis of bone matrix, which is subsequently mineralized as outlined above.

Following initial deposition, the bone matrix and the struts forming trabecular bone are remodelled, the remodelling of struts being determined by local mechanical stresses so that the bone matrix is aligned to resist local shearing and compressive stresses.

Modelling is achieved by:
- new bone deposition by active osteoblasts;
- selective resorption of formed bone by osteoclasts (Fig. 14.19).

Selective resorption of formed bone

Bone resorption occurs where the osteoclast is in contact with the bone. Osteoclasts are highly mobile and resorb bone as they move along the bone surface.

In some bone diseases, the osteoclasts are stimulated into inappropriate resorptive activity, and at the same time appear to lose their mobility, so that they remain localized to one area of the bone surface. In this situation they bore deeply into the bone at one site (tunnelling resorption) instead of sweeping bone away from a large area.

Resorption is believed to proceed as follows:
- lysosomal enzymes are released from the osteoclast cytoplasm where it is in contact with bone;
- the released enzymes hydrolyse the collagenous protein and glycosaminoglycans of the adjacent bone matrix;
- the disrupted bone matrix yields up its attached mineral salts;
- local acidic conditions, which possibly result from the secretion of organic acids such as carbonic, lactic and citric acids by the osteoclasts, break up the hydroxyapatite, thereby releasing soluble Ca^{2+} and PO_4^{2-} ions;
- some of the soluble breakdown products of demineralization and protein hydrolysis may be resorbed by the osteoclast by endocytosis.

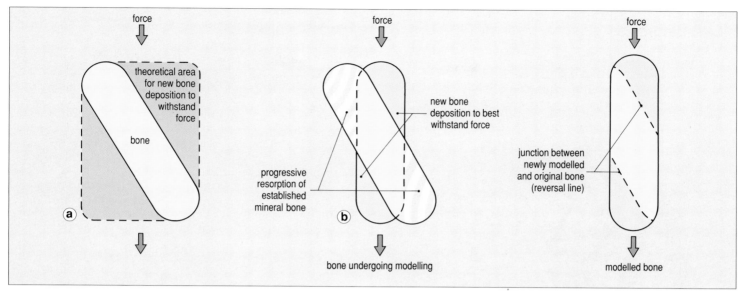

Fig. 14.19 Bone modelling.

a Diagram showing a piece of bone inappropriately orientated to best withstand the direction of the force to which it is exposed. The force could be resisted by deposition of new bone on the old in the area indicated, but this would produce a large heavy block of bone which, if repeated throughout the body as a whole, would result in such a bulky mass that movement would be impossible. A more efficient strength to weight ratio is achieved by modelling.

b Diagram to show how the bone in **a** can be modelled to become more efficient. The junctions between original bone and newly modelled bone are not easily seen in histological sections of mineralized bone, but are evident when decalcified sections are examined, particularly if the section is examined in polarized light, which accentuates the different directions of the osteoid collagen fibres.

The junctions between different phases of bone deposition in different directions are called **reversal lines,** and are particularly numerous and haphazard when bone modelling has been random and uncontrolled, as in Paget's disease (see page 242).

EFFECT OF PARATHORMONE

Osteoclast resorption of bone can be stimulated by parathormone. This hormone is secreted by the parathyroid glands, which maintain a constant level of Ca^{2+} ions in the blood by increasing their output of parathormone in response to a low serum Ca^{2+} ion concentration (see page 258).

Parathormone increases the serum Ca^{2+} ion level by stimulating osteoclastic activity, the increased resorption of bone resulting in the release of Ca^{2+} ions into the blood. In addition, parathormone can increase blood Ca^{2+} by reducing Ca^{2+} ion loss by the kidney, and by increasing Ca^{2+} absorption by the small intestine.

The effect of parathormone activity in the bone is not usually detectable histologically unless there is a prolonged and excessive parathormone secretion.

The elevation of blood Ca^{2+} produced by osteoclast-driven bone resorption is not matched by a rise in serum PO_4^{2-} because parathormone also stimulates PO_4^{2-} excretion by the kidney.

EFFECT OF CALCITONIN

Osteoclast activity and bone resorption is inhibited by calcitonin, a hormone produced by thyroid C cells (see Fig. 15.19). Calcitonin antagonizes parathormone and is secreted in response to a high serum Ca^{2+} level.

Balance between osteoblast and osteoclast activity

In normal healthy bone, osteoblast and osteoclast activity are well controlled so that the overall mass of bone remains constant and there is neither overall loss nor gain of bone once the mature bone mass has been achieved after its active growth in childhood and adolescence.

At the same time, both osteoblasts and osteoclasts are capable of increasing their activity in response to either an increased physiological demand, such as increased physical activity, or to bone fracture, requiring repair and remodelling processes.

OSTEOPOROSIS

Osteoporosis (Fig. 14.20) can occur as a result of disuse (e.g. prolonged bed rest, limb paralysis), and also in people who are otherwise healthy, particularly post-menopausal women. It results in an increased tendency to bone fracture, particularly compression fractures of vertebrae.

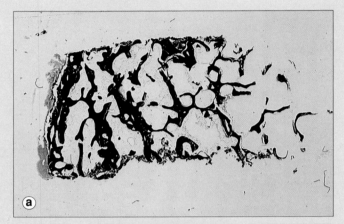

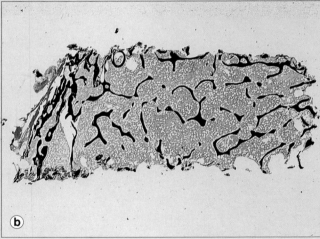

Fig. 14.20 Osteoporosis.
a Micrograph of a resin section of a bone biopsy from the iliac crest (see Fig. 1.1) showing normal cortical and trabecular bone, stained with a silver method, which stains calcified bone black
b Micrograph of bone from a patient with osteoporosis. When compared with **a**, which shows bone mass of a normal patient of the same age, it is clear that the cortical zone is narrower, and that the trabeculae are thinner and less numerous.

PAGET'S DISEASE

Paget's disease is of unknown cause, but probably results from uncontrolled osteoclast activity, leading to resorption of bone and osteoblastic attempts to fill in the resulting erosions (Fig. 14.21).

When the wave of osteoclastic resorption dies down or moves elsewhere, the osteoblasts continue to produce new bone in an attempt to repair the damage, thus paradoxically the affected piece of bone usually ends up larger than it was originally.

The repaired bone is, however, less able to resist physical stress because the new bone deposition is haphazard and reparative, rather than organized and constructive; it is therefore more prone to fracture.

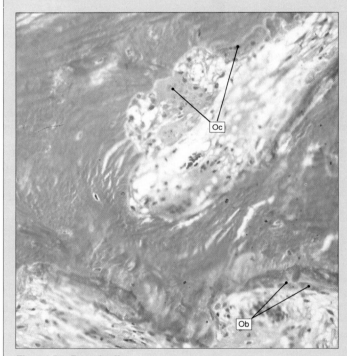

Fig. 14.21 Paget's disease.
Micrograph of a resin embedded, Goldner stained section from a patient with active Paget's disease. There is uncontrolled osteoclast (Oc) resorption of a bone, and osteoblasts (Ob) are attempting to fill in sites of recent osteoclast erosion in an adjacent site.

Fetal bone development

Bone develops in the fetus by:
- condensation from sheets of mesenchymal cells, which act as bone-forming membranes (**intramembranous ossification**);
- transformation of previously deposited cartilage (**endochondral ossification**).

Intramembranous ossification

Intramembranous ossification results in the formation of flat bones such as those of the skull, and also contributes to some of the cortical bone shafts of long bones. Intramembranous ossification (Fig. 14.22) proceeds as follows.

- Some of the primitive mesenchymal spindle cells of the mesenchymal membrane enlarge and develop abundant rough endoplasmic reticulum to become active osteoprogenitor cells and eventually osteoblasts.
- The resulting osteoblasts begin to deposit bone in isolated islands, and remodelling begins instantly by combined osteoblast and osteoclast activity to form a network of trabecular bone.
- Intervening residual mesenchymal tissue develops prominent blood vessels, and some mesenchymal cells eventually develop into haemopoietic bone marrow (see page 67).
- Further development is associated with increased bone formation on the outer and inner surfaces to form complete plates of bone (the outer and inner tables).

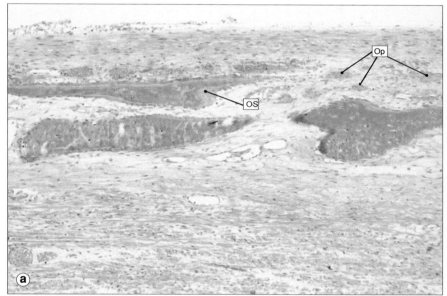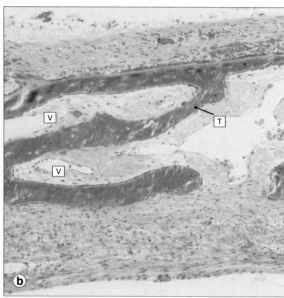

Fig. 14.22 Intramembranous ossification.

a Micrograph of an acrylic resin Goldner stained section from the skull of a developing fetus. Within the fibrocollagenous membrane, islands of primited mesenchymal cells develop into clusters of osteoprogenitor cells (Op, see Fig. 14.13), which mature into osteoblasts. The osteoblasts then lay down osteoid (OS), which becomes mineralized (green).

Although the initial bone islands are irregular in shape, remodelling by synchronized osteoblast and osteoclast activity produces flattened sheets of bone.

b Micrograph of fetal skull showing a slightly later stage in the same process. The bone is now roughly fashioned in the shape of a plate with almost continuous outer and inner layers bridged by trabeculae (T). The spaces between the bone are occupied by primitive mesenchymal tissue, developing fibrocollagenous tissue, and a system of interconnecting vascular channels (V). Later still the bone plates thicken and haemopoietic marrow populates the spaces.

Endochondral ossification

Endochondral ossification is the method whereby the fetus forms long and short bones. In this process hyaline cartilage (see Fig. 4.15) is deposited in the shape of the required bone and is subsequently transformed into bone by mineralization.

Endochondral ossification permits elongation and thickening of the bone as the fetus grows, and continues throughout childhood until bone growth ceases.

Endochondral ossification proceeds as follows.

• Hyaline cartilage develops from a mass of immature mesenchymal tissue, and assumes the approximate shape of the bone. In the case of a long bone this will include a shaft (**diaphysis**) with club-shaped expansions (the **epiphyses**) at either end (Fig. 14.23).

• A layer of spindle-shaped mesenchymal cells, chondroblasts (see page 52) and some osteoprogenitor cells, surrounds the hyaline cartilage model and forms a **perichondrium**. Later, as osteoprogenitor cells outnumber chondroblast precursors this layer is termed the **periosteum**.

• At the mid-shaft of the diaphysis, osteoprogenitor cells transform into osteoblasts and lay down osteoid, which becomes mineralized to form a collar of bone around the diaphysis. Concurrently, the chondrocytes in the cartilage model multiply so that it increases in length and breadth; chondroblasts in the perichondrium/periosteum produce new cartilage. Calcium salts are then deposited in the cartilage matrix.

Once the bony collar has been formed, the diaphysis increases in diameter by bone deposition on the outer surface of the collar and resorption of bone on the inner surface.

• Capillaries grow into the diaphysis of the model by penetrating the periosteum; they carry osteoprogenitor cells, which then establish a **primary ossification centre** in the centre of the diaphysis.

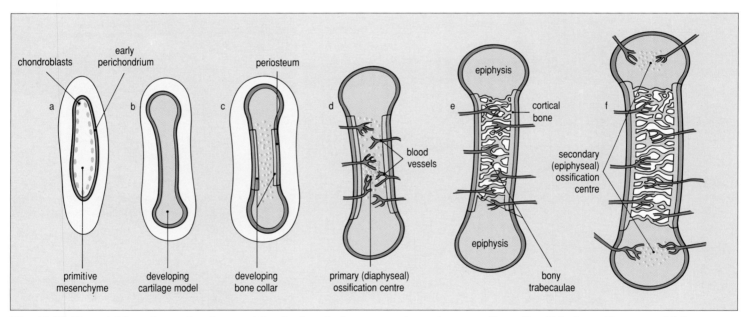

Fig. 14.23 Prenatal long bone development (endochondral ossification).

a Chondroblasts develop in primitive mesenchyme and form an early perichondrium and cartilage model.

b The developing cartilage model assumes the shape of the bone to be formed, and a surrounding perichondrium becomes identifiable.

c At the mid shaft of the diaphysis, the perichondrium becomes a periosteum through the development of osteoprogenitor cells and osteoblasts, the osteoblasts producing a collar of bone by intramembranous ossification. Calcium salts are deposited in the ever-enlarging cartilage model.

d Blood vessels grow through the periosteum and bone collar, carrying osteoprogenitor cells within them. These establish a primary (or diaphyseal) ossification centre in the centre of the diaphysis.

e Bony trabeculae spread out from the primary ossification centre to occupy the entire diaphysis, linking up with the previously formed bone collar, which now forms the cortical bone of the diaphysis. At this stage the terminal club-shaped epiphyses are still composed of cartilage.

f At about birth (the precise time varies between long bones), secondary or epiphyseal ossification centres are established in the centre of each epiphysis by the ingrowth along with blood vessels of mesenchymal cells, which become osteoprogenitor cells and osteoblasts.

• The osteoprogenitor cells in the primary diaphyseal ossification centre transform into osteoblasts and begin to deposit osteoid, which progressively replaces the calcified cartilage of the original model.

• Mineralization of the osteoid, followed by some remodelling, produces a network of trabecular bone, which progressively occupies the core of the diaphysis and merges with the denser compact bone of the peripheral bone collar.

• At about the time of birth, blood vessels and osteoprogenitor cells grow into the cartilaginous club-shaped ends of the developing bone (epiphyses) at either end of the diaphyseal shaft and form **secondary (or epiphyseal) ossification centres**.

Postnatal development of long bones

Long bones continue to grow in length and breadth throughout childhood and adolescence.

Increase in length is due to continued endochondral bone formation at each end of the long bones.

An actively proliferating plate of cartilage (the **epiphyseal plate**) remains across the junction between the epiphysis and diaphysis. This plate gives rise to apposition of new cartilage to the ends of the diaphysis, which is converted to trabecular bone, leading to a progressive increase in length (Fig. 14.24). Activity of the epiphyseal plate normally ceases after puberty.

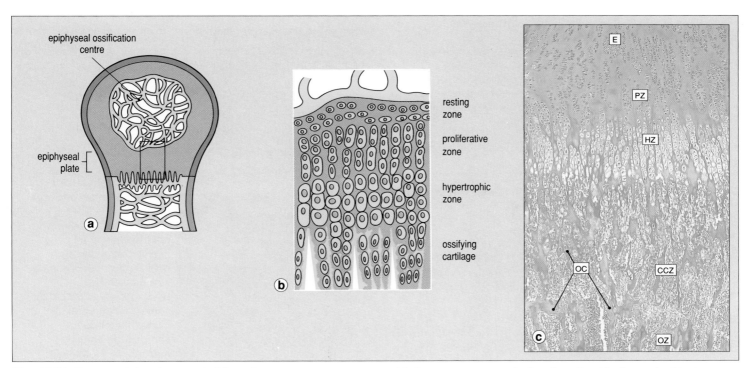

Fig. 14.24 Postnatal development of long bones (endochondral ossification).

a Diagram showing the initial enlargement of the secondary (epiphyseal) ossification centre within the epiphyseal cartilage, leaving an epiphyseal plate of cartilage and a surround of cartilage, which will ultimately become the articular cartilage.

b Diagram showing the fine detail of the epiphyseal plate between the secondary epiphyseal ossification centre on one side and the developing diaphyseal trabecular bone on the other. Chondrocytes in the epiphyseal plate proliferate in columns towards the diaphysis, becoming hypertrophied as they deposit cartilage matrix. The

matrix becomes progressively mineralized before osteoblasts deposit osteoid on the calcified matrix model.

c Low power micrograph of decalcified H&E stained epiphyseal region from a long bone of a fetus. Compare it with **b**. Epiphyseal plate cartilage (E), the proliferative zone (PZ), the hypertrophic zone (HZ), the calcified cartilage zone (CCZ) and the beginning of the ossification zone (OZ) can be seen.

At this stage there is haemopoietic marrow in the spaces between the ossifying plates of cartilage (OC).

Secondary ossification centres develop in the epiphyseal cartilage at a later stage of development than shown here.

New bone forms on the diaphyseal side of the epiphyseal plate as follows:
- cartilage on the epiphyseal face of the epiphyseal plate proliferates to produce columns of chondrocytes embedded in matrix;
- chondrocytes approaching the diaphyseal face of the epiphyseal plate become greatly enlarged and pale-staining, and begin to produce alkaline phosphatase, which facilitates calcification of the matrix;
- osteoblasts lay down osteoid on the calcified cartilaginous matrix as the first stage in the ossification of the calcified cartilaginous trabeculae;
- the deposited bone is remodelled as it is incorporated into the diaphysis.

The epiphyseal plate and the zone of ossifying cartilaginous matrix trabeculae form the **metaphysis**.

Increase in circumference of the diaphysis is achieved by formation of new bone on the outer surface of the cortical bone, which is subjected to slightly less active resorption on its inner aspect.

This not only increases the diameter of the diaphysis, but also the thickness of the cortical bone, which is necessary to cope with the increased physical demands resulting from increasing body weight and physical activity.

JOINTS

Bones are connected to each other by **joints**, which permit varying degrees of movement between the joined bones. Joints can be divided into two main groups;
- those that permit limited movement;
- those that permit free movement.

Limited movement

In joints that permit only limited movement, the bones are connected by flexible fibrocollagenous or cartilaginous tissue. Such joints generally occur between bones subserving a primary supportive or protective role, for example between;
- the flat bones of the skull, which are joined by fibrous or ligamentous tissues (**syndesmoses**);
- the ribs and the sternum, which are joined by cartilage (**synchondroses**).

In old age, the support tissue forming both syndesmoses and synchondroses tends to be replaced by bone to form a rigid immobile joint (**synostosis**).

Intervertebral disc

The bodies of the vertebrae are joined to each other to form a long uninterrupted column (the vertebral column) by the **intervertebral discs**. These are thick rubbery pads, which not only act as shock-absorbers, but also permit some movement so that the column is flexible within limits.

Intervertebral discs are composed essentially of fibrocollagenous tissue containing some chondrocytes and cartilage matrix (fibrocartilage, see page 53). The two surfaces in contact with the vertebral bodies consist of a thin layer of hyaline cartilage, which covers a concentrically lamellated rubbery structure of fibrocartilage (the **annulus fibrosus**). At the centre of the disc is a soft semi-fluid core of soft gelatinous matrix (the **nucleus pulposus**, Fig. 14.25).

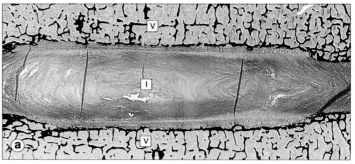

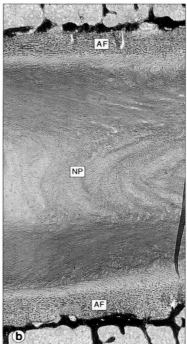

Fig. 14.25 Intervertebral disc.
a Micrograph of an acrylic resin section of an intervertebral disc (I) between two vertebrae (V) stained with H&E.
b Micrograph of part of the same intervertebral disc at higher magnification, showing the annulus fibrosus (AF) forming a compact outer region adjacent to vertebral bone and the soft, semi-fluid central nucleus pulposus (NP).

Free movement

Joints that allow free movement between adjacent bones are held together by bands of collagenous tissue (**ligaments**); these surround a fibrous capsule enclosing the heads of the bones, which are separated from each other by fluid. Such a joint is termed a **synovial joint**.

Synovial joint

In the synovial joint, the bone ends are ensheathed by a strong fibrocollagenous capsule and are separated from each other by a reservoir of slightly viscid fluid (the **synovial fluid**).

The internal lining of the joint capsule is a specialized secretory epithelium, the **synovium**, which produces the synovial fluid.

Because the bone ends move against each other, they are coated with a smooth, friction-free layer of hyaline cartilage (**articular cartilage**), and the synovial fluid provides a thin lubricant film between the opposing articular cartilages.

Structures around the joint, which prevent excess movement, include collagenous ligaments and tendinous muscle attachments (Fig.14.26).

In some complex joints, there are internal ligaments (e.g. cruciate ligaments in the knee joints) to prevent overstretching or twisting, and fibrocartilaginous menisci (also in the knee), to stabilize and guide gliding movements.

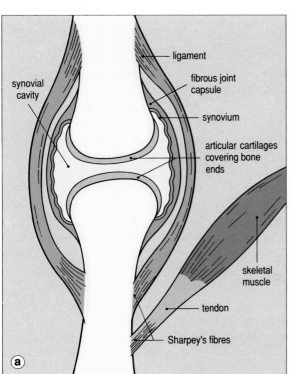

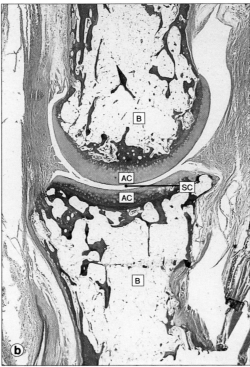

Fig. 14.26 Synovial joint.
a Diagram of a simple synovial joint showing the two articulating bone ends separated from each other by synovial fluid and enclosed within a fibrocollagenous capsule. Surrounding ligaments and tendinous muscle attachments prevent excess movement.
b Low power micrograph of an interphalageal joint of the finger. Note the ends of the articulating bone (B), the articular cartilages (AC) and the joint capsule enclosing the synovial cavity (SC), which contains synovial fluid. The synovial cavity is lined internally by synovium.

SYNOVIAL MEMBRANE

The synovium is composed of 1–4 layers of synovial cells, which merge on their deep surface with a zone of loosely arranged fibrocollagenous tissue containing adipocytes, fibroblasts, mast cells, and macrophages. This deep layer merges with the denser fibrocollagenous tissue of the joint capsule.

Synovial cells vary from flat, mesothelial-like cells through to spindle-shaped, polyhedral or cuboidal cells.

Two cell types have been defined in synovial membrane: type A cells are phagocytic and contain numerous lysosomes, while type B cells contain abundant rough endoplasmic reticulum and appear to be adapted for protein production. The synovial membrane has an abundant blood, lymphatic and nerve supply running in the loose fibrocollagenous tissue.

LIGAMENTS

Ligaments surround articular (synovial) joints, attaching one bone to the other over the outer surface of the joint capsule.

Ligaments are composed of tightly packed collagen fibres all running in the same direction, with compressed fibrocytes in between; thus they resemble tendon. They differ from tendon because they contain elastic fibres. Ligaments strengthen the joint; they permit normal movement, but prevent over-flexing or over-extension. The attachment of ligament to bone is similar to that of tendons.

ARTHRITIS

Osteoarthritis

Some synovial joints, particularly the hip and finger joints, are exposed to persistent wear and tear over many years. This leads to degeneration of the articular cartilage, which loses its normal complement of hydrated glycosaminoglycans and is unable to resist compressive forces. This leads to erosion of the bones and rubbing together of adjacent bare bone surfaces.

Eventually the surface bone becomes highly compacted and ivory-like; this is called eburnation.

The constant bone-to-bone trauma and excessive movement at the joint leads to a painful swollen joint with:
- thickening of the joint capsule;
- irregular protuberances of abnormal new bone at the edges of the articular surfaces (**osteophytes**);
- reduction in the synovial space.

These are the changes of osteoarthritis.

Rheumatoid arthritis

Another common form of arthritis is rheumatoid arthritis, which is an autoimmune disease causing immune-mediated damage to the synovial membrane and articular cartilage.

The synovial membrane becomes thick and extensively infiltrated by cells of the immune system (mainly lymphocytes and plasma cells), whilst the damaged articular cartilage is replaced by vascular fibrocollagenous tissue (**pannus**).

15. ENDOCRINE SYSTEM

Cell communication is vital for any multicellular organism to function efficiently.

At a local level, cells communicate via cell surface molecules and gap junctions (see page 32), while remote communication is mediated by the secretion of chemical messengers, which activate cells by interacting with specific receptors. Such secretion may be one of four types: autocrine, paracrine, endocrine or synaptic (Fig. 15.1).

• **Autocrine secretion** occurs when a cell secretes a chemical messenger to act on its own receptors. This is particularly evident in the local control of cell growth by growth factors such as epidermal growth factor.

• **Paracrine secretion** describes the secretion of chemical messengers to act on adjacent cells. This is also mainly concerned with the local control of cell growth and is also a mode of action of many of the cells of the diffuse neuroendocrine system (see page 266).

• **Endocrine secretion** is the secretion of chemical messengers (hormones) into the blood stream to act on distant tissues.

• **Synaptic secretion** refers to communication by direct structural targeting from one cell to another via synapses, and is confined to the nervous system.

The chemical messengers belong to four main molecular classes:

• amino acid derivatives (e.g. adrenaline, noradrenaline, thyroxine);
• small peptides (e.g. encephalin, vasopressin, thyroid releasing hormone);
• proteins (e.g. nerve growth factor, epidermal growth factor, insulin, growth hormone, parathormone, thyroid stimulating hormone);
• steroids (e.g. cortisol, progesterone, oestradiol, testosterone).

Most chemical messengers are water-soluble, hydrophilic molecules that diffuse freely and usually interact with a cell surface receptor protein. However, steroids and thyroxine are hydrophobic; after carriage to a cell by special proteins in the blood, they pass through its membrane to interact with receptor proteins inside.

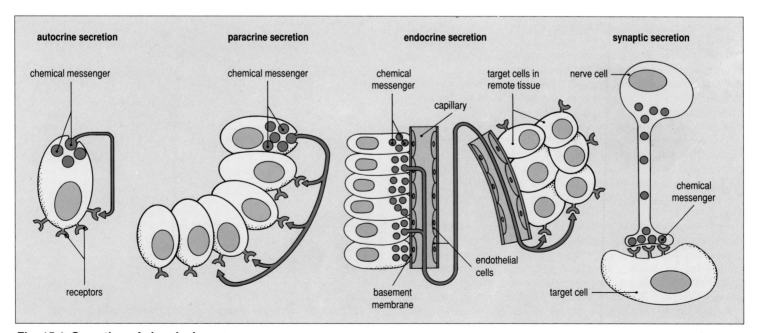

Fig. 15.1 Secretion of chemical messengers.
Diagram showing the four mechanisms of chemical messenger secretion.

ENDOCRINE CELL AND TISSUE SPECIALIZATION

Cells whose main role is to secrete messenger substances are termed **endocrine cells** and it is possible to consider three anatomical distributions:
- endocrine cells gathered together in one specialized organ to form an **endocrine** gland (e.g. adrenal, pituitary and pineal glands);
- endocrine cells forming discrete clusters in another specialized organ (e.g. ovary, testis, pancreas);
- endocrine cells dispersed singly amongst other cells in epithelial tissues, particularly in the gut and respiratory tract, and referred to as the **diffuse neuroendocrine system**.

Endocrine cells and tissues have certain characteristics related to their secretory function as follows.
- Certain cells termed **neuroendocrine** cells have **membrane-bound vesicles,** which are granules containing the chemical messenger. Secretion is achieved by exocytosis in which the membrane of the vesicle fuses with the cell membrane, thereby discharging its contents outside the cell. Certain neuroendocrine cells transiently store the messenger as specific **neuroendocrine granules**, which can be identified in cells using immunohistochemical staining techniques.
- Endocrine tissues are usually vascular to facilitate rapid dissemination of secreted products into the blood stream. In contrast to other types of secretory cell, the secretory pole of endocrine cells is adjacent to the capillary vessel wall, while the nucleus is found at the opposite pole.
- Autocrine and paracrine messengers do not enter the blood stream, but act on local cell receptors within a fraction of a mm away and are rapidly destroyed once secreted, thereby limiting their activity.
- Endocrine messengers act relatively slowly, having to diffuse into the blood stream, circulate to a target organ, and then enter a target cell.
- Many neuroendocrine cells secrete amines or peptides and have common metabolic features, involving the uptake of amines which then undergo decarboxylation in the process of hormone synthesis. This has led to the term **APUD cells** (amine precursor uptake and decarboxylation).
- Cells containing neuroendocrine granules and of neuroendocrine lineage have a restricted set of specific metabolic isoenzymes and structural proteins, which can be detected histochemically. $\gamma\gamma$-enolase is an isoenzyme in the glycolytic pathway that is present in high concentration in neuroendocrine cells together with PGP 9.5 (ubiquitin-C-terminal hydrolase). In the neuroendocrine granules, chromogranin is a component of the core protein and synaptophysin is a glycoprotein in their membrane. Histochemical detection of these substances can be used as markers of neuroendocrine differentiation.

PITUITARY

The pituitary is a multi-functional endocrine gland that secretes a large number of hormones to activate many peripheral endocrine cells, for example those in the adrenal, thyroid, testis and ovary.

Anatomy and development

The pituitary is a bean-shaped gland approximately 12 x 10 x 9 mm in size and weighing 0.4–0.9 g in the adult. It is sited beneath the brain, to which it is linked by the pituitary stalk, and is surrounded by the bone of the base of the skull in a structure termed the sella turcica (Fig. 15.2). Anatomically the pituitary is divided into two parts.

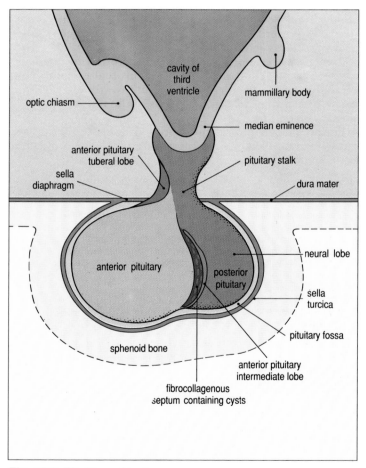

Fig. 15.2 Pituitary gland.
Diagram showing the pituitary gland and its relationships to surrounding structures.

- The **anterior pituitary (adenohypophysis)** is an epithelial-derived tissue with three distinct components; the distal lobe (**pars distalis**) forming the major portion of the gland, the intermediate lobe (**pars intermedia**), which is a rudimentary zone in man but prominent in other mammals, and the tuberal lobe (**pars tuberalis**), which is a layer of cells running up the pituitary stalk.
- The **posterior pituitary (neurohypophysis)** is composed of neuronal processes and glia and has three components; the **neural lobe (pars nervosa, infundibular process)** lying behind the anterior pituitary in the sella turcica, the **pituitary stalk (infundibular stem)** in which axons run from the brain above, and the **median eminence (infundibulum)**, which is a funnel-shaped extension of the hypothalamic portion of the brain.

Embryologically, the anterior pituitary is thought to be derived from an outgrowth of the foregut endoderm called Rathke's pouch. This connects with a downgrowth of the developing hypothalamus, which forms the posterior pituitary and comes to lie in the base of the skull.

Arterial supply

The vascular anatomy of the pituitary (Fig. 15.3), is essential to its functional integration into the nervous system; a special network of vessels (**pituitary portal system**) carries hormones from the hypothalamus of the brain to stimulate or inhibit the hormone secretion of the anterior pituitary.

The major blood supply to the anterior pituitary is derived from vessels that run down the pituitary stalk which are easily damaged in severe head injury, resulting in death of the anterior pituitary and consequent ablation of its endocrine function.

Anterior pituitary

Neuroendocrine cells of the anterior pituitary are arranged in small clusters surrounded by a fine capillary network, which brings blood from the hypothalamus and contains both stimulatory and inhibitory hormones (Fig. 15.4). Secretions from these cells diffuse into the venular capillary network, which drains into the pituitary veins and thence into the carotid venous sinus and systemic circulation.

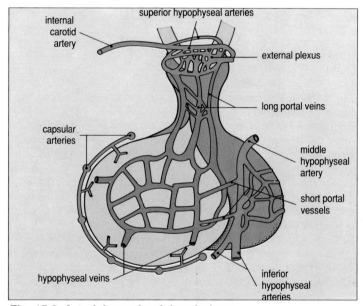

Fig. 15.3 Arterial supply of the pituitary.
The blood supply of the pituitary arises from three paired arteries originating from the internal carotid arteries. The superior hypophyseal arteries enter the median eminence and form the external plexus close to nerve endings from neuroendocrine cells in the hypothalamus. This gives way to a parallel capillary network, which surrounds larger central muscular vessels and run down the pituitary stalk to form the long portal vessels. Arising from the portal vessels, capillary vessels run forwards into the anterior pituitary, providing a direct vascular link between the hypothalamic area of the brain and the neuroendocrine cells of the anterior pituitary.

Additional arterial supply to the posterior pituitary is derived from the small middle and inferior hypophyseal arteries. A minor blood supply to the peripheral portions of the anterior pituitary is derived from small blood vessels in the capsule of the gland.

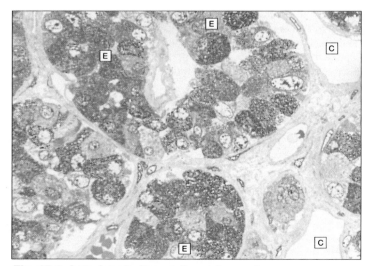

Fig. 15.4 Anterior pituitary cells and vessels.
Toluidine blue resin section showing pituitary endocrine cells (E) arranged in groups and surrounded by capillaries (C).

251

The anterior pituitary contains five distinct types of endocrine cell which vary in their distribution within the gland (Figs 15.5 & 15.6); each type has the same basic ultrastructure (Fig.15.7).

- **Somatotrophs** (Fig. 15.8) secrete **growth hormone (GH)**.
- **Lactotrophs** (Fig. 15.9) secrete **prolactin (PRL)**.
- **Corticotrophs** (Fig. 15.10) secrete **adrenocorticotrophic hormone (ACTH)**, β-**lipotropin** (β-**LPH**), α-**melanocyte stimulating hormone** (α-**MSH**), and β-**endorphin**.
- **Thyrotrophs** secrete **thyroid stimulating hormone (TSH)**.
- **Gonadotrophs** (Fig. 15.11) secrete the gonadotrophic hormones, **follicle stimulating hormone (FSH)** and **luteinizing hormone (LH)**.

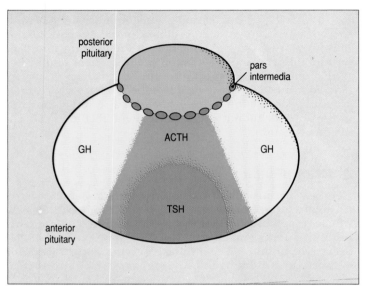

Fig. 15.5 Regional distribution of anterior pituitary cells.
Diagram of a horizontal cross-section of the distal lobe of the pituitary. The lateral wings contain mainly somatotrophs, which secrete GH, while corticotrophs, which secrete ACTH, β-lipotropin, α-MSH and β-endorphin are concentrated in the median portion of the gland just in front of the posterior pituitary. Thyrotrophs, which secrete TSH, are concentrated anteriorly. Lactotrophs secreting PRL and gonadotrophs secreting FSH and LH are uniformly scattered throughout the gland and mingle with the other cell types.

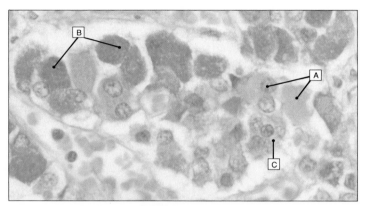

Fig. 15.6 Traditional methods for demonstrating cells of the anterior pituitary.
Traditionally cells of the anterior pituitary have been classified into three types: acidophils (cytoplasm staining with acidic dyes), basophils (cytoplasm staining with basic dyes and the periodic acid Schiff (PAS) method), and chromophobes (cells with no cytoplasmic staining). In the PAS orange-G haematoxylin stain shown here, acidophils (A) stain bright yellow, basophils (B) stain purple, and chromophobes (C) do not stain. Nuclei are stained black by the haematoxylin.

It is now customary to classify cells according to their hormone content, which is demonstrable by immunohistochemical staining using antibodies to each hormone type. It is also possible to distinguish the cells of the anterior pituitary by electron microscopy.

These techniques have shown that acidophils are cells secreting GH or PRL (i.e. somatotrophs and lactotrophs), and that basophils are thyrotrophs, corticotrophs, and gonadotrophs. All of these cells contain abundant dense core granules. Basophils stain well with haematoxylin and PAS, which detect glycosyl groups, because TSH, LH, and FSH are glycoproteins and the ACTH precursor protein is glycosylated. Chromophobes fail to stain because they contain very few granules, but may be lactotroph, somatotroph, thyrotroph, gonadotroph or corticotroph in nature. Some cells contain sparse dense-core granules with no recognizable immunostaining and have been termed null cells.

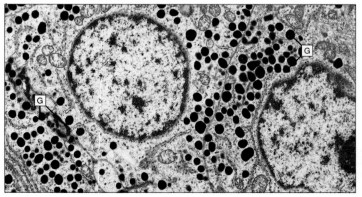

Fig. 15.7 Ultrastructure of anterior pituitary cells.
Electronmicrograph of anterior pituitary cells showing their numerous hormone-containing dense-core granules (G).

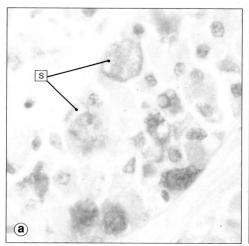

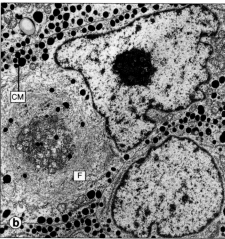

Fig. 15.8 Somatotrophs.

a Somatotrophs make up about 50% of the anterior pituitary and are generally large, ovoid or polygonal in shape, as shown in this section stained to show GH by an immunoperoxidase method.

b Electronmicrograph of a somatotroph. Note the numerous granules 300–500nm in diameter ranged along the cell membrane (CM), and the whorled structure termed a fibrous body (F), which is composed of intermediate filaments and contains degenerate cell organelles.

Fibrous bodies are a feature of somatrophs, especially in those that form benign tumours (adenomas) of the pituitary (see Fig. 15.12).

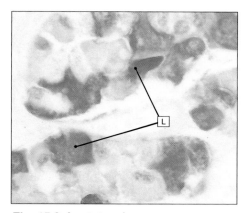

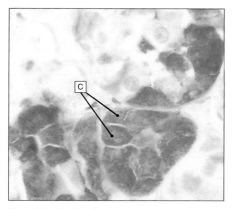

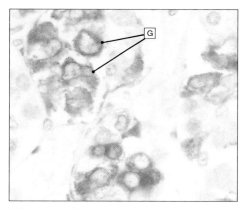

Fig. 15.9 Lactotrophs.

Lactotrophs (L) make up about 25% of the anterior pituitary. While some are rounded and polygonal, most are compressed by adjacent cells into narrow angular profiles as shown in this section of gland stained by an immunoperoxidase method to show PRL. They increase in size and number during pregnancy and lactation.

Ultrastructurally, lactotrophs have a prominent Golgi compared to all other anterior pituitary cells and their granules measure 200–350 nm in diameter.

Interestingly, exocytosis may be seen at their lateral borders (misplaced exocytosis) as well as in the usual site adjacent to capillary basement membrane. This feature can be used in the diagnostic assessment of tumours of the pituitary gland as it is limited to lactotroph-derived tumours.

Fig. 15.10 Corticotrophs.

Accounting for 15–20% of the anterior pituitary, corticotrophs (C) are large and polygonal in shape, as shown in this micrograph stained to show ACTH by an immunoperoxidase technique.

Many corticotrophs possess an unstained perinuclear vacuole called the enigmatic body, which is derived from secondary lysosomes.

Granules in corticotrophs are large and typically measure 250–700 nm in diameter.

Large perinuclear bundles of intermediate cytokeratin filaments are prominent ultrastructurally and these become even more prominent in glucocorticoid excess when they are visible under the light microscope as pink-staining inclusions (Crooke's hyaline).

Fig. 15.11 Gonadotrophs.

Constituting around 10% of anterior pituitary cells, gonadotrophs (G) are scattered as single cells or small groups throughout the gland, as seen in this section which has been stained to show the β-subunit of FSH by an immunoperoxidase technique. Both FSH and LH may be evident within the same cell.

Ultrastructurally the granules are 150–400 nm in diameter. Following ablation of the ovaries or testis, gonadotrophs develop extensive cytoplasmic vacuolation. This is due to dilation of the endoplasmic reticulum by stored product and caused by the loss of feedback inhibition by gonadal steroids. Such cells are large, rounded, and vacuolated on light microscopy and are called castration cells.

PITUITARY ADENOMA

Adenomas are benign tumours of pituitary neuroendocrine cells and are commonly functional, causing endocrine syndromes. They are usually treated by surgical removal.

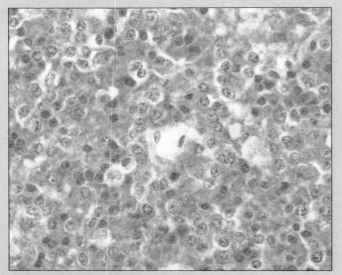

Fig. 15.12 Pituitary adenoma.
Micrograph of pituitary showing proliferation of somatotrophs. The resulting excessive GH secretion caused acromegaly.

Intermediate lobe

The intermediate lobe of the anterior pituitary is located between the posterior pituitary and the distal lobe (see Fig. 15.2). It is poorly developed in humans compared to other mammals, consisting of a series of gland-like acini lined by a cuboidal epithelium. These cells are usually immunoreactive for corticotrophic hormones and it has been suggested that they may be producing one of the minor subunits of the pre-pro-opiomelanocortic peptide such as β-LPH, α-MSH, or β-endorphin, rather than ACTH.

Tuberal lobe

The tuberal lobe is an upward extension of the anterior pituitary consisting of a thin layer of cuboidal epithelial cells lying around the pituitary stalk. Immunohistochemically most of the cells are gonadotrophs.

Occasionally nests of squamous cells can be seen, from which cysts and even tumours may develop, it has been assumed that they are embryological remnants of the endodermal Rathke's pouch.

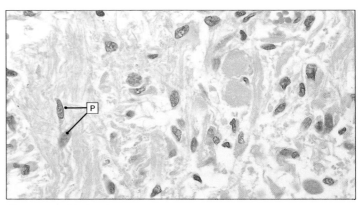

Fig. 15.13 Posterior pituitary.
The posterior pituitary is composed of axons, which originate from cells in the hypothalamus and possess numerous neurosecretory granules containing either oxytocin or vasopressin, together with a carrier protein termed **neurophysin**, and ATP. Where axons are adjacent to capillaries they form fusiform swellings filled with neurosecretory granules (Herring bodies). The posterior pituitary also contains specialized stellate-shaped glial cells called pituicytes.

In this micrograph the axons are seen as a pale fibrillary background in which the nuclei of pituicytes (P) and small capillary vessels are present.

Posterior pituitary

The posterior pituitary is a continuation of the hypothalamic region of the brain into the pituitary stalk and sella turcica (see Fig. 15.2) and secretes **oxytocin** and **antidiuretic hormone** (**vasopressin**).

It is composed of the axons of neuronal cells lying in the supraoptic and paraventricular nuclei of the hypothalamus, together with supporting glial cells termed **pituicytes** (Fig. 15.13). The axons terminate in the posterior pituitary adjacent to a rich network of capillary vessels

HYPOTHALAMUS

The actions of the endocrine and nervous systems are coordinated by the hypothalamus, a region of brain composed of several clusters of neurones that secrete hormones. These hormones act as either releasing or inhibiting factors for the hormones secreted by the anterior pituitary, and are transported to the pituitary gland by two routes as follows.
• A specialized system of blood vessels transports hypothalamic hormones to act locally on neuroendocrine cells in the anterior pituitary (Fig. 15.14).
• Axons project down from the hypothalamus to form the pituitary stalk, which terminate as the posterior pituitary.

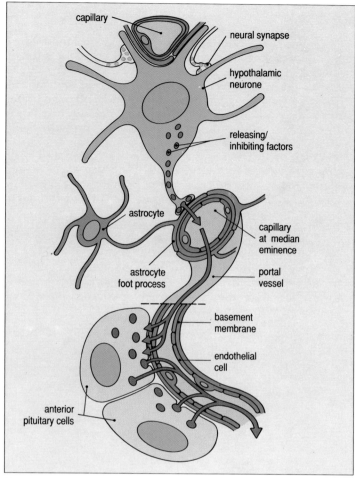

Fig. 15.14 Hypothalamic control of anterior pituitary hormone production.

Hypothalamic neurones secrete releasing/inhibiting factors in response to chemoreceptive and neural inputs. These hormones diffuse into capillaries at the median eminence and are carried to the anterior pituitary in the portal vessels. Astrocyte foot processes which surround the capillary vessels form part of their diffusion barrier.

PINEAL

The pineal gland is located just below the posterior end of the corpus callosum of the brain and is a flattened conical stucture 6–10 mm long and 5–6 mm wide; it is covered by leptomeninges and composed of lobules of specialized cells, which are separated by septa containing unmyelinated nerves and blood vessels (Fig. 15.15). The gland consists of two major cell types: pinealocytes and glial cells

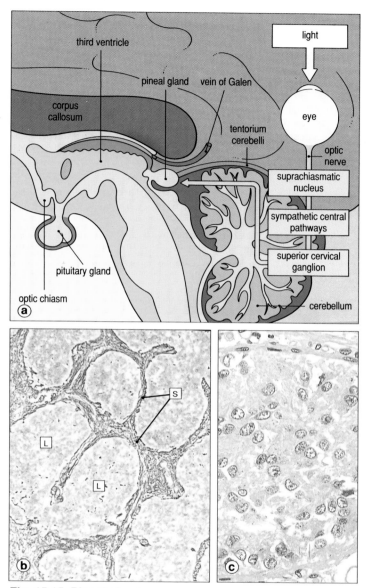

Fig. 15.15 Pineal gland.

a Diagram to show the location of the pineal gland. Output of pineal melatonin is modulated by light through nervous pathways which input as sympathetic innervation to the gland.

b Low power micrograph of a reticulin stained section of pineal showing the septa (S) which divide it into discrete lobules (L) of pinealocytes.

c High power micrograph of an H&E stained section of pineal showing a single pineal lobule surrounded by septa composed of glial processes and small vessels. In the centre of the lobule pinealocyte cell bodies are found in a background of pink-staining cell processes, some of which form a rosette structure.

• **Pinealocytes** are neurone-like cells that produce melatonin, which induces rhythmic changes in the secretions of the hypothalamus, pituitary and gonads, and is said to act as an endocrine transducer. They have pink-staining cytoplasm and dark-staining rounded nuclei, and are often arranged in rosettes, where several cells surround a central fibrillary area composed of cell processes directed towards a small capillary vessel.

• **Glial cells** tend to be bipolar elongated cells that run between nests of pinealocytes. They are indistinct unless specially stained.

A common age-related change in the pineal is the accumulation of calcium particles, which are visible on a skull radiograph; thus the gland can be used as a radiological midline landmark.

The pineal gland is innervated by sympathetic and parasympathetic nervous systems. In addition, signals from the retina arrive indirectly, as shown in Fig. 15.15a.

THYROID

The thyroid gland secretes two hormones, **thyroxine,** and **calcitonin**. Thyroxine has a major role in the regulation of the basal metabolic rate, while calcitonin is involved in calcium homeostasis.

Anatomy and development

The thyroid gland consists of two lateral lobes arranged on either side of the thyroid cartilage and upper trachea in the anterior portion of the neck. These lobes are joined near their lower poles by an isthmus crossing in front of the lower larynx; occasionally a small triangular pyramidal lobe projects upwards from the midpoint of the isthmus.

Each lateral lobe is about 5 cm long, 3–4 cm wide and 2–3 cm deep. In the normal healthy adult, the thyroid weighs 15–20g and is slightly heavier in males, though many factors influence its weight at any one time, for example pathological abnormalities.

The thyroid is enclosed by a thin collagenous capsule from which internal septa penetrate the parenchyma, dividing it into irregular lobules.

Embryologically the thyroid develops from a downgrowth of endoderm arising near the root of the tongue and called the thyroglossal duct, which atrophies and leaves a nodule of thyroid tissue at its correct anatomical site.

THYROGLOSSAL DUCT CYST

Ocasionally the thyroglossal duct fails to atrophy completely, and thyroglossal duct tissue persists in the midline of the neck, usually as a cyst or a sinus track (thyroglossal duct cyst).

Cytology

The glandular component of the thyroid is composed of epithelium arranged as tightly-packed spherical units called acini (Fig. 15.16).

Each acinus is lined by a single layer of specialized thyroid epithelium, which rests on a basement membrane and encloses a lumen filled with thyroid colloid, which is a pink-staining (eosinophilic) homogeneous proteinaceous material rich in thyroglobulin.

Thyroglobulin is the storage form of thyroxine and is an iodinated glycoprotein (Fig. 15.17). The size of an acinus depends on whether it is in a secretory or a storage phase.

During an active secretory phase the thyroid follicular cells show the following changes:
• the endoplasmic reticulum becomes more prominent;
• free ribosomes become more prominent;
• the Golgi enlarges;
• the surface microvilli increase in number and length;
• intracytoplasmic droplets (representing colloid in endocytotic vesicles generated by pseudopodial extensions of cytoplasm at the luminal surface) appear.

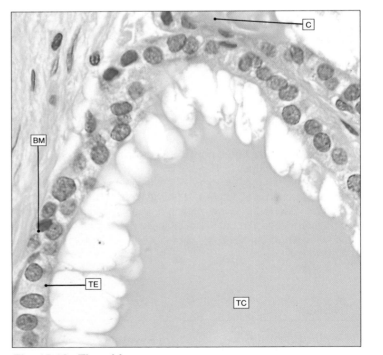

Fig. 15.16 Thyroid.
Micrograph showing thyroid acinus composed of specialized thyroid epithelium (TE) resting on a basement membrane (BM). These epithelial cells enclose a lumen filled with thyroid colloid (TC), and are surrounded by a fine network of capillaries (C) associated with thin fibrous septa.

Control of Hormone Secretion

The synthesis and breakdown of thyroglobulin is controlled by the hypothalamus and pituitary gland. Low blood thyroxine levels stimulate the hypothalamus to produce thyrotropin releasing hormone (TRH), which then stimulates the anterior pituitary to produce thyroid stimulating hormone (TSH). In turn, TSH stimulates both thyroglobulin synthesis and breakdown, with a consequent increase in thyroxine release into the capillary circulation. When the thyroxine levels rise, TRH and TSH production decreases.

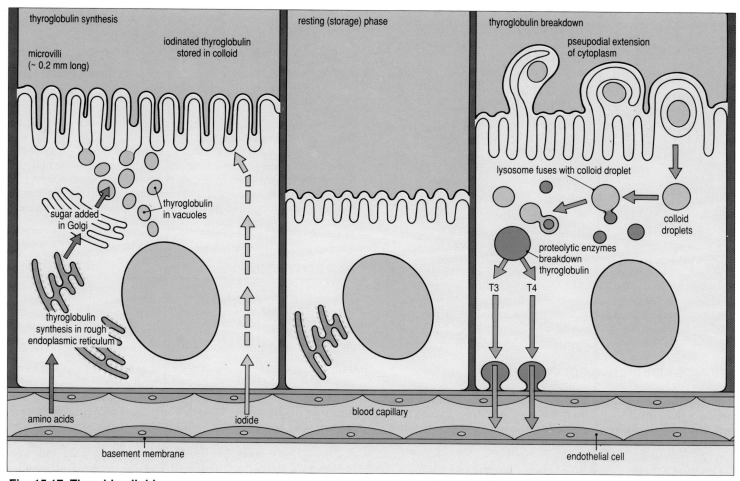

Fig. 15.17 Thyroid colloid.

a Thyroglobulin is synthesized by the thyroid epithelial cells, its protein component being synthesized in the rough endoplasmic reticulum and transported to the Golgi where most of its sugar component is added by glycosylation.

Thyroglobulin leaves the exit face of the Golgi in small vacuoles, which are transported to the luminal surface. It is then released into the lumen by exocytosis.

Shortly after this release iodine is added to its tyrosine component, the iodine having been formed in the epithelial cell cytoplasm by the oxidation of iodide. (The thyroid epithelial cell is not only able to transport iodide against a concentration gradient from the capillary blood into the lumen of the follicle, but is also able to convert iodide into iodine).

b Thyroglobulin acts as a reservoir from which thyroxine can be produced and secreted into the capillary circulation when required.

c To release thyroxine from the stored colloid, the thyroid epithelial cell extrudes pseudopodial extensions of cytoplasm from its luminal surface; these enclose small droplets of colloid, which are then incorporated into its cytoplasm.

Lysosomes fuse with the small vacuoles, and hydrolysis and proteolysis of the thyroglobulin occurs, breaking it into smaller units, the most important of which is tetraiodothyronine (T4) or thyroxine. Another product is triiodothyronine (T3). Both are iodinated amino acids.

THYROTOXICOSIS

In thyrotoxicosis the thyroid epithelial cells increase in size and number, and their work rate increases, so that excessive thyroxine is produced (Fig. 15.18).

This is manifest clinically by weight loss and heat intolerance (due to an increased basal metabolic rate), tremor, rapid pulse, and bulging of the eyes (exophthalmos), due to an increase in the orbital support tissues.

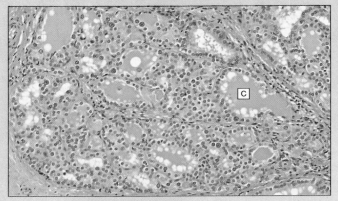

Fig. 15.18 Thyrotoxic hyperplasia.
Micrograph showing the characteristic features of hyperplastic thyroid. An increased number of thyroid epithelial cells is shown by the development of papillary folds of acinar epithelium; in addition each epithelial cell is large and columnar and the edges of the colloid (C) are scalloped indicating active removal of stored colloid for processing into thyroxine.

C (calcitonin-producing) cells

The thyroid also produces the hormone calcitonin, which inhibits calcium resorption from bones by osteoclasts, thus antagonizing the action of parathormone (see below), and lowering blood calcium levels. It may increase the rate of osteoid mineralization.

Calcitonin-producing cells (C cells) are scattered between the thyroid acinus (follicle) lining cells, but are occasionally seen in small clusters in the wall of an acinus or as larger clusters in the interstitial spaces between adjacent acini. This latter location is most common in animals such as the dog, and explains their old name 'parafollicular cells'.

C cells are small pale-staining cells, which are difficult to see by routine light microscopy but can be identified either by electron microscopy, or by immunoperoxidase techniques (Fig. 15.19). Ultrastructurally they contain the dense-core neurosecretory granules that are characteristic of neuroendocrine cells.

Calcitonin secretion seems to be controlled directly by blood calcium levels.

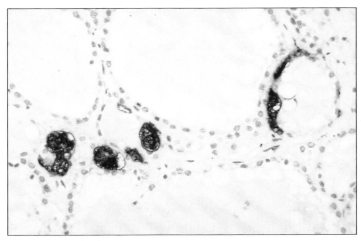

Fig. 15.19 Thyroid C cells.
Micrograph showing the distribution of thyroid C cells (identified using an immunoperoxidase method for calcitonin) in the adult human thyroid; they are scattered between the thyroid acinus lining cells singly, in clumps, and as interstitial clusters. Cells in the acini tend to be sited on the basement membrane, apparently having no contact with the colloid-filled lumen.

PARATHYROID

The parathyroid glands secrete parathormone, which is involved in calcium homeostasis.

Anatomy and development

The parathyroid glands, of which there are at least four and in some people up to eight, are small pale coffee-coloured endocrine glands. They are usually ovoid in shape, but are occasionally flattened by moulding from adjacent organs or tissues.

Each gland is approximately 5 mm long, 3 mm wide and 1–2 mm thick, although size varies considerably with age and calcium metabolic status. In adults each gland weighs approximately 130mg, those in women being slightly heavier than those of men.

Parathyroid glands are sited in the neck in the region of the thyroid gland, but their precise location is variable. They are derived from the third and fourth branchial pouches, the glands from the third pouch being located near the lower pole of the thyroid, while those from the fourth lie close to the upper pole, either behind it or at the cricothyroid junction; those behind the upper pole are often sited inside the thyroid capsule, and are therefore apparently intrathyroidal.

The parathyroids at the lower pole have a much more variable location. Approximately half are sited on the

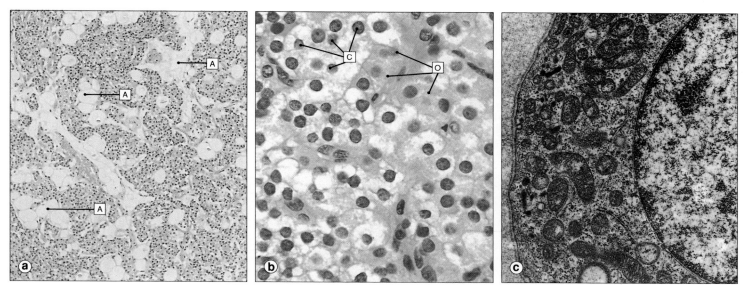

Fig. 15.20 Parathyroid.
a Low power micrograph of an H&E stained section of parathyroid. Note the adipocytes (A), which are seen as non-staining areas.
b High power micrograph of an H&E stained section of parathyroid showing chief cells (C) and oxyphil cells (O).
c Electronmicrograph of parathyroid showing the edge of an oxyphil cell and its nucleus (N). Note the neurosecretory granules (G) and numerous mitochondria (M).

anterior or posterior surface of the lower pole of the lateral lobes, the other half being located in the thymic tongue just beneath the lower pole. Occasionally parathyroid glands may be found in the mediastinum within thymic remnants.

Cytology

The normal adult human parathyroid is surrounded by a thin fibrous capsule and is composed of three cell types: chief cells, which produce parathormone, oxyphil cells, and adipocytes.

ADIPOCYTES
Adipocytes appear in the parathyroid at puberty and gradually increase in number up to about the age of 40, from then on remaining a fairly constant proportion of the entire gland, though their number may decrease in old age. They form a background stroma in which the chief and oxyphil cells are arranged in cords and nests close to a fine network of capillary vessels.

CHIEF CELLS
Parathyroid **chief cells** are about 8–10 μm in diameter and are roughly spherical in shape. Their nuclei are small, round, dark-staining and central, and their cytoplasm is usually pale pinkish-purple (Fig. 15.20), although at certain stages of their activity they become vacuolated with

glycogen and lipid, when they are sometimes referred to as 'clear cells'.

As chief cells are the endocrinologically active component of the parathyroid, their ultrastructural appearance depends largely on whether they are in a resting, synthesizing or secreting stage of hormone response. They contain membrane-bound neuroendocrine granules of parathormone commonly arranged towards the periphery of the cell, and in the synthesizing phase, there are stacks of rough endoplasmic reticulum and an active Golgi. In the resting phase, the neuroendocrine granules are still present, but the Golgi is small and the rough endoplasmic reticulum less prominent; glycogen granules and small lipid droplets are also seen. This glycogen and lipid becomes less apparent during hormone synthesis, but reappears when the cells are secreting the packaged hormone.

In the normal adult with a normal calcium balance approximately 80% of the chief cells are in the resting phase. If hypercalcaemia develops this proportion increases to 100% (and the cells contain numerous fine lipid droplets), but decreases with transient or permanent hypocalcaemia. At light microscopy, a synthesizing or secreting chief cell can be identified by its purplish cytoplasm and the absence of fine lipid droplets.

OXYPHIL CELLS
Oxyphil cells are larger than chief cells (i.e. greater than 10 μm in diameter) and possess comparatively more

cytoplasm, which is markedly eosinophilic and granular due to the presence of many mitochondria; their nuclei are small, spherical and dark-staining.

Ultrastructurally, oxyphil cell cytoplasm is packed with large active mitochondria, with intervening cytoplasm containing only scanty free ribosomes and glycogen granules; endoplasmic reticulum and neurosecretory vacuoles are uncommon indicating that the cells are not endocrinologically active. Transitional cell forms with features of both oxyphil and active chief cells are occasionally seen.

Oxyphil cells are rare before puberty, but appear in increasing numbers in early adult life, either singly or in clumps. In the elderly, they are often numerous and sometimes form variably sized oval or rounded tumour-like nodules within a normal sized parathyroid.

DISORDERS OF PARATHORMONE SECRETION

Parathormone maintains the serum calcium level by mobilizing calcium from the pool located in mineralized bone, thus excess parathormone has a destructive effect on bone. Such hyperparathyroidism may be primary or secondary.

- **Primary hyperparathyroidism** results from a benign tumour (adenoma) of one of the parathyroid glands (Fig. 15.21).
- **Secondary hyperparathyroidism** is due to generalized hyperplasia of all of the parathyroid glands in response to a low serum calcium resulting from excessive loss of calcium in the urine. This is usually caused by a primary disease of the kidneys (renal hyperparathyroidism).

Persistent **hypercalcaemia** can produce severe systemic symptoms including muscular weakness, dizziness, lethargy and extreme thirst, and predisposes to the deposition of calcium salts in the tissues, particularly in blood vessel walls (**heterotopic calcification**).

Hypocalcaemia is usually caused by surgical removal of most or all of the parathyroid glands, but can also result from excessive loss of calcium from the kidney or from inadequate dietary calcium absorption.

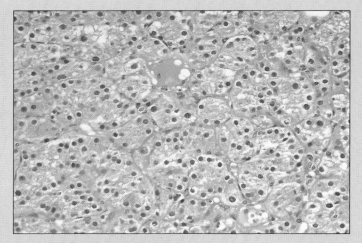

Fig. 15.21 Parathyroid adenoma.
Micrograph showing a benign tumour (**adenoma**) of the parathyroid gland. The tumour is composed of sheets of chief cells (CC) secreting parathormone.

Such tumours are treated by surgical removal.

ADRENAL

The adrenal glands are located on the upper poles of the kidneys and combine two distinct neuroendocrine systems within one organ.

- The **adrenal cortex** synthesizes and secretes steroid hormones produced from cholesterol.
- The **adrenal medulla** is a neuroendocrine component, synthesizing and secreting the vasoactive amines, adrenaline and noradrenaline.

Adrenal cortex

Anatomy and development

The adrenal cortex forms the outer layer of the adrenal gland and in the adult is composed of three distinct zones, the zona glomerulosa, zona fasciculata and zona reticularis. These zones are bounded externally by a thin fibrous capsule, and delimited internally by the adrenal medulla (Fig. 15.22).

- The outer **zona glomerulosa** (Fig. 15.23) synthesizes and secretes mineralocorticoids, mainly **aldosterone** and **deoxycorticosterone**.

• The middle **zona fasciculata** (Fig. 15.24) secretes glucocorticoids, mainly **cortisol** and **corticosterone**, and also small amounts of the androgenic steroid **dehydroepiandrosterone** (DHA).

• The inner **zona reticularis** (Fig. 15.25), produces androgenic steroids and some glucocorticoids, but normally only in small amounts.

In the fetus and neonate, the adrenal cortex is proportionately much larger than in the adult and has an additional external cortical zone, which involutes after birth, the three layers of the adult cortex developing from the remaining cells. The cells that involute have the appearance of steroid-secreting cells, possessing a large Golgi and many lipid droplets; furthermore they have round mitochondria with tubular cristae very similar to those of the adult zona fasciculata.

Activity of the fetal adrenal cortex is partly controlled by the fetal pituitary through the feedback of cortisol on pituitary ACTH secretion, and partly controlled by the placenta.

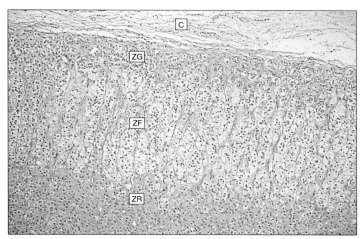

Fig. 15.22 Adrenal cortex.
Micrograph showing the three distinct zones of the adrenal cortex: the zona glomerulosa (ZG), the zona fasciculata (ZF) and the zona reticularis (ZR), which are enclosed by a capsule (C).

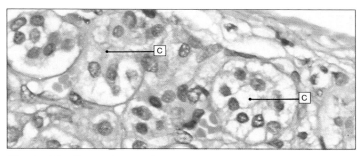

Fig. 15.23 Zona glomerulosa.
The zona glomerulosa is the thin subcapsular zone of adrenal cortex that merges imperceptibly on its inner surface with the middle zona fasciculata. It is not always a complete layer and has a patchy distribution.

The zona glomerulosa is composed of small compact cells (C) arranged in clumps and separated by stroma composed largely of thin-walled capillaries. the cells contain scanty lipid droplets associated with well developed smooth endoplasmic reticulum and comparatively little rough endoplasmic reticulum.

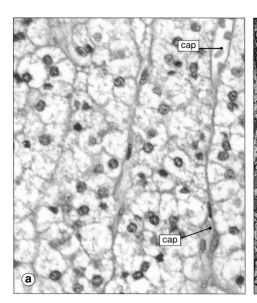

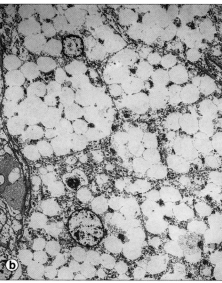

Fig. 15.24 Zona fasciculata.
a The zona fasciculata occupies most of the adrenal cortex and is composed of large rectangular cells with light-staining clear or finely vacuolated cytoplasm due to intracytoplasmic accumulation of lipid droplets containing cholesterol and intermediate lipids, as well as formed glucocorticoids. These cells are arranged in vertical columns, which are usually 2–3 cells wide, the columns being separated by capillaries (cap)(see Fig.15.22).
b Ultrastructurally, the cells have prominent rough endoplasmic reticulum, characteristic small round or ovoid mitochondria with tubular cristae (see page 13) and extensive lipid vacuoles. The surface of cells adjacent to capillaries may show small microvilli extending to the capillary wall.

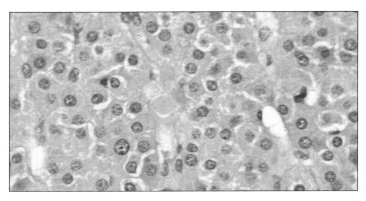

Fig. 15.25 Zona reticularis.
This inner zone of the adrenal cortex is thinner than the zona fasciculata, but thicker than the zona glomerulosa. It is composed of cells with eosinophilic cytoplasm arranged in an anastomosing network of clumps and columns with a capillary network closely apposed to the cell membranes. A characteristic feature of this layer when stained with H&E is the presence of brown pigment (lipofuscin). To the naked eye the layer appears pale brown, whereas the zona fasciculata is bright yellow.

Ultrastructurally, the cells possess prominent smooth endoplasmic reticulum, and electron-dense irregular aggregations of lipofuscin, as well as lysosomes and oval or long mitochondria with tubular cristae, similar to those seen in the cells of the zona fasciculata.

DISORDERS OF THE ADRENAL CORTEX

The most common disorders of the adrenal are hypoadrenalism and hyperadrenalism, resulting from a deficiency or an excess of all of the adrenal cortical steroid hormones, respectively; their clinical manifestations are, however, largely due to the hormones produced by the zona fasciculata, the glucocorticoids.

The most common cause of **hypoadrenalism (Addison's syndrome)** is destruction of both adrenals by disease, leading to insufficient adrenal cortex for hormone production. This usually results from autoimmune disease, but can also be due to tuberculosis.

In addition hypoadrenalism can be induced by giving large doses of glucocorticoids therapeutically; this suppresses ACTH by the pituitary so that the adrenal cortex produces no native steroid hormone. If in this situation the therapeutic steroid is suddenly discontinued, the patient may develop an acute hypoadrenal crisis.

Hypoadrenalism is manifest clinically by hypotension, hyponatraemia and brown skin pigmentation, and may present as a crisis with sudden collapse associated with severe shock.

Hyperadrenalism usually results from hyperplasia of the adrenal cortex or from a hormone-secreting tumour. If the tumour produces glucocorticoids, the patient develops Cushing's syndrome, whereas mineralocorticoid production results in Conn's syndrome.
- **Cushing's syndrome** is manifest clinically by Cushingoid facies, hirsutism, acne, central obesity, striae, osteoporosis, diabetes mellitus, hypertension, hypokalaemia, muscle weakness and mental disturbance.
- **Conn's syndrome** is associated with hypertension, hypokalaemia causing polyuria and muscle weakness, and alkalosis.

Adrenal medulla

Anatomy and development

The adrenal medulla occupies the centre of the adrenal gland and is surrounded by adrenal cortex; it usually has a brown colour.

The adrenal medulla is derived from the neural crest and is part of the neuroendocrine system, secreting **adrenaline, noradrenaline**, and assorted peptides, including **enkephalins**. Adrenaline and noradrenaline synthesis is controlled by sympathetic and parasympathetic nerve twigs present in the gland.

Cytology

Adrenal medullary cells have large, commonly pale-staining nuclei and their cytoplasm is usually finely granular with a purplish staining reaction. They are polyhedral in shape and arranged in clumps, cords or columns, surrounded by a rich network of capillaries (Fig. 15.26a).

Ultrastructurally, the cells contain neuroendocrine granules which vary in size and appearance, ranging from 150–350 nm in diameter.
- Cells secreting adrenaline have small spherical neuroendocrine granules, almost entirely occupied by electron-dense material with a narrow clear halo between the central material and the thin surrounding membrane.
- Cells secreting noradrenaline have larger neuroendocrine granules with a more obvious electron-lucent layer inside the membrane, the granules containing irregular and often angulated electron-dense material (Fig. 15.26b).

Adrenal medullary cells synthesize and store their respective peptide hormones, and normally release only small amounts at a time, though during periods of acute stress or excitement larger quantities are secreted under the influence of the autonomic nervous system.

Because of their high catecholamine content, adrenal medullary cells develop an intense brown colour when exposed to air or to a strong oxidizing agent, such as potassium dichromate, due to the formation of brown pigment when the amines are oxidized. This is the basis of their antiquated name 'chromaffin cells'.

Adrenal blood supply

The adrenal glands receive a rich arterial supply, which forms an arterial plexus of capsular arteries over their surface. Two types of vessel are derived from these arteries: cortical arterioles and medullary arterioles (Fig. 15.27).

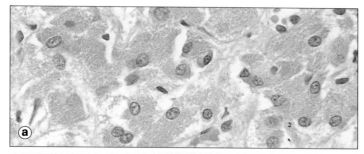

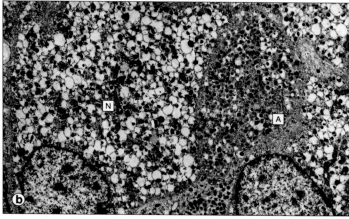

Fig. 15.26 Adrenal medulla.
a Micrograph of adrenal medullary cells showing their large nuclei, and finely granular cytoplasm.
b Electronmicrograph showing large dense-core granules corresponding to noradrenaline (N) and adrenaline (A) granules.

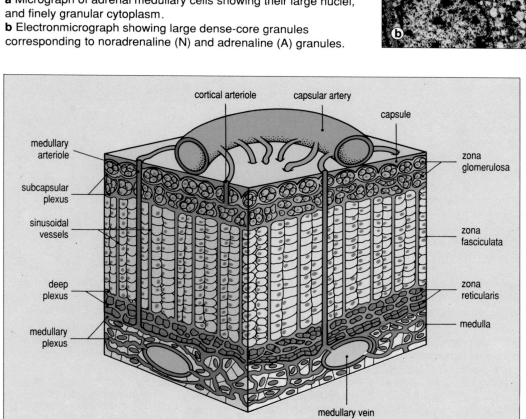

Fig. 15.27 Vascular anatomy of the adrenal gland.
Cortical arterioles form a subcapsular plexus, which gives rise to sinusoidal vessels running down between the columns of the zona fasciculata of the adrenal cortex, before forming a further deep plexus in the zona reticularis. This deeper plexus communicates with the plexus of vessels supplying the medulla.

Medullary arterioles arise directly from the capsular arteries and run straight down through the cortex into the medulla where they form a medullary plexus. The deep medullary plexus drains by small venous vessels into the large medullary vein.

PANCREAS

The neuroendocrine component of the human pancreas exists in three forms.
- Islets of Langerhans are distinct structures accounting for most of the hormone-producing cells.
- Isolated nests or clumps of neuroendocrine cells form a minority population of cells gathered into small groups, which are distinct from islets.
- Single cells are scattered within the exocrine (see page 168) and ductular component of the pancreas and are demonstrable by immunocytochemical methods.

Islets of Langerhans

Islets of Langerhans are discrete rounded clusters of cells scattered throughout the pancreatic tissue and embedded in its exocrine component. They are most numerous in the tail region and vary considerably, both in size and in the number of cells they contain. Individual cells within the islets are smaller and paler than the exocrine cells and assume spherical or polygonal shapes from moulding by adjacent cells. Each islet has a capillary network which is in contact with each cell (Fig. 15.28).

Pancreatic islets develop as cellular buds from the same small ducts which ultimately supply the exocrine pancreatic component, and occasionally in man, variably sized islets can be seen in association with a pancreatic duct in the supporting fibrous tissue.

Each pancreatic islet contains a number of different neuroendocrine cells, each of which is mainly concerned with the secretion of a single hormone. The nomenclature of these individual cell types is confusing, and many different names have been used. In this book we adopt the simple straight-forward method of identifying a cell by its main hormone, other nomenclatures being given in brackets.

There are five main cell types, and at least two minor cell types. Of the total number of pancreatic endocrine cells, the proportions of the main cell types are as follows.
- Approximately 70% are insulin and amylin-secreting cells (B or β cells) (Fig. 15.29).
- Approximately 20% are glucagon-secreting cells (A or α cells) (Fig. 15.30).
- Approximately 5–10% are somatostatin-secreting cells (D, δ or type III cells) (Fig. 15.31).
- Approximately 1–2% are pancreatic polypeptide secreting cells (PP or F cells). These cells, which are comparatively scanty when a random block of the pancreas is examined, are found in greater numbers in the posterior lobe of the pancreas in the head and neck region. They are also found as scattered cells in duct walls. Their neurosecretory vacuoles are spherical with a central electron-dense core surrounded by a wide electon-lucent area.

The minor cell types are:
- vasoactive-intestinal peptide (VIP)-secreting cells (D1 or type IV cells);
- mixed secretion cells (EC or enterochromaffin cells).

Minor cell types are present in small numbers in the islets and scattered in the exocrine and ductular components. The mixed secretion cells have been reported to produce a number of active peptides, including serotinin, motilin and substance P.

An apparent anomaly is that the gastric hormone, gastrin, is secreted in excess by some islet cell tumours, but has not been satisfactorily demonstrated in the normal pancreatic islet. .

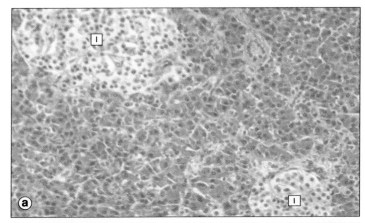

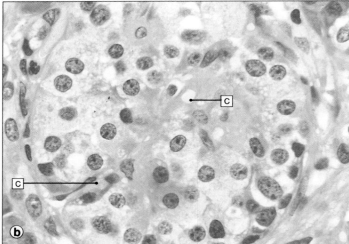

Fig. 15.28 Islets of Langerhans.
a Low power micrograph showing the discrete rounded clusters of islet cells (I) scattered throughout the pancreatic tissue and embedded in its exocrine component.
b High power micrograph showing islet cells; note that each cell is in contact with the capillary network (C).

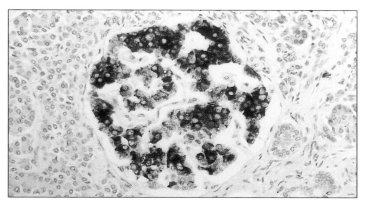

Fig. 15.29 Insulin-secreting cells.
Insulin/amylin-secreting cells occupy the central area of the pancreatic islets and are the most common cell type. This micrograph shows an islet stained by an immunoperoxidase method for insulin.

These cells have well-developed rough endoplasmic reticulum, a prominent Golgi, and numerous neurosecretory vesicles about 300 nm in diameter. The vesicles have a central electron-dense core in the form of a rhomboidal or polyhedral crystalline structure surrounded by an electron-lucent halo and bounded by a narrow membrane. In a few vesicles the core is missing, possibly due to the recent discharge of insulin (the central core is thought to be composed of insulin complexed with zinc). The peptide amylin is thought to modulate the action of insulin.

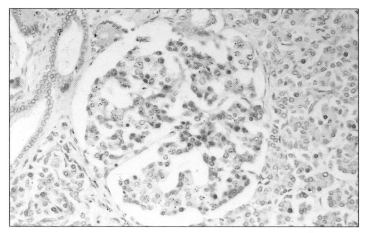

Fig. 15.30 Glucagon-secreting cells.
Glucagon-secreting cells are located mainly at the periphery of the pancreatic islet as shown in this micrograph of a section stained to show glucagon by an immunoperoxidase technique.

Glucagon-secreting cells possess similar ultrastructural features to those of insulin-secreting cells, except the secretory vesicles are smaller and have a more spherical electron-dense core, which is usually eccentrically located.

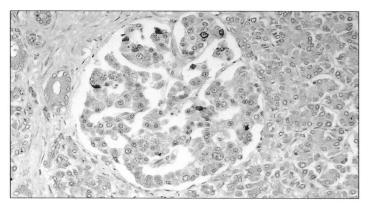

Fig. 15.31 Somatostatin-secreting cells.
Somatostatin-secreting cells are a minority population and, in man, are scattered apparently randomly throughout the pancreatic islets, as shown in this micrograph stained to show somatostatin by an immunoperoxidase technique. Some islets contain substantial numbers of these cells, while others contain none at all.

Somatostatin-secreting cells contain larger neurosecretory vesicles than insulin-secreting and glucagon-secreting cells, being up to 350 nm in diameter, and also their dense core is much less electron-dense.

Vascular and nerve supply

The islets contain a complex network of capillaries which, as in many other endocrine organs, have fenestrated endothelium. These capillaries arise from small arterioles outside the islet and after penetrating the islet merge with capillaries supplying the exocrine component of the pancreas.

Pancreatic islets are innervated by the autonomic nervous system, with both sympathetic and parasympathetic twigs contacting the surfaces of about 10% of all of the cells directly. There are well developed gap junctions between adjacent islet cells, which may provide the mechanism whereby the neural stimulus is passed to all cells. The autonomic nervous system also innervates the blood vessels and possibly affects perfusion.

Parasympathetic stimulation increases insulin and glucagon output, whereas sympathetic stimulation inhibits insulin release.

OVARY AND TESTIS

Although their main function is to produce female and male gametes, the ovary and testis also act as endocrine organs (see Chapter 17, pages 305–314, and Chapter 18, pages 333–339).

DIFFUSE NEUROENDOCRINE SYSTEM

So far, only those neuroendocrine cells that are gathered together to form distinct endocrine glands have been discussed. There is however, an extensive system of scattered neuroendocrine cells producing hormones and active peptides, many of which act on the local environment rather than having a distant systemic impact. Almost all of these cells belong to the so-called APUD or diffuse neuroendocrine system and have the following common characteristics.
• Uptake and decarboxylation of amine precursor compounds, producing active amines, peptides and hormones (**Amine Precursor Uptake and Decarboxylation, APUD cells**).
• Possession of characteristic cytoplasmic organelles, known as **dense-core granules, neurosecretory vesicles**, or **rimmed vacuoles**. These have a common basic structure of a variably electron-dense core (usually spherical, but occasionally angulated), a clear electron-lucent halo around the dense core, a thin distinct membrane surrounding the halo, and irrespective of the shape of the central dense core, the entire vesicle is usually spherical or oval. The vesicles vary in size (usually 100–600 nm in diameter), shape (spherical or oval), width of electron-lucent halo, and electron density of the central core, depending on the nature of the amine, peptide or hormone produced. In some cases their secretion is under neural control.

Examples of neuroendocrine cells have already been described in this chapter, for example, adrenal medullary cells (see page 262), calcitonin-secreting C cells (see page 258) and pancreatic islet cells (see page 264). Further examples will be met in other chapters, for example renin-producing juxtaglomerular cells (see page 294).

The important cells of the diffuse neuroendocrine system are gut-associated endocrine cells and respiratory-associated endocrine cells.

Gut-associated endocrine cells

Throughout the alimentary tract the lining epithelium contains scattered endocrine cells termed **gut-associated endocrine cells** or **enteroendocrine cells**. These are mainly concentrated in the stomach and small intestine (see Figs 10.25 & 10.40), but are also present in the lower oesophagus and large intestine, and in the ducts of organs draining into the gut (i.e. the bile and pancreatic ducts).

In general enteroendocrine cells are small, with a round spherical nucleus and pale-staining cytoplasm, and lie in contact with the basement membrane on which the mucosal epithelial cells sit (Fig. 15.32); many are not in contact with the lumen. Neurosecretory vesicles are concentrated mainly in the basal portion of these cells.

Enteroendocrine cells are difficult to identify by routine H&E staining, but can be highlighted by certain silver stains, hence their antiquated former name of argentaffin or argyrophil cells. Another old synonym, enterochromaffin cells, is based on their reaction with potassium dichromate to produce a brown pigment. Immunocytochemical methods have demonstrated many more enteroendocrine cells than are visible by current silver methods, and also

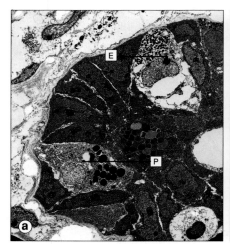 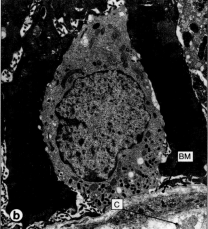 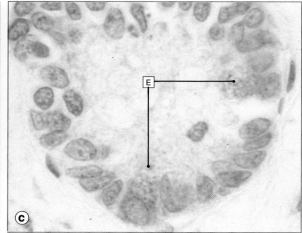

Fig. 15.32 Enteroendocrine cell.
a Low power electronmicrograph an enteroendocrine cell (E) in the base of a small bowel gland. This contrasts with a Paneth cell (P) (see Fig. 10.39).
b High power electronmicrograph showing neuroendocrine vesicles facing the basement membrane (BM) of the gland, and an adjacent capillary vessel (C).
c Micrograph showing enteroendocrine cells (E) demonstrated by an immunoperoxidase method to detect synaptophysin, a glycoprotein specific to the neuroendocrine vesicle membrane.

indicate their main secretion; they have therefore effectively replaced empirical silver methods for demonstrating such cells.

The ultrastructural features of enteroendocrine cells, particularly the size, shape and number of neurosecretory vesicles, vary according to the amine or peptide hormone produced, more than 20 of which have been identified. Most of these hormones cannot be accurately matched with an ultrastructurally characteristic cell type, and it is likely that some or all of the cells can produce more than one active secretion.

Respiratory-associated endocrine cells

Pulmonary neuroendocrine cells in humans exist in two forms.

- Individual neuroendocrine cells are scattered throughout the trachea, intrapulmonary airways and occasionally in the alveolar wall. These cells are pale when stained by H&E and are difficult to distinguish without the aid of special methods such as immunocytochemical techniques. Most of the cell sits on the epithelial basement membrane in a manner similar to that of enteroendocrine cells (see Fig. 15.32a), but a cytoplasmic process extends towards the lumen between adjacent epithelial cells.
- Small aggregates of neuroendocrine cells form small mounds protruding into the airway lumen or alveoli. These aggregates, which are particularly prominent where airways branch, receive unmyelinated axons from peribronchial and peribronchiolar nerves and have been called **neuroepithelial bodies** (see Fig. 9.11).

The cytoplasm of both individual and clumped pulmonary neuroendocrine cells contains numerous neurosecretory vesicles. Serotonin, bombesin, calcitonin and leucine-enkephalin have all been demonstrated within these cells.

In humans, respiratory-associated neuroendocrine cells are most numerous and prominent at birth, decreasing rapidly in number thereafter, whereas in some other animals, particularly rodents, they remain in significant numbers throughout life.

PARAGANGLIA

The paraganglia are specialized neuroendocrine glands associated with the autonomic nervous system, each consisting of prominent neuroendocrine cells containing neurosecretory vesicles. Those which have been adequately investigated have been shown to contain active amine or peptide hormones and are therefore regarded as part of the neuroendocrine system.

In many cases, their precise function and the nature of their secretions is not clear, but it is known that some of the larger paraganglia in the thorax and neck (e.g. aortic body and carotid body) act as chemoreceptors.

Paraganglia vary in size from clumps of a few cells associated with nerves, visible only with microscopy, to structures up to 3 mm in diameter, which are anatomically distinct. The largest paraganglia are the intercarotid paraganglia (carotid bodies) and the aortico-sympathetic paraganglia (organ of Zuckerkandl)

General structure

Histologically, paraganglia are composed mainly of so-called **chief cells**, which are neuroendocrine cells containing neurosecretory vesicles, arranged into roughly round clumps or nests (zellerballen). Each clump is surrounded by an intimate network of capillaries with fenestrated endothelium and a basement membrane. Between the neuroendocrine cells and the capillaries are occasional flattened support cells, the sustentacular cells (Fig. 15.33).

Sustentacular cells, which account for 35–45% of paraganglion cells, have elongated spindle-shaped nuclei and pale-staining cytoplasm with ill-defined cell borders. Concentrated at the periphery of the clumps of neuroendocrine cells, they send cytoplasmic processes into the

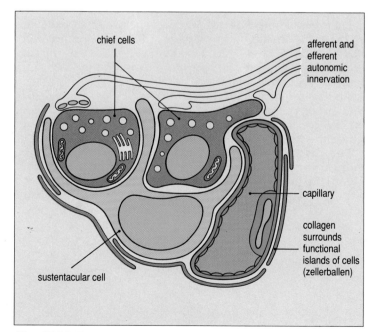

Fig. 15.33 Paraganglion.
Diagram to illustrate a paraganglion, showing that it is composed of chief cells arranged into clumps, which are surrounded by sustentacular cells and capillaries.

clumps and also around nerve axons, thus behaving in a similar manner to Schwann cells (see page 210), which they closely resemble, histologically and ultrastructurally.

The neuroendocrine cells are of two types.

• Most are termed **light cells** and have pale vacuolated cytoplasm containing moderate numbers of spherical electron-dense neurosecretory vesicles about 100–150 nm in diameter.

• A minor proportion are termed **dark cells** and have darker staining cytoplasm containing large numbers of pleomorphic, often angulated, neurosecretory vesicles 50–250 nm in diameter.

Paraganglia are richly innervated by both the sympathetic and parasympathetic nervous systems.

Carotid and aortic bodies

A single oval carotid body lies in the fibrocollagenous support tissue between the bifurcation of each common carotid artery into internal and external branches. Each carotid body measures about 3x2x2 mm and weighs 5–15 mg.

Carotid bodies are most prominent in children and teenagers, becoming progressively less obvious with increasing age, except in people with chronic hypoxia due to lung disease, or those living in low oxygen tension at high altitudes; in these people the carotid bodies increase in size as a result of hyperplasia (an increase in cell number), and may reach 40 mg in weight.

The carotid body has the general structure of all paraganglia (see Fig. 15.33) and in humans the only peptides identified in it are enkephalins. In other species, such as the cat, other active peptides are also found, including VIP, substance P, and catecholamines.

Similar in structure to the carotid bodies, but smaller, are the aortico-pulmonary paraganglia (aortic bodies), located on the concave surface of the arch of the aorta, close to where the right pulmonary artery passes beneath it.

The carotid and aortic bodies act as chemoreceptors monitoring the arterial oxygen tension and pH of the blood, the precise mechanism of which is not known.

Aortico-sympathetic paraganglia

There are a large number of small paraganglia situated around the abdominal aorta from above the level of origin of the renal arteries to the iliac bifurcation and beyond. On the anterior surface of the aorta they are particularly numerous around the coeliac axis and around the origin of the inferior mesenteric artery. Although prominent in infants, they are much less obvious in adults and are rarely discernable naked eye. Collectively they are known as the organs of Zuckerkandl, particularly the cluster around the origin of the inferior mesenteric artery.

Histologically, aortico-sympathetic paraganglia have the same general structure of paraganglia, but the neuroendocrine cells have larger neurosecretory granules than those in the carotid body and more closely resemble those of the adrenal medulla (Fig. 15.34).

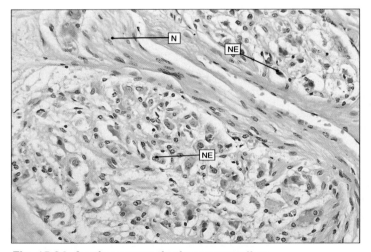

Fig. 15.34 Aortico-sympathetic paraganglion.
Low power micrograph showing a small aortico-sympathetic type paraganglion. Note the afferent nerve fibres (N) and the nests of neuroendocrine cells (NE).

PRACTICAL HISTOLOGY

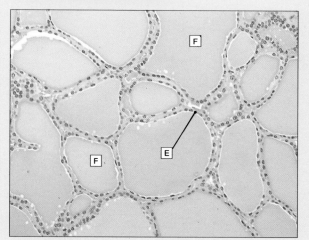

Fig. 15.35 Thyroid.
Micrograph showng normal human thyroid composed of variable sized follicles (F) filled with pink-staining thyroid colloid. In this illustration, the thyroid follicles are in a storage phase, so the lining epithelium (E) is cuboidal or flat, and the stored colloid fills the follicle. There is a complex intimate capillary network between adjacent follicles.

The details of the thyroid epithelial cell in an active phase are illustrated in Figs 15.17 and 15.18, and the calcitonin-secreting component of the thyroid in Fig. 15.19.

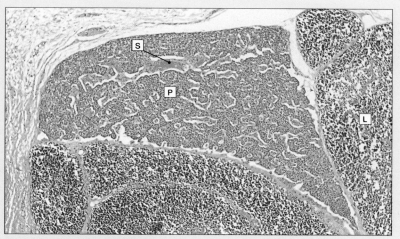

Fig. 15.36 Parathyroid gland.
Micrograph showing a parathyroid gland (P) closely associated with lymphoid tissue (L). In this parathyroid (from a child), the gland is almost entirely composed of endocrine cells separated by fibrocollagenous septa (S) rich in blood vessels. With increasing age, progressively more adipose tissue develops in the parathyroid gland (see page 259). The details of the cell types present in the parathyroid are illustrated in Fig. 15.20.

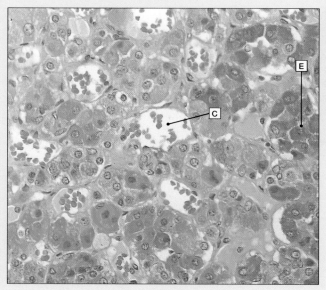

Fig. 15.37 Pituitary gland.
Micrograph of human anterior pituitary (adenohypophysis) stained by the H&E method showing clusters of endocrine cells with varying degrees of cytoplasmic staining by eosin. The cells with the strongest eosin staining (E) are responsible for the secretion of growth hormone; the identity of the other cell types can only be accurately established by immunocytochemical methods (see Figs 15.8–15.11), although other special staining methods enable some of them to be classified further (see Fig. 15.6).

The spaces between clumps of pituitary endocrine cells are occupied by a complex capillary network (C).

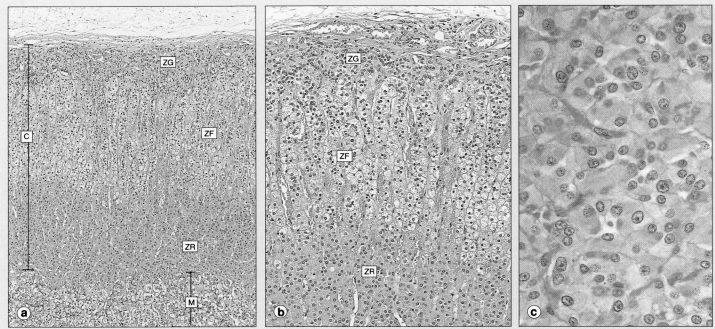

Fig. 15.38 Adrenal gland.

a Low power micrograph showing adrenal cortex (C) and medulla (M). Three distinct zones can be seen in the cortex, the zona glomerulosa, (ZG), zona fasciculata (ZF) and zona reticularis (ZR).

b Micrograph showing the adrenal cortex at higher magnification. Note the zona glomerulosa (ZG), zona fasciculata (ZF) and zona reticularis (ZR). The zona fasciculata is the middle zone, and is composed of pale-staining cells rich in lipid droplets. The histological details of the cells in these zones are shown in greater detail in Figs 15.23–15.25.

c Medium power micrograph of adrenal medulla, which is composed of irregularly shaped cells with granular cytoplasm. These cells contain abundant neuroendocrine vesicles, and secrete adrenaline and noradrenaline (see Fig. 15.26). There is an intimate capillary supply.

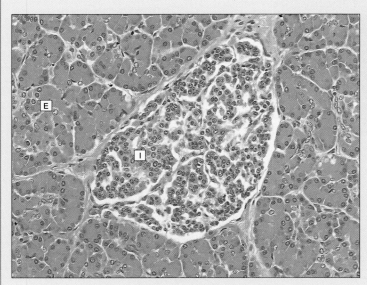

Fig. 15.39 Pancreatic islets of Langerhans.

Micrograph of H&E stained section of an islet of Langerhans (I) embedded in the exocrine component (E) of the pancreas. The islets are roughly spherical and are composed of much smaller cells than the exocrine pancreas from which they are separated by a fine fibrocollagenous capsule. The cytological detail of islet cells is shown in Fig. 15.28b. The use of immunhistochemistry enables the various cell types to be accurately identified (see Figs 15.29–15.31).

16. URINARY SYSTEM

The main function of the urinary system is the production, storage and voiding of urine.

Urine is an aqueous solution of excess anions and cations, and many of the breakdown products of the body's metabolic processes, particularly those which would be toxic if allowed to accumulate.

The most important toxic metabolites are the nitrogen-containing products of protein breakdown, such as urea and creatinine. Both the composition and concentration of urine can be varied to maintain internal homeostasis.

Urine production and the control of its composition, is the responsibility of the kidney, while storage and voiding is performed by the bladder.

The pelvicalyceal systems and ureters transfer urine from the kidney to the bladder, and the urethra is the channel through which stored urine is voided from the bladder.

As befits their comparatively simple roles, the pelvicalyceal systems, ureters, bladder and urethra have a relatively uncomplicated structure (see page 300).

The kidney, however, performs a wide range of biochemical and physiological tasks during the production of urine, and its structure is accordingly complex.

OUTLINE OF THE URINARY SYSTEM

The general arrangement of the interconnecting components of the urinary system is illustrated in Fig. 16.1.

The **kidneys** are solid bean-shaped organs located high on the posterior abdominal wall beneath the peritoneum. The concave aspect of each bean faces towards the midline where the major channel of arterial supply (the aorta) and venous drainage (the inferior vena cava) run. This concave area is called the **hilum**, and is the site of entry of the renal arterial supply, and of the emergence of the renal venous drainage and urine transport system.

The **pelvicalyceal system** and **ureters** are hollow muscular tubes lined by a specialized epithelium, which is resistant to damage by the variable osmolarity of urine, and by the concentration of toxic solutes within it. The wall of the tubes is composed of smooth muscle capable of pushing the fluid towards the bladder by alternate coordinated contraction and relaxation; this process is called **peristalsis** (see page 158).

The **bladder** has basically the same structure as the pelvicalyceal system and ureters, but its arrangement of muscle fibres is more sophisticated to allow it to act as both a capacious reservoir for urine, and as a pump to force out the urine through the urethra under voluntary control.

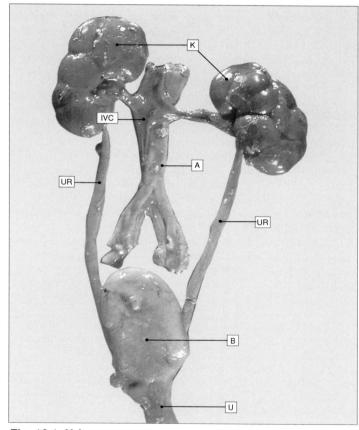

Fig. 16.1 Urinary system.
Photograph of dissected urinary system from a term male stillbirth demonstrating the interrelationships between the aorta (A), the inferior vena cava (IVC), the kidneys (K), the ureters (UR), the bladder (B), and the urethra (U). In the adult the bladder is more spherical.

KIDNEY STRUCTURE

Each kidney has two distinct zones, an outer **cortex** and an inner **medulla** (Fig. 16.2).
• The cortex forms an outer shell, and also forms columns (the so-called columns of Bertin), which lie between the individual units of the medulla.
• The medulla is composed of a series of conical structures (**medullary pyramids**), the base of each cone being continuous with the inner limit of the cortex, and the pointed peak of the pyramid protruding into part of the urine collecting system (the **calyceal system**) towards the hilum of the kidney. This pointed tip of the medullary pyramid is known as the **papilla**.

Each human kidney bears 10–18 medullary pyramids, thus 10–18 papillae protrude into the collecting calyces.

Each medullary pyramid, with its associated shell of cortex, comprises a functional and structural lobe of the kidney. This lobar architectural arrangement is clearly visible in the fetal kidney (see Fig. 16.1), but becomes less obvious as the kidney increases in size with increasing age.

KIDNEY FUNCTION

Urine is produced in the kidney by the selective removal of substances from the blood plasma. Subsequent controlled reabsorption of water, ions, salts, sugars and other carbohydrates, and small molecular weight proteins allows the kidney to produce urine, the composition of which is appropriate to the body's internal environment and requirements at the time.

For example, if the plasma volume is expanded and diluted by a substantial ingestion of water, the kidney will then excrete the excess water by producing large quantities of a dilute urine. Conversely, if fluid ingestion is restricted, the kidney will produce a small amount of highly concentrated urine.

Whatever the quantity and concentration of the urine, it will contain the required amount of waste products and ions to maintain internal biochemical homeostasis.

An inability to produce concentrated or dilute urine is an important feature of kidney failure, as is evidence of inadequate excretion of nitrogenous waste products and other substances, for example potassium ions (see page 295).

It is important to realize that the kidneys (and lungs) differ from most other organs in one important respect. In most organs, the blood vascular supply is the servant of the parenchymal tissues, providing them with oxygen and other raw materials required for the tissue's metabolic processes,

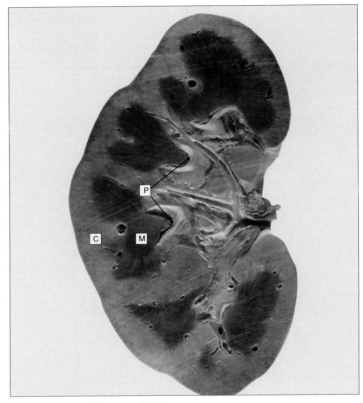

Fig. 16.2 Adult human kidney.
Photograph of adult human kidney cut longitudinally to show the arrangement of the cortex (C), medulla (M), and papilla (P).

and carrying synthesized cell products and waste materials away from the organ. In the kidney however, the parenchymatous components of the organ are the servants of the blood supply, since the function of the kidney, in broad terms, is the filtration and cleansing of the blood.

Thus, the parenchymal unit of the kidney, the **nephron,** which is composed of the **glomerulus** and **cortical** and **medullary tubular systems**, can be regarded as an appendage of the renal blood vascular system, attached to it for servicing purposes. It is not surprising, therefore, that the blood vascular system of the kidney is both substantial and structurally unusual, reflecting its central role; the two kidneys receive 25% of the total cardiac output. Consequently, most of the important and common diseases of the kidney result from an abnormality in the blood vascular component (see page 295).

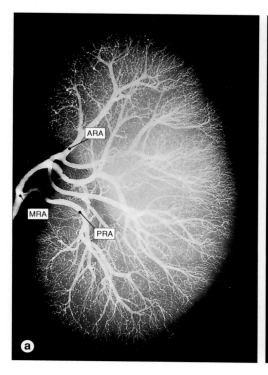

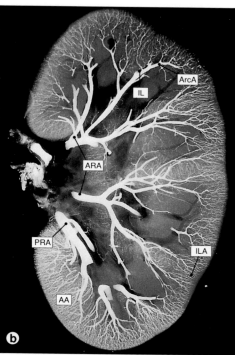

Fig. 16.3 Arterial system of the kidney.

a Arteriogram of a whole postmortem human kidney showing the division of the main renal artery (MRA) into two branches, a comparatively minor posterior branch (PRA), and a more substantial anterior branch (ARA).

The posterior branch supplies the lower pole, whilst the larger anterior branch divides, in this case, into four segmental arteries, which together supply the mid-zone and upper pole of the kidney.

b In this section the posterior (PRA) and anterior (ARA) branches of the renal artery can be seen, although some segments are missing due to the tortuosity of the arteries at the hilum.

Note the interlobar arteries (IL), the arcuate arteries (ArcA), and the fine network of interlobular arteries (ILA).

The faint haziness (AA) in some areas of the cortex indicates filling of the afferent arterioles.

KIDNEY VASCULATURE

Arterial supply

The major arteries to the kidney often vary although the pattern within the kidney is fairly constant. A common variant is the presence of a separate artery arising directly from the aorta, and supplying one or other pole. In most cases, however, the arterial supply to each kidney comes from a single renal artery, which is a substantial direct lateral branch of the abdominal aorta, and its course is as follows.

• The **renal artery** runs towards the concave hilum of the kidney and divides into two main branches, one anterior, one posterior (Fig. 16.3), each of which divides into a number of **interlobar arteries** that run between the medullary pyramids, one branch to each developmental lobe.

• At about the midpoint of the thickness of the kidney parenchyma, where the cortex abuts on the broad base of the medullary pyramid (the **cortico-medullary junction**), the interlobar artery divides into several lateral **arcuate arteries,** which run laterally.

• The arcuate arteries then give rise to a series of side branches (**interlobular arteries**), which run vertically upwards into the cortex.

• Interlobular arteries give rise laterally to a series of arterioles, called **afferent arterioles**, usually directly, but sometimes via a short **intralobular artery**, and terminate at the periphery of the kidney, just beneath the capsule, where each divides into a stellate **subcapsular arteriola**r and **capillary plexus**.

Thus far, the arterial supply has been like the arterial supply of almost every organ. From the afferent arterioles onwards, however, the renal vascular system becomes unique.

Renal microcirculation

The renal microcirculation is the key to renal function, and has a number of unusual features, most notably it consists of two capillary systems. In almost every other case the capillary network lies between the terminal part of the arterial/arteriolar system and the proximal part of the venular/venous system, and is the major site of oxygen/carbon dioxide exchange. In contrast, the renal vascular system has:

- a highly specialized preliminary capillary network, the **glomerular tuft**, which receives blood from an afferent arteriole and is the site of filtration of blood to extract waste products from plasma;
- a second capillary system arising from the efferent arteriole, which varies in structure and function according to its location within the kidney (Fig. 16.4).

In most cases (see Fig. 16.6), after leaving the glomerulus the efferent arteriole divides into a complex capillary system which runs in the interstitial spaces between the components of the system of cortical tubules. Each capillary is in intimate contact with these tubules, and is thus ideally placed to take up any substances reabsorbed from the glomerular filtrate by tubular epithelial cells (see page 284).

On the other hand, the capillary system originating from efferent arterioles leaving glomeruli situated deep in the cortex, close to the cortico-medullary junction (**juxta-medullary glomeruli**), is different (see Fig. 16.4). These efferent arterioles divide into a series of long thin-walled vessels, the **vasa recta**, which run straight down into the medulla alongside the medullary components of the tubular systems. These vessels play an important role in the ionic and fluid exchanges occurring in the medulla (see page 290). Some vasa recta arise as direct, vertically running, side branches of the arcuate artery.

The first capillary system, the glomerular tuft, does not transfer its contained oxygen to the tissues, nor does it take up a significant amount of carbon dioxide. The major exchange of dissolved gases takes place in the second capillary system; oxygen is supplied to the cortical and medullary parts of the renal parenchyma, which have the highest demand because of their high metabolic activity.

Venous drainage

In general, the renal venous drainage mirrors the arterial supply, except that there is no venous equivalent of the glomerular capillary tuft.

The subcapsular arteriolar and capillary plexus drains into a **subcapsular venular** and **venous plexus** of **stellate veins** which form the origin of the **interlobular veins**. As they proceed towards the cortico-medullary junction the interlobular veins receive venous tributaries from the peritubular capillary network, and as the juxtamedullary zone is approached, from some of the venous tributaries from the medulla, which are the venous equivalent of the arterial vasa recta.

Many of the medullary venous vessels drain directly into the **arcuate veins**, which run laterally with the equivalent artery at the cortico-medullary junction. These in turn drain into large interlobular veins lying between adjacent medullary pyramids and then into the major vein tributaries at the renal hilum. The major renal vein opens end-to-side into the inferior vena cava.

NEPHRON

The functional unit of the kidney parenchyma which serves the blood supply is called the **nephron** and has two main components:

- the **glomerulus**, which is associated with the first capillary system;
- the **cortical** and **medullary tubular systems**, which are associated with the second capillary system.

The glomerulus is the site of initial blood filtration, and the tubular systems are the site where the concentration and chemical content of blood returned to the general systemic circulation, and hence the concentration and content of the urine to be voided from the body, is controlled.

Within the renal cortex, the nephrons are organized in a distinct repeated lobular pattern. The glomeruli, and proximal and distal tubules, are aligned mainly on either side of the interlobular arteries, which supply them with blood (see Fig. 16.4).

At the midpoint between adjacent interlobular arteries is a vertically running arrangement of tubules and ducts known as the **medullary ray**, (see Fig. 16.25), at the centre of which is a main collecting duct, which collects all of the largely unconcentrated urine from the nephrons on either side. The other tubular components of the medullary ray are the straight collecting tubules carrying urine from the end of the distal tubule to the main cortical collecting duct. The duct systems of the medullary rays run vertically downwards into the medulla.

The subunit of cortex, comprising a centrally placed medullary ray and the nephrons on either side of it is called the **renal lobule** and each interlobular artery runs upwards in the cortex between adjacent lobules. This lobular arrangement and the medullary ray system can be seen in Fig. 16.25.

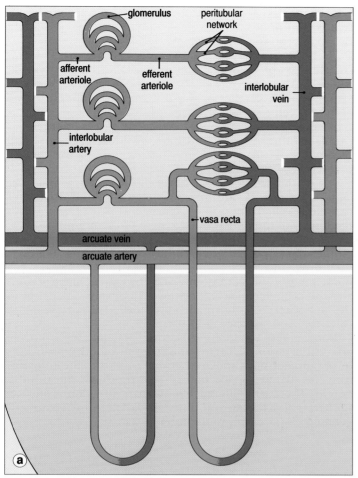

Fig. 16.4 Renal microcirculation.

a Diagram illustrating the principles of the renal microcirculation. The afferent arteriole, which is a branch of the interlobular artery, enters the glomerular capillary tuft at the vascular hilum. The emerging vessel, the efferent arteriole normally divides into a complex system of capillaries, the peritubular capillary network, which surrounds the cortical tubules. The venous tributaries arising from the PCN drain into small veins opening into the interlobular vein, which runs vertically alongside the interlobular artery, and drains into the arcuate vein running alongside the arcuate artery at the cortico-medullary junction.

Close to the cortico-medullary junction, some of the efferent arterioles give rise to vertically running vessels, the vasa recta, which pass down into the medulla alongside the medullary duct and tubular systems. Some vasa recta arise as direct branches of the arcuate artery and drain directly into the arcuate vein.

b A carmine-gelatin injection specimen showing a vertically running interlobular artery (ILA) in the renal cortex, with glomerular capillary tufts (G) arising from lateral branches of the artery, and the afferent arterioles (AA). Some peritubular capillary networks (PCN) can also be seen.

c A carmine-gelatin injection specimen showing the interlobular artery (ILA), the afferent (AA) and efferent (EA) arterioles, the glomerular tuft (G), and the peritubular capillary network (PCN).

d A carmine-gelatin injection specimen of the cortico-medullary junction. Note the arcuate artery (ArcA), an interlobular artery (ILA), glomeruli (G), and a number of peritubular capillary networks (PCN) in the cortex. The medulla contains parallel bundles of straight blood vessels, the vasa recta (VR), some of which arise as direct vertical branches of the arcuate artery, and others from the efferent arterioles of some glomeruli close to the cortico-medullary junction.

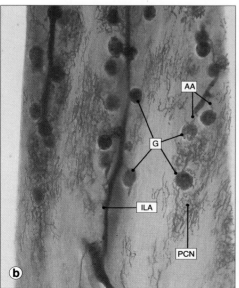

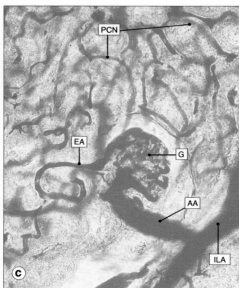

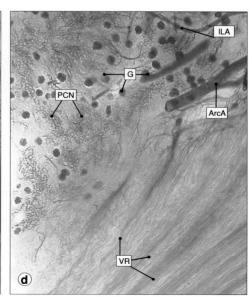

GLOMERULUS

The first functional component of the nephron encountered by the microcirculation is the glomerulus, which is the site of initial filtration of the blood arriving by the afferent arterioles.

The afferent arteriole enters the glomerular structure at the vascular pole, and splits up into about five main branches. Each branch then subdivides into its own capillary network (see Fig. 16.4), the short main branch and its capillaries being supported by its own strip or stalk of mesangium (see page 281).

The division of the glomerular capillary network into about five independent segments gives the glomerular tuft an implicit lobularity, which is rarely apparent by routine light microscopy in health, but becomes evident in some forms of primary glomerular disease, particularly when the mesangial component of each segment is enlarged (see Fig. 16.14). The independence of each glomerular segment is also demonstrated by disease affecting only one segment (e.g. segmental glomerulonephritis).

The glomerular capillaries converge to form a single efferent arteriole, which leaves the glomerulus at the same vascular pole as the afferent arteriole enters.

In simple terms, the structure of the glomerulus is best conceived as a globular capillary network intruding into a hollow sphere of epithelial cells called **Bowman's capsule**, which represents the bulbous, distended, closed end of a long hollow tubular system (Fig. 16.5). This means that the glomerular capillary system, which is lined internally by endothelial cells, acquires an outer layer of epithelial cells that is continuous at the vascular pole with the cells lining Bowman's capsule.

The epithelial cells of Bowman's capsule are flat and simple, except near the opening of the tubular system, where they become more cuboidal and acquire some of the cytoplasmic organelles of the proximal convoluted tubule epithelial cells (see page 284).

In contrast, the epithelial cells coating the glomerular capillary tuft are larger and have a highly specialized and unusual structure, which has led to their being named **podocytes** (see page 280).

The epithelial-lined space between the coated glomerular capillary network and the parietal shell of Bowman's capsule is called the **urinary space**, and is continuous with the lumen of the long tubular system of the nephron.

As well as the outer epithelial (podocyte) coating, the glomerular capillary network has other unusual features, including the possession of an unusually thick basement membrane (the **glomerular basement membrane**), and the presence of a supporting strip or stalk analogous to the mesentery of the small bowel, called the mesangium (Fig. 16.6 and see page 281).

Blood enters the glomerular capillary network from the afferent arteriole. Ultrafiltration of the blood then occurs in the glomerular capillary network, and the filtrate passes into the urinary space before passing down the tubular system. The partly filtered blood leaves the glomerulus via the efferent arteriole and flows onwards to provide an oxygenated blood supply to the tubular systems.

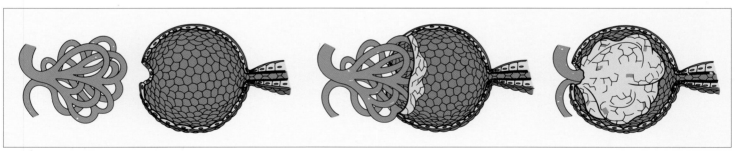

Fig. 16.5 Relationship between the glomerular capillary tuft and Bowman's capsule.
Although the glomerulus and Bowman's capsule do not in fact develop in this way, the relationships between the two are best conceived by imagining the intrusion of the glomerular tuft into the spherical, distended and closed end of the tubular system. This is particularly helpful in conceptualizing the glomerular tuft with its outer coating of epithelial cells, which is continuous with the cells lining Bowman's capsule.

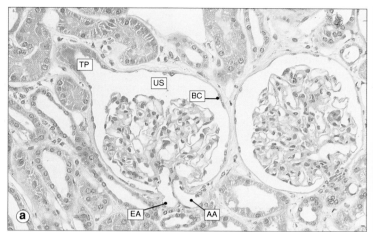

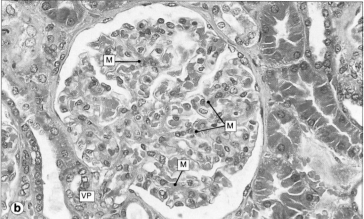

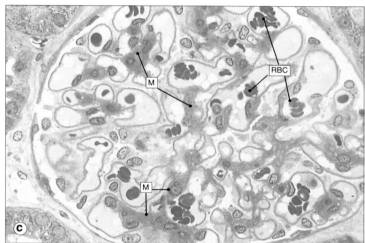

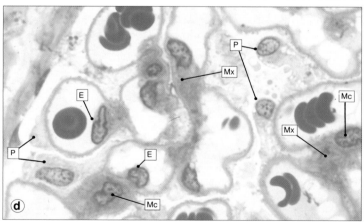

Fig. 16.6 Normal human glomerulus.

a An H&E paraffin section of normal human kidney, which has been inflation fixed to distend the blood vessels. Note the afferent arteriole (AA) and efferent arteriole (EA) at the vascular pole.

Opposite the vascular pole is the tubular pole (TP) where the urinary space (US) empties into the first part of the tubular system.

Although fine details of the glomerular structure are not apparent in this micrograph, the suggestion of glomerular lobularity is evident. The flattened epithelial lining of Bowman's capsule (BC) is easily seen.

b Special stains reveal more detail of glomerular structure, particularly if methods are selected which highlight the glomerular basement membrane and mesangium.

This micrograph of a glomerulus sectioned through the vascular pole and stained by the MSB method shows the mesangium (M) on which the glomerular capillaries sit. Such a section shows how the mesangium radiates from the vascular pole (VP) in a distinct lobular pattern.

c A thin epoxy resin section of a normal human glomerulus stained with toluidine blue. This technique permits much greater resolution of the structure of the glomerulus. The dilated capillary loops contain red blood cells (RBC) and are supported by the darkly stained mesangium (M).

d High power micrograph of a thin epoxy resin section of a segment of the glomerular tuft, stained with toluidine blue. At this magnification, details of the glomerular capillary wall, endothelial and epithelial cells, and mesangium, become apparent.

The capillary loops are supported by darkly stained mesangial stalks comprising acellular matrix (Mx) and nucleated mesangial cells (Mc). The capillary basement membrane is lined internally by endothelial cytoplasm and endothelial cell nuclei (E) are apparent.

External to the glomerular basement membrane are the epithelial podocytes (P).

Glomerular filtration barrier

The barrier between circulating blood and the urinary space is occupied by the unusually modified glomerular capillary wall, which comprises the structurally visible glomerular filtration barrier (Fig. 16.7). It is composed of:
- the capillary endothelial inner layer;
- the unusually thick glomerular capillary basement membrane;
- the podocyte (the outer epithelial) layer.

Glomerular capillary endothelial cells are flattened and their nuclei are usually located near the mesangium. The cytoplasm forms a thin sheet broken by numerous small circular pores or fenestrations, each about 70 nm in diameter.

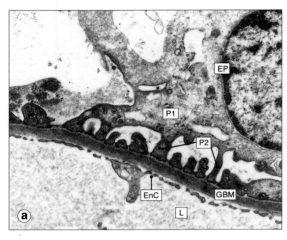
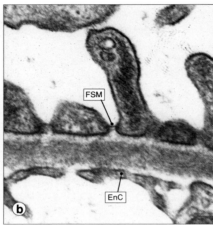

Fig. 16.7 Glomerular capillary wall.
a Electronmicrograph showing the relationship between the glomerular basement membrane (GBM), capillary lumen (L), endothelial cytoplasm (EnC), and the epithelial podocyte (EP) with its primary (P1) and secondary (P2) foot process system.
b High power electronmicrograph of the glomerular filtration barrier, comprising fenestrated endothelial cytoplasm (EnC), glomerular basement membrane and podocyte foot processes. Note the filtration slit membrane (FSM, see page 280).

GLOMERULAR ENDOTHELIAL ABNORMALITIES

In some primary glomerular diseases, there is a great increase in the size and number of the endothelial cells, and the glomerular capillary lumina become blocked (Fig. 16.8). This produces the **acute nephritic syndrome**, which is characterized by:
- an increase in blood pressure due to the increased peripheral resistance following blockage of the vast glomerular capillary network;
- a rise in the blood levels of nitrogenous waste products, due to the failure of filtration by the abnormal glomeruli;
- haematuria (loss of red blood cells in the urine), the mechanism of which is not known.
- oedema (fluid accumulation in support tissues).

Primary structural abnormalities of the glomerulus, such as that illustrated here, are known by the name **glomerulonephritis**. The micrograph shows an example of acute **endocapillary glomerulonephritis**.

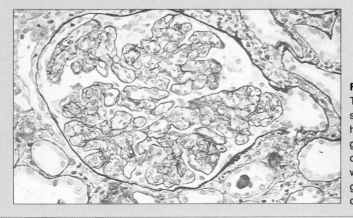

Fig. 16.8 Acute nephritic syndrome.
This paraffin section of kidney from a child with the acute nephritic syndrome has been stained by the Jones methenamine silver technique to highlight the basement membranes and mesangium of the glomerular capillary loops (brown-black). The capillary lumina are obliterated by proliferations of cells within the basement membrane, which are therefore largely endothelial cells. If this occurs in all of the glomeruli, as is usually the case, blood flow through the glomerular capillary network is reduced.

Glomerular basement membrane is much thicker than normal capillary basement membranes and measures approximately 310–350 nm in healthy young adults, being slightly thicker in males. Both the inner endothelial and outer epithelial cell populations contribute to its production. It has three layers:

- a central electron-dense **lamina densa**;
- electron-lucent **lamina rare interna** on the endothelial or capillary lumen side;
- electron-lucent **lamina rara externa** on the epithelial podocyte, or urinary space side.

This layered structure is clearly seen in rodents and children, but becomes less apparent in most adults.

The lamina densa is partly composed of type IV collagen (see page 44), and the fibril network acts as a physical barrier to the passage of large molecules from the blood into the urinary space.

The lamina rara layers, and the surfaces of some podocyte secondary foot processes, contain fixed negatively charged (polyanionic) sites, composed of glycosaminoglycan (see page 42). In the basement membrane this is heparan sulphate, and on the foot process surfaces it is a sialic acid-rich substance named **podocalyxin**. When demonstrated ultrastructurally using a cationic substance such as ruthenium red or polyethyleneimine (Fig. 16.9),

such sites appear to be organized to form fairly regular lattice with a spacing of approximately 60 nm.

It is thought that the polyanionic sites act as a charge barrier, preventing the passage of cationic molecules.

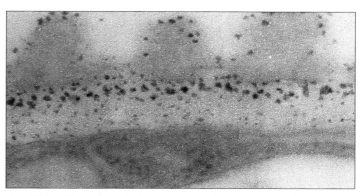

Fig. 16.9 Glomerular basement membrane–polyanionic sites (polyethyleneimine method).
Electronmicrograph of the glomerular filtration barrier identifying the sites of high polyanionic charge in both the basement membrane and on the surfaces of the podocyte foot processes. Loss of this surface anionic charge leads to leakage of excess protein.

BASEMENT MEMBRANE ABNORMALITIES IN GLOMERULAR DISEASE

Abnormalities in the structure of the glomerular basement membrane are responsible for some important kidney diseases, which are characterized by an excessive loss of protein in urine (**proteinuria**). Sometimes so much protein is lost in the urine that the capacity of the liver to synthesize fresh protein (particularly albumin) is outstripped. The patient then develops a low blood albumin (**hypoalbuminaemia**), and **oedema** due to the low oncotic pressure of the blood.

The combination of proteinuria, hypoalbuminaemia and oedema is called the **nephrotic syndrome**.

There are many causes of the nephrotic syndrome, but all appear to be related to a structural or functional abnormality of the glomerular basement membrane.

Diseases in which the abnormality is structural include **diabetes mellitus** and **membranous nephropathy**.

- In nephrotic syndrome associated with diabetes mellitus, the glomerular basement is thickened 3–5 fold and the demarcation into three laminae is lost (Fig. 16.10a).
- In membranous nephropathy, the basement membrane is damaged by the deposition of antigen–antibody complexes within it (Fig. 16.10b).

Although in these examples the basement membrane is physically thickened, it is functionally leaky, and many large molecules pass into the urinary space, including large molecular weight proteins.

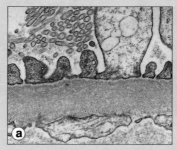 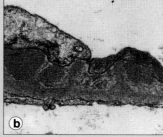

Fig. 16.10 Patterns of basement membrane thickening in disease.
a Electronmicrograph of a uniformly thickened basement membrane from a patient with diabetes mellitus who presented with the nephrotic syndrome. Photographed at same magnification as Fig. 16.7a.
b Electronmicrograph of a basement membrane thickened by deposition of antigen–antibody complexes on the epithelial side of the basement membrane, from a patient with membranous nephropathy who presented with the nephrotic syndrome. Photographed at same magnification as Fig. 16.7a.

The combination of layers in the glomerular basement membrane produces both a physical and electrical barrier to the passage of large molecules (e.g. over 70,000 daltons) and highly cationic molecules of many sizes. Nevertheless, certain large molecules, including some proteins, may pass through into the urinary space and require reabsorption in the tubular system.

The full thickness of the glomerular basement membrane does not completely surround the circumference of the capillary wall, but instead occupies about three-quarters of it, being partly deficient at the site of the attachment of the capillary to the mesangium. The lamina rara externa and lamina densa are reflected onto the surface of the mesangium, (see Fig. 16.13). The lamina rara interna continues as an ill-defined layer lying between the endothelial cytoplasm and the cytoplasmic and matrix components of the mesangium.

The podocyte layer, which is continuous at the vascular hilum with the flat, relatively inert epithelium lining Bowman's capsule, is highly specialized in structure, and presumably in function as well, though much of its functional detail is not known.

The podocyte is so-named because the main body of the cell hovers above the external surface of the glomerular capillary and sends down cytoplasmic extensions (foot processes), which make contact with the basement membrane (see Figs 16.7 & 16.10).

Between adjacent foot processes on the glomerular basement membrane is a fairly consistent gap of 30–60 μm, the **filtration slit**. A thin membrane, the **filtration slit membrane**, bridges the gap between adjacent foot processes.

The functional aspects of this complex cytoplasmic arrangement are not understood, but it obviously plays an important role in preventing certain molecules from passing into the urinary space. Loss of the podocyte foot process pattern in some renal diseases is associated with such excessive protein loss (mainly albumin) that the patient develops the nephrotic syndrome (see page 279).

PODOCYTE ABNORMALITIES IN GLOMERULAR DISEASE

In children, the most common cause of the nephrotic syndrome is the so-called **minimal change nephropathy**. By light microscopy the glomerulus appears normal, but electron microscopy reveals loss of the foot process pattern, with the outer surface of the glomerular capillaries being covered by an almost continuous sheet of podocyte cytoplasm, probably representing primary process remnants (Fig. 16.12). The abnormality is usually only temporary; structure and function return to normal in time. The podocyte abnormalities are associated with loss of the polyanionic charge (see page 279), which possibly explains the protein leak.

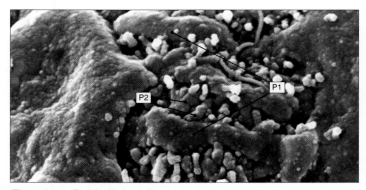

Fig. 16.11 Epithelial podocyte.
Scanning electronmicrograph of the epithelial podocyte and its foot processes in a healthy human adult.

Arising from the main cell body of each epithelial cell are a number of broad cytoplasmic processes, the primary processes (P1), which extend along and wrap around the capillary, giving rise at regular intervals to a series of smaller processes, the secondary processes (P2), which rest on the glomerular basement membrane. There is interdigitation of secondary processes so that adjacent foot processes may be derived from different podocytes. The foot process pattern in the adult human is not so neatly arranged as it is in the neonate or the rodent.

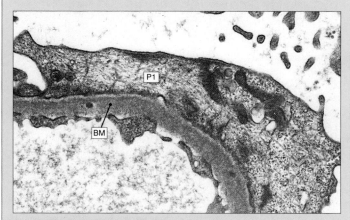

Fig. 16.12 Foot process fusion.
Compare the foot process arrangement in this electronmicrograph with that seen normally (Fig. 16.7). In this kidney from a child with the nephrotic syndrome due to minimal change nephropathy, the complex secondary foot process arrangement is lost and the primary foot processes (P1) lie directly on the basement membrane (BM). Minimal change nephropathy is the commonest cause of the nephrotic syndrome in childhood and spontaneously resolves with no long term renal impairment.

MESANGIUM

The mesangial support to the glomerular capillary network has two components: **mesangial cells** and **extracellular mesangial matrix**. The role of the mesangium as a support for the glomerular capillary system can be seen in Fig. 16.6, while Fig. 16.13 illustrates the details of the structure of the mesangium, and its relationship to the glomerular capillary and the glomerular basement membrane.

Mesangial cells

Mesangial cells are irregular in shape, and have a number of cytoplasmic processes, which run in an apparently haphazard fashion through the extracellular mesangial matrix.

The mesangial cell nucleus is round or oval, and is larger than the endothelial cell nucleus (see Fig. 16.6). There is a dense rim of nuclear chromatin inside the nuclear membrane, and numerous small chromatin clumps are scattered throughout the nucleoplasm.

The mesangial cell cytoplasm contains myosin-like filaments and bears angiotensin II receptors. In the experimental animal, contraction of mesangial cell filaments has been shown to be stimulated by angiotensin II.

Mesangial matrix

Mesangial matrix is an acellular material produced by the mesangial cell and largely enclosing it, but permeated by mesangial cell cytoplasmic processes. Ultrastructurally it is

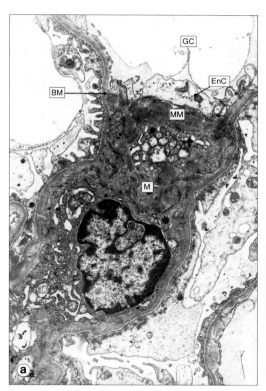
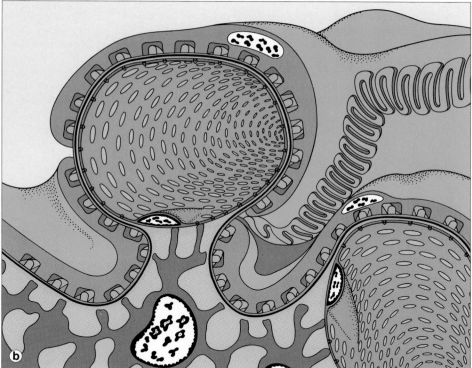

Fig. 16.13 Mesangium.
a Electronmicrograph of mesangium (M) and its relationship with the glomerular capillary (GC).

The capillary wall is deficient in basement membrane (BM) at the site of attachment to the mesangium, the wall being composed of endothelial cell cytoplasm (EnC) lying directly on mesangial matrix (MM).

The basement membrane continues over the surface of the mesangium to the next capillary loop.

b The podocytes with their foot processes (green) are separated

from the fenestrated endothelium (red) by the glomerular basement membrane. Note the supporting role of the mesangium (matrix−beige, cytoplasm−brown).

The lamina densa (black) and lamina rara externa (blue) of the basement membrane (see Fig. 4.11) are not continuous around the capillary, but are reflected over the mesangial surface to the next capillary.

The lamina rara interna (orange) appears to blend with the mesangial matrix where the capillary is attached to the mesangium.

of variable electron density, the more electron-lucent parts closely resembling the lamina rara interna of the glomerular basement membrane, with which it is in continuity where the glomerular capillary and mesangium meet.

Role of the mesangium

The precise mechanisms of action of the mesangium in humans are not known, but it has four postulated functions.
• Support of the glomerular capillary loop system.
• Possible control of blood flow through the glomerular loop by the myosin-angiotensin mechanism described above.

• Possible phagocytic function, as intravenously injected particulate matter (e.g. colloidal carbon, ferritin, etc.,) in the experimental animal, and circulating immune complexes in man, appear in the mesangium in some disease states. The incompleteness of the basement membrane over the area of attachment to the mesangium would facilitate this function.
• Possible maintenance of the glomerular basement membrane. Note the close resemblance and continuity of mesangial matrix and lamina rara interna. The importance of the mesangium in human glomerular disease suggests that it is a vital functional component of the glomerulus, and that it has been neglected.

MESANGIAL ABNORMALITIES

Abnormalities of the mesangium are an important component of many glomerular diseases.
• In some forms of immunological damage to the glomerulus, there is a proliferation of mesangial cells which leads to compression of the glomerular capillaries (**mesangial glomerulonephritis**); this is often associated with the deposition of immune complexes within the mesangium (Fig. 16.14).

• In diabetes mellitus, the mesangial cells of one or more of the glomerular segments produce excessive amounts of acellular matrix to form spherical nodules known as **Kimmelstiel-Wilson nodules** (Fig. 16.15).
• In permanently damaged glomeruli, whatever the cause, excessive formation of mesangial matrix in all segments eventually converts the glomerular tuft into an acellular spherical mass (**hyalinization**, see end-stage kidney, Fig. 16.27).

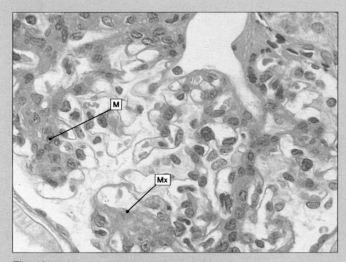

Fig. 16.14 Mesangial glomerulonephritis.
A paraffin section of kidney showing proliferation of the mesangial cells (M), and excessive production of mesangial matrix (Mx) expanding the lobules of the glomerular tuft and beginning to compress the glomerular capillary lumina. This pattern of disease is called mesangial glomerulonephritis.

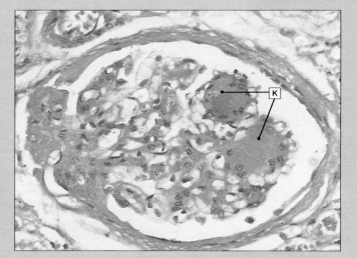

Fig. 16.15 Kimmelstiel-Wilson nodule.
An H&E stained paraffin section of kidney from a patient with diabetes mellitus showing a localized nodule of mesangial matrix (Kimmelstiel-Wilson nodule, K) in two of the glomerular lobules.

TUBULAR AND COLLECTING SYSTEM

The course of the glomerular filtrate after leaving the urinary space at the tubular pole of the glomerulus, on its way to the pelvicalyceal system, is illustrated in Fig. 16.16.

The convoluted parts of both proximal and distal tubules are found close to the glomeruli, which are usually clustered around the ascending interlobular arteries, from which their afferent arterioles are derived.

In contrast the straight parts of the tubular system and the cortical parts of the collecting duct system are concentrated together in the segments of cortex virtually devoid of glomeruli; these segments are inaccurately called **medullary rays**.

Such zoning divides the cortex into lobules. Each lobule is the segment of cortex between adjacent interlobular arteries and has a medullary ray at its centre.

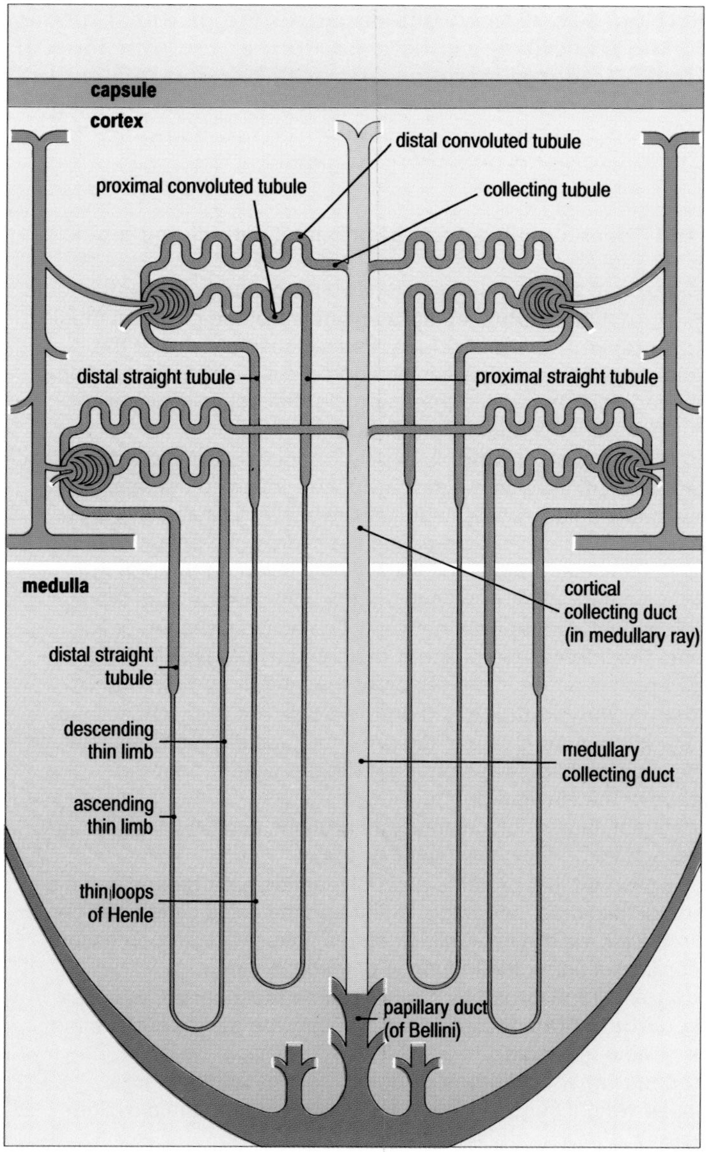

Fig.16.16 Tubular and collecting system of the nephron.
The first part of the tubular system is the **proximal tubule**, which is a continuation of Bowman's capsule and initially pursues a convoluted course (the **proximal convoluted tubule**), remaining close to the glomerulus from which it arises.

The proximal tubule then straightens and descends towards the medulla (**proximal straight tubule**, or the **thick descending limb of the loop of Henle**), merging with a thin-walled part of the tubular system (**thin limb of the loop of Henle**). This runs down in the cortex, and then in the medulla, towards the papillary tip (**descending thin limb**). It then loops back on itself (**ascending thin limb**) and re-enters the cortex. The wall then becomes thicker, forming the straight segment of the distal tubule (the **thick ascending limb of the loop of Henle** or the **distal straight tubule**).

In the cortex, close to the glomeruli, the distal tubule becomes convoluted (**distal convoluted tubule**), and empties into a collecting tubule, which in turn empties into a collecting duct lying within a medullary ray.

The collecting ducts descend into the medulla where a number of collecting ducts converge to produce large diameter ducts in the papillae (**papillary ducts** or **ducts of Bellini**). These ducts open into the calyces at the tips of the papillae, the concentration of the openings producing a sieve-like surface appearance to the papillary tip (the **area cribrosa**).

The length of the various components of the tubular system varies, mainly according to the location of the glomerulus from which each is derived. The main variation in length occurs in the thin ascending and descending limbs of the loop of Henle. The proximal convoluted tubule is longer than the distal convoluted tubule.

283

Proximal tubule

In the proximal tubule there is extensive reabsorption of various components of the glomerular filtrate (Fig. 16.17).

The cells that line the proximal tubule are continuous with the cells lining Bowman's capsule, and there is an abrupt transition of cell form at the tubular pole of the glomerulus.

Proximal tubule cells are cuboidal or columnar, and have a centrally placed nucleus and a well developed luminal brush border composed of numerous closely packed microvilli about 1 μm in length. At the base of the microvillous brush border are pinocytotic vesicles which lie close to lysosomes. Each cell rests on a basement membrane, which is continuous with the basement membrane of Bowman's capsule.

The basal membrane of each tubule cell shows extensive basal interdigitation and some lateral interdigitation, which makes the lateral borders irregular and difficult to define except apically, where the intercellular space is sealed off from the tubule lumen by a tight junction (Fig. 16.18).

Although the lateral intercellular space of proximal tubule cells is narrow and difficult to define throughout its length from apex to base, it is often easy to distinguish points where the space is distended into roughly spherical saccules.

In the lower half of each proximal tubule cell, numerous elongated mitochondria are closely associated with the basal interdigitations from adjacent cells and are arranged in parallel with the interdigitating basal cytoplasmic membranes.

The membrane and cytoplasmic specializations are most developed in the convoluted part of the proximal tubule. In the straight descending portion, as the thin loop of Henle is approached, the microvilli become smaller and less numerous, the degree of basal and lateral interdigitation less marked, and mitochondria and lysosomes fewer. The cells also become more cuboidal.

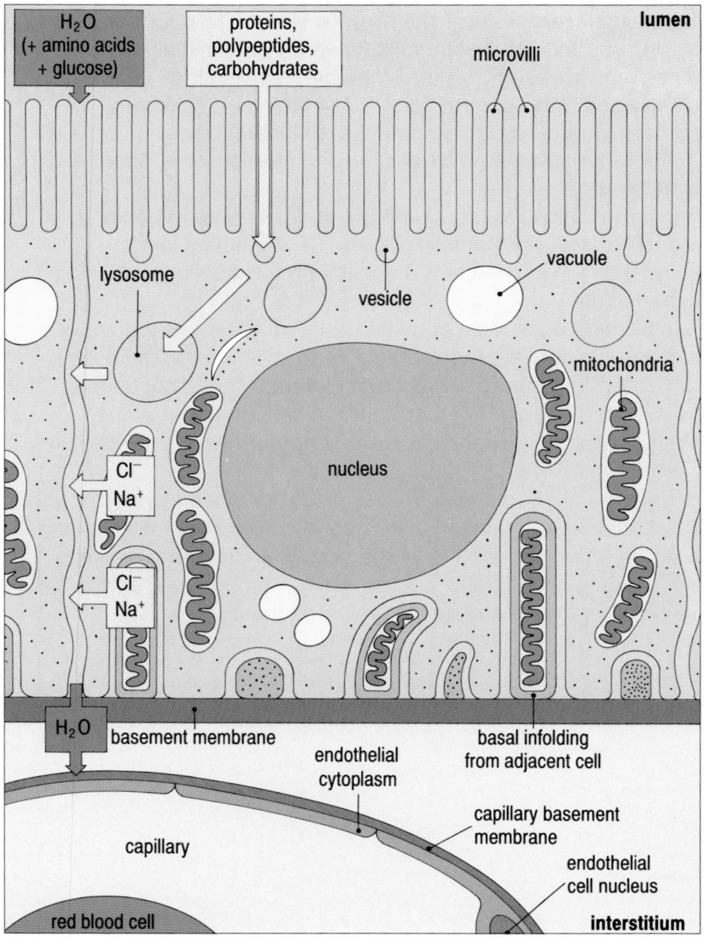

Fig. 16.17 Functional aspects of proximal convoluted tubule cells.

In the proximal tubule there is extensive reabsorption of components of the glomerular filtrate. The apical microvilli of the proximal tubule cells provide an immense surface area for absorption, and the mitochondria, which are particularly numerous and prominent in the convoluted portion, provide the energy for the active transport of various components against gradients.

The reabsorption of **water** is largely a secondary osmotic consequence of the active transport of Na^+ ions into the lateral spaces between adjacent tubule cells, which is followed by passive diffusion of Cl^- ions. This increases the hydrostatic pressure in the lateral intercellular space, and watery fluid is forced through the tubule basement membrane into the interstitial tissue, and thence into the peritubular capillary network. The active transport of Na^+ ions into the intercellular space is mediated by the Na^+/K^+ ATPase pump, which is active in the region of the lateral cell membranes.

Proteins, polypeptides and **amino acids** are also reabsorbed from the glomerular filtrate in the proximal tubule region. Soluble amino acids probably pass through with the water under the influence of the Na^+ ion pump.

In contrast, large molecular weight proteins and polypeptides are reabsorbed by endocytosis (see Fig. 2.4).

It is presumed that proteins and polypeptides are broken down by lysosomal enzymes (see page 16) into amino acids, which then enter the circulation via the intercellular space, interstitial support tissue and capillaries under the influence of the Na^+ pump.

Glucose is reabsorbed by the Na^+ pump mechanism, whereas **larger carbohydrate** molecules may follow the same route as the larger protein molecules.

Enzymes capable of breaking down proteins and the larger molecular weight sugars can be demonstrated at the microvillous surface.

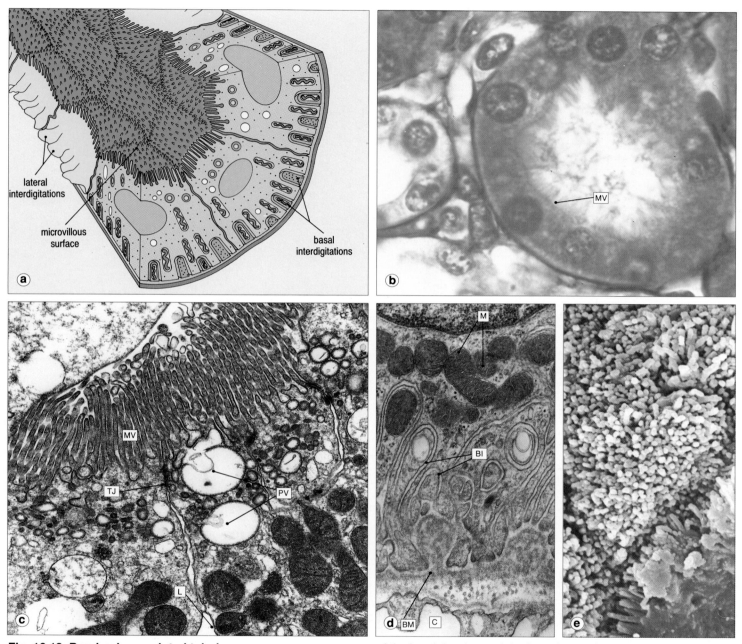

Fig. 16.18 Proximal convoluted tubule.

a Diagram showing the microvillous surface, the complex basal interdigitations, and the lateral interdigitations of proximal convoluted tubule cells.

b High power micrograph showing the microvillous (Mv) brush border lining the lumen of the Azan stained proximal tubule.

c High power electronmicrograph of the microvillous brush border (Mv) and the system of pinocytotic vesicles (PV).

Note the tight junction (TJ) joining adjacent cells near the base of the brush border, and the lateral saccular space (L) between adjacent cells.

d Electronmicrograph showing the system of basal interdigitations (BI) at the site of attachment of the proximal convoluted tubule cell to its basement membrane (BM). Note the abundant large mitochondria (M) and the proximity of an interstitial capillary (C).

e Scanning electronmicrograph of the lumen of a proximal convoluted tubule showing the complex microvillar system.

Loop of Henle

Traditionally the loop of Henle is regarded as having thick descending and ascending components, and a thin walled part in between. It is better however to regard the thin walled part as a distinct functional and structural entity for the following two reasons.
• The thick descending and ascending components are ultrastructurally closely identifiable with the proximal and distal convoluted tubules respectively.
• The transitions between thick and thin tubules are abrupt, whereas the thick ascending and descending parts merge gradually with the proximal and distal convoluted tubules.

Thin limb of loop of Henle

The thin limbs of the loop of Henle vary in length; those associated with juxtamedullary glomeruli are long and extend deep into the medulla towards the papillary tip, whereas those associated with mid-cortical or subcapsular glomeruli extend only partway into the medulla. Thus thin Henle loops may be found in the cortex and medulla, and in the human kidney a few loops of Henle are located entirely within the cortex.

The thin limbs, both ascending and descending, have flat lining epithelium showing very little cytoplasmic specialization (Fig. 16.19). At its simplest, the thin loop resembles a dilated capillary by light microscopy and can be difficult to distinguish in routine paraffin sections.

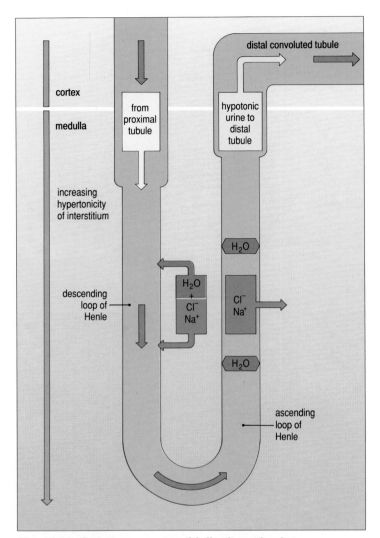

Fig. 16.20 Countercurrent multiplier hypothesis.
The descending thin loop of Henle is freely permeable to water, Na^+ and Cl^- ions, whereas the ascending thin limb actively pumps Cl^- ions out from the lumen into the interstitium and is impermeable to water; Na^+ ions follow the Cl^- ions to maintain ionic neutrality.

Thus the ascending limb pumps Na^+ and Cl^- ions out into the interstitium, but retains water within its lumen. Some of the Na^+ and Cl^- ions diffuse back into the tubular lumen at the descending thin limb but are pushed out again when they reach the ascending limb.

This produces the multiplier effect, and leads to hypertonicity of the interstitial tissue in relation to the fluid in the tubular lumen, particularly near the papillary tip. The fluid emerging from the end of the ascending limb of the loop of Henle into the distal tubule system is hypotonic.

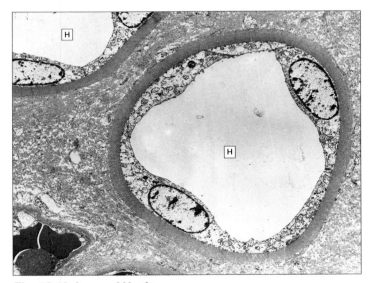

Fig. 16.19 Loop of Henle.
This electronmicrograph shows the structural simplicity of the thin loops of Henle (H) in the medulla.

In other areas however, the epithelium, though flat, is rather more prominent, and ultrastructurally has short microvilli and some of the basal and lateral interdigitations seen to a greater degree in proximal tubules. In some rodents this taller, more specialized epithelial pattern is consistently found in the descending thin limb of short-looped nephrons from more superficial glomeruli, but such consistent placement is not apparent in man.

Function. The thin limb of loop of Henle creates a gradient of hypertonicity from the cortico-medullary junction to the tip of the renal papilla, by the variable passage of sodium and chloride ions between the lumen of the Henle loop and the interstitium. It allows concentration of the urine in the collecting duct system as it passes through the medulla. The widely accepted hypothesis of this mechanism is called the countercurrent multiplier hypothesis (Fig. 16.20).

Distal tubule

The ascending thin limb of the loop of Henle opens into the short straight part of the distal tubule, which passes into the cortex running in a medullary ray, and then becomes convoluted before opening into the collecting tubule. At about the junction between the straight and convoluted parts, the distal tubule runs close to the glomerular hilum to form a specialized segment called the macula densa (see page 292).

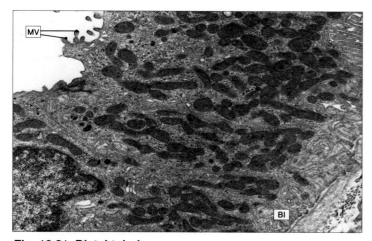

Fig. 16.21 Distal tubule.
Electronmicrograph showing the features of a distal convoluted tubule cell. Note that it exhibits similar basal interdigitations (BI) to those of the proximal convoluted tubule cell, but that the luminal microvilli (Mv) are scanty and poorly formed. Compare with Fig. 16.7

The distal tubule is lined by cuboidal epithelial cells with extensive basal and lateral interdigitations which are similar to those seen in the proximal tubule, but the microvilli on the luminal surface are less well formed and comparatively scanty (Fig. 16.21). Mitochondria are numerous and mainly situated close to the lateral and basal interdigitations. There are none of the luminal invaginations and vesicles seen close to the microvillar border in the proximal convoluted tubule.

The structure of the distal tubule is virtually identical in the convoluted and straight segments (ascending thick limb of loop of Henle), but the macula densa shows a local variation in structure.

Function. The distal tubule is crucial in the control of acid-base balance, and is also important in urine concentration.

As can be deduced from its rich mitochondrial content, the distal tubule cell has the ability to pump ions against concentration gradients.

In the distal tubule:
- sodium ions are reabsorbed from the dilute urine in the lumen and potassium ions are excreted;
- bicarbonate ions are reabsorbed and hydrogen ions are excreted, thus rendering the urine acidic.

These functions are dependent on the presence of the hormone **aldosterone**, a mineralocorticoid secreted by the adrenal cortex (see page 260).

Role of ADH. **Antidiuretic hormon**e(ADH), which is secreted by the posterior pituitary (see page 254), acts on the last part of the distal convoluted tubule to increase its permeability, thus permitting the absorption of water to produce a more concentrated urine.

ADH also acts on the collecting ducts in a similar manner, permitting the absorption of water from the duct lumen into the hypertonic interstitium, and thence into the blood system (vasa recta). This movement of water is dependent on the countercurrent exchanger system (see Fig. 16.25).

DIABETES INSIPIDUS

In the permanent absence of ADH, as occurs in the disease **diabetes insipidus**, vast volumes of dilute urine are formed because of the failure of water reabsorption at the distal convoluted tubule.

Fatal body water depletion is only prevented by drinking large quantities of water, which is stimulated by a constant feeling of thirst.

ABNORMALITIES OF TUBULAR FUNCTION

The renal tubular and duct system is almost entirely dependent for its oxygen supply on the integrity of the glomerular capillary network and the arterial vessels supplying the glomeruli, since they receive oxygen from the peritubular capillary networks, which are branches of the efferent arterioles leaving the glomeruli (see Fig. 16.4).

Thus the tubular epithelial cells can become significantly hypoxic if there is arterial or glomerular disease that reduces the blood flow into the efferent arterioles. For example, obliteration of the glomerular capillary lumina by proliferation of the lining endothelial cells (see Fig. 16.6) leads to impaired oxygenation of the tubular epithelial cells; the clinical and biochemical picture is however usually dominated by features resulting from retention of nitrogenous waste products and the increase in peripheral vascular resistance (acute nephritic syndrome, see page 278).

If such damage to the glomeruli persists, then the tubular epithelial cells become so depleted of oxygen that their enzyme systems and various pumping mechanisms are unable to function, and biochemical abnormalities develop as a result of the loss of the sensitive homeostatic mechanisms.

The most important biochemical abnormalities resulting from impaired tubular function are due to failure of excretion of H^+ and K^+ ions. The blood therefore contains a high concentration of H^+ ions (acidosis) and K^+ ions (hyperkalaemia). These, along with the retention of nitrogenous waste material due to failure of glomerular function, are features of **chronic renal failure** (see page 295).

Acute tubular necrosis

Failure of tubular function due to poor oxygenation can also occur in the absence of any significant disease of arteries or glomeruli. The most common cause is a central failure of blood circulation due to poor cardiac output, usually due to either low blood volume (hypovolaemia), for example, following massive blood loss through haemorrhage, or low blood pressure (hypotension), for example, following a myocardial infarction.

Poor perfusion through the peritubular capillary network leads to inadequate oxygen supplies for the tubular epithelial cells, and this leads to failure of enzyme systems and pump mechanisms, with consequent biochemical abnormalities, particularly acidosis and hyperkalaemia. Because the glomeruli are not being perfused with arterial blood at an adequate pressure, little filtration takes place, so the production of urine falls or may even cease (oliguria and anuria, respectively). The syndrome of **acute renal failure** comprises:

- oliguria or anuria (partial or total cessation of urine production);
- hyperkalaemia (raised K^+ ion level in the blood);
- acidosis (raised H^+ ion level in the blood).

When the tubular failure is due to a central cause such as hypovolaemia or hypotension, the tubular epithelial cells degenerate (Fig. 16.22), their histological appearance being due to accumulation of water within the cytosol.

If hypovolaemia or hypotension are treated promptly, tubular epithelial cells can recover normal structure and function, but if they persist, the tubular epithelial cells die (**acute tubular necrosis**). Loss of large numbers of tubular epithelial cells is not irrevocable; if adequate oxygenation is reestablished, the tubules become repopulated with epithelial cells.

In renal transplants, the tubular epithelial cells of the donor kidney die almost immediately after the kidney is removed. When the kidney is transplanted (usually many hours after its removal) and its arterial supply is reestablished, the tubules are eventually repopulated with functioning epithelial cells, and normal homeostatic control is regained.

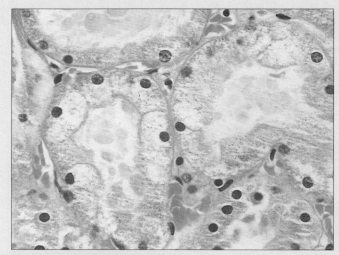

Fig. 16.22 Acute tubular damage.
Micrograph of an H&E stained paraffin section from a patient with early acute renal failure.

The proximal convoluted tubule epithelium shows early degenerative changes resulting from inadequate oxygenation following a prolonged fall in blood pressure. The individual cells are swollen with water as a result of failure of the Na^+/K^+ ATPase pump at the lateral walls of the cells, leading to inadequate excretion of water into the interstitium. Note that the microvilli are largely lost. Compare with Fig. 16.18.

COLLECTING TUBULES AND DUCTS

The convoluted segment of the distal tubule opens into the collecting system of tubules and ducts. This transition is not abrupt as there is a variable segment (sometimes called the **connecting segment**) where the epithelial lining contains both distal tubule and collecting tubule cell types in an apparently random fashion.

The collecting tubule (Fig. 16.23) is lined by two types of cell: **clear cells** (the majority) and **intercalated dark cells**.

• The clear cells are cuboidal or rather flat in the proximal part of the collecting system, and have light, poorly staining cytoplasm, which contains few cytoplasmic organelles, (mainly randomly arranged small round mitochondria). Basal membrane infoldings are present in the proximal part of the collecting system but become less apparent further along, while microvilli are short and sparse.

• The intercalated or dark cells are richer in cytoplasmic organelles, possessing numerous mitochondria. Their luminal surface has a well-developed microvillar system, with vesicles in the cytoplasm at the base of the microvilli. There are normally no basal infoldings.

The collecting tubules in the cortex pass towards the medullary rays, and open into collecting ducts which run vertically within the rays into the medulla. All of the medullary collecting ducts merge near the papilla to form large straight papillary ducts, which run to the tip of the papilla where they open out into the pelvicalyceal system.

The collecting ducts are lined initially by epithelium that is identical in type to that of the collecting tubules. As they pass down the medullary rays and into the medulla however, the number of intercalated dark cells decreases and the clear cells become progressively taller and more prominent, so that as the papilla is approached, the ducts are lined by regular straight-sided columnar clear cells (Fig. 16.24).

In humans, the basement membrane of the collecting duct system becomes progressively thicker as it nears the papillary tip. This feature becomes exaggerated with age.

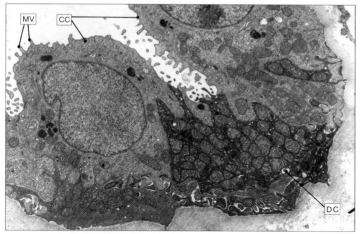

Fig. 16.23 Collecting tubule.
Electronmicrograph of collecting tubule, which connects the end of the distal convoluted tubule and the collecting duct in the medullary ray of the cortex. Note the intercalated dark cell (DC), which is rich in mitochondria, and the sparse, short microvilli (Mv) of the clear cells (CC).

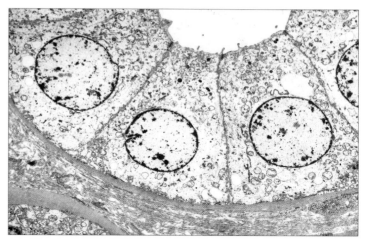

Fig. 16.24 Collecting duct.
Electronmicrograph of a large collecting duct in the medulla. Note the lining of regular cuboidal or columnar clear cells and the sparsity of organelles.

Functions of collecting tubules and ducts. The collecting tubules and ducts are not solely conduits for the transfer of urine into the pelvicalyceal system, but play an important role in the final concentration of the urine. This is achieved by interplay between the collecting tubules and ducts, the interstitium and the vasa recta, to produce a countercurrent exchanger system (Figs 16.25 & 16.26).

Role of ADH. Controlled water transport is made possible by the variable permeability of the collecting duct under the influence of ADH (see page 287). The amount of ADH released depends on the body's requirement for water excretion or retention.

In the presence of high levels of ADH, water is lost from the collecting duct lumen into the interstitium from where it passes into the blood circulation via the ascending vasa recta. This results in the production of a small amount of highly concentrated urine. When low levels of ADH are present, water remains within the collecting duct lumen and is lost in the form of copious dilute urine.

Role of vasa recta. The vascular networks of the vasa recta also play a role in the concentration of urine in the medulla. On the descending (arterial) side of the looped vessels, the walls are permeable to water and salts; water passes out into the interstitium, and sodium and chloride ions pass in. Thus, blood in the vasa recta is more or less in equilibrium with the hypertonic medullary interstitium.

On the ascending (venous) side of the vascular loop, sodium and chloride ions pass from the vessel lumen to the interstitium, and water is reabsorbed into the venous blood from the interstitium.

DISORDERS OF COLLECTING DUCTS

The most important disorders of the collecting ducts are:
- **infection**, which usually results from the ascent of bacteria into the kidney from an infection in the bladder;
- **papillary necrosis**, in which the tips of the papillae undergo necrosis and drop off;
- **deposition of insoluble crystals**, which may occur in gout (urate crystals) or in hypercalcaemia (calcium crystals).

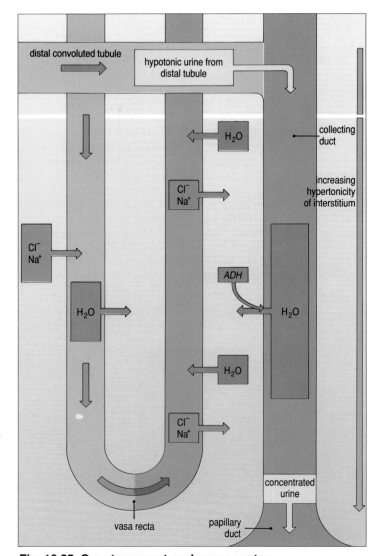

Fig. 16.25 Countercurrent exchanger system.
Dilute urine in the collecting tubule and duct system is progressively concentrated by the osmotic transfer of water from the lumen into the hypertonic medullary interstitial tissue, from whence it is reabsorbed into the vasa recta. The hypertonicity is due to the high concentration of Na^+ and Cl^- ions in the medulla resulting from the countercurrent multiplier activity of the loops of Henle. Thus an increasingly concentrated urine is produced.

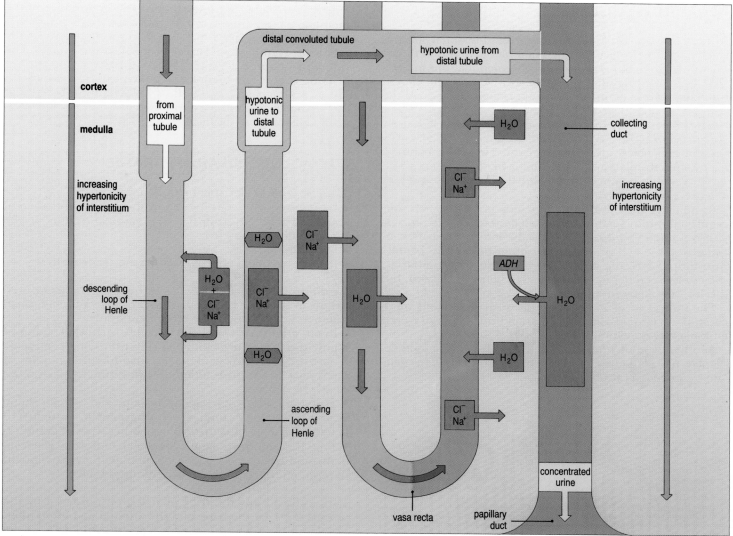

Fig. 16.26 Interrelationships between countercurrent multiplier and exchanger systems.

Movement of water and ions across the walls of the thin loops of Henle (countercurrent multiplier, see Fig. 16.20) creates a hypertonic milieu in the interstitium, the tonicity increasing progressively as the tip of the papilla is approached.

The resulting hypertonicity of the interstitium encourages the absorption of water from the dilute urine passing down the collecting duct (countercurrent exchanger, see Fig. 16.25). The amount of water absorbed, and hence the final concentration of the urine excreted, is controlled by the level of circulating antidiuretic hormone (ADH), which alters the collecting duct permeability to water.

RENAL INTERSTITIUM

In the cortex of the human kidney the interstitial space is small and largely occupied by small blood vessels and lymphatics (Fig. 16.30). However, in the medulla, the interstitium becomes a significant component, both in bulk and in function, increasing in size and importance as the tip of the papilla is neared (Figs 16.35 & 16.36).

Ultrastructurally, the medullary interstitium is largely composed of loose electron-lucent acellular material, partly protein and partly glycosaminoglycans, in which collagen fibres, lipid droplets and basal lamina-like material are scattered. Variable numbers of interstitial cells are also present (Fig. 16.27).

In humans, the most frequently seen interstitial cell is irregular in outline with narrow stellate cytoplasmic processes extending in all directions into the interstitial matrix. In rodents, these cell processes can often be seen to contact thin loops of Henle and adjacent medullary capillaries, sometimes seeming to act as a bridge between the two, but this is rarely apparent in man.

The cytoplasm of interstitial cells in man contains mitochondria, lysosomes, lipid droplets and small runs of rough endoplasmic reticulum.

Another type of interstitial cell, which is often spindle shaped and contains abundant rough endoplasmic reticulum, resembles a fibroblast.

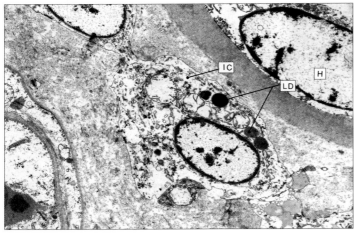

Fig. 16.27 Medullary interstitial cell and matrix.
Electronmicrograph showing a typical human medullary interstitial cell (IC), located in the loose matrix near to the loop of Henle (H). The characteristic cytoplasmic feature is the presence of electron-dense spherical lipid droplets (LD), but there is abundant rough endoplasmic reticulum and a few mitochondria.

Function of medullary interstitium. The importance of the medullary interstitium in salt and water homeostasis has already been described in relation to the functions of the loops of Henle, vasa recta and collecting ducts. The function of the interstitial cells is however not known. Although the renal medulla is known to be an important site of prostaglandin synthesis, it is currently believed that the epithelial cells of the collecting ducts, and not the interstitial cells, are responsible.

JUXTAGLOMERULAR APPARATUS

The juxtaglomerular apparatus comprises:
- renin-producing cells located in the walls of the afferent and efferent arterioles at the vascular hilum of the glomerulus;
- lacis cells;
- the macula densa area of distal tubule (Fig. 16.28).

Renin-producing cells. In man, these are concentrated mainly in the walls of the afferent arteriole, although small numbers are present in the efferent arteriole.

Renin-producing cells have the ultrastructural features of highly specialized myoepithelial cells with some contractile filaments. They also contain neuroendocrine granules of many shapes and sizes although two distinct types can be clearly recognized.
- Type I granules are irregular in shape and contain rhomboidal crystalline bodies (**protogranules**) which are believed to be the precursors of the other types of granules.
- Type II granules are larger, spherical, uniformly electron-dense and have an ill-defined membrane; they are thought to represent the **mature renin-secreting granules**.

Lacis cells occupy the triangular region bordered by the macula densa at the base, and the afferent and efferent arterioles at the sides; the apex is formed by the base of the glomerular mesangium. Lacis cells have a network (lacis) of thin interwoven processes, which are separated by an acellular matrix of basement membrane-like material.

Because of their apparent continuity with the glomerular mesangium at the vascular pole of the glomerulus, these cells have also been called **extraglomerular mesangial cells**. Their function is not known.

The macula densa is a specialized zone of the distal tubule where it is in close contact to the vascular hilum of the glomerulus.

In this region the epithelial cells of the distal tubule are taller and more tightly packed than elsewhere in the tubule, and the nuclei lie closer to the luminal surface; the Golgi is located between the nucleus and the basement membrane.

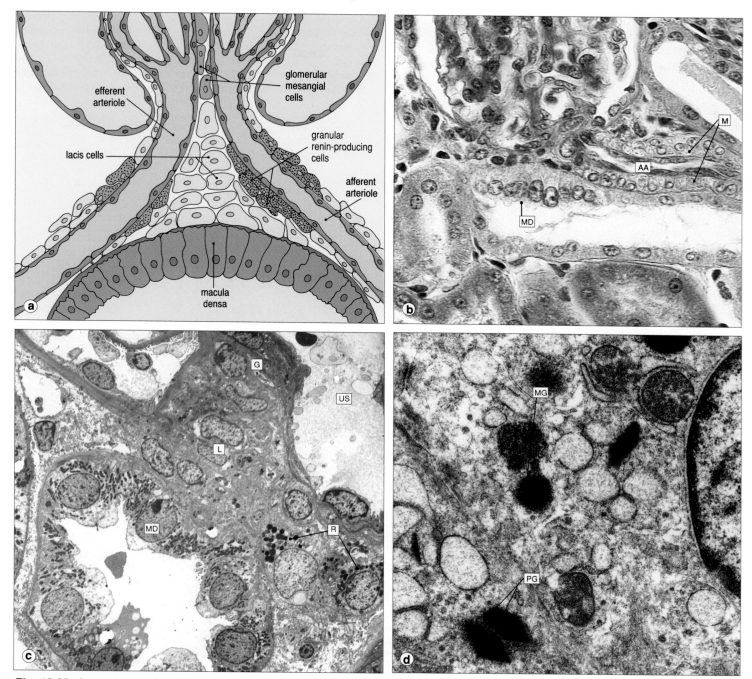

Fig. 16.28 Juxtaglomerular apparatus.

a Diagram of the juxtaglomerular apparatus, which consists of the macula densa, lacis cells, and the afferent and efferent arterioles. Within the walls of the arterioles are granular renin-secreting cells.
b Masson trichrome stain showing the macula densa (MD) and afferent arteriole (AA) with prominent muscle cells (M) containing renin granules.

The efferent vessel and lacis cells are not visible in this section.
c Electronmicrograph of human juxtaglomerular apparatus. Note the macula densa (MD), renin-producing cells (R), lacis cells (L), glomerular mesangial cells (G), and urinary space (US).
d High power electronmicrograph of the renin-secreting granular cells in the afferent arteriole wall. Note the protogranules (PG) (Type I) and mature granules (MG) (Type II).

The precise function of this specialized zone of distal tubule is not known but it may act as a sensor, regulating juxtaglomerular function by monitoring sodium and chloride ion levels in the distal tubule lumen.

Renin produced in the juxtaglomerular apparatus catalyses the conversion of inactive **angiotensinogen**, an α-2 globulin produced in the liver, to the decapeptide **angiotensin I**. Angiotensin I is then converted to **angiotensin II**, which stimulates the secretion of **aldosterone** by the zona glomerulosa of the adrenal cortex (see page 260).

Aldosterone is a mineralocorticoid hormone which regulates body sodium and potassium ion levels through its effect on the sodium pump mechanism at cell membranes.

In the distal tubule of the kidney, aldosterone promotes the reabsorption of sodium ions and water from the glomerular filtrate (Fig.16.29), and thereby contributes to the maintenance of plasma volume and blood pressure.

Control of renin secretion

Two possible mechanisms have been proposed for the feedback control of renin synthesis and release; it is probable that both may operate.
• One proposal is that the macula densa cells monitor the sodium concentration (or some other parameter) in the distal tubule lumen contents, and effect some form of control over renin release by the granulated juxtaglomerular cells in the arteriole walls.
• The other postulated mechanism is that the juxtaglomerular cells act as sensory receptors by monitoring arteriolar stretching caused by an increase in blood volume.

Erythropoietin synthesis

Another function which has been ascribed to the juxtaglomerular apparatus in the past is the synthesis of the erythrocyte-stimulating hormone, **erythropoietin,** but there is no substantial evidence for this, other than the proven neuroendocrine function of the apparatus.

Despite the application of modern techniques, the precise site of erythropoietin formation within the kidney remains a mystery. Based on tissue culture studies, claims have been made for its synthesis by mesangial cells, but gene probe analysis seems to indicate that erythropoietin messenger RNA is confined to the cortical tubules and interstitium.

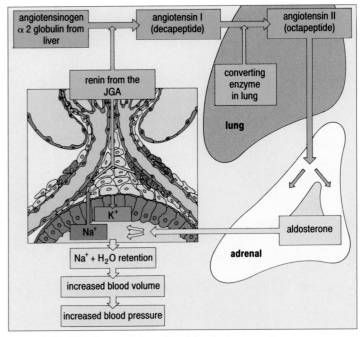

Fig. 16.29 Renin-angiotensin-aldosterone system.
Renin secreted by the juxtaglomerular apparatus (JGA) catalyses the production of angiotensin I from its inactive precursor, angiotensinogen. Angiotensin I is then converted in the lung into the active octapeptide, angiotensin II, which stimulates the release of aldosterone from the adrenal cortex. Aldosterone mediates the absorption of sodium and water from the glomerular filtrate at the distal tubule.
The feedback control of renin secretion is not known.

KIDNEY FAILURE

Since the blood circulatory system in the kidney is its most important component, it is not surprising that many renal diseases are the result of abnormalities in this system. Common vascular diseases, such as systemic hypertension, diabetes mellitus and atherosclerosis, frequently damage the kidney leading to impaired excretory and homeostatic functions.

Chronic renal failure

Decreased blood flow through the glomerular capillary system because of thickening of the arterial and arteriolar walls, and the consequent reduction in the lumina of these vessels, produces chronic ischaemia of the tubular system and reduces glomerular filtration. If prolonged, this leads to disuse shrinkage of the components of the glomerulus (**glomerular hyalinization**), and atrophy of the tubules (Fig.16.30). When these changes affect most of the glomeruli and their associated tubular systems, all of the functions of the kidney are impaired, and the patient develops symptoms of **chronic renal failure**.

Failure of the kidney's excretory function leads to retention in the blood of toxic metabolic waste materials, particularly urea and creatinine, from the endogenous breakdown of body protein; this is called **uraemia**, and the accumulation of urea and creatinine can be measured chemically. Eventually, without treatment, this intoxication leads to coma, fitting, and death. Failure of homeostatic functions carried out by the renal tubules leads to a loss of control of the body's water and electrolyte concentration, and hydrogen and potassium ions accumulate in the blood producing **acidosis** and **hyperkalaemia**, respectively.

The kidneys are unable to produce a urine with a concentration or dilution commensurate with the body's needs. Instead a urine of constant specific gravity is produced, irrespective of the degree of haemoconcentration or haemodilution.

These biochemical disorders are the result of a slow inexorable destruction of all of the activities of all nephrons, hence the name chronic renal failure, and the condition is irreversible.

Acute renal failure

In **acute renal failure**, there is a sudden transient cessation of all nephron activity, which is usually due to sudden damage to all tubules, or all glomeruli, or both. Depending on the cause, some recovery is usually possible if the patient can be sustained through the period of intense metabolic upset whilst the nephrons are inactive.

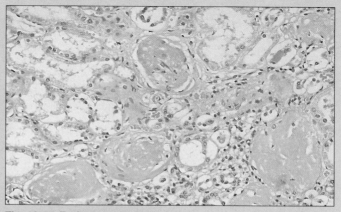

Fig. 16.30 End-stage kidney.
This H&E section shows the kidney from a patient with long-standing chronic renal failure due to progressive disease of the renal arterial supply. Little remains of the normal structure of the nephron. The glomeruli have been converted into acellular spheres containing no capillary network, and the tubules have atrophied, the epithelial cells being flattened or cuboidal.

PRACTICAL HISTOLOGY

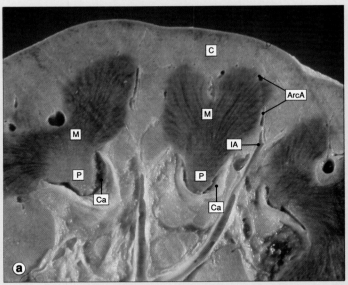

Fig. 16.30 Anatomy of adult kidney.

a Photograph of sectioned adult kidney, which has been fixed in formalin and the near natural colour restored in alcohol. Note the cortex (C), the medullary pyramid (M) culminating in the papillary tip (P), which protrudes into the lumen of a calyx (Ca). Interlobar arteries (IA) and arcuate arteries (ArcA) can also be seen. Little detail of cortical structure is visible with the naked eye, but the vertical linearity of the components of the medulla is highlighted by clusters of prominent blood vessels (vasa recta).

b In this H&E stained paraffin section prepared from the tissue block shown in **a**; the distinction between cortex (C) and medulla (M) can be easily seen. This section also shows the vertical linearity of the components of the medulla, both tubules and vessels.

At this low magnification, glomeruli can be seen as small dots in the cortex. Note that some areas of the cortex are free of glomeruli, but contain vertically running duct systems; these areas are known as medullary rays and represent the sites where cortical tubules drain into the collecting ducts.

c In this micrograph of cortex at a higher magnification than in **b** it can be seen that the medullary ray (MR) area is devoid of glomeruli and that the interlobular arteries (ILA) run in the glomeruli-rich area.

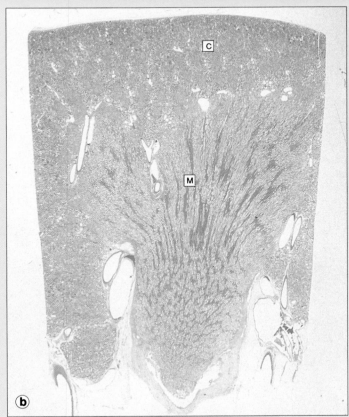

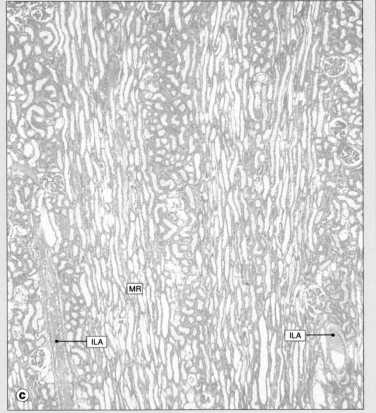

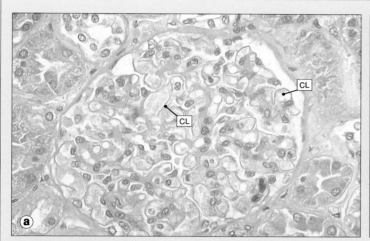

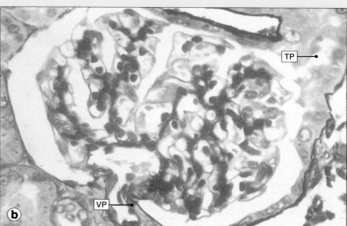

Fig. 16.31 Glomerulus.

a The details of the structure of the glomerular tuft are not easily seen in routine paraffin sections without the assistance of special stains to delineate capillary basement membranes. In this high power micrograph occasional capillary lumina (CL) can be seen, but it is difficult to distinguish clearly between endothelial, mesangial and epithelial podocyte cells.

b A glomerulus stained by the Jones methenamine silver method to show the mesangium and capillary basement membranes. Clear delineation of the capillary basement membrane permits the recognition of endothelial cells (inside the membrane) and epithelial podocytes (outside the membrane). Note that this fortuitous section shows both the vascular (VP) and tubular (TP) poles.

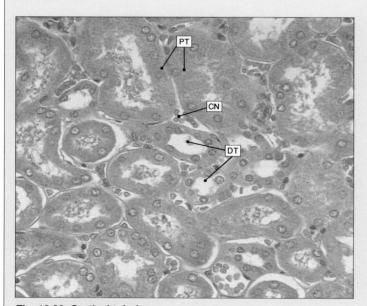

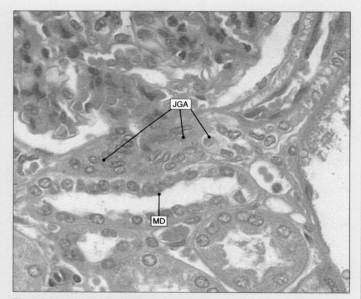

Fig. 16.32 Cortical tubules.

In this high power micrograph of cortical tubules, the proximal tubules (PT) are most numerous and prominent, having tall epithelium and small lumina. Distal tubules (DT) are smaller, have a cuboidal epithelium and proportionately larger lumina. Note the intimate capillary network (CN). Collecting ducts on their way to the medullary ray, and thick and thin loops of Henle are also visible.

Fig. 16.33 Juxtaglomerular apparatus.

Any glomerulus sectioned through the vascular hilum may show part of the juxtaglomerular apparatus (JGA), though the detailed structure is rarely apparent. The most easily seen component in a paraffin section is the macula densa (MD), and the afferent and efferent arterioles are sometimes visible. Without the assistance of special stains, the juxtaglomerular and lacis cells cannot be specifically identified

297

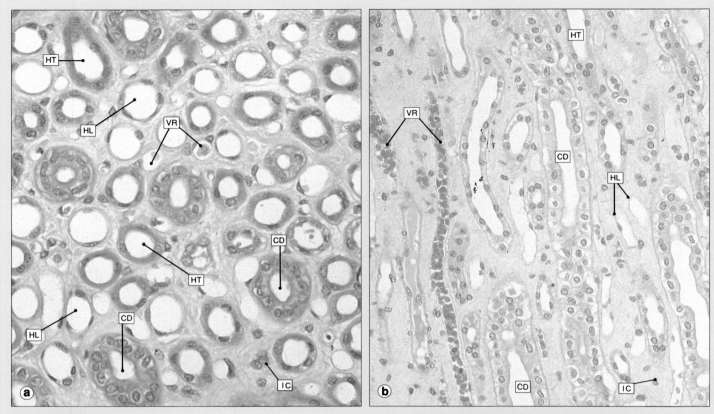

Fig. 16.35 Medulla.
In the medulla, all the various tubules, ducts and vessels run in the same direction towards the papillary tip. The appearance on histological examination depends on whether the section has been cut longitudinally to the axis of the tubules (in which case the tubules and ducts are cut in longitudinal section), or transversely. In most randomly selected tissue blocks, the section is usually oblique to the longitudinal plane of the medulla to a greater or lesser extent.

a In this micrograph of outer medulla, just below the cortico-medullary junction, the tubules and ducts are seen in transverse section. The outer medulla contains a mixture of thick descending and ascending portions of Henle loops (HT), which are histologically very similar to proximal and distal convoluted tubule, thin loops of Henle (HL), small collecting ducts (CD) and vasa recta (VR). In this region there is a small amount of interstitium in which a few interstitial cells (IC) can be seen.

b Micrograph of the same area of outer medulla shown in **a** sectioned almost longitudinally.

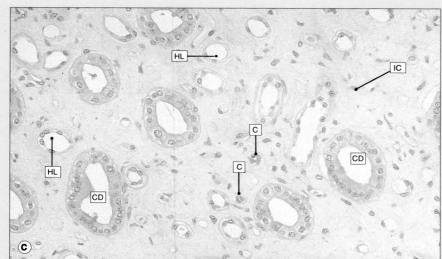

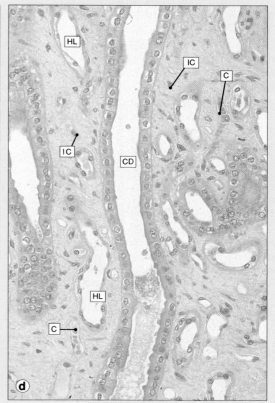

c In this micrograph of lower medulla note the difference in the content of tubules and ducts to that of outer medulla shown in **a** and **b**. There are now no thick portions of Henle loops, but thin Henle loops (HL) are numerous as are thin-walled capillaries (C).

The collecting ducts (CD) are larger and lined by distinct clear-celled cuboidal epithelium. The pale-staining interstitium now forms a substantial part of the bulk of the tissue, and scattered small stellate and spindle-shaped interstitial cells (IC) are numerous. In this micrograph the Henle loops, vessels and collecting ducts are in transverse section.
d Micrograph of same area of lower medulla shown in **c** sectioned longitudinally. Note the prominent straight collecting ducts running down towards the papilla; the nearer the tip of the papilla, the larger the ducts become.

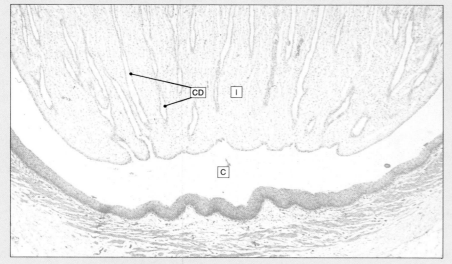

Fig. 16.36 Papilla.
The large collecting ducts (CD), are few in number as a result of fusion, and open into the calyx (C) at the papillary tip. At the papilla, the distal medulla consists almost entirely of large collecting ducts embedded in bulky interstitium (I), with very few thin Henle loops, and a number of vasa recta vessels. Interstitial cells are numerous.

Lymphatic drainage and nerve supply of the kidney

The lymphatic drainage of the cortex of the kidney is mainly by a series of lymphatics which run in parallel with the cortical blood vessels; the main channels follow the interlobular, arcuate and interlobar blood vessels and emerge at the kidney hilum. A minor lymphatic system runs in the renal capsule and receives small tributaries from the outer cortex. There is some communication between these two systems within the cortex.

The nerve supply to the kidney arises mainly from the coeliac plexus, and both adrenergic and cholinergic fibres have been demonstrated. In general, these nerves have been seen to follow the course of blood vessels throughout the cortex and the outer medulla.

The importance of the lymphatic drainage and nerve supply of the kidney for normal function is probably minimal, since both are destroyed during renal transplantation with no serious side-effects.

LOWER URINARY TRACT

The lower urinary tract is a functional rather than a geographical entity, since it extends from an intrarenal component high in the loins to the tip of the urethra. It comprises:

- the calyceal collecting system into which the large collecting ducts of Bellini in the medullary papillae disgorge the urine;
- the renal pelvis, which is the reservoir at the hilum of the kidney into which the various calyces pass the urine;
- the ureter, which is a long muscular tube that conducts the urine down to the bladder;
- the bladder, which acts as a major reservoir, holding the urine until there is sufficient for voiding at a convenient time and in socially acceptable circumstances;
- the urethra, through which the urine stored in the bladder is voided to the exterior.

These excretory passages have essentially the same basic structure, being hollow tubes with muscular walls. With the exception of part of the urethra, they are lined by a specialized epithelium that is capable of withstanding contact with a fluid of variable concentration containing a number of toxic substances. This specialized lining is a form of stratified epithelium known as **transitional epithelium** or, in this site, the **urothelium** (Fig. 16.37).

At various points there are sphincters capable of closing off parts of the lower urinary tract so that it can act as a reservoir. The most important of these muscular sphincters are located at the junction between the bladder and urethra, and are under voluntary control.

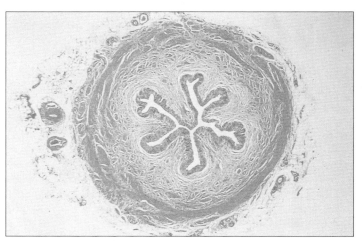

Fig. 16.37 Basic structure of lower urinary tract.
Low power micrograph of a transverse section of human ureter showing the basic structure of the lower urinary tract. The walls are muscular and there is an internal lining of specialized urothelium.

Urothelium

The **urothelium** is a multilayered epithelium which varies in thickness at various sites in the lower urinary tract. In the small calyces it is only 2–3 cell layers thick, but in the empty bladder it can usually be seen to contain up to 5 or 6 layers; presumably this reflects the different degrees of distension to which the two components are usually subjected. As these epithelial cells have the ability to stretch, shift on each other, and flatten, a distended bladder may appear to be lined by only a 2–3 cell layer of stretched flat cells.

In the non-distended state, urothelium has a rather compact cuboidal basal layer, polygonal-celled middle layers, and a surface layer composed of tall, rather columnar cells, which are often binucleate, with a convex luminal surface bulging into the lumen.

By light microscopy the luminal surface of urothelium often appears fuzzy in the undistended bladder, due to the relaxation of the complex and convoluted cell surface membrane (Fig. 16.38).

Ultrastructurally, the surface layer appears to be highly specialized. The luminal aspect of each cell is convoluted, with deep clefts running down into the cytoplasm, which also contains fusiform vesicles lined by cell membrane identical to that seen on the luminal surface (Fig. 16.39).

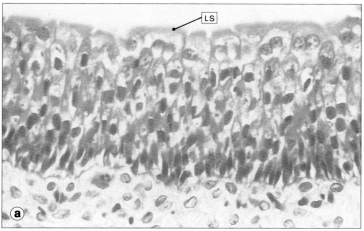

Fig. 16.38 Urothelium.
a High power micrograph showing the characteristic appearance of the H&E stained urothelium in the undistended state. When the lumen is distended with urine the cells flatten and form a thinner layer. Note the 5–6 layers, the occasional binucleate surface cell,

and the indistinct luminal surface (LS).
b Masson trichrome stain showing the lateral cell borders of urothelium and its stratified nature. Note the indistinct luminal membrane (LS).

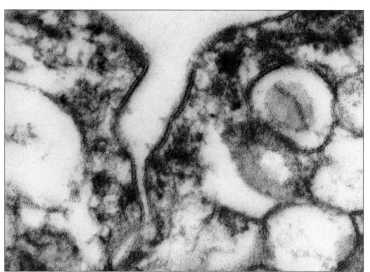

Fig. 16.39 Urothelial cell surface.
Electronmicrograph of a non-distended human bladder post mortem, showing something of the unique structure of the surface of the urothelial cell. The luminal surface shows areas of a three-layered cell membrane (**asymmetric membrane**), most clearly seen in the invagination forming **membrane plaques**.

The membrane has a central lucent lamina between a thick electron-dense outer lamina and a thinner dense inner lamina. Immediately beneath the surface, the cytoplasm contains numerous round or oval **vesicles (multilaminate vesicles)** lined by identical **trilaminar** membrane. These vesicles become incorporated onto the luminal surface by fusing with the frequent invaginations as the bladder fills and the surface urothelium stretches.

It is not yet clear whether all of these vesicles communicate with the lumen (i.e. represent clefts which have been sectioned obliquely) or whether they represent reserve segments of surface membrane which can be incorporated into the surface layer when the lumen is distended with urine and a greater surface area is required.

In conditions of distension, the tall cells of the surface layer become flattened and lose their convex apical bulge, and ultrastructurally the deep clefts and multilaminate vesicles largely disappear. Throughout most of the lower urinary tract the urothelium stands on a thin indistinct basement membrane supported by a variable layer of dense subepithelial support tissue which is mainly collagen (the lamina propria).

Beneath the lamina propria are the layers of smooth muscle which, in the pelvicalyceal system and ureters, are responsible for the peristaltic contractions forcing urine down into the bladder in one direction only.

301

Muscle layers

In the simple tubular ureter there appear to be two distinct layers of muscle: an inner longitudinal layer, and an outer circular layer (Fig. 16.37). However, three-dimensional studies suggest that both muscle layers are in fact helical arrangements, with a loosely spiralled internal helix and a more tightly spiralled outer helix (Fig. 16.40), which appear to be longitudinal and circular, respectively, when the ureter is sectioned transversely.

In the architecturally more complex pelvicalyceal system, and in the virtually spherical bladder, arrangement of the muscle layers is less clearly defined. Nevertheless the bladder is considered to have three muscle layers:
- an inner layer continuous with the inner longitudinal layer of the ureter;
- a middle layer continuous with the outer circular layer of the ureter;
- an additional outer layer in which the fibres run in approximately the same direction as the innermost layer (i.e. approximately longitudinal).

Since the bladder is roughly spherical instead of cylindrical, and the bladder musculature is, in any case, a distorted continuation of the helical arrangement seen in the ureter, the terms longitudinal and circular have little meaning.

The arrangement of muscle often appears rather haphazard in histological sections, except at the narrow bladder neck where the layers again become more distinct (Fig. 16.41).

Micturition

In the normal ureter, which is a narrow bore tube, urine is forced downwards by peristalsis so that none refluxes back towards the kidney. In the larger spherical bladder however this cannot be achieved, since the lumen of the fully distended reservoir is too big for a segment of it to be closed off by muscle contraction; thus when the bladder musculature contracts during micturition urine could reflux back up the open ureters, and damage the kidney.

Although there are no anatomical valves at the junction of the ureters and bladder, potentially damaging reflux is prevented by a physiological valve, which results from the oblique path by which the ureters enter the posterolateral wall of the bladder through the bladder wall musculature.

As the bladder distends and enlarges, the ureteric openings close, partly due to compression of the ureter lumen by extrinsic pressure from the musculature of the bladder wall, and partly by acute angulation at the site of opening produced by bladder distension.

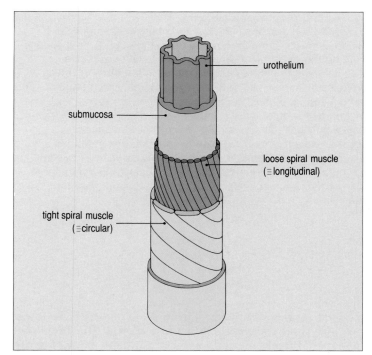

Fig. 16.40 Musculature of the lower urinary tract.
The arrangement of the muscle layers in the ureter is shown, emphasizing that the muscles are not truly circular and longitudinal, but are tight spirals and loose spirals, respectively.

urothelium

submucosa

loose spiral muscle
(≡ longitudinal)

tight spiral muscle
(≡ circular)

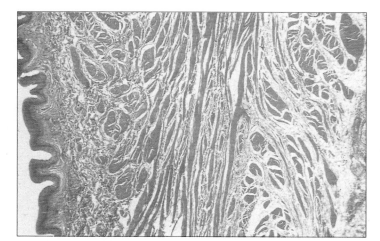

Fig. 16.41 Bladder wall.
Beneath the urothelium is a fibrocollagenous submucosal region. The bulk of the wall is composed of smooth muscle which is loosely organized into three layers. This arrangement is most clearly seen at the bladder neck, as in this micrograph.

At the junction between the bladder and the urethra is a muscular sphincter, the **internal sphincter**, which when closed permits the bladder to act as a reservoir of urine. When this sphincter relaxes micturition occurs.

Nerve supply

The bladder nerve supply is from the autonomic nervous system, and both sympathetic and parasympathetic nerves are found.
• Sensory fibres from the bladder transmit signals of the degree of bladder distension to the sacral spinal cord.
• Parasympathetic fibres ending in the muscles and adventitia of the bladder act as the effector nerves for micturition.
• Sympathetic nerves innervate the blood vessels to the bladder.

URETHRA

The urethra is the final conduit through which urine passes to the exterior and differs in the male and female.

Female

The human female urethra is short being approximately 5 cm long. It runs from the bladder and opens to the exterior in the midline of the genital vestibule just between the clitoris and superior border of the vaginal introitus.

The urethra is lined mainly by stratified squamous epithelium and its lamina propria contains many vascular channels as well as a few small mucus-secreting glands.

Although the urethral muscular wall is a continuation of the involuntary smooth muscle of the bladder, there is a sphincter, the **external sphincter**. This is composed of striated muscle and is under voluntary control; it is found around the mid-portion of the urethra where it passes through the striated muscles of the pelvic floor.

Male

The male urethra is 20–25 cms long and is more complex than the female urethra since it serves two purposes. Not only is it the final conduit of the urinary system, but it is also the terminal conduit of the male reproductive system (see Fig. 17.1). It can be divided into three segments: the prostatic urethra, the membranous urethra, and the penile urethra.
• The **prostatic urethra** begins at the bladder neck and runs through the prostate gland from which many peri-urethral glands open into it through short ducts. It also receives the openings of the ejaculatory ducts.
• The **membranous urethra** is the short segment (i.e. approximately 1 cm long), which runs through the pelvic floor muscles. This is the site of voluntary control of micturition since it is here that a sphincter, the **external sphincter**, of striated muscle surrounds the urethra.
• The **penile urethra** is the distal part of the urethra, and runs through the corpus spongiosum of the penis, opening to the exterior at the external meatus of the glans penis; small mucous glands, analogous to those in the female, open into the penile urethra.

The male urethra is lined proximally by transitional epithelium similar to that in the remainder of the lower urinary tract, but this becomes progressively less urothelial in character in the membranous and penile segments, where it changes to a rather unspecialized, pseudostratified, columnar epithelium. This finally changes to a stratified squamous epithelium at the distal penile urethra close to the external urinary meatus where the epithelium merges with the stratified squamous epithelium of the glans penis.

17. MALE REPRODUCTIVE SYSTEM

The male reproductive system is responsible for:
- production, nourishment and temporary storage of the haploid male gametes (**spermatozoa**);
- intromission of a suspension of spermatozoa (**semen**) into the female genital system;
- production of male sex hormones (**androgen**s).

Whereas the first two functions are important only during the years of sexual maturity, hormone production is required throughout life, even *in utero*.

The male genital system (Fig. 17.1) comprises:
- **testes,** which produce spermatozoa, and synthesize and secrete androgens;
- **epididymis, vas deferens**, **ejaculatory duct** and part of the male **urethra,** which form the ductal system responsible for the carriage of spermatozoa to the exterior;
- **seminal vesicles, the prostate gland and the bulbo-urethral glands** (**of Cowper**), which are secretory glands providing fluid and nutrients to support and nourish the spermatozoa, and forming the bulk of the semen;
- **penis,** which is an organ capable of becoming erect for insertion into the female vagina during sexual intercourse.

The testes, epididymis, and vas deferens are located in the scrotal sac, which is a skin covered pouch enclosing a mesothelial lined cavity continuous with the peritoneal cavity at the inguinal canal.

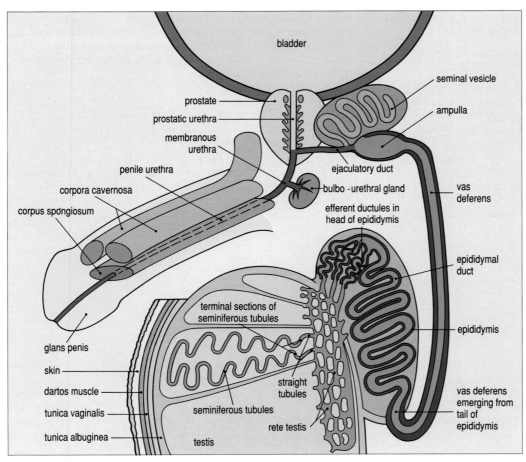

Fig. 17.1 Diagram of the male genital system.
Spermatogenesis occurs in the seminiferous tubules, and the resulting spermatozoa pass into the rete testis at the hilum (mediastinum) of the testis.

From the rete testis, spermatozoa are transported by about a dozen efferent ductules into the head of the epididymis, where the ductules fuse to form the single highly coiled epididymal duct. Within this duct they acquire their motility.

The spermatozoa then pass into a long straight tube, the vas deferens, which transports them from the scrotal sac into the short ejaculatory duct, receiving abundant secretions from the seminal vesicles.

The ejaculatory ducts from the right and left side run through the tissue of the prostate gland and open into the prostatic urethra.

Prostatic secretions and the secretions of the bulbo-urethral glands (of Cowper) accompany or precede the semen along the penile urethra.

TESTES

Anatomy and development

The testes are paired organs located outside the body cavity in a pouch of highly specialized skin, the scrotum (Fig. 17.2), which means that they are maintained at a temperature approximately 2–3°C below body temperature; this lower temperature is essential for normal spermatogenesis.

Embryologically, the testes develop high on the posterior abdominal wall and migrate to the scrotum, usually arriving there in the seventh month of intrauterine life. When the testes fail to migrate into the scrotum, they fail to produce spermatozoa (cryptorchidism).

Each mature adult testis is a solid ovoid organ, approximately 4–5 cm long, 3 cm deep and 2.5 cm wide, and usually weighs 11–17g. The right testis is commonly slightly larger and heavier than the left.

Each testis has epididymis (see page 311) attached to its posterior surface, and is suspended in the scrotal sac by the spermatic cord containing the vas deferens (see page 312), the arterial supply, and the venous and lymphatic drainage.

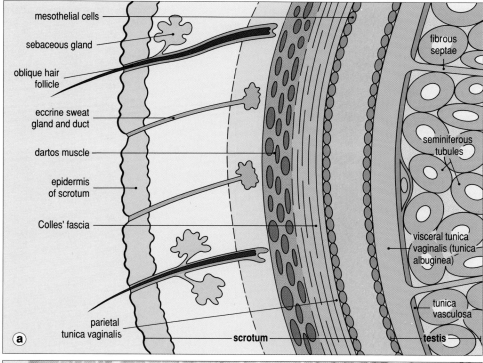

Fig. 17.2 Scrotum and tunica vaginalis.
a The scrotum is covered externally by skin with oblique hair follicles (producing curly hair) and numerous eccrine sweat glands.

In the deeper layers of the skin, smooth muscle fibres arranged in a rather haphazard manner form the poorly defined dartos muscle, contraction of which produces wrinkling of the scrotal skin.

Beneath the dartos muscle lies fibrocollagenous fascia (Colles' fascia), the deepest layer being compacted to form the dense parietal layer of tunical vaginalis, which is lined internally by flattened mesothelial cells similar to those lining the peritoneal cavity with which it is continous. This smooth mesothelial-coated parietal tunica vaginalis forms the inner layer of the scrotal sac, and is separated from the external surface of the testis by a potential space containing a watery fluid, which acts as a lubricant, allowing the testis to move smoothly within the scrotal sac without friction.

The testis is covered externally by a thick collagenous capsule, the visceral layer of the tunica vaginalis (the tunica albuginea), the outer surface being coated with flattened mesothelial cells. Beneath the tunica albuginea lies a narrow variable layer of loosely arranged collagen containing superficial blood vessels, and internal to this are the seminiferous tubules.
b Micrograph of the tunica albuginea of the testis. Note the scrotal cavity (C), the collagenous tunica albuginea (T) covered externally by small mesothelial cells, the narrow vascular layer (V), which is sometimes called the tunica vasculosa, and the seminiferous tubules (S).

The testis is completely enclosed by the tunica albuginea, which is thickened posteriorly to form the mediastinum of the testis, projecting some way into the body of the testis (see Fig. 17.3). Blood and lymphatic vessels, and the channels carrying spermatozoa pass through this area (rete testis, see page 312). Fibrous septa from the mediastinum divide the body of the testis (Fig. 17.3), into 250–350 lobules, each lobule containing 1–4 seminiferous tubules.

Seminiferous tubules

Each seminiferous tubule is approximately 150 µm in diameter, and 80 cm long. (It has been calculated that the combined total length of all of the seminiferous tubules in each testis is 300–900 m).

A seminiferous tubule is a coiled, unbranching closed loop, both ends of which open into a system of channels (the **rete testis**) at the posterior hilum of the testis, close to the mediastinum.

In a sexually mature man, each seminiferous tubule has a central lumen lined by an actively replicating epithelium, the **seminiferous** or **germinal epithelium**, mixed with a population of supporting (sustentacular) cells, the **Sertoli cells**.

The lining cells sit on a well defined basement membrane lying inside a collagenous layer containing fibroblasts and other spindle-shaped cells, which are contractile myoid cells, containing intermediate filaments and desmin, like smooth muscle cells. In some animals these myoid cells form a continuous peritubular layer and contract rhythmically, possibly propelling the non-motile spermatozoa towards the rete testis (spermatozoa only acquire their motility after

they have passed through the epididymis). In human testis, the myoid cells form a less distinct layer and are not usually circumferential.

The outer wall of the tubule, comprising basal lamina, collagen layer and myoid cell layer is sometimes called the **tunica propria**.

Blood vessels and clumps of hormone-producing **interstitial (Leydig) cells** are found in the interstices between adjacent seminiferous tubules (Fig. 17.4).

Germinal epithelium and spermatogenesis

The germinal epithelium lining the seminiferous tubules produces the haploid male gametes (spermatozoa) by a series of steps called, in sequence, spermatocytogenesis, meiosis and spermiogenesis (Fig. 17.5).

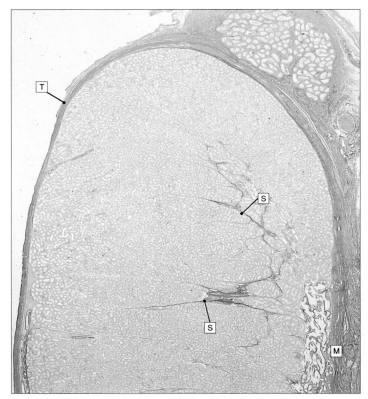

Fig. 17.3 Testis.
Low power micrograph of a sagittal section through testis stained by the van Gieson method, which stains collagen red. Note the tunica albuginea (T), which is thickened posteriorly to form the mediastinum testis (M). From the mediastinum, fibrous septae (S) enter the testis, separating it into lobules.

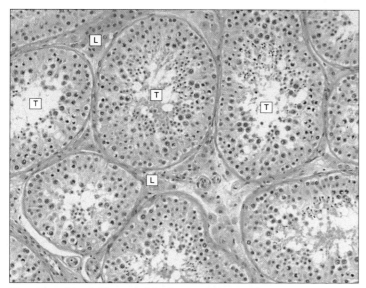

Fig. 17.4 Seminiferous tubules and interstitium.
Micrograph showing seminiferous tubules (T) cut in transverse, longitudinal and oblique section, lined by germinal epithelium and enclosed by tunica propria. In the interstices are blood vessels and clumps of Leydig (interstitial) cells (L).

Fig. 17.5 Spermatocytogenesis and meiosis.
Spermatocytogenesis begins with the development of spermatogonia of which three types are recognized: the type A dark (Ad) cell, the type A pale (Ap) cell, and the type B cell.

It is thought that the Ad cells are the precursor cells, which divide to produce new Ad cells and some Ap cells, the latter giving rise to type B cells, which subsequently pass through a meiotic phase to produce spermatocytes.

The B cells pass through several stages of maturation before the first meiotic division, and in these early stages are known as primary spermatocytes. The preleptotene cell is similar to the type B cell, but is not in contact with the basement membrane of the seminiferous tubule. The cell then undergoes its first meiotic division to produce a secondary spermatocyte, which is smaller than its parent primary spermatocyte, and has fine granular chromatin. This immediately undergoes a second meiotic division to produce the haploid spermatids from which the spermatozoa will develop.

The spermatids are located towards the lumen of the seminiferous tubule and have spherical central nuclei with finely granular chromatin and occasional larger chromatin masses. Their nuclear diameter is about half that of the primary spermatocytes from which they are derived.

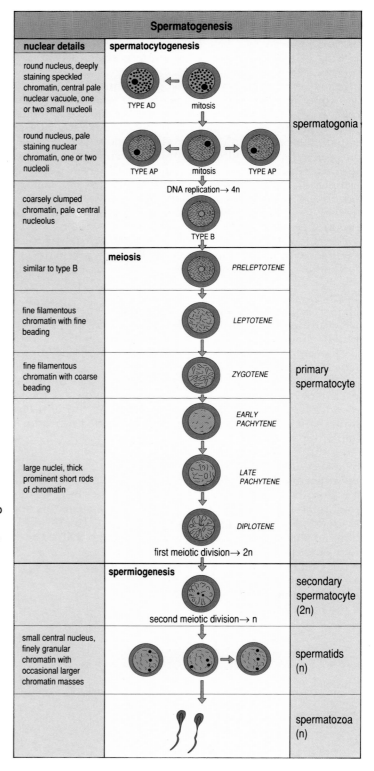

SPERMATOCYTOGENESIS

In **spermatocytogenesis** the stem cells (spermatogonia) undergo mitosis (see Fig. 2.23) to produce not only more spermatogonia, but also cells that differentiate into primary spermatocytes (Fig. 17.6).

In man, spermatogonia can be divided into three groups according to their nuclear appearances: **type A dark (Ad) cells**, **type A pale (Ap) cells**, and **type B cells**. It is thought that Type Ad spermatogonia are the stem cells of the system, their mitotic division producing more Type Ad cells and some Type Ap cells, which further replicate by mitosis to form clusters of daughter cells linked to each other by cytoplasmic bridges. These Type Ap spermatogonia mature into Type B cells, which divide mitotically to produce further Type B cells; these cells then mature in a cluster to produce primary spermatocytes.

Primary spermatocytes replicate their DNA shortly after their formation (i.e. they are 4n). Primary spermatocyte formation marks the end of spermatocytogenesis.

MEIOSIS

Meiosis is described on page 24. Primary spermatocytes pass through a long prophase lasting about 22 days, during which changing patterns of nuclear chromatin enable preleptotene, leptotene, zygotene, pachytene and diplotene stages to be identified (see Fig. 17.5).

The first meiotic division occurs after the late pachytene/diplotene stages, with the formation of diploid secondary spermatocytes, which rapidly (i.e. within a few hours) undergo the second meiotic division to produce haploid spermatids.

SPERMIOGENESIS

Spermiogenesis is the process by which haploid spermatids are transformed into spermatozoa. It can be divided into four phases, all of which occur while the spermatids are embedded in small hollows (see Fig. 17.6) in the free luminal surface of the Sertoli cells (see page 309). These four phases (Fig. 17.7) are:

• the Golgi phase;
• the cap phase;
• acrosome phase;
• the maturation phase.

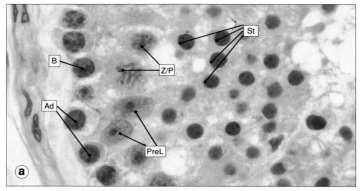

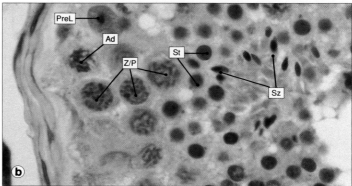

Fig. 17.6 Spermatocytogenesis and spermiogenesis in seminiferous tubule.

Spermatogenesis occurs in waves along the length of the seminiferous tubules, thus adjacent areas of the same tubule show spermatocytogenesis and spermiogenesis at various stages.

a Micrograph showing spermatogonia of various types including Ad and B types, and preleptotene (PreL), zygotene/pachytene (Z/P) stages of primary spermatocytes. Some spermatids (St) are also present.

b Micrograph showing a later stage in which there is spermiogenesis as well as spermatocytogenesis. Ad spermatogonia, preleptotene (PreL) and zygotene/pachytene (Z/P) stages of primary spermatocytes, and spermatids (St) are shown, as well as developing spermatozoa (Sz) embedded in Sertoli cell cytoplasm. Sertoli cells are poorly defined in light microscopic sections of human testis.

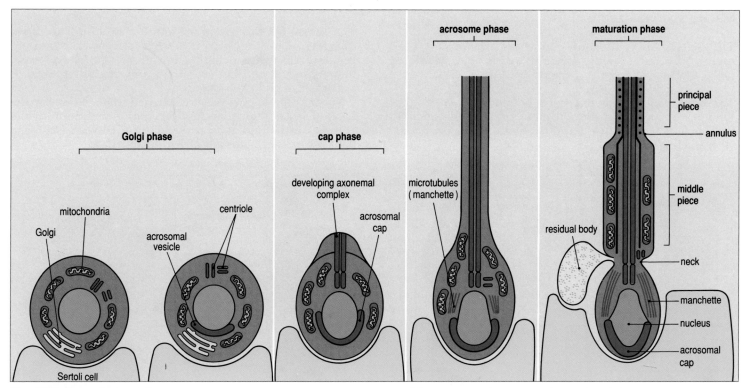

Fig. 17.7 Spermiogenesis.

In the **Golgi phase**, PAS-positive granules (pre-acrosomal granules) appear in the Golgi and fuse to form a membrane-bound acrosomal vesicle close to the nuclear membrane. This vesicle enlarges, and its location marks what will be the anterior pole of the spermatozoon.

The two centrioles migrate to the opposite (posterior) pole of the spermatid, the distal centriole becoming aligned at right angles to the cell membrane. It then begins the formation of the axoneme complex of the sperm tail.

In the **cap phase**, the acrosomal vesicle changes shape to enclose the anterior half of the nucleus and become the acrosomal cap. The nuclear membrane beneath the acrosomal cap thickens and loses its pores, and the nuclear chromatin becomes more condensed.

In the **acrosome phase**, the increasingly dense nucleus flattens and elongates; an anterior pole, capped by the acrosomal cap, and a posterior pole, closely related to the developing axonemal complex, can be identified. With the changed shape of the nucleus, the cytoplasm between the acrosomal cap and the anterior cell membrane migrates to the posterior part of the cell.

The entire cell orientates itself so that the anterior pole is embedded in the luminal surface of the Sertoli cell, pointing down towards the base of the seminiferous tubule; the cytoplasm-rich posterior pole of the spermatid protrudes into the tubule lumen. At the same time, a sheath of microtubules extends from the posterior part of the acrosomal cap towards the developing tail, and is called the **manchette**.

The centrioles (see Fig. 2.20), which have migrated posteriorly, form the neck of the developing spermatozoon, which is the connecting piece between the head (containing the nucleus and acrosomal cap) and the developing tail.

One centriole continues to synthesize the axonemal complex of the sperm tail, producing a regular tubular complex comprising two central microtubules surrounded by a ring of nine peripheral doublets. In the neck region, nine coarse fibres are produced, which extend down into the tail around the microtubules of the axonemal complex.

Prominent mitochondria aggregate in and below the neck to surround the nine coarse fibres; this forms the segment known as the middle piece. The mitochondria finish abruptly at a ring (annulus) demarcating the middle piece from the main parts of the tail (the principal piece and end piece).

The **maturation phase** is characterized by the pinching off of surplus cytoplasm, particularly from the neck and middle piece regions, and its phagocytosis by Sertoli cells. The immature spermatozoa then become disconnected from the Sertoli cell surface and lie free in the seminiferous tubule lumen, marking the end of spermiogenesis. The immature male gametes are later modified in the ductular systems leading to the penis.

The duration of spermatogenesis from spermatogonium type Ad to released immature spermatozoon is about 70 days.

Mature spermatozoon

The mature spermatozoon comprises a head and a tail region, the latter being composed of a neck, a middle piece, a principal piece and an end piece (Fig. 17.8).

The head, which is flattened and pointed, is composed of the nucleus covered by the acrosomal cap; the chromatin of the nucleus is condensed and broken only by occasional clear nuclear vacuoles.

The **acrosomal cap** covers the anterior two-thirds to three-quarters of the nucleus; it is a glycoprotein containing numerous enzymes including a protease, acid phosphatase, neuraminidase and hyaluronidase, and can be regarded as a specialized giant lysosome.

The acrosomal enzymes are released when the spermatozoon contacts the ovum, and facilitate penetration of the corona radiata and zona pellucida of the ovum (see page 336) by the spermatozoal nuclear head.

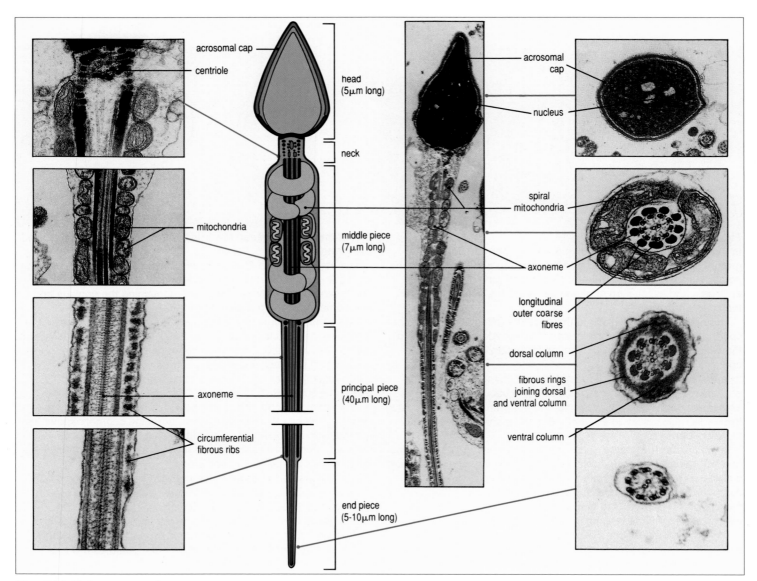

Fig. 17.8 Mature spermatozoon.
Diagram of a mature spermatozoon accompanied by electronmicrographs confirming its structure.

Neck. The proximal part of the tail is the neck. This is a short narrow segment containing the pair of centrioles and connecting piece, which forms the nine fibrous rings surrounding the axoneme.

Middle piece. The axoneme runs through the centre of the middle piece and is surrounded by the nine coarse longitudinal fibres from the connecting piece in the neck, and an outer zone of tightly packed elongated mitochondria. The lower limit of the middle piece is marked by a sudden narrowing sometimes associated with an annular thickening of the cell membrane, the annulus.

Principal piece. The principal piece is the longest part of the tail and comprises the axoneme surrounded by the nine coarse longitudinal fibres, which are in turn enclosed by numerous external sheath fibres orientated circumferentially. As one of the anterior and one of the posterior longitudinal fibres are fused with the circumferential fibres, the remaining seven fibres are distributed asymmetrically, four in one lateral compartment and three in the other.

End piece. At the junction between the principal piece and the short end piece, the longitudinal and circumferential fibres cease, thus the end piece is composed of axoneme only.

Sertoli cells

Sertoli cells are the main cell type until puberty, after which they comprise only about 10% of the cells lining the seminiferous tubules. In elderly men however, a decrease in the number of germinal epithelial cells is common, so Sertoli cells again become a significant component of the tubule cell population.

Sertoli cells are not affected by any of the factors that injure the sensitive germinal epithelium. For example, they do not degenerate when exposed to normal body temperature, and can therefore survive in the undescended testis.

The Sertoli cell is a tall columnar cell, which sits on a basement membrane with its irregular apex extending into the lumen of the seminiferous tubule (Fig. 17.9). Its nucleus is irregular with deep folds, but tends towards an oval shape, with the long axis at right angles to the basement membrane. The nucleus has a vesicular chromatin pattern and a prominent nucleolus.

The Sertoli cell outline is irregular, with many ramifying cytoplasmic extensions, which make contact with those from neighbouring Sertoli cells to form a meshwork of cytoplasm. This encloses the developing cells of the germinal epithelium and forms tight junctions (see Fig. 3.6), which roughly divide the seminiferous tubule lining into basal and adluminal compartments.

Spermatogonia and preleptotene spermatocytes occupy the basal compartment, while remaining primary spermatocytes, secondary spermatocytes and spermatids are located in the adluminal compartment. These compartments are clearly distinguishable in some animal species including primates, but not in man.

Other forms of intercellular junctions (see Chapter 3) between Sertoli cells, including gap junctions and (occasionally) desmosomes, have been described, and intercellular junction-like structures have been seen between Sertoli cells and developing germinal epithelial cells.

Sertoli cell cytoplasm is eosinophilic and finely granular, and may contain lipid vacuoles. Ultrastructually it has abundant endoplasmic reticulum, often arranged as flat stacked cisternae (**annulate lamellae**) with associated ribosomes. The lipid vacuoles are usually found close to the larger cisternae.

Endoplasmic reticulum is also prominent in the cytoplasmic processes interdigitating between the developing germ cells, while clusters of free ribosomes are numerous at the base of the cell. Microfibrils and microtubules are common in areas of cytoplasm close to the developing spermatids.

FUNCTION
Sertoli cells were originally though to be supporting or sustentacular cells, but are now known to be polyfunctional, having supportive, phagocytic and secretory functions.

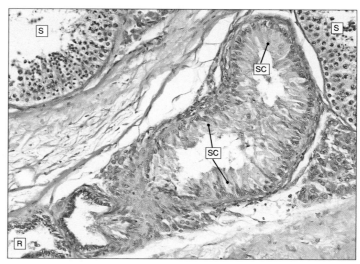

Fig. 17.9 Sertoli cells.
Sertoli cells (SC) are rarely clearly identifiable in the lining of seminiferous tubules (S) in which active spermatogenesis is occurring, but form the entire lining of the tubule for a short distance at its distal end shortly before it drains into the rete testis system (R) at the mediastinum testis. This micrograph is taken from such an area.

Supportive functions probably include the provision of nutrients to developing germinal cells via their intimate cytoplasmic processes, and the transport of waste materials from spermiogenesis to the blood and lymph vascular systems surrounding the seminiferous tubules.

Phagocytic functions. It has long been assumed that Sertoli cells phagocytose any residual cytoplasm (residual bodies) shed by the maturing spermatids during spermiogenesis. They may also phagocytose any effete cellular material derived from degenerate germinal cells that fail to complete spermatogenesis.

Secretory functions vary with sexual maturity. In the male embryo at about the 8th or 9th week of fetal development, Sertoli cells secrete Müllerian inhibitory substance (MIS), which is thought to suppress further development of the Müllerian duct system, and in the prepubertal testis, they may secrete a substance preventing meiotic division of the germinal epithelial cells.

In the sexually mature testis, Sertoli cells secrete androgen binding protein (ABP), which binds testosterone and hydroxytestosterone produced outside the seminiferous tubule; high concentrations of these testosterones are required within the germinal epithelium and tubule lumen for normal germ cell maturation.

ABP secretion is dependent on follicle stimulating hormone (FSH) secretion by the pituitary, and FSH receptors are present on Sertoli cells. FSH promotes spermatogenesis, probably by inducing Sertoli cells to produce varying amounts of ABP.

Sertoli cells also secrete the hormone inhibin, which inhibits the secretion of FSH by the pituitary gland, and therefore plays an important feedback role in controlling the rate of spermatogenesis.

Testicular interstitium

The interstitial tissue lying between the seminiferous tubules is a loose network of fibrocollagenous tissue composed of:
- fibroblasts;
- collagen, in which occasional macrophages and mast cells are present;
- blood and lymphatic vessels;
- clumps of interstitial or Leydig cells (see page 319).

Rete testis

Spermatozoa formed in the seminiferous tubule loops pass to the terminal portions, which are lined entirely by Sertoli cells, and thence via the short straight tubules into the rete testis (Fig. 17.10).

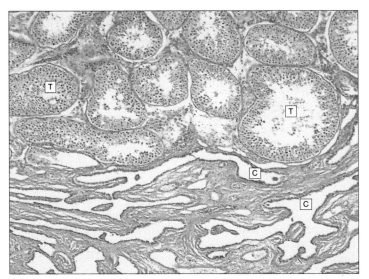

Fig. 17.10 Rete testis.
The rete testis is a network of interconnecting channels (C) into which the seminiferous tubules (T) empty. Spermatozoa are transferred from the rete testis to the epididymis via the efferent ductules.

Both straight tubules and rete testis are lined by a simple epithelium of cuboidal or low columnar cells bearing microvilli on their luminal surface. Most of the rete testis epithelial cells bear a single long central flagellum. The rete testis is a complex arrangement of interconnecting channels located at the mediastinum of the testis, and embedded in a fibrous stroma continuous with the tunica albuginea.

Efferent ductules

Channels of the rete testis fuse to form about a dozen efferent ductules that emerge from the upper end of the mediastinum of the testis, penetrating the tunica albuginea (see Fig.17.1), and entering the head of the epididymis. Here they gradually merge to become a single tube, the epididymal duct.

The efferent ductules are lined by a mixed epithelium of tall ciliated columnar cells and non-ciliated cuboidal or low columnar cells with microvilli on their luminal surface (Fig. 17.11). The cilia beat towards the epididymis and propel the spermatozoa onwards, while the non-ciliated cells absorb some of the testicular fluid, which is the transport medium for the immature and still immotile spermatozoa.

The efferent ductules are highly convoluted and have a narrow sheath of circumferential smooth muscle cells interspersed with elastic fibres; peristaltic contractions of this muscle enhance the progression of the spermatozoa.

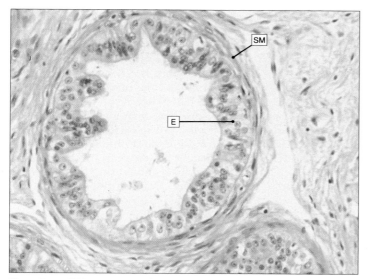

Fig. 17.11 Efferent ductules.
Note the mixed columnar and cuboidal epithelium (E), the typical fringed internal lumen, and the circumferential ring of smooth muscle (SM) fibres.

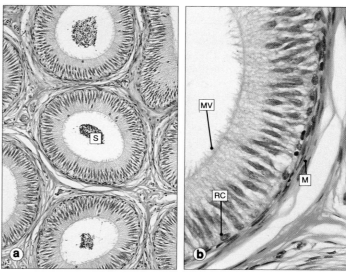

Fig. 17.12 Epididymal duct.
a Micrograph of epididymal duct lined by tall columnar epithelium with basal nuclei; the lumina contain clumps of spermatozoa (S).
b High power micrograph showing a single duct. Note the unusually tall microvilli (MV), the scattered small round cells at the base of the columnar epithelium (RC) and the narrow band of circular muscle fibres (M).

EPIDIDYMIS

The epididymal duct (**ductus epididymis**) formed by the fusion of the efferent ductules is a single highly convoluted tube about 5 m long. It is embedded in a loose vascular supporting stroma of fibroblasts, collagen and glycosaminoglycan matrix, and is surrounded by a dense fibrocollagenous capsule, to form the comma-shaped body called the epididymis.

The epididymis can be divided into head, body and tail regions, with the efferent ductules entering the head, and the distal end of the epididymal duct emerging at the tail to become the vas deferens.

The human epididymis is usually 5 cm long and 1 cm wide, and as the entire 5 m of epididymal duct is contained within it, it is clear that the duct is enormously convoluted.

The epididymal duct is lined by a tall columnar epithelium bearing numerous very long atypical microvilli (Fig. 17.12), which are largely immotile and inaccurately named stereocilia; they neither contain the internal microtubular structures of cilia (see Fig 3.17), nor function like cilia. These giant microvilli are about 80 μm long in the epididymal head and 40 μm long in the tail. The cells also possess coated vesicles and lysosomes, rough endoplasmic

reticulum and a prominent Golgi, and have the following absorptive/phagocytic and secretory functions.
• Absorption of testicular fluid commenced by the efferent ductules.
• Phagocytosis and digestion of degenerate spermatozoa and residual bodies.
• Secretion of glycoproteins, sialic acid and a substance called glycerylphosphorylcholine, which is believed to play a role in the maturation of the spermatozoa, though the precise mechanism is unknown. The glycoproteins bind to the surface membranes of the spermatozoa, but their function is also unknown.

In addition to the tall columnar cells, there is a population of small round cells with a high nucleus:cytoplasm ratio, which lie on the epithelial basement membrane and are thought to be the precursors of the tall cells.

The entire epididymal duct is surrounded by a narrow sheath of circular muscle similar to that in the efferent ductules, but in the tail there is also a longitudinal layer internal to the circular layer, and an outer longitudinal layer.

All of the muscle layers thicken within the epididymal tail, becoming significant layers where the duct emerges to become the vas deferens.

VAS DEFERENS

The **ductus (vas) deferens** is a straight tube running vertically upwards behind the epididymis within the spermatic cord, which also contains arteries, veins, lymphatics and nerves. The veins form a complex anastomotic plexus called the pampiniform plexus. Externally the spermatic cord contains longitudinal fibres of voluntary striated muscle, the cremaster muscle.

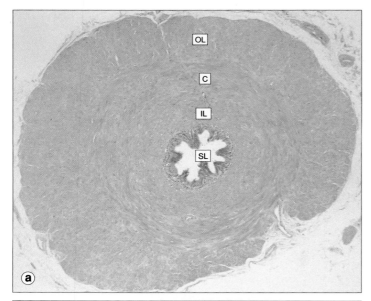

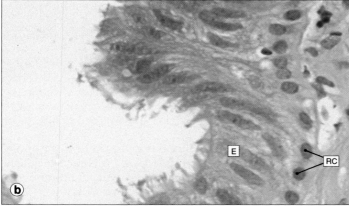

Fig. 17.13 Vas deferens.
a Low power micrograph showing the three muscle layers (a central circular (C) layer between outer (OL) and inner longitudinal (IL) layers) and the stellate lumen (SL).
b High power micrograph showing the tall ciliated columnar epithelium (E), the basal layer of small regular round cells (RC), and the pattern of folds.

The vas deferens has a thick muscular wall composed of a middle circular layer, and outer and inner longitudinal layers. Internal to the inner layer is a fibro-elastic lamina propria covered with a tall columnar epithelium almost identical to that of the epididymis, but thrown up into longitudinal folds by the lamina propria; this produces a small stellate lumen (Fig. 17.13). Peristalsis of the thick muscular wall propels spermatozoa forwards during emission.

Each vas deferens enters the pelvic cavity via the inguinal canal and then passes downwards and medially to the base of the bladder. Near its distal end, close to the base of the bladder, each vas deferens has a dilatation (the **ampulla**) where the muscle layer becomes thinner; the mucosal layer in the ampulla appears thicker because the folds, some of which are branched, are taller.

At the distal end of the ampulla the vas deferens is joined by a short duct from the seminal vesicles.

SEMINAL VESICLES

Each **seminal vesicle** arises as a highly convoluted, 15 cm long, unbranched tubular diverticulum of the vas deferens, which is coiled on itself to form a body about 5–6 cm long. This tube is surrounded by an inner circular and an outer longitudinal smooth muscle layer, and an external layer of fibrocollagenous tissue containing many elastic fibres.

Seminal vesicle mucosa is composed of a fibroelastic lamina propria thrown up into tall narrow complicated folds (Fig. 17.14), covered by non-ciliated tall columnar epithelial cells, and a population of non-specialized basal round cells similar to those seen in the proximal ducts and ductules. The tall cells have the characteristics of secretory cells with large secretory vacuoles near their luminal surface and abundant rough endoplasmic reticulum; they may also contain small yellow–brown lipofuscin granules.

The complexity of the mucosal folding produces a vast surface area for secretion, and 70–80% of the human ejaculate is thick, creamy-yellow secretion of the seminal vesicles. This secretion contains abundant fructose and other sugars, prostaglandins, proteins, amino acids, citric acid and ascorbic acid. Fructose is the major nutrient of spermatozoa.

Contraction of the seminal vesicle smooth muscle propels accumulated secretion into the **ejaculatory duct**, formed by the merging of the short duct from the seminal vesicle with the vas deferens distal to the ampulla.

Each ejaculatory duct is only 1 cm long and is lined by an epithelium of tall columnar and small round cells identical to that of the ampulla; there is no smooth muscle in its wall. The right and left ejaculatory ducts run through the prostate gland and open into the prostatic urethra at the prostatic utricle.

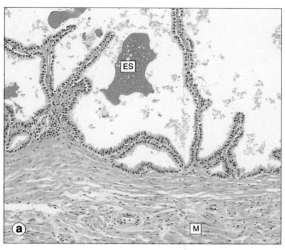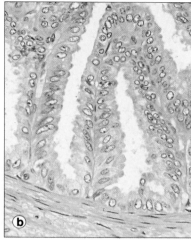

Fig. 17.14 Seminal vesicle.
a Micrograph of seminal vesicle showing part of the muscular surround (M), and the pattern of tall mucosal folds. The lumen contains blobs of eosinophilic secretion (ES).
b Micrograph showing the tall columnar secretory epithelium at high magnification.

PROSTATE

The prostate is composed of secreting glands that open into the urethra, which runs through its body. These prostatic glands and ducts are embedded in a supporting stroma of fibroblasts, collagen and smooth muscle.

The entire prostate gland is surrounded by a fibrocollagenous capsule from which septa extend partway into its body, dividing it into ill-defined lobes.

The prostate gland progressivley enlarges from about 45 years of age, and may become very large in elderly men.

Prostatic glands

The prostatic glands are arranged in three concentric groups (Fig. 17.15):
- a small group of **mucosal gland**s open directly into the urethra;
- a larger group of **submucosal gland**s open into the urethra via short ducts;
- a substantial outer group of so-called **main prostatic glands** open into the urethra via long ducts.

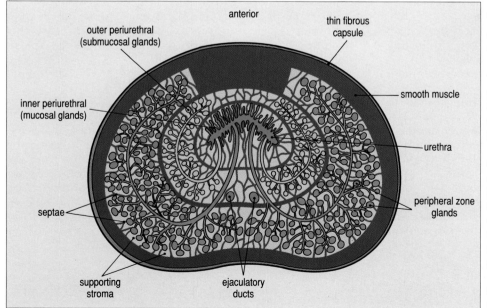

Fig. 17.15 Prostate.
The prostate is surrounded by a thin fibrous capsule internal to which is a substantial layer of smooth muscle, giving rise to septa (mainly muscular, but with a fine fibrocollagenous component), which penetrate the organ to provide an intimate stroma supporting and demarcating the glandular elements. Division into central and peripheral zones is indistinct.

The inner periurethral (mucosal) glands are small and open directly into the urethra around its entire surface; the outer periurethral glands are more numerous and open into the urethra through short ducts that enter the posterolateral urethral sinuses on their posterior surface, on either side of the central ridge, the urethral crest. These two groups of glands comprise the central zone.

The glands of the peripheral zone empty their secretions into the urethra by long ducts opening alongside the urethral crest.

315

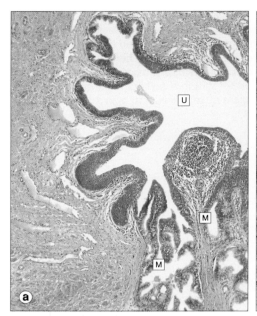

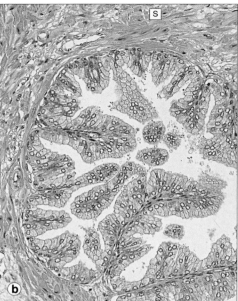

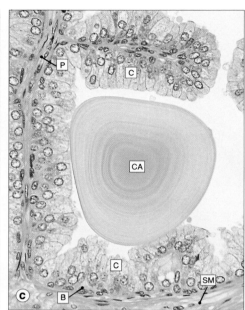

Fig. 17.16 Prostatic glands.

a Micrograph of prostatic mucosal glands (M) opening directly into the urethra (U).

b Micrograph showing the general architecture of a typical prostatic gland with its papillary pattern of ingrowths. Note the smooth muscular and fibrocollagenous stroma (S).

c Micrograph showing the cytological detail of prostatic gland lining epithelium. It is is composed of tall pale-staining columnar cells (C) and occasional small basal cells (B) with darker staining nuclei.

Note the delicate supporting stroma of the papillary ingrowth (P) and the narrow periglandular layer of smooth muscle fibres (SM).

The lumen contains an uncalcified, concentrically laminated corpus amylaceum (CA).

The ducts of the submucosal and main prostatic glands open posteriorly into the urethral sinuses on either side of a longitudinal ridge called the **urethral crest**.

The epithelium lining the prostatic glands is thrown up into complex folds, accompanied by a narrow supporting lamina propria. There are two types of epithelial cell:

• tall columnar or cuboidal cells with pale foamy cytoplasm and basal pale-staining nuclei;

• scanty flat basal cells with small dark-staining nuclei in contact with the basement membrane (Fig. 17.16).

Ultrastructurally the tall columnar cells have a prominent Golgi located between the basal nucleus and the luminal surface, and lysosomes, secretory granules and rough endoplasmic reticulum are numerous.

The secretory products of these cells include acid phosphatase (produced in large quantities by the lysosomes), citric acid, fibrinolysin, amylase and other proteins. The gland lumina usually contain some stored secretion; in older men small spherical **corpora amylacea**, which are mainly condensed glycoprotein and often calcified, are found.

The ducts of the prostatic glands may also be lined by tall columnar epithelium, but as they near the urethra this becomes progressively more cuboidal, and even transitional, like that of the urethra itself.

Hormone dependency

The prostatic epithelium depends on adequate testosterone levels to maintain its structural and functional integrity; any inadequacy is manifest by a change of epithelium from tall secretory to cuboidal, with loss of, or reduced secretory activity. This change is seen increasingly from middle age onwards, and in extreme cases the epithelium may be converted to a stratified squamous pattern, often with keratin formation.

BENIGN PROSTATIC HYPERPLASIA

The most common disorder of the prostate occurs in elderly men and is benign prostatic hyperplasia. This is characterized by considerable enlargement of the prostatic glands in the mucous and submucosal gland groups due to an increase in the number and size of the glands and ducts, and an increase in the bulk of the supporting fibromuscular stroma. Many glands are over-distended with secretion (Fig. 17.17).

The increase in bulk of the prostatic tissue leads to compression of the urethra and micturition difficulties, which include retention of urine.

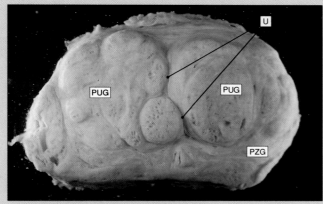

Fig. 17.17 Benign prostatic hyperplasia.
Micrograph showing the low power view of typical benign prostatic hyperplasia. There is nodular overgrowth of the periurethral glands (PUG), which is causing compression and distortion of the urethra (U). Note that the peripheral zone glands (PZG) are not involved.

CARCINOMA OF PROSTATE

Cancer in the prostate gland almost always originates in the main glands arranged around the periphery and is often advanced before producing symptoms by blocking the urethra (Fig. 17.18).

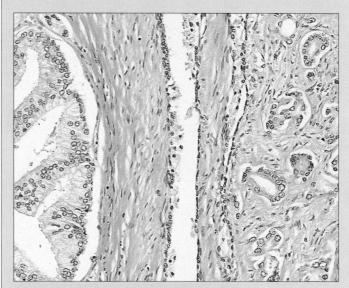

Fig. 17.18 Adenocarcinoma of the prostate.
Micrograph showing cancerous transformation of the prostatic glands. Those on the left have a normal arrangement with regular tall columnar epithelium. The cancerous prostatic glands on the right have lost their tall columnar pattern as well as their regular architecture.

BULBO-URETHRAL GLANDS

Seminal fluid enters the prostatic urethra from the right and left ejaculatory ducts, and passes through the short membranous urethra and then the penile urethra before entering the vagina during sexual intercourse. Opening into the membranous urethra are the long narrow ducts from the paired small bulbo-urethral glands.

The bulbo-urethral glands are about 5 mm in diameter, and are lined by tall mucus-secreting epithelium, which produces a watery, slightly mucoid, fluid containing abundant sugars (mainly galactose) and some sialic acid. This fluid precedes the thicker semen along the penile urethra during emission and may have a lubricatory function.

PENIS

The penis is composed of erectile tissue arranged into two dorsal cylinders (**corpora cavernosa**) and a smaller central ventral cylinder (**corpus spongiosum**), through which the penile urethra runs. The cylinders are each surrounded by a dense fibrocollagenous sheath, the tunica albuginea, which also holds them together (Fig. 17.19).

The erectile tissues are essentially interconnecting vascular spaces, which are empty when the penis is flaccid (Figs. 17.20 & 17.21), but fill with blood during erection to form an enlarged rigid organ.

The arterial supply to the penis is provided by the **dorsal** and the **deep artery**. From the deep arteries arise arteries supplying the tunica albuginea, and the **helicine arteries**, which supply the erectile tissue.

The helicine arteries are so-named because they are spiral in the flaccid penis, but during erection they straighten and dilate, and fill the corpora with blood.

This filling effect is partly due to closure of the arteriovenous shunts existing between the helicine arteries and deep veins, which are the normal route of helicine artery blood flow in the flaccid state.

Parasympathetic nerve discharges cause the closure, leading to diversion of the helicine artery blood into the cavernous spaces, while increased pressure in the corpora compresses the thin-walled veins, preventing emptying.

After ejaculation the parasympathetic stimulation ceases, the arteriovenous shunts open and blood passes from the corpora into the veins.

During erection the two corpora cavernosa become more turgid than the corpus spongiosum. The pressure exerted by the corpus spongiosum on the urethra running through it is not sufficient to prevent passage of the semen, which is forcibly ejected by contraction of the smooth muscle, but is usually sufficient to prevent successful pain-free micturition.

The erectile component of the penis is surrounded by skin, which has a very loose subcutis, permitting it to move considerably during intercourse.

At the distal end of the penis the corpus spongiosum terminates on the **glans penis**, which is covered with non-keratinizing squamous epithelium containing sebaceous glands. The penile urethra opens to the exterior at the meatus at the centre of the glans penis.

For most of its length the penile urethra is lined by non-secreting columnar epithelium into which small mucus glands embedded in the corpus spongiosum drain. Within the glans penis, however, the urethra dilates

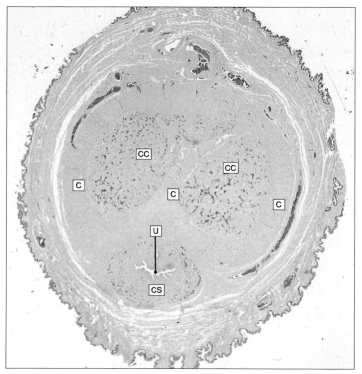

Fig. 17.19 Penis.

Transverse section of penis showing the arrangement of the vascular erectile tissue into two dorsal corpora cavernosa (CC) and a single ventral corpus spongiosum (CS) through which the penile urethra (U) runs.

Small mucus glands in the corpus spongiosum are particularly concentrated around the penile urethra into which they open.

The corpora are enclosed within, and divided by, a broad fibrocollagenous capsule (C). The erectile core is surrounded by a sheath of skin to which it is connected by a very loose subcutis containing a number of blood vessels including the small paired dorsal arteries and the midline superficial and deep dorsal veins.

(**navicular fossa**) and becomes lined by non-keratinizing statified squamous epithelium identical to that covering the glans.

The end of the penis is normally covered by an overlap of penile skin (the **prepuce**), which is rich in elastic fibres and permits it to retract over the glans penis during intercourse.

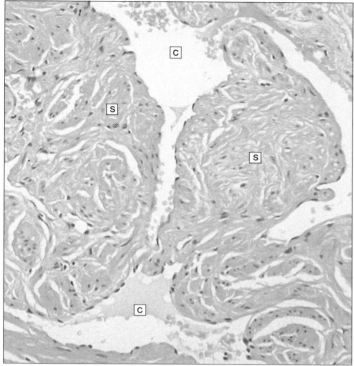

Fig. 17.20 Corpus spongiosum.
Micrograph of corpus spongiosum, showing large irregular interconnecting vascular channels (C) lined by flat endothelium, and separated by a fibrocollagenous stroma (S) containing some smooth muscle bundles.

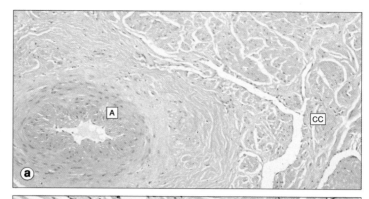

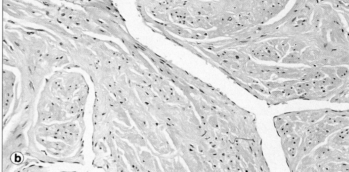

Fig. 17.21 Corpora cavernosa.
a Micrograph of part of the corpora cavernosa (CC) with the central deep artery (A).
b Micrograph showing the system of interconnecting vascular channels (V) of the corpora cavernosa in the non-erectile state.

ENDOCRINE CONTROL

The male sex hormone **testosterone** is essential for the male reproductive system to function successfully.

In the embryo, testosterone and other androgens produced by the developing testes are responsible for development of the penis and accessory sex glands, such as the prostate and epididymis.

With the onset of puberty, male secondary sexual characteristics develop under the influence of testosterone, which also induces maturation and division of spermatogonia in the seminiferous tubules, leading eventually to full spermatogenesis with the production of mature spermatozoa.

In addition, testosterone is responsible for the maturation of the characteristic epithelia of the male genital ducts, and the accessory glands which discharge secretions into them.

In the adult male, continued production of spermatozoa, and maintenance of the normal structure and function of the ducts and accessory glands, is dependent on continued testosterone production.

Failing testosterone production in old age leads to partial or complete cessation of spermatogenesis, and alteration of the specialized secretory, absorptive and microvillous epithelium of the ducts and accessory glands to a more simplified cuboidal or squamous epithelium, which is unable to perform its previous functions.

319

Thus testosterone is the hub of the structure and function of the male genital system. It is produced by Leydig (interstitial) cells from cholesterol under the influence of luteinizing hormone secreted by the gonadotroph cells of the pituitary (see page 252).

The secretion of testosterone is controlled by an efficient feedback mechanism based on the monitoring of circulating testosterone levels by the hypothalamus, which secretes gonadotrophin releasing hormone. In order to maintain a high concentration of testosterone within the lumina of the seminiferous tubules and genital ducts, the Sertoli cells produce **androgen-binding protein** (ABP) under the influence of follicle stimulating hormone. Like luteinizing hormone, FSH is also produced by the pituitary following stimulation by gonadotrophin releasing hormone secreted by the hypothalamus.

ABP binds testosterone and its release is believed to be controlled by negative feedback through the production of a polypeptide called **inhibin**, which is also produced by Sertoli cells (Fig. 17.22).

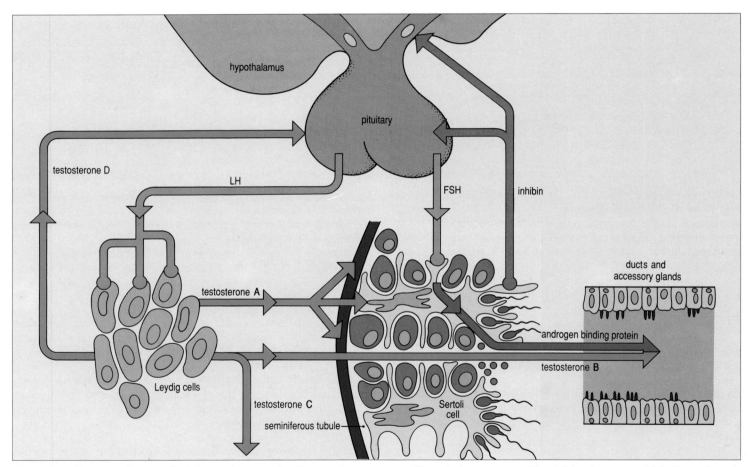

Fig. 17.22 Hormonal control of the male reproductive system. Testosterone stimulates spermatogenesis in seminiferous tubules (A), maintains structure and function of the ducts and accessory glands (B), stimulates and maintains secondary sexual characteristics (C), and provides a feedback mechanism (D) controlling pituitary output of luteinizing hormone (LH). Secretion of testosterone by Leydig cells is stimulated by LH.

Sertoli cells secrete androgen-binding protein (ABP) under the influence of follicle stimulating hormone (FSH) from the pituitary, and also produce inhibin, which is responsible for feedback control.

Leydig cells

Leydig cells synthesize testoserone and, although they are most common in the tubular interstitium, they can occasionally be found in the mediastinum of the testis, the epididymis, or even in the spermatic cord. They are often closely related to nerves, like their female equivalent, the hilus cells of the ovary (see page 333).

Leydig cells have round vesicular nuclei with prominent nuclear membranes and one or two nucleoli. Some of the cells are small and spindle shaped, and are thought to be immature forms, but most are round or polygonal.

Leydig cells have granular eosinophilic cytoplasm containing lipases, oxidative enzymes, esterases and a number of steroid dehydrogenases.

A characteristic feature of Leydig cells is the Reinke crystalloid, which is an intracytoplasmic, eosinophilic, elongated, rectangular or rhomboid mass, approximately 3 µm thick and up to 20 µm long (Fig. 17.23).

Reinke crystalloids are not seen before puberty, and increase in number during the years of sexual maturity, becoming most common in old age.

Yellow-brown lipofuscin pigment is present in most Leydig cells.

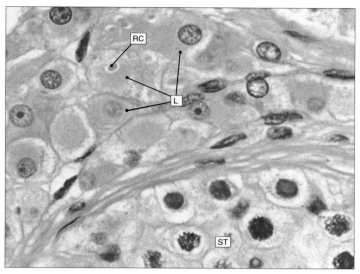

Fig. 17.23 Leydig (interstitial) cells.
Micrograph showing a cluster of Leydig cells (L) situated in the interstitium between seminiferous tubules (ST). They have abundant eosinophilic cytoplasm, and some of the cells contain Reinke crystalloids (RC).

18. FEMALE REPRODUCTIVE SYSTEM

The female reproductive system:
- produces haploid female gametes (ova);
- receives haploid male gametes (spermatozoa) prior to fertilization;
- provides a suitable environment for fertilization of ova by spermatozoa;
- provides a suitable physical and hormonal environment for implantation of the embryo;
- accommodates and nourishes the embryo and fetus during pregnancy;
- expels the mature fetus at the end of pregnancy.

The structure of the human female reproductive system changes considerably from childhood into reproductive maturity, and later the menopause, under the control of trophic hormones.

Furthermore, the various components undergo structural and functional modification at different stages in the monthly cycle.

The system (Figs 18.1 & 18.2) comprises the ovaries, fallopian tubes, uterus and vagina (collectively referred to as the **internal genitalia**), together with the mons pubis, vulva (labia majora and labia minora) and clitoris (referred to as the **external genitalia**).

Unlike many other mammals, the human female ovulates at regular intervals (approximately every 28 days) throughout the year.

As tissues from other animals do not accurately reflect the changes seen in the human, only human tissues are described and shown in this chapter.

MONS PUBIS, LABIA MAJORA AND LABIA MINORA

The mons pubis, labia majora and labia minora all consist of modified skin (see Chapter 19) as follows.
- The **mons pubis** (**mons veneris**) is skin superimposed on a substantial pad of subcutaneous fat overlying the symphysis pubis, and is characterized by the presence of unusually oblique hair follicles, which produce the coarse curly pubic hair common to most races.

- Posterolateral extensions of the mons pubis on either side of the vaginal introitus form the **labia majora**, which are similarly richly endowed with subcutaneous fat and oblique hair follicles (Fig. 18.1c). There are smooth muscle fibres in the subcutaneous fat.

The accumulation of subcutaneous fat and the development of the oblique hair follicles and pubic hair is hormone-dependent and begins with the onset of sexual maturity, usually between the ages of 10 and 13 years.

This area is also rich in apocrine glands and prominent sebaceous glands, both of which mature and become active at the onset of sexual maturity, while eccrine sweat glands, which are present from birth, show no change.
- The **labia minora** are thin flaps of skin devoid of adipose tissue, but with abundant blood vessels and elastic fibres. Although hair follicles are absent, there are many sebaceous glands, which open directly onto the epidermal surface (Fig. 18.1d).

The outer, lateral aspect of the labia minora is usually more pigmented than the inner medial aspect, and the epidermis has a well developed rete ridge system.

On the inner aspect, the melanin pigmentation becomes progressively reduced as the vaginal introitus is approached, and the keratinized, stratified, squamous epithelium becomes thinner, with flattening of the rete ridges and thinning of the keratin layer.

This keratinized epithelium extends into the vaginal vestibule as far as the **hymen**, which is a thin fibrous membrane that is rarely completely intact and usually appears as an irregular 'frill' in the lining of the lower vagina, the hymeneal tegmentum. On its exterior (vulval) surface, the hymen is covered with the keratinized stratified squamous epithelium, whereas the inner (vaginal) surface is covered with non-keratinized, stratified, squamous epithelium, rich in glycogen, which is similar to that lining the vagina (see Fig. 18.3).

Characteristically, the epidermis of both the labia majora and minora becomes pigmented by melanin with the onset of puberty.

The hymen can be regarded as the junction between the internal and external genitalia.

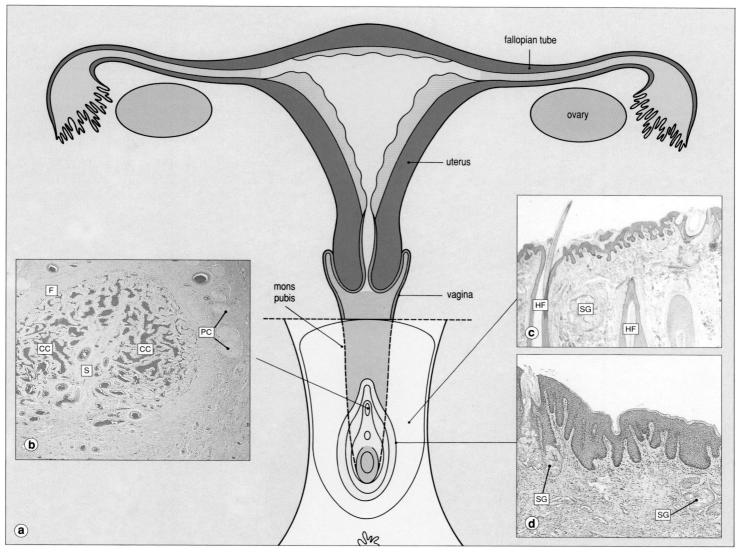

Fig. 18.1 Internal and external genitalia.

a Diagram showing the relationship between the external and internal genitalia.

b Micrograph of clitoris; note the two corpora cavernosa (CC) arranged side by side, and engorged with blood, the incomplete central septum (S), and the fibrocollagenous sheath (F), outside which are prominent nerve endings (mainly Pacinian touch corpuscles (PC) see Chapter 19).

c Micrograph of labia majora. The skin contains many hair follicles (HF), sebaceous glands (SG), and eccrine sweat glands and ducts.

d Micrograph of labia minora. The skin is devoid of hair follicles, but rich in sebaceous glands (SG), which open directly onto the surface. Note that the dermis is highly vascular.

CLITORIS

The **clitoris** is located below the mons pubis, and is the female equivalent of the penis. It is composed of two corpora cavernosa of erectile vascular tissue which lie side by side, surrounded by a fibrocollagenous sheath; an incomplete central septum partly separates the two corpora (see Fig. 18.1b).

The clitoris is covered by thin epidermis that is devoid of hair follicles, sebaceous glands, eccrine and apocrine glands, but is richly equipped with sensory nerves and a variety of receptors.

Over the superior surface of the clitoris the skin forms an incomplete hood (the clitoral prepuce), and on the inferior surface, a thin midline frenulum. At the base of the clitoris, the corpora cavernosa diverge to lie along the pubic rami, where they contain fibres of the ischio-cavernosus muscle.

The clitoris, which is small before puberty, enlarges to a greater or lesser extent with the onset of sexual maturity. During sexual arousal it becomes engorged in a manner similar to that of the penis.

URETHRAL MEATUS, PARAURETHRAL GLANDS AND BARTHOLIN'S GLANDS

The urethral meatus opens to the exterior in the midline below the clitoris.

On either side of the meatus are the openings of the **paraurethral glands (of Skene)**. These glands are located around the urethra, mainly posteriorly and laterally, and are lined by pseudostratified columnar epithelium.

Bartholin's (vulvovaginal) glands are located around the lower vagina and are composed of acini lined by tall columnar mucus-secreting cells with pale cytoplasm and small basal nuclei.

These glands open into the vagina posterolaterally at the level of the hymeneal remnants through a duct lined by a transitional epithelium with a surface mucin-secreting layer.

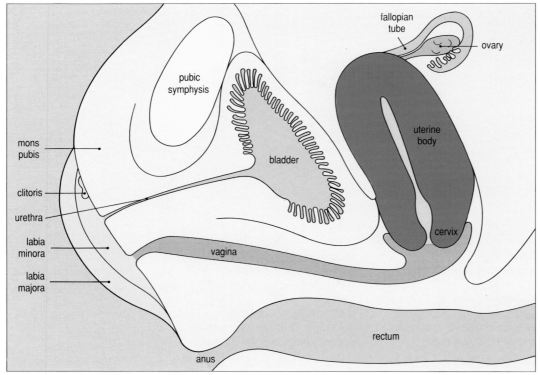

Fig. 18.2 Lateral view of female genitalia.
Note the angle of insertion of the uterus into the vagina.

VAGINA

The **vagina** is a fibromuscular tube extending from the vestibule to the uterus (see Fig. 18.1), and in the mature female is 7–9 cm long. It forms an angle of more than 90° with the normal anteverted uterus(see Fig. 18.2).

At its inner end the vagina forms a cuff around the protruding cervix of the uterus, forming anterior, posterior and lateral pouches, known as the fornices.

The vagina has four layers (Fig. 18.3) as follows.
• Stratified squamous epithelial mucosa.
• Lamina propria (subepithelial region), which is rich in elastic fibres and thin-walled blood vessels, mainly veins and venules.
• A fibromuscular layer containing ill-defined bundles of circularly arranged smooth muscle and a more prominent outer layer of longitudinally arranged smooth muscle. At the lower end this layer also contains some skeletal muscle, which is found mainly around the vaginal introitus in the hymeneal region.
• Adventitia, which is composed of fibrocollagenous tissue containing numerous thick elastic fibres, large blood vessels, nerves and clumps of ganglion cells.

The rich meshwork of elastic fibres in the vaginal wall is responsible for its elasticity and permits the great temporary distension required during parturition; the extensive submucosal plexus of thin-walled blood vessels is thought to permit the diffusion of watery fluid across the epithelium and contribute to the vaginal fluid.

Although structurally a tube, at rest the vagina is collapsed so that the anterior wall is in contact with the posterior wall, and for much of its length there are shallow longitudinal grooves in the midline of both of these walls. In addition, the vaginal mucosa is rugose, being thrown up into a series of closely packed transverse mucosal folds or ridges.

The structure of the vagina varies with age and hormonal activity, the main changes occurring in the non-keratinizing, stratified, squamous epithelium which lines it.

Before puberty, the epithelium is thin, a state to which it reverts after the menopause, but during the reproductive years the epithelium responds to the activity of oestrogens, and thickens. The basal cells and the distinct parabasal layer show increased mitotic activity, while the more superficial cells increase not only in number, but also in size as a result of the accumulation of stored glycogen and some lipid within the cytoplasm.

Glycogen content is maximal at the time of ovulation, and some glycogen-rich surface squames are shed into the vaginal cavity after ovulation, during the secretory phase of the menstrual cycle.

Breakdown of the glycogen by commensal lactobacilli in the vaginal cavity produces lactic acid resulting in an acid pH. This restricts the vaginal bacterial flora to acid-loving commensals and deters invasion by bacterial pathogens and fungi such as *Candida albicans*, which is the cause of vaginal 'thrush'.

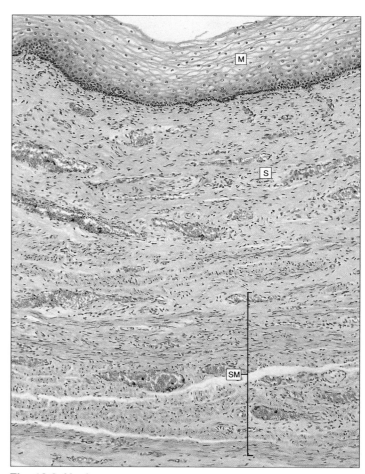

Fig. 18.3 Vagina.
Micrograph of vaginal wall showing glycogen-rich stratified squamous epithelial mucosa (M), a highly vascular submucosa (S), and irregular smooth muscle (SM).

UTERUS

The uterus is a muscular organ and receives the right and left fallopian tubes. It is lined by columnar epithelium and at its lower end it opens into the vagina.

The uterus can be divided into three parts, the fundus, the body and the cervix (Fig. 18.4). Whereas the fundus and body have the same histological structure (see page 329), that of the cervix is different.

Cervix

The **cervix** is the lower part of the uterus, part of which protrudes into the vagina. The junction between it and the uterine body is the **internal os**, and at this point the nature of the lining epithelium and the uterine wall changes.

The cervical lumen opens into the vaginal cavity at the **external os**, where again there is an important change in the nature of the lining epithelium. This zone is the site of many important pathological changes (see Fig. 18.8).

The cervix is cylindrical and symmetrical, being about 3 cm long and 2–2.5 cm in diameter, but becomes more barrel-shaped after pregnancy and parturition. After childbirth, the external os becomes a transverse slit dividing the distal end of the cervix into anterior and posterior lips, whereas the external os of the nulliparous cervix is circular.

Cervical stroma is composed mainly of fibrocollagenous tissue and some smooth muscle; blood vessels are numerous (Fig. 18.5).

Ectocervix

The external surface of the part of cervix that protrudes into the vagina, the **ectocervix**, is covered by non-keratinizing, stratified, squamous epithelium, continuous with that of the vagina at the vaginal fornices.

Like vaginal squamous epithelium, the ectocervical epithelium is rich in glycogen in the sexually mature period (Fig. 18.6) and undergoes cyclical changes during the menstrual cycle under the influence of oestrogens and progesterone.

Before the menarche and after the menopause the epithelium is much thinner with fewer layers and smaller cells containing less glycogen.

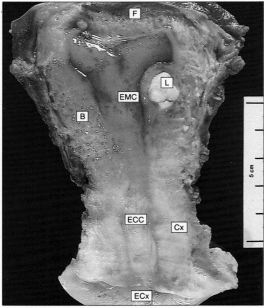

Fig. 18.4 Uterus.
Section through the uterus of a 35-year-old woman showing the fundus (F), body (B) and cervix (Cx). Note the endometrial cavity (EMC), endocervical canal (ECC) and ectocervix (ECx). The smooth muscle of the body contains a small tumour, a leiomyoma (L) (see Fig. 18.11).

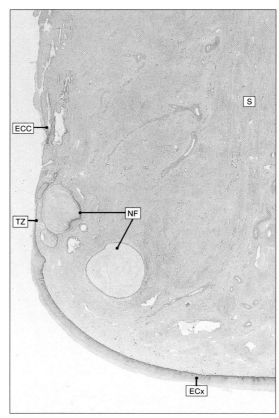

Fig. 18.5 Cervix.
Low power micrograph of cervix. The stroma (S) is composed of smooth muscle fibres embedded in collagen, the proportions of muscle and fibrous tissue varying according to age and parity; blood and lymphatic vessels are prominent and numerous. The ectocervix (ECx) is covered with stratified squamous epithelium, while the endocervical canal (ECC) is lined by tall columnar epithelium.

The junction between the squamous and columnar epithelium is located in the region of the external os. In this example, there is a transformation zone (TZ) (see page 328) of squamous epithelium which has extended into the endocervical canal; note the Nabothian follicles (NF).

Endocervix

The **endocervical canal** runs between the uterine and vaginal cavities, and is lined by a single layer of tall columnar mucus-secreting epithelium (Fig. 18.7a).

Longitudinal or transverse histological sections of the cervix have given the impression that there are glandular structures (endocervical mucus glands) extending into the underlying stroma. Three-dimensional studies indicate however that the structures are in fact deep slit-like invaginations of the surface epithelium, with blind-ended tubules arising from the clefts (Fig. 18.7b). Thus, there is a large surface area for the production of cervical mucus, which fills the endocervical canal. Before puberty and after the menopause, the amount of cervical mucus is greatly reduced.

As well as contributing to vaginal lubrication during sexual intercourse, the mucin in the endocervical canal acts as a protective barrier, preventing bacterial ascent into the endometrial cavity.

Movement of endocervical mucus into the vaginal canal is facilitated by a few ciliated columnar epithelial cells scattered among the mucus-secreting endocervical cells, particularly at the upper end of the canal, close to the junction with the endometrium.

Both the mucin-secreting and ciliated cells have fine microvilli which are only visible ultrastructurally.

During the menstrual cycle, the physicochemical properties of cervical mucin are subject to marked changes, but the endocervical columnar epithelium shows little microscopic variation, although ultrastructural changes in cytoplasmic organelles have been noted.

During the proliferative (follicular, oestrogenic) phase, the mucin is thin, watery and abundant, and has an alkaline pH (features which may facilitate movement of spermatozoa). It is composed of a micellar network of glycoprotein molecules, the spaces in between being occupied by plasma rich in Na^+, K^+ and Cl^-. The high ionic concentration is responsible for its ability to crystallize ('ferning' or 'arborization' pattern) in this ovulatory phase.

After ovulation the mucus becomes viscid and scanty, and has an acidic pH, deterring penetration by spermatozoa, and sealing the uterus in preparation for possible embryo implantation.

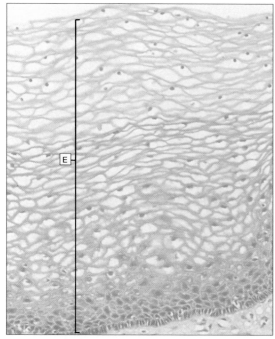

Fig. 18.6 Ectocervix.
Stratified squamous epithelium (E) covers the ectocervix. Like that of the vagina, the cells are rich in glycogen during the period of sexual maturity.

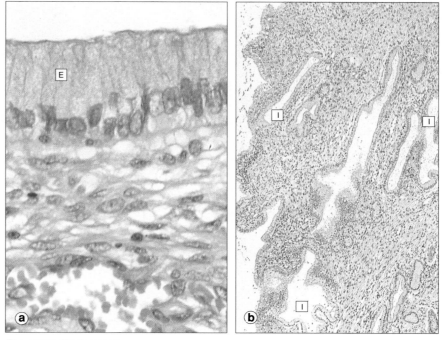

Fig. 18.7 Endocervix.
a The endocervical canal is lined by a single layer of tall columnar mucus-secreting epithelium (E).
b Numerous deep invaginations (I) of the mucus-secreting epithelium extend into the cervical stroma and greatly increase the surface for mucus production.

Squamo-columnar junction of cervix

The **squamo-columnar junction** of the cervix is the line where the columnar epithelium of the endocervical canal meets the squamous epithelium of the ectocervix, and is important in disease.

The original squamo-columnar junction is usually located in the region of the external os, but its precise location at birth is influenced by maternal hormone exposure *in utero*.

At about puberty, hormonal influences lead to extension of the columnar epithelium onto the ectocervix forming an **ectropion** or **cervical erosion** (Fig. 18.8), which is augmented by a first pregnancy, particularly when this occurs shortly after menarche.

Before puberty the pH of the vagina and cervix is alkaline, but afterwards bacterial breakdown of the glycogen in the vaginal and cervical squamous epithelium renders an acidic environment, with a pH of about 3.

Exposure of the sensitive columnar epithelium of the ectropion to the postpubertal acidic environment of the vagina induces squamous metaplasia and a transformation zone between the endocervical columnar epithelium and the ectocervical squamous epithelium.

This zone is composed of new squamous epithelium in an area previously occupied by columnar epithelium.

Thus the squamo-columnar junction is of variable size, but its site always approximates to the external os. In older women it may retreat into the endocervical canal.

One almost invariable consequence of squamous metaplasia near the external os is that the openings of some of the deep crypts of previously everted endocervical mucous glands become obliterated so that mucin produced deep in the crypts cannot be excreted into the endocervical lumen or vagina. Instead, it accumulates within the blocked clefts and produces spherical cystic masses of inspissated mucus lined by flattened endocervical mucus-secreting epithelium; these are called **Nabothian follicles**. Other consequences of this constant change of epithelium include the development of abnormal epithelium, which may progress to cancer.

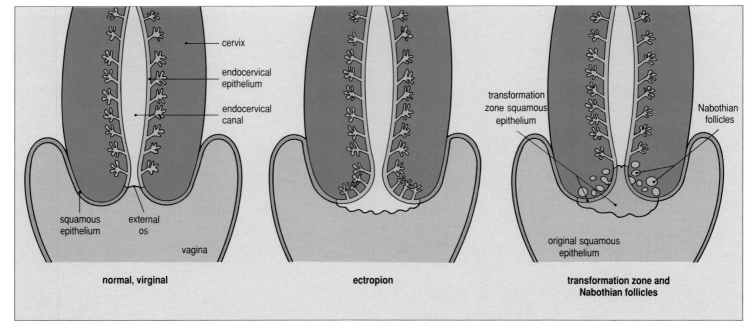

normal, virginal

ectropion

transformation zone and Nabothian follicles

Fig. 18.8 Squamo-columnar junction of the cervix.
Diagram illustrating the mobility of the squamo-columnar junction, the development of ectropion, and the formation of the transformation zone.
a The squamo-columnar junction is originally situated in the region of the external os.

b At puberty the endocervical epithelium extends distally into the acid environment of the vagina, and forms an ectropion.
c A transformation zone forms as squamous epithelium regrows over the ectropion. The openings of the crypts may be obliterated in the process, and result in the formation of mucus-filled Nabothian follicles (see Fig. 18.5).

CARCINOMA OF THE CERVIX

The transformation zone of the cervical epithelium is the most common site of origin of carcinoma of the cervix, the development of which is usually preceded by histological abnormality of the squamous epithelial cells in this zone. The abnormal cells:

- lose their regular stratified pattern;
- have a high nucleus-to-cytoplasm ratio;
- show variation in shape and size, and increased mitotic activity.

These cytological features are characteristic of malignant tumour cells, and are usually associated with evidence of invasive behaviour. However, in the cervix, the cytological changes of malignancy may be present for years before the abnormal epithelium begins to invade the underlying stroma; and are referred to as **carcinoma-in-situ** or **cervical intraepithelial neoplasia** (**C.I.N.**) (Fig. 18.9a).

Eventually the abnormal epithelial cells breach the basement membrane and invade the cervical stroma (Fig. 18.9b), gaining access to blood and lymphatic vessels, which are their route for spread to other sites, such as the lymph nodes around the iliac arteries. This is **invasive carcinoma**.

Early diagnosis of C.I.N. can be obtained by cervical cytology (cervical smear); cells are scraped from the epithelial surface in the region of the external os, and examined microscopically for abnormal cells. Abnormal areas can then be treated, usually by surgical removal, thus preventing the future development of invasive cancer.

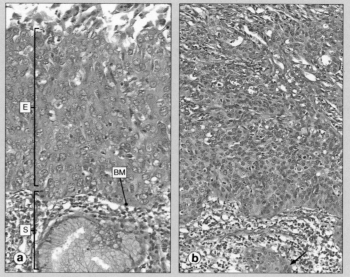

Fig. 18.9 Carcinoma of the cervix.
a The cervical epithelial cells (E) have lost their regular stratified pattern, have high nucleus–cytoplasm ratios and show increased mitotic activity (compare with Fig. 18.7a). As the basement membrane (BM) between the epithelium and underlying stroma (S) is intact, this is carcinoma-in-situ or cervical intraepithelial neoplasia (C.I.N.).
b Some of the abnormal epithelial cells have breached the basement membrane and invaded the cervical stroma (arrow); this is invasive carcinoma.

Uterine body

Myometrium

The body and fundus of the uterus have thick walls composed of smooth muscle (**myometrium**), which is arranged into three ill-defined layers.

Myometrium is hormone-sensitive and undergoes both **hypertrophy** (an increase in cell size) and **hyperplasia** (an increase in cell numbers) during pregnancy (Fig. 18.10), progressively returning to its normal size (involuting) in the weeks after delivery.

Within the myometrium are prominent blood vessels, both arterial and venous, which undergo marked dilation and thickening of their walls during pregnancy.

With cessation of hormonal stimulation after the menopause, the myometrial cells atrophy and the uterus shrinks. The fibrocollagenous tissue between the muscle bundles, which is comparatively insignificant when the myometrial smooth muscle is prominent during sexual maturity, then becomes obvious.

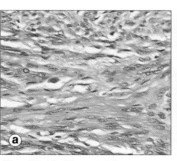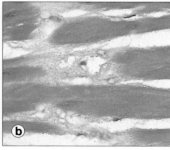

Fig. 18.10 Myometrium.
a Normal myometrium from a non-pregnant 35-year-old woman. The muscle cells are small and tightly packed.
b Myometrium from a 28-year-old woman in the 8th month of pregnancy, photographed at the same magnification as **a**. Note the enormous increase in size of the individual muscle fibres, almost entirely due to an increase in cytoplasm. This is an example of physiological hypertrophy, and is a common response of muscle cells to an increased work load, in this case the need to increase the propulsive power of the uterus to expel the fetus at childbirth.

LEIOMYOMA

The myometrium is the site of one of the most common benign tumours, the **leiomyoma** or **fibroid** (Fig. 18.11, see also Fig. 18.4), which is derived from smooth muscle of the uterine wall.

Like normal uterine smooth muscle, leiomyomas are hormone dependent and progressively enlarge until the menopause, after which time they regress.

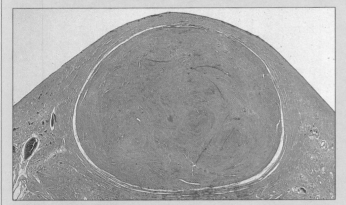

Fig. 18.11 Leiomyoma.
Micrograph of a typical small leiomyoma.

Endometrium

The body and fundus of the uterus have a highly specialized mucosal lining, the **endometrium**, which is composed of glands and supporting stroma.

Before puberty, the endometrium is simple and composed of low cuboidal epithelium supported by a scanty spindle-celled stroma. Downgrowths of epithelium into the stroma produce a small number of rudimentary tubular glands.

Between the menarche (the first menstrual period) and the menopause the endometrium can be differentiated into two layers; a deep basal layer at the junction with the myometrium, and a superficial functional layer lining the lumen. It is the functional layer which is hormone-responsive and undergoes the monthly cycle of proliferation, secretion, necrosis and shedding (see page 339).

If fertilization and successful implantation of an ovum occurs, the endometrium remains unshed and forms the decidua (see page 346).

The basal layer, which is not shed at menstruation, provides a cellular reserve from which a new functional layer develops after menstrual shedding. The endometrium

does not respond evenly to ovarian hormonal stimulation; functional endometrium in the lower segment close to the junction with the cervix, and patches around the entrances of the fallopian tubes, may show little proliferative or secretory activity, and often resembles the basal layer. As the menopause approaches, more and more of the endometrium may fail to respond fully to the hormonal stimulus.

At the menopause, when hormonal stimulation ceases, the endometrium reverts to the simple prepubertal pattern, although the tubular downgrowths may undergo cystic distension and the stroma may become compact (**atrophic cystic endometrium**).

FALLOPIAN TUBES

The **fallopian tubes** (or **oviducts**) convey ova from the ovary to the body of the uterus, and are the site of their fertilization by spermatozoa. After fertilization, the tube transmits the fertilized ovum to the endometrial cavity where implantation can take place.

Each fallopian tube is 10–12 cm long and extends from a dilated open end close to the ovary to a narrow portion which passes through the myometrial wall of the uterus before opening into the uterine cavity. There are four recognizable tubal segments (Fig. 18.12), each differing histologically, particularly in their proportions of muscle and epithelium, and the degree of convolution of their epithelium.
• The **infundibulum** is surrounded by a fringe of epithelial-coated **fimbriae**, some of which may become adherent to the nearby ovary.
• Medial to the infundibulum is a thin-walled zone called the **ampulla** where ovum fertilization usually takes place.
• The ampulla leads into a narrower, thick-walled segment called the **isthmus**.
• In turn, the isthmus is continuous with the short **intramural segment**, which opens into the uterus.

The fallopian tube is essentially a muscular tube lined by specialized epithelium which is variably folded and plicated, and differs in appearance at different sites.

Tubal muscle and lamina propria

The smooth muscle wall of the fallopian tube is composed of two layers; the inner layer, which appears to be circular in histological sections, and the outer layer, which appears to be longitudinal. In reality these layers are almost certainly arranged as a tight spiral (circular) and a loose spiral (longitudinal) as seen in the ureter (see page 301). Close to the uterus, a third muscular layer is also present.

Internal to the muscle layers, a delicate vascular lamina propria supports the tubal epithelial lining.

PRIMORDIAL FOLLICLES

The primary oocytes which survive degeneration in the second trimester enter the prophase of the first meiotic division (see page 24). They remain in this phase for many years and acquire a single layer of flat surrounding cells (**granulosa cells**); these structures are called **primordial** **follicles** (Fig. 18.18a). At birth the ovarian cortex is packed with large numbers of primordial follicles embedded in cellular cortical stroma, and some of these persist in the ovarian cortex throughout the period of sexual maturity (Fig. 18.18b).

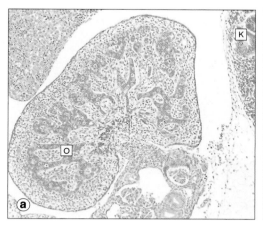

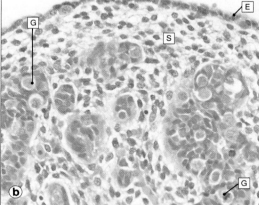

Fig. 18.17 Ovary in embryo.
a The developing ovary (O) in a 9-week-old embryo is shown close to the developing kidney (K).
b At this stage of development the columns of primordial germ cells (G) are embedded in a mesenchymal stroma (S) surrounded by a layer of cuboidal surface cells (E).

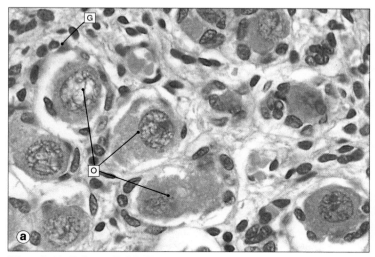

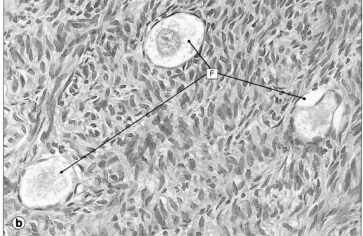

Fig. 18.18 Primordial follicles.
a Ovarian cortex from a 32-week-fetus; it is packed with primordial follicles, each comprising a large primary oocyte (O) with a single surrounding layer of flat granulosa cells (G). Most primordial follicles undergo continuing atresia throughout infancy, childhood and the years of sexual maturity.
b Ovarian cortex from a 25-year-old woman showing persistence of some primordial follicles (F).

PRIMARY FOLLICLE

At puberty, the cyclical secretion of follicle stimulating hormone (FSH) from the pituitary stimulates the further development of a small number (probably 30–40) of the primordial follicles.

The first step is enlargement of the oocyte, which is associated with an increase in size of the surrounding granulosa cells so that they become cuboidal or columnar; at this stage the structure is called a **unilaminar primary follicle**.

Continuing FSH secretion then induces the granulosa cells to divide to produce a multilayered surround to the enlarging oocyte, while a distinct glycoprotein layer of eosinophilic (PAS-positive) material forms between the oocyte and these cells (Fig. 18.19a). This layer is called the **zona pellucida** and is traversed by microvilli protruding outwards from the oocyte and by thin cytoplasmic processes from the inner layer of the granulosa cells. The follicle is now known as a **multilaminar primary follicle**.

Meanwhile ovarian stromal cells come to lie in roughly concentric layers around the enlarging follicle to form a capsule-like arrangement. At about this stage, most follicles then degenerate by a process called atresia (see page 339). A small number of follicles however continue to develop, although atretic degeneration still occurs at all subsequent stages; thus only a few follicles reach full maturity.

SECONDARY FOLLICLES

With continuing follicle maturation the granulosa cell layers increase in thickness, and the outer capsule of ovarian stromal cells begins to differentiate into two layers.

The inner layer of stromal cells (the **theca interna**) increases in size as the cells develop prominent smooth endoplasmic reticulum and mitochondria with tubular cristae (features characteristic of cells producing steroid hormones), and begin to secrete oestrogens; this layer also acquires a prominent capillary network.

The outer layer of stromal cells (the **theca externa**) remains small and compact and has no known secretory function. The follicle is now known as a **secondary follicle** (Fig. 18.19b).

TERTIARY (GRAAFIAN) FOLLICLES

A small fluid-filled split appears in the layers of granulosa cells surrounding the oocyte, and enlarges to form a fluid-filled cavity (the **antrum**), which progressively increases in size; the fluid is slightly viscous and is rich in hyaluronic acid.

The oocyte lies to one side of the by now large follicle, and is separated from the follicle fluid by a coat of granulosa cells called the cumulus oophorus.

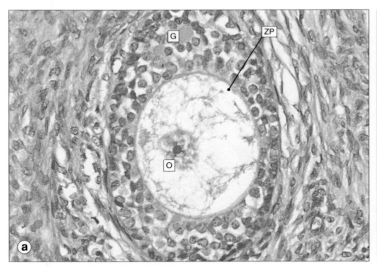
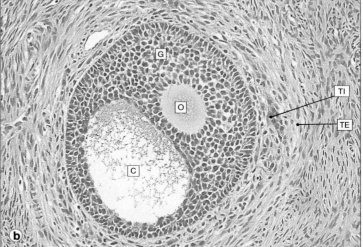

Fig. 18.19 Follicle maturation.
a Micrograph of a multilaminar primary follicle. The granulosa cells (G) have divided to produce a layer 3–5 cells thick, and the pink-staining zona pellucida (ZP) becomes apparent between the oocyte (O) and the granulosa cells.
b Further maturation to a secondary follicle occurs by continuing proliferation of the granulosa cells (G), the appearance of a fluid-filled cavity (C) within them, and condensation of stromal cells around the follicle to form an inner layer of plump cells (theca interna, TI), and an outer layer of smaller spindle-shaped cells, (theca externa, TE).

The follicle is now known as a **tertiary** or **Graafian follicle**, and is ripe for ovulation (Figs 18.20a&b).

The first stage of meiosis is then completed to produce a haploid gamete and a small polar body, which can sometimes be seen attached to the oocyte (now called a **secondary oocyte**). Follicle maturation takes approximately 15 days, by which time the mature follicle is ready for ovulation.

The theca interna secretes increasing amounts of oestrogen to stimulate proliferation of the endometrium (see Fig. 18.24) in preparation for possible implantation of a fertilized ovum.

Ovulation

At ovulation, the Graafian follicle is usually so large that it distorts the surface of the ovary; it appears to the naked eye as a small cystic mass bulging from the ovarian surface, covered only by a thin layer of germinal epithelium and membrane, and an attenuated zone of cortical stromal cells.

The stimulus to ovulation is probably a surge of luteinizing hormone (LH) from the pituitary, which induces completion of the first stage of meiosis, and probably leads to disruption of the structure of the follicle as well.

Before leaving the ovary, the oocyte may break free from its attachment in the follicle wall, and float freely in the follicle fluid, surrounded by an irregular ring of granulosa cells which remain attached to it (the **corona radiata**).

The area of follicle wall in intimate contact with the germinal epithelial covering of the ovarian surface breaks down, and the follicular fluid containing the oocyte is disgorged into the peritoneal cavity.

The oocyte with its surrounding corona radiata is then drawn into the infundibular opening of the fallopian tube, possibly by the waving action of the fimbriae at the infundibular margin.

With rupture of the follicle, there is bleeding from the decompressed lining (particularly from the highly vascular theca interna), filling the follicle with blood clot. Small quantities of blood may pass into the peritoneal cavity.

The disgorgement of blood and follicular fluid onto the pain-sensitive peritoneal surface is thought to be responsible for the transient mid-cycle (day 14–16) lower abdominal pain experienced by some women.

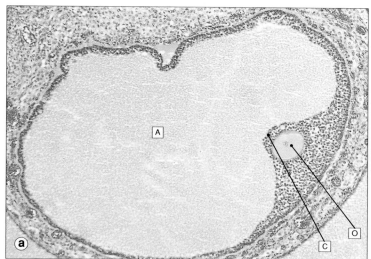

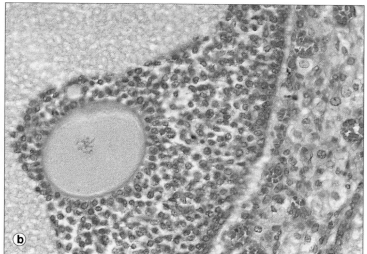

Fig. 18.20 Tertiary (Graafian) follicle.

a A mature tertiary follicle. Note the fluid-filled antrum (A), the eccentrically located oocyte (O) and the cumulus oophorus (C) of granulosa cells around the oocyte.

b Micrograph of the oocyte, cumulus oophorus and granulosa cell layer at higher magnification. The theca layer is highly vascular.

Formation of corpus luteum

After ovulation the remains of the follicle change under the influence of continuing LH secretion by the pituitary gland. The clot-filled lumen of the follicle (**corpus haemorrhagicum**) undergoes progressive organization and fibrosis over the following weeks.

The main changes occur in the granulosa and theca interna cells. In these cells, LH induces changes (**luteinization**), which convert the effete follicle into an endocrine structure known as the **corpus luteum**.

Thus the granulosa cells enlarge, acquire a substantial network of smooth endoplasmic reticulum, become distended with lipid (**granulosa lutein cells**), and secrete progesterone (Fig. 18.21a).

Some of the theca interna cells, already well equipped with smooth endoplasmic reticulum, also accumulate lipid and persist as **theca lutein** or **paralutein** cells, and continue to secrete oestrogens as they did before ovulation. However, many theca interna and externa cells involute, becoming small, compact and spindle-shaped.

The formed corpus luteum therefore has a central area of fibrosing blood clot surrounded by a broad zone of yellow, lipid-rich granulosa lutein cells, with scantier collections of smaller theca lutein cells scattered around the periphery.

Fibrous septa partly separate the granulosa lutein masses, and clusters of theca lutein cells are particularly prominent in the regions of these septa (Fig. 18.21b).

At its maximum size (usually on about day 20 of the menstrual cycle), a corpus luteum is commonly an ovoid structure up to 2 cm long and 1.5 cm wide; it then begins to involute, unless the cycle has been interrupted by fertilization of the oocyte in the fallopian tube (see page 342).

Formation of corpus albicans

Normally, involution of the corpus luteum begins by a decrease in the size of the granulosa and theca lutein cells, with the appearance of vacuoles in their previously uniformly eosinophilic cytoplasm. Progression of this change leads to reduced secretion of progesterone and oestrogen by the two cell types.

At the same time the spindle-shaped cells of the theca externa, and the spindle-shaped fibroblasts forming the fibrous septa, rapidly produce collagen, which replaces the involuting lutein cells.

By about the 26th day of the cycle the hormone-secreting cells are completely eliminated, and the progesterone and oestrogen levels fall dramatically with a significant impact on the endometrium (see Fig.18.24g).

The end result of corpus luteum involution is a small ovoid mass of relatively acellular (hyaline) collagenous tissue, with the general physical configuration of the corpus luteum. This structure is a corpus albicans (Fig. 18.22) and remains in the ovary, decreasing in size with the passing years, but never disappearing.

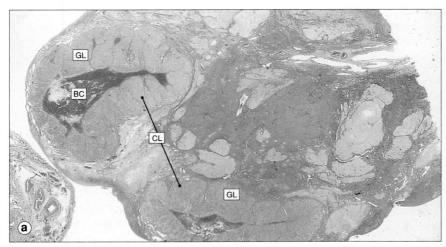

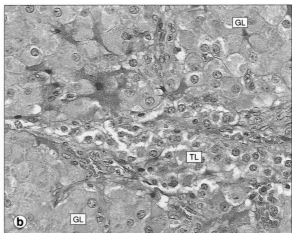

Fig. 18.21 Corpus luteum.
a Micrograph of an ovary containing two corpora lutea (CL), two follicles having ripened to maturity in the same ovary in the same menstrual cycle providing the potential for non-identical twins. Each corpus luteum shows central blood clot (BC) surrounded by a thick layer of lipid-rich granulosa lutein cells (GL).
b Micrograph of the large pale-staining granulosa lutein (GL) cells and the small compact theca lutein (TL) cells, which are mainly concentrated along fibrous septa at the periphery of the corpus luteum.

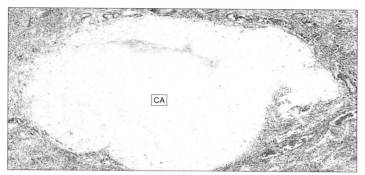

Fig. 18.22 Corpus albicans.
The corpus luteum involutes to form a shrunken mass of collagenous tissue, the corpus albicans (CA), which approximately maintains the shape of the original corpus luteum. Incomplete involution of a corpus luteum may produce a luteal cyst, which is a cyst lined by attenuated granulosa and theca lutein cells.

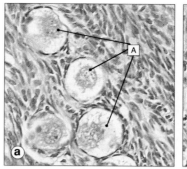
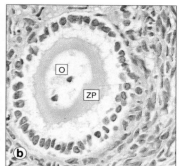

Fig. 18.23 Follicle atresia.
a Micrograph showing a cluster of four primordial follicles, of which three are undergoing atresia (A); they will leave no scar.
b Micrograph showing a primary follicle undergoing atresia, which is mainly manifest by a degenerate oocyte (O) and a collapsing zona pellucida (ZP).

Follicle atresia

Of the vast number of oogonia formed *in utero* by mitotic division of primitive germ cells, only about 500–600 reach full maturity and ovulation during a woman's reproductive life. Some fail to develop, whilst others undergo a process called **atresia**.

Atresia can occur at any stage, but is most marked during intrauterine life when primary oocyte numbers are enormously reduced. As atresia continues throughout infancy, childhood, and the reproductive years, degenerating primary and secondary oocytes can be seen on histological examination of any ovary.

Atresia can supervene at any stage of follicle development. When the follicles are small (primary and secondary stages), the components of the follicle undergo cellular degeneration and complete resorption, leaving no scar (Fig. 18.23a). However larger follicles (tertiary stage) with a substantial cellular component undergo gradual disintegration and replacement by hyaline fibrous tissue. The oocyte disintegrates and the granulosa cells separate and degenerate, while the zona pellucida collapses and wrinkles but remains identifiable.

Often a glassy membrane develops between the degenerating granulosa cells and the outer thecal layers, and may proliferate transiently, perhaps providing the source of the fibrocollagenous fibrous tissue, which ultimately replaces the atretic follicle.

When a large follicle has undergone atresia, a substantial collagenous scar may form, a **corpus fibrosum**, which resembles a small corpus albicans in shape.

MENSTRUAL CYCLE

During the reproductive years, the histological appearance of the superficial functional zone of the endometrial lining varies from day to day on a regular cyclical basis, the **menstrual cycle**.

A complete cycle normally takes about 28 days, but there is considerable variation between women, and also some variation in individual women at different times, for example the first few cycles after the menarche and after a pregnancy tend to be irregular, and increasing irregularity of the cycle is common prior to the menopause.

At the end of every cycle the superficial functional endometrium undergoes necrosis and is shed via the cervix and vagina with bleeding (**menstruation**), leaving only the basal endometrium to act as a reservoir for the development of a new functional layer during the next cycle.

Menstruation lasts for about 4 days, and the day it starts is taken as the first day of the menstrual cycle.

The cyclical changes in the functional endometrium are governed by the changing pattern of hormone secretion by the ovaries, which in turn is influenced by the cyclical secretion of hormones (FSH and LH) by the pituitary gland. The secretion of the gonadotrophic hormones is in turn controlled by the secretion of gonadotrophin-releasing hormones by the hypothalamus. Thus the histological appearance of endometrial curettings can be used to stage (within a few days on either side) the endometrial cycle.

The sequence of changes in the menstrual cycle, is repeated throughout the period of sexual maturity, from the menarche to the menopause, and is interrupted only by pregnancy or hormone therapy, for example oestrogen and progesterone given as a contraceptive.

Proliferative (oestrogenic or follicular) phase

During menstruation the entire superficial functional zone of endometrium is shed, leaving the compact basal endometrium behind.

At the same time, a new cycle of ovarian follicle maturation begins the resulting increasing oestrogen secretion by the developing follicle stimulating mitotic activity in the basal endometrial glands and stroma (Figs 18.24a&b). Continued proliferation of these cells over 10–12 days re-establishes a substantial functional endometrial layer comprising straight tubular endometrial glands embedded in stroma.

As the levels of oestrogen continue to rise in the latter stages of this phase the glands usually become slightly tortuous and their lumina may distend, while continued mitotic proliferation of endometrial gland columnar cells may produce some heaping up of cells, and therefore a pseudostratified appearance. This proliferative phase of the menstrual cycle lasts from day 4 to about day 15 or 16.

Ovulatory (interval) phase

Ovulation occurs at about day 14–16, and is accompanied by the development of **subnuclear vacuolation** in the endometrial glands (Fig. 18.24c), which coincides with peak levels of LH secretion by the pituitary gland. Eventually all of the glands show this change.

Secretory (luteal) phase

The onset of the next (secretory or luteal) phase in the menstrual cycle is marked by the appearance of supranuclear secretory vacuoles at the apical poles of the endometrial gland cells. Secretory material is shed into the gland lumen by the apocrine method (see Fig. 15.1) and the luminal surfaces of the gland cells become irregular and ill-defined. The glands themselves become tortuous (Fig. 18.24d) and their lumina distend with secretion (Fig. 18.24e).

This phase of gland secretion occurs in response to progesterone secreted by the corpus luteum and lasts from about day 16 to day 25 or so.

Premenstrual phase

At about day 22 the secretory activity of the endometrial glands declines and they begin to show involutional changes; the luminal secretion diminishes and that which remains becomes inspissated. The glands become irregular and begin to collapse, and there are significant changes in the stroma, including prominent spiral arterioles (Figs 18.24f&g) and swelling of the stromal cells, particularly around the arterioles.

These changes are precipitated by the sudden fall in progesterone and oestrogen secretion due to involution of the corpus luteum. This premenstrual phase lasts from about day 25 to menstruation at day 28.

Menstruation

At menstruation, increased coiling of the spiral arterioles decreases blood flow, and further constriction of the arterioles leads to significant ischaemia of the functional endometrium. Subsequent dilatation of deeper vessels, combined with necrosis of the walls of the more superficial vessels, then leads to haemorrhage into the stroma.

The necrotic endometrial glands and stroma, together with the stromal accumulations of blood, are then shed as menstrual debris, usually piecemeal with the most superficial endometrium shed first; the deeper layers are lost over the next 4–5 days until only basal endometrium remains. During this time the endometrium begins to regenerate, with re-epithelialization of the naked surface of remaining basal endometrium. This healing process is not hormone dependent.

Fig. 18.24 Menstrual cycle.
Diagram showing the cyclical release of pituitary hormones in response to releasing factors from the hypothalamus. These hormones (FSH and LH) control ovarian maturation and ovulation. In turn the developing follicle cells secrete oestrogen and progesterone, which control uterine endometrial activity.
a Micrograph showing a new layer of functional endometrium (F) developing from the compact basal layer (B) at approximately day 10. The functional endometrium (**proliferative endometrium**) is not much thicker than the basal layer at this stage.
b High power micrograph of proliferative endometrium.
c At about day 16 of a normal cycle (i.e. coinciding with ovulation) the previously straight tubular endometrial glands begin to convolute, and vacuoles (V) appear in a subnuclear location (**early secretory endothelium**).
d Micrograph showing increasing convolution of the tubular endometrial glands (G) stimulated by progesterone secreted by the corpus luteum.
e High power micrograph showing supranuclear vacuolation (V) and accumulation of secretion (S) in the tubular lumina (**late secretory endometrium**).
f Micrograph showing early decidual change in some of the endometrial stromal cells, particularly near the surface (DC) and around spiral arteries (**premenstrual endometrium**).
g High power micrograph of premenstrual endometrium showing contracting, thick-walled spiral arteries (SA).

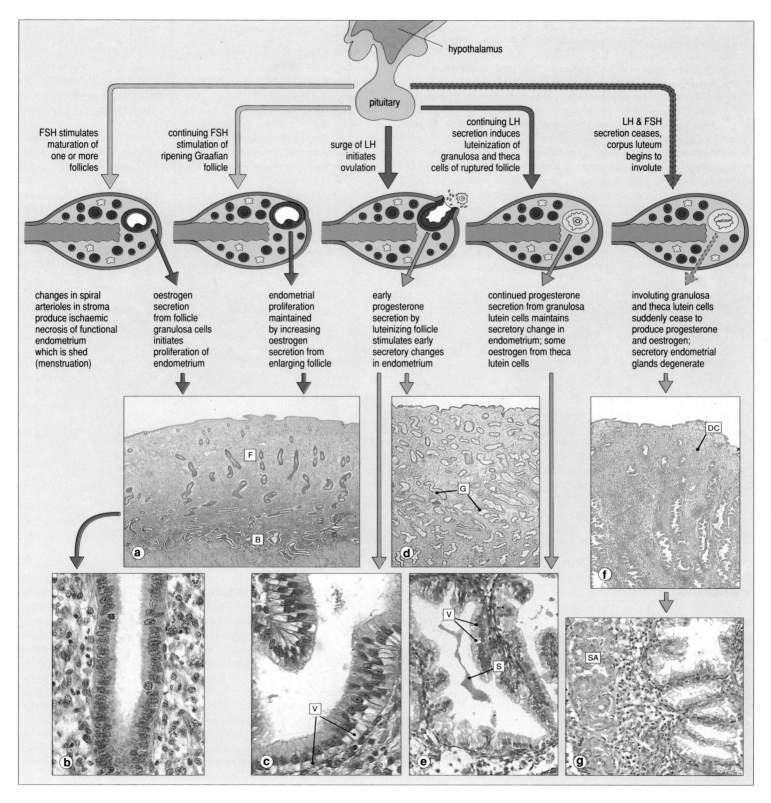

hypothalamus

pituitary

FSH stimulates maturation of one or more follicles

continuing FSH stimulation of ripening Graafian follicle

surge of LH initiates ovulation

continuing LH secretion induces luteinization of granulosa and theca cells of ruptured follicle

LH & FSH secretion ceases, corpus luteum begins to involute

changes in spiral arterioles in stroma produce ischaemic necrosis of functional endometrium which is shed (menstruation)

oestrogen secretion from follicle granulosa cells initiates proliferation of endometrium

endometrial proliferation maintained by increasing oestrogen secretion from enlarging follicle

early progesterone secretion by luteinizing follicle stimulates early secretory changes in endometrium

continued progesterone secretion from granulosa lutein cells maintains secretory change in endometrium; some oestrogen from theca lutein cells

involuting granulosa and theca lutein cells suddenly cease to produce progesterone and oestrogen; secretory endometrial glands degenerate

ENDOMETRIAL DISORDERS

There are many abnormalities which can occur in endometrium, most resulting from inappropriate ovarian hormone stimulation, and causing abnormal patterns of menstruation.

Since the endometrium is largely shed once a month, many abnormalities are transient, but persisting endometrial abnormalities are important.

- **Benign cystic hyperplasia** (Fig. 18.25a) of the endometrium is the result of unopposed oestrogen secretion and may occur in the presence of an oestrogen-secreting ovarian tumour.

- **Atypical endometrial hyperplasia** is marked by hyperplastic endometrial glands, which show disorganization of architectural arrangement, while the epithelial cells show atypical dysplastic features similar to those seen in malignant tumours of endometrial glands. This condition (Fig. 18.25b) is considered capable of conversion into an invasive endometrial tumour.

- The typical malignant tumour of the endometrium, the **endometrial adenocarcinoma** (Fig. 18.25c), occurs mainly in post-menopausal women and presents as post-menopausal bleeding.

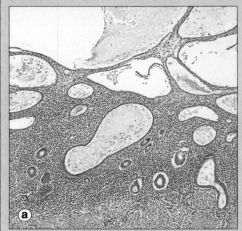 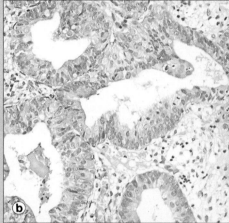 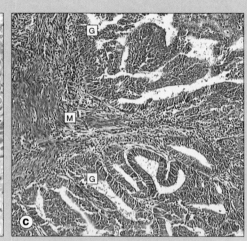

Fig. 18.25 Disorders of endometrium.
a Micrograph of a benign cystic hyperplasia of the endometrium, showing marked cystic dilation of endometrial glands.

b Micrograph of atypical endometrial hyperplasia, showing disorganized, hyperplastic endometrial glands.

c Micrograph of endometrial adenocarcinoma, showing cancerous endometrial glands (G) invading the myometrium (M).

PREGNANCY

The cyclical changes in the ovary and endometrium described above are seen either when fertilization of the ovum does not occur, or if fertilization is followed by death of the zygote or failure of implantation into the endometrium.

In the event of successful fertilization and implantation, the cyclical changes are suspended until some time after childbirth, and almost all of the tissues of the female genital tract undergo structural changes.

The structural changes in the vagina, cervix, myometrium and fallopian tube have been described on pages 326, 329 & 332.

Fertilization and implantation (Fig. 18.26)

When the ovum is disgorged from the ovary at ovulation it enters the open infundibular end of the fallopian tube and passes into the dilated ampullary portion, which is the most common site for its fertilization.

The second meiotic division of the ovum is only completed once the ovum has been successfully penetrated by a spermatozoon. The nuclear material of the penetrating spermatozoon then joins with that of the ovum, forming a diploid zygote, which immediately begins a series of mitotic divisions to produce a solid ball of cells, the morula. The morula migrates down the fallopian tube and arrives in the endometrial cavity about 4–5 days after fertilization.

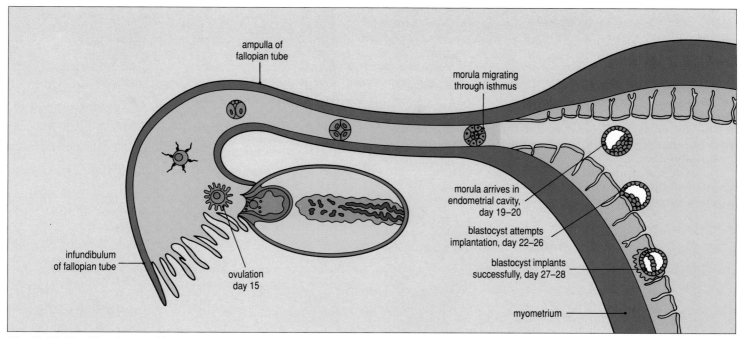

Fig.18.26 Fertilization and implantation.
Diagram illustrating the main features of fertilization and implantation.

Further divisions rapidly produce a cystic mass called the **blastocyst** comprising a fluid-filled cavity (the **blastocoele**) surrounded by a cellular wall (the **trophoblast**). A solid collection of cells, internal to the trophoblast at one pole of the blastocyst, is called the **inner cell mass** and gives rise to the embryo.

After a day or so floating free in the endometrial cavity, the blastocyst must implant in the secretory endometrium if the pregnancy is to continue. Attempts at implantation begin about 6 days after fertilization, which is usually 7–8 days after ovulation, and on day 21–22 of the menstrual cycle. If unsuccessful, the blastocyst degenerates and is expelled with the degenerate endometrium and blood with the onset of menstruation at 28 days.

Sometimes implantation occurs, but cannot be maintained; menstruation eventually supervenes, often after some delay, and the menstrual loss may be greater than usual.

When implantation is successful, the blastocyst gains access to the endometrial stroma, probably directly across the endometrial surface, and by about 11 days after fertilization (i.e. day 27 of the cycle) is completely embedded in endometrial stroma.

From about the time of ovulation, the corpus luteum secretes progesterone. If fertilization and implantation

occur it does not regress, but increases in size up to 3–4 cm in diameter (the **corpus luteum of pregnancy**). This persists throughout the first trimester of pregnancy and is a constant source of progesterone, which is necessary to sustain the pregnancy; thereafter the placenta takes over this function, and the corpus luteum of pregnancy involutes.

At the time of implantation, the endometrium is in its late secretory phase (see Fig. 18.24e), being characterized by bulky tortuous secretory glands and a stroma which may be demonstrating early decidual change (see Fig. 18.24f).

Implantation stimulates the development of true decidual change under influence of the continuing progesterone secretion from the corpus luteum of pregnancy.

Because of the progesterone secretion, the endometrial glands develop exaggerated secretory appearances, which taken in conjunction with the stromal decidual change produces the appearance known as **pregnancy pattern endometrium**.

Further development of the trophoblast and some of the decidualized endometrial stroma produce the **placenta**, which is responsible for continued nourishment of the developing embryo, and also for continued secretion of hormones necessary for maintaining the pregnancy.

Further development of the embryo from the inner cell mass is beyond the scope of this book.

343

Trophoblast

On implantation the single layer of trophoblast, which forms the outer wall of the blastocyst, becomes a double layer.

• The outer layer is characterized by the loss of its lateral cell margins so that it forms a thin syncytial layer, the **syncytiotrophoblast**.

• The inner layer begins as a continuous monolayer of cuboidal cells with pale staining cytoplasm, the **cytotrophoblast**.

The syncytiotrophoblast has numerous surface microvilli, and the ability to erode or invade adjacent tissue, which ensures successful erosion of the endometrial tissues and

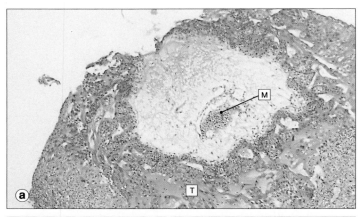

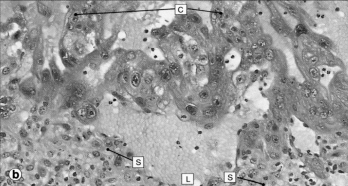

Fig. 18.27 Implantation site.
a Low power micrograph showing an early human implantation site. The blastocyst has infiltrated the superficial endometrium and the trophoblast (T) is beginning to infiltrate the endometrial stroma. Part of the inner cell mass (M) can be seen.
b High power micrograph from the area of trophoblast infiltration. Cords of syncytiotrophoblast (S) have eroded blood vessels and produced lakes of maternal blood (L). Islands of cytotrophoblast (C) are extending into the syncytial masses.

vessels at implantation. The blastocyst initially attaches to the surface epithelium of the endometrium by adhesion. Individual trophoblast cells then intrude between the epithelial cells, so that the blastocyst can insinuate itself through the epithelium and into the endometrial stroma, where erosion of an endometrial capillary ensures it of an adequate blood supply (Fig. 18.27a).

The breach in the endometrial surface is covered by a small blood clot and the surface is quickly re-epithelialized.

The presence of the blastocyst within the endometrial stroma induces early decidualization of the stromal cells, which rapidly involves all of the endometrium and leads to marked thickening.

Once the blastocyst is embedded in the endometrial stroma, the trophoblast rapidly proliferates and the outer syncytial layer extends as irregular protrusions into the surrounding stroma, eroding the walls of small blood vessels as it goes.

Lakes of maternal blood form between the protrusions (Fig. 18.27b), and the surface microvilli of the syncytiotrophoblast probably assist in transferring oxygen and nutrients from the maternal blood to the developing blastocyst.

Chorionic villi

The cytotrophoblast grows into the syncytial protrusions as finger-like extensions, such solid masses of cytotrophoblast covered by syncytium forming the **primary** or **stem chorionic villi**.

With the development of a loose mesenchymal core, the orgin of which is uncertain, the villi are known as **secondary villi**, and soon acquire a system of capillaries which become part of the blood circulatory system of the embryo.

Fully vascularized villi are referred to as **tertiary villi** (see Fig. 18.29a).

As the villi mature, the mesenchymal core contains interlacing vascular channels, fibroblasts, some smooth muscle cells and large pleomorphic cells with vacuolated cytoplasm (**Hofbauer cells**). These cells have some of the ultrastructural and immunocytochemical features of macrophages, and are believed to be motile macrophages with a particular facility for protein ingestion and pinocytosis.

The early chorionic villi subdivide in an arborizing pattern to form a complex system which provides an immense surface area for exchange between the maternal and fetal circulations.

After the complex branching of the villi, the terminal villi contain small thin-walled capillaries, all of which connect with larger vessels in the larger 'twigs', 'branches' and 'trunks' of the tree-like proliferation; these vessels ultimately combine to form the two arteries and single vein that run in the umbilicus to the blood circulation of the embryo (Fig. 18.28).

The appearances of the chorionic villi change with time.
• In early pregnancy the villi contain central capillaries embedded in bulky mesenchyme, but later the capillaries proliferate and come to lie close to the trophoblast surface. As the capillaries become more numerous and dilated, the mesenchyme is reduced in bulk, and its cellular component is reduced, in particular Hofbauer cells become scarce.
• Initially the cytotrophoblast cells predominate and the syncytiotrophoblast is a thin layer. Division of cytotrophoblast probably maintains the syncytial cell mass throughout gestation. As the pregnancy progresses, the syncytiotrophoblast becomes the predominant layer and the cytotrophoblast appears to partly regress, becoming a

discontinuous layer, then collections of scattered cells beneath the syncytiotrophoblast.
• At term (Fig. 18.29b), the villi show increasing hyalinization of the mesenchymal stroma, and fibrin is deposited in the blood-filled intervillous spaces, often coating the outer surface of the villi.

The arrangement of complex chorionic villi of fetal origin intruding into a constantly blood-filled intervillous space of maternal origin provides an efficient means of transferring oxygen, nutrients, maternal antibodies and hormones from the mother to the fetus, and waste metabolites from the fetus to the mother (see Fig. 18.28).

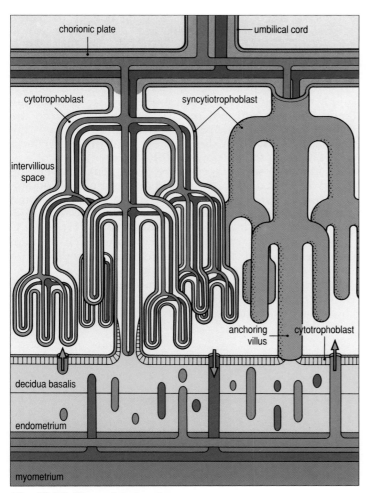

Fig. 18.28 Placental structure.
This diagram illustrates the basic structure of the placenta, and the relationship between the fetal and maternal blood circulations.

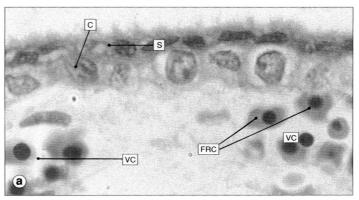

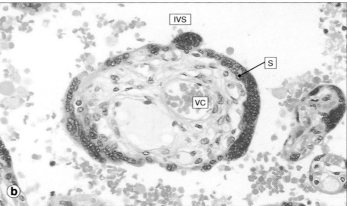

Fig. 18.29 Chorionic villi.
a Micrograph showing part of an early chorionic villus, which is covered by a layer of cuboidal cytotrophoblast (C) and an outer layer of syncytiotrophoblast (S). Note the villus capillaries (VC) filled with nucleated fetal red cells (FRC).
b Micrograph of chorionic villi close to end of pregnancy; note the prominent heaped up syncytiotrophoblast (S), maternal blood in the intervillous space (IVS), and fetal blood in the villous capillaries (VC).

Endocrine functions of the placenta

In addition to being a site of exchange, the placenta also acts as an endocrine organ.

• The syncytiotrophoblast secretes **human chorionic gonadotrophin** (**HCG**) (Fig. 18.30), which is responsible for maintaining the corpus luteum of pregnancy (see page 343) after cessation of the LH stimulus from the pituitary gland.

• The syncytiotrophoblast secretes **human chorionic somatomammotrophin** (**HCS**), which is believed to stimulate lactogenesis.

• The placenta secretes **progesterone** and **oestrogens**; oestrogen precursors produced by the adrenal cortex and liver of the fetus are converted into active oestrogens in the placenta.

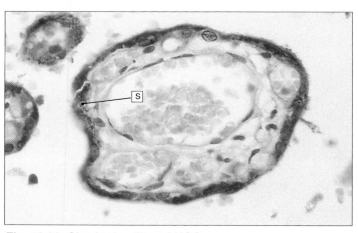

Fig. 18.30 Chorionic villi and HCG.
Micrograph showing a chorionic villus from a term placenta demonstrating localization of human chorionic gonadotrophin (HCG) to the syncytiotrophoblast (S).

Decidua

After implantation, the normally small compact cells of the endometrial stroma undergo remarkable enlargement; this process is known as **decidualization**.

Decidualization begins in the stromal cells around the implanted blastocyst, but soon spreads to involve the rest of the pregnancy endometrium. As the stromal cells enlarge they dominate the endometrium, and the glandular component becomes insignificant. The thickened superficial endometrial layers become the **decidua** as follows (Fig. 18.31).

• The endometrium immediately beneath the implantation site, into which the major trophoblast growth occurs, becomes the **decidua basalis**.

• The thin rim of endometrial stroma overlying the blastocyst becomes the **decidua capsularis**.

• The endometrium lining the rest of the uterine cavity is called the **decidua parietalis.**

Of the decidua, the decidua basalis is the most important since the vessels in this part of the modified endometrium supply maternal arterial blood to the lacunae between the fetal chorionic villi and receive venous blood from the lacunae. The villous trophoblast (from the fetus) and the decidua basalis (from the mother), and the intervillous spaces between them, comprise the placenta.

Decidualized stromal cells have prominent pale-staining round or ovoid nuclei, often with finely granular chromatin and one or two nucleoli; their cytoplasm is bulky, and usually eosinophilic, and granular or slightly foamy, although some cells may have a basophilic tinge (Fig.18.31c).

Ultrastructurally the decidualized stromal cells contain prominent, often long, mitochondria, together with variable amounts of rough endoplasmic reticulum.

The eosinophilia or basophilia of the cytoplasm in individual cells depends on the relative proportions of mitochondria (eosinophilic) and rough endoplasmic reticulum (basophilic).

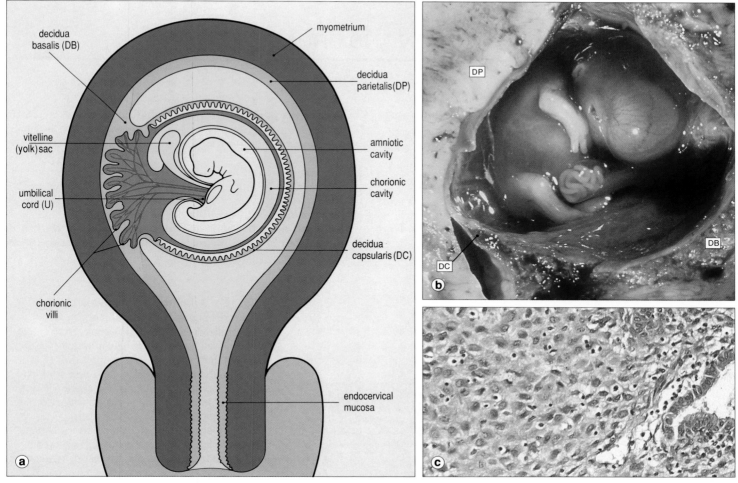

Fig. 18.31 Decidua.

a Diagram showing the decidua and their relationships with the developing fetus and placenta.

b Photograph showing the decidua defined in **a**. Note the decidua parietalis (DP), decidua capsularis (DC) and decidua basalis (DB).

c Micrograph of decidual cells. They are large polygonal cells with pale-staining nuclei and granular eosinophilic cytoplasm.

19. SKIN AND BREAST

The skin is an extensive organ covering the exterior of the body, and varies in structure from site to site according to specific functions, which include:
- protection from external damaging agents;
- thermoregulation;
- sensation (touch, heat, pressure, pain);
- secretion of protective lipids, milk, etc.

The **breast** is a highly modified area of skin with specialized sweat glands to produce nutritious secretions under hormonal influences.

The skin is composed of two main layers, the epidermis and dermis, and a variable third layer, the subcutis.

- **Epidermis** is the surface epithelial layer in contact with the external environment. Downgrowths of this layer produce sweat glands, hair follicles and other **epidermal appendages**.
- **Dermis** is a middle supporting layer containing the epidermal appendages, blood vessels, nerves and nerve endings, which are embedded in an elastocollagenous stroma produced by fibroblasts.
- **Subcutis** is the deepest layer, and varies in size and content, but is usually composed mainly of adipose tissue (Fig. 19.1).

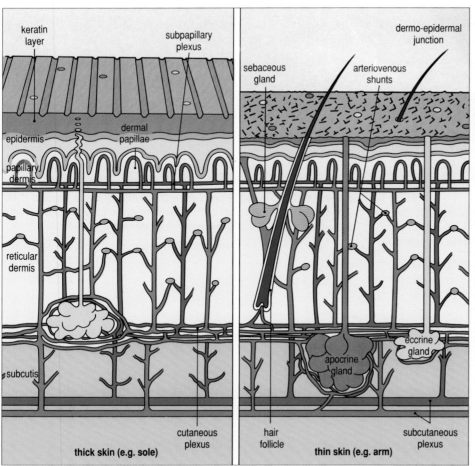

thick skin (e.g. sole)

thin skin (e.g. arm)

Fig. 19.1 Architecture of the skin.
The most superficial layer of the skin is the epidermis. This varies in thickness from site to site and is covered by acellular keratin, which is thick in thick skin and thin in thin skin.

Beneath the epidermis is the dermis, which has two components: a more superficial loose papillary dermis, and a denser reticular dermis, which comprises the bulk of the layer.

The deepest layer of the skin, the subcutis, has a variable structure; when prominent it is composed largely of adipose tissue, intersected by fibrocollagenous septa.

The subcutis contains the main subcutaneous network of arteries and veins from which vessels extend upwards and form a network (the **cutaneous plexus**) at the dermo-subcutaneous junction. From here, smaller vessels penetrate the dermis, giving branches to the skin appendages and culminating in a superficial network of small venules and arterioles (the **subpapillary plexus**). Capillary loops from this plexus extend upwards into the dermal papillae to lie close to the dermo-epidermal junction.

Blood vessels do not penetrate the epidermis.

EPIDERMIS

Epidermis is the protective skin layer in contact with the external environment. It is a stratified epithelium (see page 27), the surface layer being composed of closely packed flat plates of protein (**keratin**), which form a tough, water-repellent layer (**stratum corneum**).

Keratin is produced by the main cell type in epidermis, the **keratinocyte**. Note that despite traditional teaching, the stratum corneum is not cellular, but composed entirely of intracytoplasmic keratin remnants deposited on the surface after the death of the keratinocytes that produced them (see Fig. 3.27), each keratin plate conforms roughly to the shape of the keratinocyte shortly before its death.

Although usually thin, the stratum corneum is very thick in skin exposed to constant trauma, such as that on the soles and palms.

Epidermis is traditionally regarded as a stratified squamous epithelium, but in fact only the most superficial two or three living cell layers of the epidermis approach a squamous or flat configuration, most keratinocytes being cuboidal or polyhedral.

The surface plates of keratin, and the flat dying keratinocytes which precede them, are known as **squames**, and result from the maturation of the other layers of keratinocytes comprising the epidermis. These layers are the basal layer, the prickle cell layer and the granular layer (Fig. 19.2).

Basal layer

The basal layer is the deepest layer of the epidermis and is responsible for the constant production of keratinocytes.

The basal layer cells are cuboidal or low columnar in shape and are attached to the basement membrane, which separates it from the underlying dermis, by hemidesmosomes, and to adjacent basal cells by true desmosomes.

Basal cells have round or oval nuclei (Fig. 19.3) with prominent nucleoli, and their cytoplasm is rich is ribosomes and mitochondria; tonofibrils are present in small numbers. In pigmented skins the cytoplasm also contains melanin granules and lysosomes.

It is in the basal layer that cells in mitosis are seen, as well as scattered non-keratinocyte cells, melanocytes and Merkel cells (see page 354).

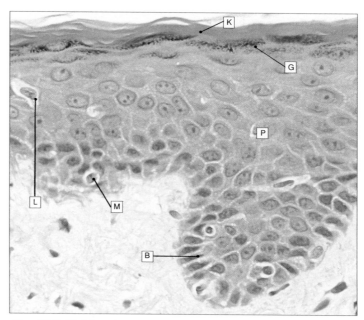

Fig. 19.2 Epidermis.
The three cell layers of the epidermis are most clearly seen in thick skin, as shown here; the basal layer (B) sits on the basement membrane, and is covered by the prickle cell layer (P) and then the granular layer (G), which is characterized by its content of dark-staining keratohyaline granules. In thick skin, there is a thick layer of dense acellular keratin (K).

Two non-keratinocyte cells of the epidermis, a melanocyte (M) and a Langerhans' cell (L) (see page 354) are also evident.

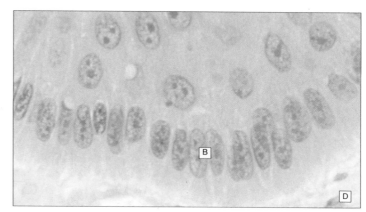

Fig. 19.3 Basal cells.
The basal cells (B) are smaller than the other keratinocytes and may show a regular, regimented arrangement (palisading). They have rounded or oval nuclei, and rest on the basement membrane marking the junction between epidermis and dermis (D).

Dermo-epidermal junction

The junction between the dermis and epidermis is an important area, tethering the two layers together, and structured to minimize the risk of dermo-epidermal separation by shearing forces as follows.

• Tethering fibres connect the dermis and epidermis to intervening basement membrane.

• The basal cell membrane of individual basal cells, and the underlying basement membrane are convoluted (see Fig. 19.6).

• There is a system of **rete ridges** (i.e. downgrowths of epidermis into dermis), which varies markedly from site to site. In protected areas, where the skin is not normally subjected to shearing stress (e.g. the trunk), rete ridges are barely evident and the dermo-epidermal junction appears flat, but in areas constantly exposed to shearing stress (e.g. tips of the fingers, palms and soles), the rete ridge system is highly developed (see Figs. 19.1 & 19.19–19.23).

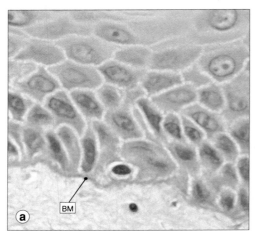

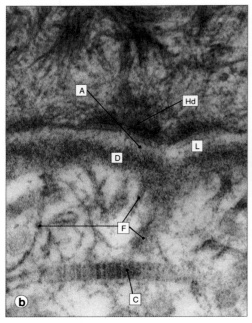

Fig. 19.4 Dermo-epidermal junction.
a By light microscopy, basement membrane (BM), which separates the epidermis and dermis, is difficult to see unless a special stain is used, such as PAS shown here; PAS stains the abundant glycoprotein in the basement membrane (see Fig. 4.11).
b In this electronmicrograph of dermo-epidermal junction, the basement membrane can be seen to consist of three three main layers: a superficial electron-lucent lamina lucida (L), an electron-dense lamina densa (D) and an ill-defined fibroreticular lamina.

The basal cells are tethered to the lamina densa by hemidesmosomes (Hd) from which anchoring proteins (A) cross the lamina lucida. On the dermal aspect fine anchoring fibrils (F) of type VII collagen attach the lower surface of the lamina densa to collagen fibres (C) in the papillary dermis, while fibrillin microfibrils attach it to elastic fibres. In addition, the zone immediately beneath the lamina densa contains abundant fibronectin (see page 46).
c Diagram of dermo-epidermal junction showing the components of the basement membrane and its attachments to basal cells and dermal fibres.

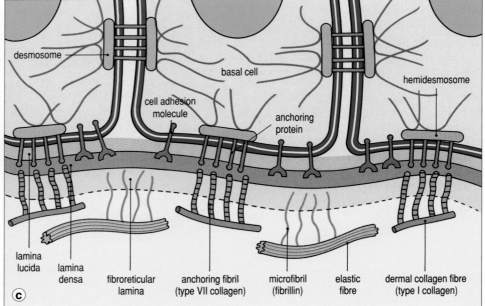

BASAL BLISTERS

The dermo-epidermal junction is a site where fluid can accumulate in sufficient quantity to lift the epidermis away from the dermis, thus forming a basal blister. This can result from:
- excessive shearing force;
- structural abnormality.

Excessive shearing forces are the most common cause and are usually due to constant shearing friction, such as occurs with tight-fitting shoes.

Structural abnormalities may be primary or secondary.
- The most important primary cause is the rare inherited skin disease **epidermolysis bullosa**, in which the dermo-epidermal junction is intrinsically weak and unable to resist even minimal shearing trauma. There are a number of different types of epidermolysis bullosa, depending on the site of separation, which can be ascertained by electron microscopy.
- Secondary causes are more common and usually result from inflammatory skin disease that damages the basal layer and its underlying basement membrane, for example the blistering diseases **pemphigoid** and **dermatitis herpetiformis**.

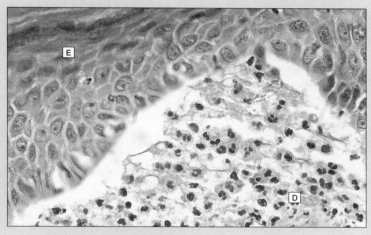

Fig. 19.5 Dermatitis herpetiformis.
Micrograph showing a secondary cause of basal blistering, **dermatitis herpetiformis,** in which patients develop an intensely itchy blistering eruption.

In dermatitis herpetiformis the immunoglobin IgA becomes deposited in the tips of the dermal papillae close to the basement membrane. This activates the complement cascade via the alternative pathway, and neutrophil polymorphs (see page 71) are attracted to the site by the release of chemotaxins. As a result the dermis (D) is damaged just below the dermo-epidermal junction, and the epidermis (E) separates, leaving a basal blister containing fluid and some remnants of neutrophil polymorphs. Note the numerous neutrophils in the small early blister shown here

Prickle cell layer

The keratinocytes above the basal cells form the prickle cell layers and are polyhedral with central round nuclei and pinkish-staining cytoplasm.

Prickle cells are in contact with each other by a system of intercellular bridges, formed from small cytoplasmic projections from the cell surface terminating in desmosomal junctions (Fig. 19.6, also see Fig. 3.11).

The cytoplasm of the prickle cells contains many tonofilaments (see Fig. 3.27), which are particularly concentrated in the cytoplasmic projections leading into the desmosomes, and are more numerous in the cell layers closest to the granular layer.

The cells of the upper prickle cell layer are flatter than the polyhedral cells of the deeper layers. The narrow interstices between the prickle cells are partly occupied by the cytoplasmic projections of melanocytes and Langerhans' cells.

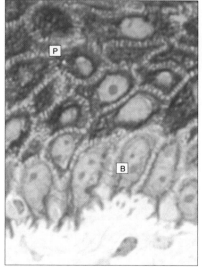

Fig. 19.6 Prickle cell layer.
A thin epoxy resin section of skin stained with toluidine blue showing the basal layer (B) and the prickle cell layer (P) above it.

Prickle cell cytoplasm stains more intensely than the basal cell cytoplasm because of its high content of tonofilaments. The characteristic intercellular bridges to which the prickle cells owe their name, are easily seen and are the site of desmosomal attachments between adjacent prickle cells.

351

Granular cell layer

The granular keratinocytes contain small or oval haematoxyphilic round bodies (**keratohyaline granules**) composed of proteinaceous material containing abundant sulphur-rich amino acids (e.g. cysteine). They also contain abundant tonofibrils and small round lamellated **keratinosomes** or **Odland bodies**.

In the upper layer the cytoplasm of granular keratinocytes is largely composed of masses of keratohyaline material and tightly packed tonofibrils, with little cytosol or cytoplasmic organelles, and at this level the cells are flat. Death of the nucleus and cytoplasm leaves the keratohyaline and tonofibrils, which combine to form the keratin (see Fig. 3.27) of the acellular surface layer, the stratum corneum (Fig. 19.7).

Keratinosomes produce a complex hydrophobic glycophospholipid, which is released when the superficial granular keratinocytes die, and probably acts as a glue,

cementing together the flakes of keratin. This substance also renders the skin surface relatively non-wettable, although prolonged exposure will wash it away, permitting the keratin to absorb water, swell and soften.

Epidermal turnover

Surface keratin is constantly lost due to normal wear and tear from surface friction, washing and scrubbing, etc. It is therefore constantly replenished from the granular layer, which in turn is constantly repopulated by cells from the prickle layer. The prickle cells are produced by proliferation of cells in the basal layer.

Turnover, from basal cell to desquamated keratin varies from site to site, being faster (i.e. 25–30 days) in traumatized areas (e.g. soles); slow turnovers range from 40–50 days. The turnover period is considerably shortened in some skin diseases, particularly psoriasis.

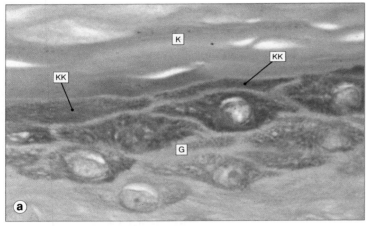

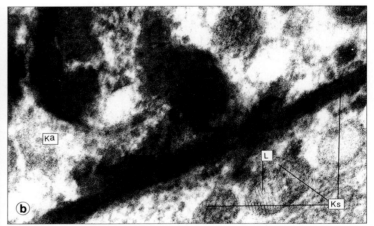

Fig. 19.7 Granular cell layer.
a Micrograph showing the granular layer (G) of the epidermis with acellular keratin (K) above it. The cytoplasm becomes progressively darker staining near the surface due to its increasing content of keratohyaline granules. The most superficial cells have lost their nuclei and are flat plates of keratohyaline and keratin (KK).
b Electronmicrograph showing part of the cytoplasm of a cell in the granular layer; it is packed with irregular masses of electron-dense keratohyaline (Kh) and round or oval keratinosomes (Ks), some of which show lamellation (L).

Non-keratinizing epidermal cells

In addition to keratinocytes, the epidermis also contains melanocytes, Langerhans' cells and Merkel cells.

Melanocytes

Melanocytes are thought to be neuroectodermally-derived cells whose main function is to produce the pigment melanin, which is largely responsible for skin colour and minimizes tissue damage by ultraviolet radiation.

Melanocytes are located in the basal layer of keratinocytes and are in contact with the basement membrane. They are pale-staining with large ovoid nuclei and abundant cytoplasm, from which numerous long cytoplasmic processes extend into the spaces between the keratinocytes. Melanocyte cytoplasm contains characteristic membrane-bound ovoid granules (**premelanosomes** and **melanosomes**),

which have a striated electron-dense core and produce melanin (Fig. 19.8). In the production of melanin, tyrosine is converted into DOPA (dihydroxyphenylalanine) by the action of the enzyme tyrosinase, the DOPA then being converted into an intermediate pigment which polymerizes into melanin.

Melanin binds to proteins to form the active melanoprotein complex, which appears ultrastructurally as spherical masses of homogeneous electron-dense material, and often obscures the premelanosomes.

Melanoprotein complexes pass along the cytoplasmic processes of the melanocyte and are transferred into the cytoplasm of basal and prickle cell layer keratinocytes, the highest concentration being in the basal layers.

Melanocyte numbers remain more or less constant, but their degree of activity is genetically variable accounting for racial and individual variation in skin colour.

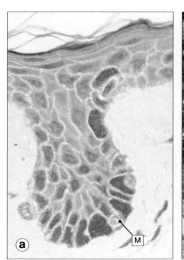 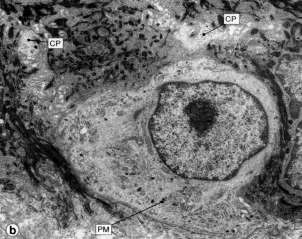 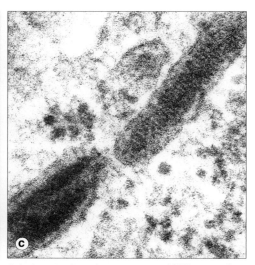

Fig. 19.8 Melanocyte.
a Micrograph showing a melanocyte (M) with its pale-staining cytoplasm. In this section of black skin it can be clearly seen against the pigment-laden basal cells.
b Ultrastructurally melanocytes contain premelanosomes (PM) and melanosomes, and their cytoplasmic processes (CP) extend between keratinocytes of the basal and lower prickle cell layers.
c High magnification electronmicrograph showing the characteristic boat shape of premelanosomes; both coarse longitudinal and fine transverse striations can be seen.

Langerhans' cells

Langerhans' cells are located in all layers of the epidermis but are most easily seen in the prickle cell layer. They recognize antigen and are an important component of the immune system (see page 85).

Like melanocytes, Langerhans' cells have an ovoid pale-staining nucleus surrounded by pale-staining cytoplasm, from which cytoplasmic (dendritic) processes extend between the keratinocytes.

Langerhans' cell cytoplasm contains scattered characteristic **Birbeck granules**, which are rod-like structures with periodic cross-striations, and are most numerous near the Golgi. Sometimes one end of the rod is distended to form a spherical saccule, giving the appearance of a tennis racket (Fig. 19.9).

Although present in small numbers in healthy skin, Langerhans' cells are increased both in number, and in the extent and complexity of their dendritic processes, in many chronic inflammatory skin disorders, particularly those with an allergic or immune aetiology, such as chronic atopic dermatitis.

Merkel cells

Merkel cells are scanty and difficult to demonstrate in normal skin. They are found in the basal layer and resemble melanocytes by routine light microscopy, but electron

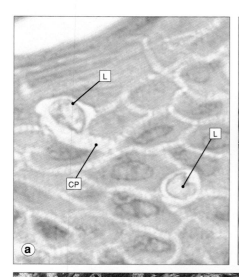
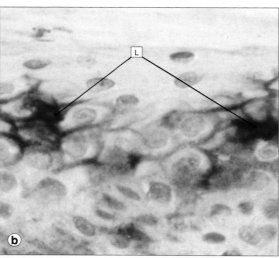
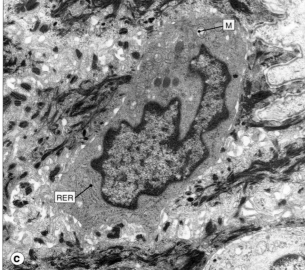
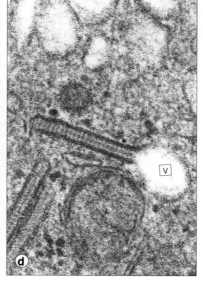

Fig. 19.9 Langerhans' cells.
a In paraffin or resin sections stained with H&E, Langerhans' cells (L) are irregular pale-staining cells in the prickle cell layer, with pale-staining oval or reniform nuclei, which are often clefted. Their numerous cytoplasmic processes (CP) pass between the keratinocytes.
b Langerhans' cells (L) carry CD1marker and can be clearly visualized by immunoperoxidase techniques.
c Ultrastructurally Langerhans' cells have an irregular clefted nucleus and are devoid of tonofilaments. They have prominent mitochondria (M), lysosomes and rough endoplasmic reticulum (RER). Birbeck granules are not seen at this magnification.
d High magnification electronmicrograph showing two characteristic Birbeck granules, one with a distended vesicle (V) at one end.

microscopy reveals rounded membrane-bound cytoplasmic neuroendocrine-type granules.

Merkel cells form synaptic junctions with peripheral nerve endings at the base of the cell, and also scanty desmosomal attachments to adjacent keratinocytes (Fig. 19.10). They occur either as scattered solitary cells, or as aggregates, when they are associated with a so-called **hair disc** located immediately beneath the basement membrane. Such aggregates are thought to be touch receptors and are sometimes called **tactile corpuscles.**

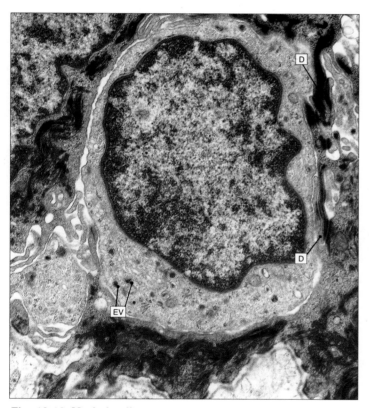

Fig. 19.10 Merkel cells.
Merkel cells can be distinguished from melanocytes by their ultrastructural features (compare with Fig. 19.8b&c). They have a convoluted nucleus, which occupies much of the cell, and no cytoplasmic processes insinuating between keratinocytes, but may have short protrusions, which contact adjacent keratinocytes at occasional desmosomes (D).

Round neuroendocrine vesicles (EV) are present in the cytoplasm, particularly at the base of the cell, close to the basal nerve terminal, which communicates with the underlying nerve disc (not shown here). The cytoplasm also contains a prominent Golgi, smooth endoplasmic reticulum and scattered ribosomes.

DERMATITIS (INFLAMMATION OF SKIN)

The skin is exposed to many damaging agents, such as chemicals and ultraviolet irradiation, which produce a wide variety of common rashes. A common type of dermatitis, **seborrhoeic dermatitis**, is shown in Fig. 19.11.

In addition, the skin reacts to internal abnormalities, and produces rashes in response to disorders such as viral infections (e.g. measles) and drug allergies (e.g. penicillin rash).

The cause of most skin diseases is not known.

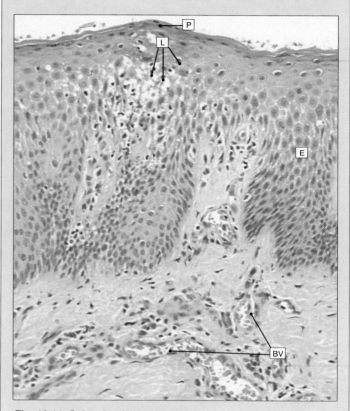

Fig. 19.11 Seborrhoeic dermatitis.
The epidermis (E) is thickened, and is disrupted by an infiltration of lymphocytes (L) associated with an accumulation of water (clear areas) between keratinocytes. Note that the surface keratin layers still contain remnants of keratinocyte nuclei. This is termed **parakeratosis** (P) and is a manifestation of disordered keratinocyte maturation in areas of epidermal damage. Blood vessels (BV) in the upper dermis are dilated and surrounded by lymphocytes and macrophages. In seborrhoeic dermatitis the damaging agent in thought to be a fungus.

SKIN APPENDAGES

The skin appendages are the pilosebaceous apparatus, isolated sebaceous glands, eccrine sweat glands and ducts, and apocrine sweat glands and ducts.

Pilosebaceous apparatus

The **pilosebaceous apparatus** produces hair and sebum, which is a non-wettable secretion that protects the hair and augments the non-wettable characteristics of the keratin.

The components of a pilosebaceous apparatus are hair follicle, hair shaft, sebaceous glands and erector pili.

HAIR FOLLICLE

The **hair follicle** is a tubular epithelial structure opening onto the epidermal surface. At its lower end, a bulbous expansion (the **hair bulb**), with a concave lower surface, contains a specialized area of dermis called the **hair papilla**. This is richly supplied with myelinated and non-myelinated nerve endings and abundant small blood vessels.

In the hair bulb numerous small actively proliferating germinative cells produce the hair shaft and the internal root sheath, which lie within the external root sheath.

Germinative hair bulb cells have dark basophilic cytoplasm with a scattering of melanocytes.

Internal root sheath is composed of three layers:
- **Henle's layer**, which is a single cell layer;
- a thicker layer characterized by the presence of large eosinophilic **trichohyaline** granules;
- **cuticle**, which consists of overlapping keratin plates.

The cuticle is continuous with the cuticle of the hair shaft (see below) in the lower regions of the hair follicle.

The internal root sheath undergoes keratinization to produce the hair shaft, and extends up from the hair bulb to about the level of the insertion of the sebaceous glands, where it disintegrates, leaving a potential space around the hair shaft into which the sebaceous gland products are secreted.

External root sheath is modified epidermis, and near the opening of the follicle onto the skin surface consists of all three epidermal layers (basal, prickle cell and granular). In the deeper parts of the hair follicle, below the point of insertion of the sebaceous glands, it is composed of highly modified prickle cells, with large pale-staining cells rich in glycogen.

Outside the external root sheath is a thick basement membrane, which is strongly eosinophilic and is known as the **glassy membrane** (Fig. 19.12).

HAIR SHAFT

Each hair shaft is composed of two or three layers of highly organized keratin; these are an inner medulla, an outer cortex and a superficial cuticle.
- The medulla is a variable component and is not present in the finer vellus and lanugo hairs. When present it is composed of layers of tightly packed polyhedral cells.
- The cortex is composed of tightly packed keratin, which is produced without the incorporation of keratohyaline granules; it is 'hard' keratin and differs in composition from the soft keratin of the epidermal surface.
- The cuticle consists of a single layer of flat keratinous scales, which overlap in a highly organized manner.

Hair shafts contain variable amounts of melanin depending on melanocyte activity in the germinative cells of the hair bulb.

SEBACEOUS COMPONENT

Sebaceous glands develop as lateral outgrowths of the external root sheath. They are largely inactive until puberty, after which they enlarge and become secretory.

Sebaceous glands are composed of lobules of large polyhedral pale-staining cells containing abundant lipid droplets and small dark-staining central nuclei. There is a single layer of cuboidal or flattened precursor cells between the basement membrane of each lobule and the central mass of cells. The sebaceous gland lobules are connected to the hair follicle, usually about two-thirds to three-quarters of the way up from the hair bulb, by short ducts lined by stratified squamous epithelium, showing all the layers seen in the normal epidermis.

The secretion of the sebaceous glands (**sebum**) is a lipid mixture, which includes triglycerides and various complex waxes. It is produced by large scale necrosis of the cells, resulting in the release of their lipid content into the ducts (Fig. 19.13) and thus into the space between the formed hair shaft and the external root sheath, following degeneration of the internal root sheath. This pattern of secretion is called holocrine secretion (see Fig. 15. 1).

The number, size and activity of sebaceous glands varies from site to site within the skin. They are particularly abundant on the face, scalp, ears, nostrils and vulva, and around the anus, but are absent from the soles and palms.

ERECTOR PILI

A further component of the pilosebaceous apparatus is a narrow band of smooth muscle, the **erector pili**, which originates in the fibrocollagenous sheath surrounding the hair follicle, and runs obliquely upwards into the upper dermis. This muscle positions the hair follicle and hair shaft, its contraction making the hair follicle and shaft more vertical, so that the hair appears to stand on end.

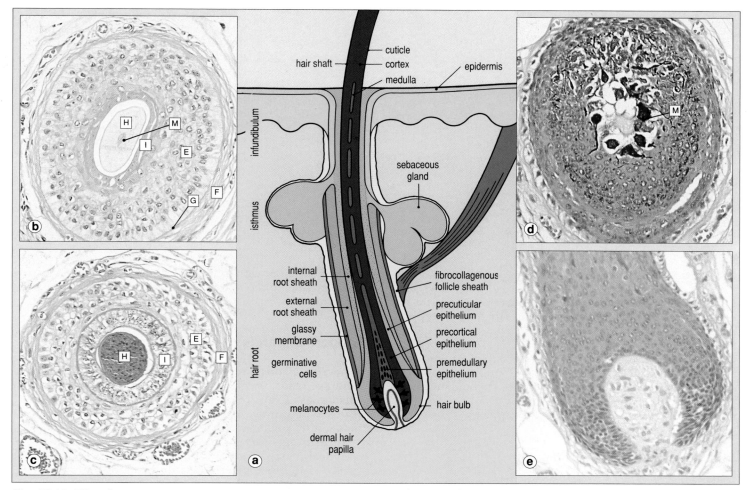

Fig. 19.12 Pilosebaceous apparatus.

a Diagram to show the general architecture of the pilosebaceous apparatus. The hair bulb is a collection of compact epithelial cells surrounding a vascularized fibrocollagenous dermal papilla, and produces the various components of the hair shaft (i.e. medulla, cortex and cuticle). In dark-haired people, abundant active melanocytes in the basal layer of the hair bulb supply melanin to the pre-cortex cells; the medulla and cuticle are not pigmented.

The outer cells of the hair bulb epithelium produce the **internal root sheath**, the middle layer of which contains numerous red-staining trichohyaline granules.

The **external root sheath** is derived from the epidermis by downgrowth, and is bound externally by a distinct homogeneous membrane, the **glassy membrane** This separates it from the **fibrocollagenous follicle sheath**, which surrounds the entire follicle and also encloses the sebaceous glands as a thin, variably distinct layer.

Attached to the fibrocollagenous follicle sheath at, or just below, the level of the sebaceous glands is the erector pili muscle, which extends obliquely upwards from this lower

attachment to its upper attachment in the papillary dermis.

The lower parts of the hair shaft consist of partly keratinized cells in which the nuclei of the progenitor epithelium can still be seen, but higher up the hair is composed of anuclear, hard compact keratin, which does not stain with eosin.

b Transverse section through a hair follicle just below the sebaceous glands. The hair shaft (H) is anucleate and composed of non-staining hard keratin; a central medullary remnant (M) can be seen. The outer fibrocollagenous root sheath (F) and glassy membrane (G) around the external root sheath (E) are well formed, but the internal root sheath (I) is acellular and degenerate.

c Transverse section through a hair follicle just above the hair bulb. The hair shaft (H) contains nuclear remnants and is strongly eosinophilic. The cellular internal root sheath (I) is well formed and contains eosinophilic trichohyaline granules. Note the external root sheath (E) and the outer fibrocollagenous root sheath (F).

d Transverse section through a hair bulb showing melanocytes (M) supplying melanin to the pre-cortex epithelium.

e Longitudinal section through a hair bulb. There are no active melanocytes in this example.

357

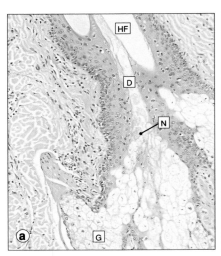

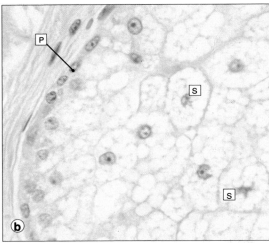

Fig. 19.13 Sebaceous gland.
a Micrograph showing a sebaceous gland (G) opening through a narrow duct (D) into the hair follicle (HF). The sebum is formed by necrosis (N) of the lipid-packed cells of the gland.
b A sebaceous gland at higher magnification showing the single layer of cuboidal or flat precursor cells (P), and the large sebaceous cells (S) distended with lipid droplets.

Isolated sebaceous glands

In certain areas of the body, the sebaceous glands do not empty into hair follicles, but open directly onto the epidermal surface. This occurs in:
- the labia minora (see page 322);
- areolar skin around the nipple, where they are known as Montgomery's tubercles (see 364);
- the eyelids, where they are known as Meibomian glands (see page 204).
- the lips and buccal mucosa (Fordyce spots).

Eccrine sweat glands and ducts

Eccrine sweat glands and ducts are found everywhere in the skin, but are particularly numerous on the forehead, scalp, axillae, palms and soles. They arise as downgrowths of the epidermis at about the 16th week of intrauterine life.

The secretory gland component, which is situated deep in the dermis or in the upper subcutis near the dermo-subcutaneous junction, communicates with the exterior via its duct. Close to the gland the duct is coiled, but then proceeds as a straight duct up to the dermo-epidermal junction. Within the epidermis the duct again becomes coiled, but this is only seen to any extent where the epidermis is thick, for example in the soles (see Fig. 19.19b).

Eccrine sweat glands are composed of two layers of cells, an inner layer of secretory cells and an outer flat layer of contractile myoepithelial cells, which is bounded by a distinct, sometimes thick, membrane. The dermal ducts consists of two layers of dark-staining cuboidal cells surrounding a distinct lumen, the surface of which is often strongly eosinophilic (Fig. 19.14).

Eccrine glands produce sweat and are controlled by the autonomic nervous system. Sweat is a hypotonic watery solution, with a neutral or slightly acid pH, containing various ions, particularly sodium, potassium and chloride ions.

Apocrine glands

Apocrine glands develop as downgrowths of the epidermis, and are scanty in man, but well developed in many other mammals. They are small and insignificant in childhood, but become more prominent and probably functionally active after puberty.

In man apocrine glands are concentrated mainly in the perineal region, around the anus and genitalia, and in the axillae. Modified apocrine glands are found in the eyelids (**Moll's glands**), in the areolar skin around the nipple, and in the external auditory canal where they form the **ceruminous glands** responsible for the production of ear wax.

Apocrine glands are composed of:
- a secretory glandular unit situated, like the eccrine gland, in the lower dermis or at the dermo-subcutaneous junction;
- a more or less straight duct, which opens into a pilosebaceous unit near the surface, usually above the entrance of the sebaceous duct.

The secretory unit of an apocrine gland is composed of an inner layer of cuboidal epithelial cells and an outer layer of discontinuous flat cells, surrounded by basement membrane. It has a large lumen (Fig. 19.15). The duct resembles the eccrine duct (see Fig. 19.14), having a double layer of cuboidal epithelium.

Apocrine glands produce a viscid slightly milky secretion in response to external stimuli such as fear, sexual excitement, etc., the function of which is not known in man ; similar glands in mammals act as scent organs for delineation of territory and sexual attraction.

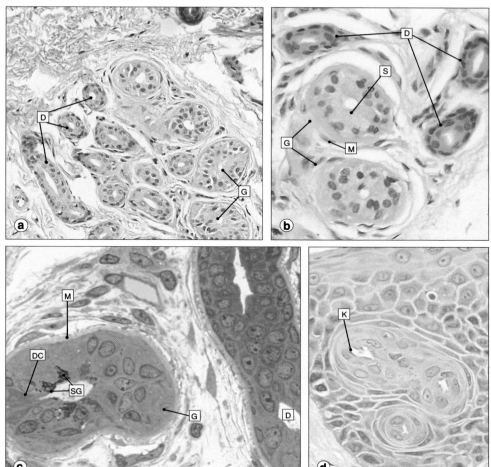

Fig. 19.14 Eccrine gland and duct.

a Micrograph showing eccrine glands (G) and ducts (D) in the deep dermis, at low magnification.

b High power micrograph showing that the glands (G) are composed of pale-staining secretory cells (S) with an outer layer of indistinct myoepithelial cells (M). The ducts (D) have a more distinct double layer of dark-staining cells.

c Thin epoxy resin section stained with toluidine blue showing that the gland (G) is composed of large pale-staining glycogen-rich cells, some of which contain dark secretory granules (SG), and a smaller number of narrow darker staining cells (DC), which secrete sialomucins. Eccrine glands are surrounded by a thick amorphous membrane (M), and their ducts (D) are lined internally by a homogeneous cuticle, which is composed of microvilli covered by an amorphous glycocalyx.

d Micrograph showing intraepidermal portion of eccrine duct, which is spiral and is sometimes called the **acrosyringium**. There is a single layer of cells lining the lumen, and two or three layers of outer cells. The lining cells develop small keratohyaline granules (K) and become keratinized where they emerge through the granular layer of the epidermis.

The spiral course continues through the keratin layer, and is most clearly seen in skin with a thick epidermis (see Fig. 19.19b).

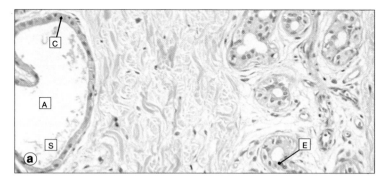

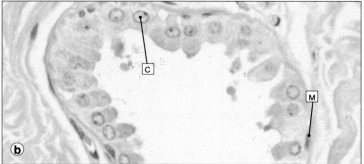

Fig. 19.15 Apocrine gland.

a Micrograph showing part of an actively secreting apocrine gland (A) from axillary skin, with part of an eccrine gland (E) for comparison. The apocrine gland has an inner layer of cuboidal epithelial cells (C) with markedly eosinophilic cytoplasm and an outer layer of discontinuous flat cells, which are thought to be myoepithelial. It is surrounded by a prominent eosinophilic

basement membrane. The lumen is large, and faintly pink homogeneous secretion (S) may be seen within it.

b High power view showing the roughly cuboidal eosinophilic lining cells (C) and the irregular luminal surface resulting from the secretory process, in which fragments of secretion-containing cytoplasm are 'pinched off' into the lumen (see Fig. 3.24). Flat myoepithelial cells (M) are present, but insignificant.

DERMIS

Dermis is the supporting tissue on which epidermis sits, and within which the epidermal appendages, blood supply, nerve supply and lymphatic drainage are situated. It is composed of:

- fibroblasts, fibrocytes and their extracellular products (see page 50);
- collagen and reticular fibres;
- glycosaminoglycan-containing matrix;
- blood vessels;
- small numbers of macrophages, lymphocytes and mast cells.

Two distinct zones of dermis can usually be identified: an upper narrow papillary dermis, which is close to the dermo-epidermal junction, and a thicker reticular dermis, between the papillary dermis and subcutaneous adipose tissue.

Reticular dermis forms the bulk of the dermis. It is composed of prominent broad bands of dense collagen with intervening long thick fibres of elastin, which usually run parallel to the skin surface. Within this tissue are the blood vessels, lymphatics and nerves of the skin.

Papillary dermis is paler than reticular dermis and contains less collagen and elastin, but more matrix. The thin collagen and elastin fibres are more randomly arranged, with a high proportion perpendicular to the skin surface. Papillary dermis contains small blood vessels of capillary size, fine nerve twigs and nerve endings (Fig. 19.16).

Vasculature

The main blood supply to the skin is located within the dermis and arises from larger vessels in the subcutaneous fat. Two distinct plexuses can be identified (see Fig. 19.1):

- a deep vascular plexus in the lower reticular dermis close to its border with the subcutis;
- a superficial vascular plexus in the upper reticular dermis close to its junction with the papillary dermis.

Loops of small vessels from the superficial vascular plexus run up into the papillary dermis, with small capillaries lying close to the epidermal basement membrane. No blood vessels penetrate the epidermis.

The dermis contains many arteriovenous anastomotic channels including highly specialized shunts (**glomus bodies**), which are found mainly the finger tips. Blood flow variation within the dermis is important to the skin's function as a thermoregulatory organ.

The skin appendages are supplied by branches from vessels connecting the deep and superficial vascular plexuses.

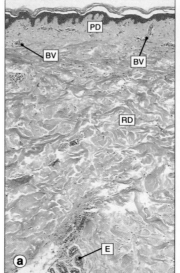
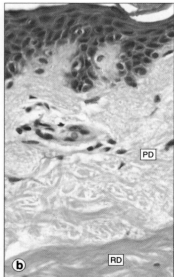
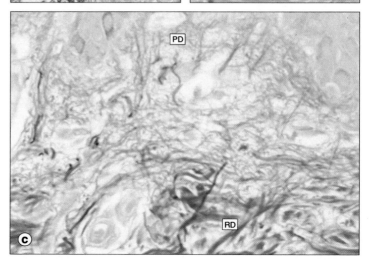

Fig. 19.16 Dermis.
a Low power view of dermis stained with H&E. It is eosinophilic because of its high content of collagen; the papillary dermis (PD), which contains less collagen, is paler. An eccrine unit (E) can be seen in the deeper part of the reticular dermis (RD). Note the concentration of small blood vessels (BV) at the junction between papillary dermis and the densely collagenous reticular dermis
b High power micrograph showing the different natures of the loose pale-staining papillary dermis (PD) and the more densely collagenous reticular dermis (RD).
c Elastic Van Gieson stained section of upper dermis demonstrating elastic (black) and collagen (red) fibres, showing the difference between papillary dermis (PD), in which both collagen and elastin are fine and vertically orientated, and reticular dermis (RD), in which the collagen and elastin fibres are thicker and coarser, and are mainly arranged longitudinally.

Nerve supply

The nerve supply of the skin is located in the dermis, and comprises:

- a rich non-myelinated supply derived from the sympathetic autonomic nervous system, which controls the skin appendages and vascular flow;
- an afferent myelinated and non-myelinated system, which detects cutaneous sensation.

Detection of cutaneous sensation is associated with a number of unspecialized and specialized nerve endings (Fig. 19.17).

- Free nerve endings (myelinated and unmyelinated) are numerous and detect pain (and its minor variant, itch) and temperature.
- **Pacinian corpuscles**, which are encapsulated nerve endings with a characteristic structure, detect pressure and possibly vibration, and are usually found in the deep dermis or subcutaneous fat of the palms and soles.
- **Meissner's corpuscles**, which are structured nerve endings confined to the dermal papillae, are most numerous on the feet and hands, and detect touch.
- **Merkel cells** and their nerve attachments (see Fig. 19.11) are slowly adapting touch receptors.

Modifications

The dermis varies in both thickness and content, and may contain bundles of smooth muscle, for example, the dartos muscle of the scrotum, and the muscle bundles in and around the nipple.

In the face, the skeletal muscle fibres of facial expression are partly located in the deep dermis.

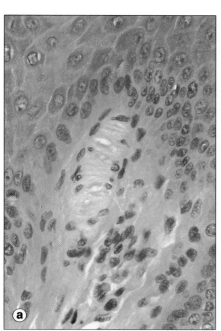
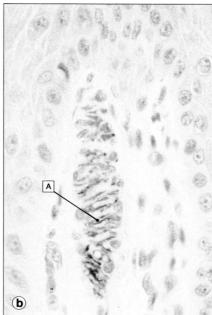
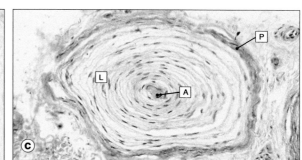
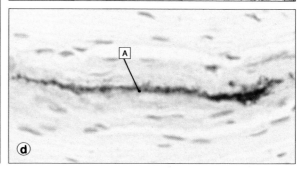

Fig. 19.17 Common nerve endings in the skin.

a Skin section stained with H&E showing a Meissner's corpuscle, which is an elongated oval body. Meissner's corpuscles are arranged vertically in the dermal papillae of hairless skin, particularly in fingers and toes, but also around lips and nipples. Internally Meissner's corpuscles are composed of spirally arranged cells surrounded by a thin fibrocollagenous capsule. In H&E sections the most commonly seen cells are flattened Schwann cells (see page 210), the axons not being visible.

b Meissner's corpuscle stained by an immunoperoxidase method for NFP to demonstrate the spirally arranged axon (A).

c Micrograph showing a Pacinian corpuscle in subcutaneous fat from the fingertip demonstrated by an immunoperoxidase method for neurofilament protein (NFP). It is a large loosely laminated structure with a central core (axon, A) surrounded by concentrically arranged lamellae (L), which are modified Schwann cells separated from each other by fluid-filled spaces. The lamellae are more tightly packed peripherally and form a dense pseudocapsule (P).

d A Pacinian corpuscle in longitudinal section stained by an immunoperoxidase method for neurofilament protein to show its longitudinally running central axon (A).

SUBCUTANEOUS TISSUE

Subcutaneous tissue may contain extensions of skin structures, for example:
- in the scalp it contains the lower parts of the long hair follicles;
- some apocrine and eccrine glands.

Subcutaneous tissue is composed largely of adipose tissue separated by fibrocollagenous septa, and contains the main blood vessels and nerves from which the overlying dermis is supplied (Fig. 19.18). It acts as an effective heat insulator, food store, and shock absorber.

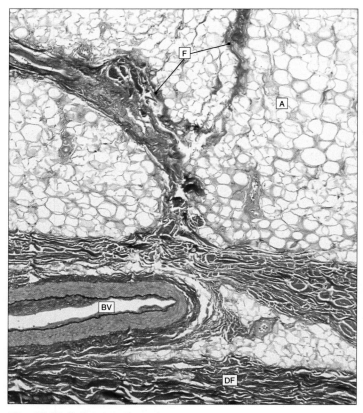

Fig. 19.18 Subcutaneous tissue.
Micrograph of subcutaneous tissue from the scalp. It is composed largely of adipose tissue (A) intersected by vertically running bands of fibrocollagenous tissue (F), which extend down from the deep dermis. In this example, the fibrous septa extend through the full thickness of subcutaneous tissue to join the dense fibrocollagenous layer (DF) covering the periosteum of the underlying skull.

Subcutaneous tissue contains the major blood vessels (BV) from which the blood supply of the dermis arises.

FEATURES OF SKIN IN DIFFERENT SITES

Most of the skin covering the body is protected by clothing and is neither excessively traumatized, nor particularly specialized. Thus skin from the back, abdomen, thighs, and arms (Fig. 19.19) has:
- a thin epidermis producing only small amounts of loosely packed keratin;
- a poorly formed rete ridge system;·
- small numbers of hair follicles producing fine hairs (large follicles and coarser hairs in men);
- variable numbers of eccrine glands.

SOLE
In contrast to the skin of the back, abdomen, thighs and arms, the skin of the sole (Fig. 19.20) is modified to withstand constant trauma, and has:
- a thick epidermis, which is covered by a thick layer of compact keratin;
- a well developed rete ridge system to prevent epidermal separation from shearing stress;
- no hair follicles;
- abundant eccrine glands and ducts.

SCALP
The characteristic feature of the scalp is the presence of tightly packed hair follicles with their associated sebaceous glands (Fig. 19.21). In straight haired people, the follicles are almost vertical, but in curly haired people they are oblique, the degree of curliness depending on the degree of obliquity.

FINGERTIP
Fingertip skin shows two structural modifications: one to minimize damage from shearing stress, the other because of its role as a tactile sensory organ (Fig. 19.22). Thus the skin in this region is characterized by:
- a thick epidermis with thick compact protective keratin;
- a well-developed rete ridge system;
- numerous Meissner's corpuscles in the dermal papillae (see Fig. 19.17);
- Pacinian corpuscles in the dermis and subcutis (see Fig. 19.17);
- specialized arteriovenous shunts (glomus bodies);
- abundant eccrine sweat glands and ducts.

AXILLA
Skin in the axillae and groin is similar, possibly because of our quadruped origins. Its most important features are:
- an abundance of highly active apocrine glands;
- numerous oblique hair follicles;
- numerous eccrine glands;
- thin epidermis (Fig. 19.23).

PRACTICAL HISTOLOGY

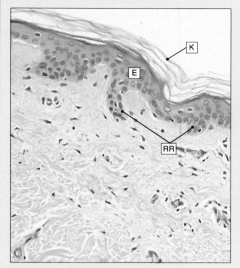

Fig. 19.19 Thin skin.
Micrograph showing the thin epidermal (E) and keratin (K) layers of thin skin, which is also characterized by a poorly developed rete ridge system (RR), small numbers of hair follicles and variable numbers of eccrine glands.

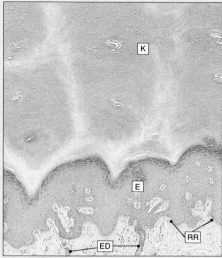

Fig. 19.20 Thick sole skin.
Micrograph showing the thick epidermal (E) and keratin (K) layers of thick skin, which is also characterized by a well developed rete ridge system (RR), and numerous eccrine glands and ducts (ED).

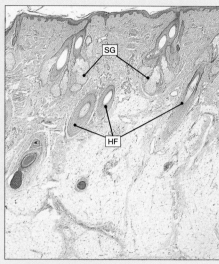

Fig. 19.21 Scalp skin.
Micrograph showing the tightly packed pilosebaceous units of scalp skin. Note the sebaceous glands (SG) and hair follicles (HF).

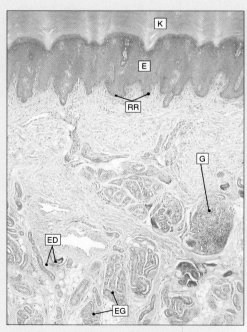

Fig. 19.22 Fingertip skin.
Micrograph showing the thick epidermis (E) and well developed rete ridge system (RR) of fingertip skin, covered by thick compact protective keratin (K). Note the glomus body (G) and the abundant eccrine sweat glands (EG) and their ducts (ED).

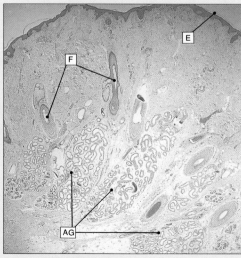

Fig. 19.23 Axillary skin.
Micrograph showing the abundant apocrine glands (AG), oblique hair follicles (HF), and thin epidermis (E) of axillary skin.

BREAST

Breasts develop as downgrowths from the epidermis along a line (**milk line** or **streak**), which runs obliquely from the axilla towards the groin on each side. In humans only one breast normally develops on each side, but occasionally there is development of an accessory breast though only the nipple component persists after birth.

Nipple

The nipple is a round raised area of modified skin with a slightly convoluted epidermis, which shows increased melanin pigmentation after the first pregnancy.

The nipple is surrounded by the **areola**, which is modified skin containing large sebaceous units forming small nodular elevations (**Montgomery's tubercles**). The areola also shows increased melanin pigmentation after the first pregnancy. At the tip of the nipple are the 12–20 small openings of the large nipple ducts (Fig. 19.24).

Breast development

The nipple and its simple system of ducts is present at birth, but full development of the epithelial downgrowth does not occur until puberty, and then usually only in females.

At puberty, and under the influence of increasing oestrogen secretion:
- the breasts increase in bulk, due initially to an increase in adipose tissue;
- the ductular system of the nipple becomes more complex with branches extending into the adipose tissue (Fig. 19.25).

Occasionally the male breast enlarges slightly at puberty, again due to increased adipose tissue and extension of the ductular system. However the enlargement is usually minimal, self-limiting and reversible, though occasionally it can progress.

Normally the male breast remains a rudimentary system of simple nipple ducts and a small amount of fibrocollagenous tissue.

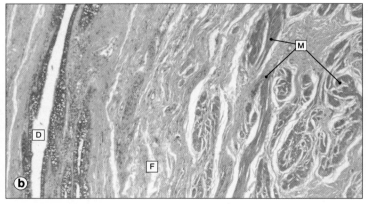

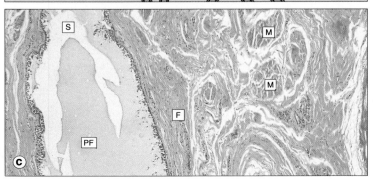

Fig. 19.24 Nipple.

a There are 12–20 openings arranged in a ring on the surface of the nipple, each being lined by keratinizing stratified squamous epithelium. In the inactive, non-lactating breast they are normally plugged by keratin. Each opening is the site of emergence of a single **lactiferous duct**, which is lined by a two-layered epithelium, the basal layer being myoepithelial cells.

Each lactiferous duct receives large mammary ducts, and there is a dilation, the **lactiferous sinus**, shortly afterwards.

The support tissue consists of fibroadipose tissue containing numerous longitudinal and circular smooth muscle bundles.
b Micrograph of a lactiferous duct (D) of the nipple, with surrounding fibrocollagenous stroma (F) and longitudinal and circular smooth muscle (M).
c Micrograph of part of a lactiferous sinus (S) just below the nipple. The sinus contains homogenous proteinaceous fluid (PF) and is surrounded by fibrocollagenous stroma (F) and muscle (M).

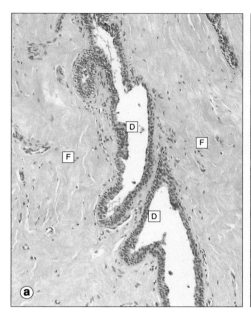

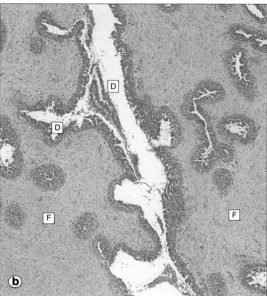

Fig. 19.25 Breast development.
a Micrograph of breast tissue from a 4-month-old female infant. All that is present is a system of scarcely branching nipple ducts (D) embedded in fibrocollagenous tissue (F).
b Micrograph of breast tissue from an 11-year-old girl at the onset of puberty. The ductular system (D) is beginning to proliferate and produce branches, and the surrounding fibrocollagenous supporting tissue (F) is actively increasing in bulk.

GYNAECOMASTIA

Excessive development of the male breast (Fig. 19.26) is called gynaecomastia and occurs under the influence of excess oestrogen secretion, which may be either endogenous (e.g. at puberty) or exogenous (e.g. stilboestrol treatment for prostatic cancer).

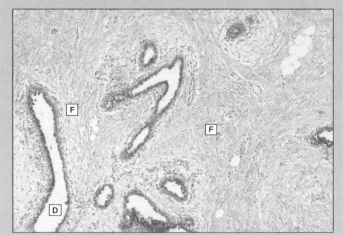

Fig. 19.26 Gynaecomastia.
Gynaecomastia is characterized by proliferation and branching of the mammary duct system, which often dilates (D), and by an increase in the periductal fibrocollagenous tissue (F).

Growth and activity of the female breast are entirely hormone dependent. Continued oestrogen secretion after the onset of puberty leads to progressive enlargement and complexity of the duct system.

The parenchyma of the breast is composed of 12–20 distinct lobes, each lobe consisting of a duct system with its own separate opening in the nipple, embedded in adipose tissue containing fibrocollagenous septa. Particularly prominent septa separate the individual lobes and are attached to overlying skin by fibrocollagenous bands, which are sometimes called the **suspensory ligaments of Astley Cooper**. On their deep surface the septa are attached to the fascia overlying the pectoralis muscle.

Mammary duct system

Each lobe of the breast is a system of ever-branching ducts, which penetrate deep into the fibroadipose tissue of the breast.

Each duct is lined by columnar or cuboidal epithelium, with a continuous surface layer of epithelial cells with oval nuclei and an outer discontinuous layer of myoepithelial cells, which have clear cytoplasm.

Each duct is surrounded by loose fibrocollagenous support tissue containing a rich capillary network. Elastic fibres are present within this fibrous sheath in all but the smallest, most peripheral branches.

Mammary gland system

The duct system terminates in a cluster of blind-ending terminal ducts, each cluster and its feeding duct comprising a **mammary lobule**, which is ovoid in shape.

The terminal ducts are embedded in a loose fibrous support tissue, which is rich in capillaries and also contains a few lymphocytes, macrophages and mast cells. This tissue is surrounded by a more dense fibrocollagenous support tissue intermingled with adipose tissue (Fig. 19.27).

Breast changes in pregnancy

Breast structure changes early in pregnancy; the vascularity and melanin pigmentation of the nipple and areola increases and the mammary lobules enlarge by hyperplastic proliferation of the terminal ducts with some vacuolation appearing in the luminal epithelial cells.

By the second trimester, there is evidence of luminal cell secretion, which is copious by the third trimester and accumulates within the hyperplastic terminal ducts (Fig. 19.28).

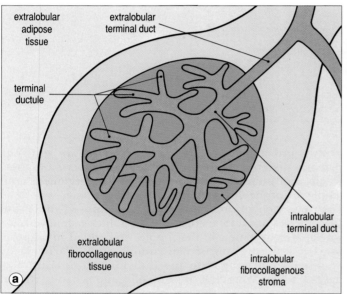

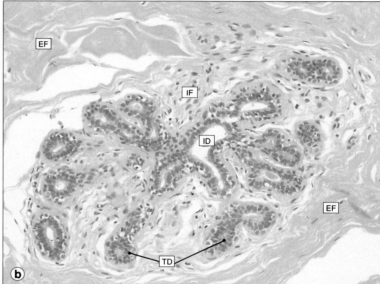

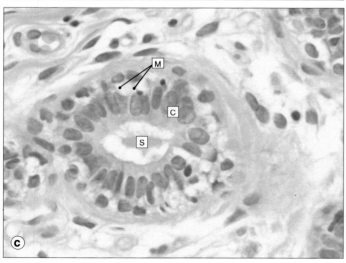

Fig. 19.27 Mammary lobule.

Diagram of a mammary lobule, which consists of a cluster of blind-ending terminal ductules together with the drainage duct system (extralobular and intralobular terminal ducts). Some lobules are located in the dense fibrocollagenous tissue of the breast whilst others are in adipose tissue.

b Micrograph of a typical mammary lobule embedded in fibrocollagenous tissue. Note the difference between the intralobular (IF) and extralobular (EF) fibrocollagenous tissue.

In this inactive lobule the epithelium of the terminal ductules (TD) is identical to that of the intralobular terminal duct (ID). The extralobular terminal duct is not visible.

c High power micrograph showing the epithelium of the intralobular terminal ductules. Essentially two-layered, the inner layer varies between a cuboidal and a low columnar pattern (C), whilst the outer layer consists of prominent myoepithelial cells (M).

Note the minute amount of secretion (S) in the lumen of the duct resulting from menstrual cycle hormone secretion.

With this expansion of the lobular units, there is an accompanying increase in the loose lobular support tissue and inflammatory cells. At term and throughout lactation the hyperplastic lobular units are distended by their lipid-rich proteinaceous secretion (milk).

The breast only reaches its full functional activity during pregnancy under the influence of pituitary and ovarian hormones secreted in high concentrations during pregnancy and breast feeding.

When breast feeding ceases, the breast returns to its normal or resting state by gradual involution over a period of some months. The luminal cells return to their former size without cytoplasmic vacuolation, and the lobular support tissue returns to its normal proportions.

Sometimes there is residual increased collagen in the involuting lobular support tissue, and this can lead to progressive distortion of the mammary lobules and persistent cystic dilation of some of the ducts.

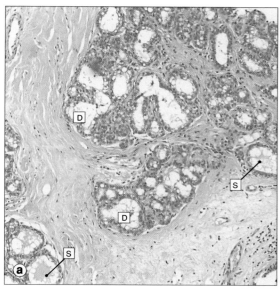
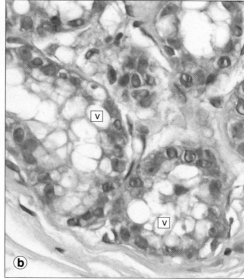

Fig. 19.28 Breast in pregnancy.
a Micrograph showing the hyperplastic breast lobules of pregnancy. The intralobular terminal ductules (D) are increased in size and complexity, and their lumina are distended by secretion (S) from the lining epithelium.
b Micrograph showing clear vacuoles (V) containing lipid-rich secretion forming on the luminal aspect of terminal ductule lining epithelium.

FIBROADENOSIS

Repeated exposure of the mammary lobules to varying oestrogen and progesterone secretions during numerous menstrual cycles can lead to disproportionate growth of various components and distortion of the normal architecture. Common changes are:
- increased duct and ductular tissue (adenosis);
- increased fibrocollagenous support tissues (fibrosis);
- dilation of the larger mammary ducts.

Such changes when they occur are most severe in multigravid women and cause increased nodularity of the breast tissue, which is sometimes associated with cyst formation (Fig. 19.29). This is the most common disorder of the breast and is variably called **fibroadenosis**, **cystic mammary dysplasia**, **benign mammary dysplasia** or **fibrocystic disease** of the breast.

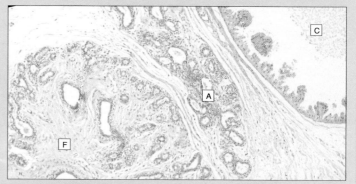

Fig. 19.29 Fibroadenosis.
Micrograph of section of breast showing the features of fibroadenosis; these are fibrosis (F), adenosis (A) and cyst formation (C).

CARCINOMA OF THE BREAST

The epithelial component of the extralobular mammary ducts, the intralobular mammary ducts and the terminal ductules, may undergo cancerous change to produce one of the most important and common cancers in women, **breast cancer**. Cancers originating in the terminal ductules are called **lobular carcinomas**, those from the ducts are called **ductal carcinomas**.

The breast is well-equipped with small blood and lymphatic vessels, so spread of the cancer away from its site of origin in the breast is common and can lead to a poor outlook.

● Spread along lymphatics is usually to the axillary group of lymph nodes on the side of the affected breast, producing metastatic deposits in the nodes (see Fig. 7.14).

● Spread via the blood stream usually occurs at a later stage, metastatic carcinoma being deposited in many organs, particularly the lungs and bones.

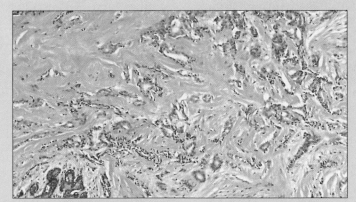

Fig. 19.30 Mammary carcinoma.
Micrograph showing the features of a typical carcinoma derived from mammary ducts. The cells have broken through into the surrounding fibroadipose tissue to produce an invasive carcinoma.

PRACTICAL HISTOLOGY

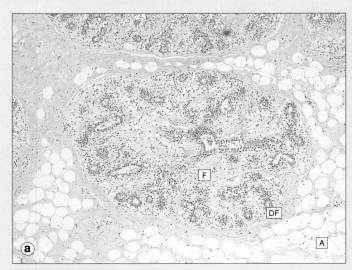

Fig. 19.31 Breast.
a Micrograph showing normal breast tissue from a 23-year-old woman. At the centre is a breast lobule in which the system of terminal ducts and ductules is embedded in loose intralobular fibrocollagenous stroma (F). There is a narrow surrounding zone of dense extralobular fibrocollagenous support tissue (DF) outside which is the soft adipose tissue (A) that forms the bulk of the breast.

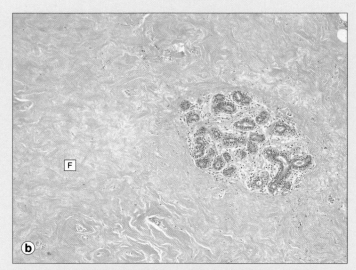

b Micrograph showing normal breast tissue from a 43-year-old woman. As women age, the amount of fibrocollagenous tissue (F) in the breast increases, replacing some of the adipose tissue. The mammary lobules become enclosed in dense collagen.

GLOSSARY OF TECHNIQUES AND STAINS

TISSUE PREPARATION TECHNIQUES

Paraffin embedding

Paraffin embedding is the standard method of preparing thin sections of biological material for histological examination by light microscopy. It is cheap, comparatively simple, and lends itself to automation.

The sample is fixed, usually in an aqueous formalin-based fixative solution, and then progressively dehydrated by passage through a series of alcohol solutions (e.g. 60% →70% →90% →100%) until all water (intrinsic tissue water and fixative water) has been removed, and the specimen is thoroughly permeated by absolute alcohol. The alcohol is then replaced by an organic solvent which is miscible with both alcohol and with molten liquid paraffin wax (alcohol is not miscible with paraffin wax). The resulting specimen is immersed in paraffin wax at a temperature just above the melting point of the wax, which is solid at normal working room temperature, and when the biological material is thoroughly permeated by the molten wax it is allowed to cool so that the wax solidifies. The wax acts as a physical support to the sample, allowing thin sections (2–7μm) to be cut without deformation of the cellular structure and architecture.

The machine used to section the sample is called a **microtome.** The thin sections are mounted on a glass microscope slide and the wax removed with an organic solvent before the section is rehydrated through increasing dilutions of alcohol. When fully rehydrated the sections are stained with any of a number of stains, some of which are outlined below.

Most of the micrographs shown in this book have been prepared from paraffin sections except where otherwise stated.

Frozen sections

The embedding of biological material in paraffin and other media (see below) may destroy certain components, particularly enzymes and some antigenic sites. If frozen water is used as the supporting medium, these are better preserved and can be demonstrated by suitable techniques. Fresh (unfixed) material is rapidly frozen to -150 to -170°C by immersion in, for example, liquid nitrogen, so that it hardens to a solid mass due to freezing of tissue water. Thin sections (5–10μm) are then cut on a special microtome housed in a refrigerated cabinet (a **cryostat**), and stained without exposure to alcohol or other organic solvents.

Frozen sections are used to demonstrate the cellular localization of enzymes and soluble lipids, and in the identification of substances using immunofluorescent and immunocytochemical methods.

In skilled hands, a stained frozen section of a sample of human tissue can be prepared and examined under the microscope within 5 minutes of its removal from the body. In this way a rapid and accurate histological diagnosis can be established whilst the patient is in the operating theatre, enabling the appropriate surgical operation to be performed.

Acrylic resin embedding

Certain acrylic resins are used in a similar way to paraffin wax as embedding media. When set, they are harder than paraffin wax and offer more support to the tissue than wax. They have two main advantages over paraffin wax for light microscopy:

- they enable good quality sections of very hard material to be cut, and are therefore used in the histological examination of mineralized bone (see Figs 14.14a & 14.18).
- with the use of a special microtome, much thinner sections (i.e. 1–2μm thick) can be obtained than with paraffin wax, giving greater resolution with the light microscope, and enabling much more detail to be seen.

Epoxy resin embedding

Epoxy resins are the hardest supporting media, offering greatest support to biological material. With special sectioning machines, sections as thin as 0.5–1μm can be cut for high resolution light microscopy, and ultrathin sections can be prepared for transmission electron microscopy.

The transmission electronmicrographs in this book have been prepared from ultrathin epoxy resin sections. These resins are resistant to the damaging effects of the electron beam in the electron microscope, and continue to support the biological material, whereas other embedding media volatilize in the electron beam.

Most of the staining methods used with paraffin and acrylic resin sections are unable to penetrate epoxy resins. Fortunately, the stain toluidine blue is an exception, and differentially stains biological components in various shades of blue. The greatest cellular detail obtainable by light microscopy is by the use of 0.5-1μm epoxy resin sections stained with toluidine blue (see Fig. 16.6d).

OUTLINE OF COMMON STAINING METHODS USED IN THIS BOOK

Haematoxylin and eosin (H&E)

The combination of the two dyes, haematoxylin (blue) and eosin (red), is the most useful stain for the examination of biological material; it is simple to perform, reliable, inexpensive and informative. Most of the micrographs in this book are stained with H&E, particularly in the **Practical Histology** sections.

Van Gieson method

The simple Van Gieson method stains collagen pinkish-red and muscle yellow (see Fig. 8.4b); it is commonly used in combination with a stain for elastic fibres.

Elastic Van Gieson (EVG)

The elastic Van Gieson stain is valuable for demonstrating and differentiating the common support cell fibres, particularly elastic fibres, which stain brown-black, and collagen fibres, which stain pinkish-red; muscle is stained yellow (see Fig. 8.16).

Trichrome methods

The trichrome methods employ a mixture of three different dyes to stain different components in different colours. There are many trichrome methods, and they can be used to demonstrate general architecture (see Fig. 16.6b), to emphasize support fibres (see Fig. 11.8), or to distinguish support fibres from muscle fibres (see Fig. 5.9b). An important use of a trichrome method is the demonstration of the cellular, osteoid and mineralized components of bone in undecalcified bone embedded in acrylic resin (see Figs 14.21 & 14.22).

Silver methods

Under appropriate conditions, certain biological components reduce silver nitrate to form black deposits of metallic silver at the site of chemical reduction. By modifying the conditions of the sliver niotrate solution used, these methods can be used to demonstrate a wide range of structures, including reticulin fibres (see Fig. 11.3b).

Periodic Acid Schiff (PAS) method

The widely used PAS method has many applications, particularly in the demonstration of vaious carbohydrates, either alone (e.g. glycogen) or combined with other molecules, such as proteins (e.g. glycoproteins). It can therefore be used to delineate basement membranes (see Figs 4.11a & 19.4a) and some neutral mucins secreted by various secretory epithelial cells (see Fig. 9.10b). The mucous cells of the stomach are strongly PAS positive.

Alcian blue method

The alcian blue dye method is used mainly to demonstrate acidic mucins secreted by some epithelial cells (see Fig. 10.43b), and can be combined with the PAS reaction to distinguish between acidic and neutral epithelial mucins (see Fig. 9.10b).

By varying the pH or other variables in the staining solution, the alcian blue method can be used to demonstrate the extracellular glycosaminoglycan matrix (see Fig. 4.13d) of support cells.

May-Gruenwald-Giemsa method

The use of the May-Gruenwald-Giemsa method is confined mainly to the examination of smear preparations of blood and bone marrow cells. Most of the micrographs in Chapter 6 show red and white blood cells stained by this method.

Toluidine blue

Toluidine blue is used to demonstrate cells and fibres in very thin epoxy resin sections (see above). It gives considerable cellular detail, staining the various components of the cells and fibres in shades of blue in a way that represents their relative electron desnsity; hence the resulting blue picture closely resembles a low power electronmicrograph.

A modification of the toluidine blue method can be applied to paraffin sections to demonstrate mast cells, and to acrylic sections of undecalcified bone to demonstrate calcification fronts and other cellular detail.

Myelin methods

Several staining techniques can be used to demonstrate normal myelin. The dye solochrome cyanin is frequently used to demonstrate myelin in paraffin sections (see Fig. 13.22b). Other methods use modified haematoxylin or osmium tetroxide.

Enzyme histochemical methods

Enzyme histochemical techniques identify and localize the sites of activity of particular enzyes. An incubating solution contains the specific substrate for the enzyme or group of enzymes to be demonstrated, together with any necessary co-factors or inhibitors so that the enzyme in the tissue reacts with the substrate to form an insoluble primary reaction product. This is then visualized by its reaction with a visualizing agent, which may be included with the incubating medium, or applied as a separate second step.

Since most biological enzyme systems are labile, they may be destroyed by fixation and tissue processing; thus most enzyme histochemical methods are carried out on frozen sections.

Immunohistological methods

Variably specific antibodies have been created against particular cell constituents, and these antibodies can be used to identify the presence and localization of the specific consituent within biological material. When the specific antibody links to its tissue antigen, the site of reaction can be identified either by **immunofluorescence** or **immunochemical** means.

In immunofluorescence, the antibody is linked to a fluorescent molecule, which can be visualized by fluorescence microscopy, whereas in immunochemistry it is linked to a chemical compound, which can subsequently be rendered visible by light microscopy.

Immunocytochemical techniques are revolutionizing the histological investigation of biological material, enabling the specific identification and localization of hormones (see Fig. 15.29), and the accurate typing of lymphocytes (see Figs 7.10b & 7.12b).

INDEX